T0337493

Core Curriculum

OSTOMY MANAGEMENT

SECOND EDITION

Wound, Ostomy, and Continence Nurses Society™ (WOCN®)

Core Curriculum

OSTOMY MANAGEMENT

SECOND EDITION

EDITED BY

Jane Carmel, MSN, RN, CWOCN
Faculty, R.B. Turnbull, Jr., MD School of WOC Nursing Education Program
Cleveland Clinic
Cleveland, Ohio

Janice Colwell, APRN, CWOCN, FAAN
Advanced Practice Nurse Ostomy Care Services
The University of Chicago Medicine
Chicago, Illinois

Margaret T. Goldberg, MSN, RN, CWOCN
Delray Wound Treatment Center
Delray Beach, Florida

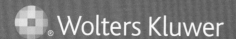
. Wolters Kluwer

Philadelphia • Baltimore • New York • London
Buenos Aires • Hong Kong • Sydney • Tokyo

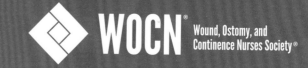

Not authorised for sale in United States, Canada, Australia, New Zealand, Puerto Rico, and U.S. Virgin Islands.

Acquisitions Editor: Jamie Blum
Development Editor: Maria M. McAvey
Editorial Coordinator: Anthony Gonzalez/Linda Christina
Production Project Manager: Kirstin Johnson
Design Coordinator: Teresa Mallon/Stephen Druding
Manufacturing Coordinator: Kathleen Brown/Beth Welsh
Marketing Manager: Linda Wetmore
Prepress Vendor: SPi Global

Second Edition

Cataloging-in-Publication Data available on request from the Publisher

ISBN: 978-1-9751-6456-0

shop.lww.com

PREVIOUS EDITION CONTRIBUTORS

Jean Asburn, MD

Janice Beitz, PhD, RN, CS, CNOR, CWOCN, CRNP, APN-C, MAPWCA, FAAN

Greta V. Bernier, MD

Ruth A. Bryant, MS, RN, CWOCN

Jane E. Carmel, MSN, RN, CWOCN

Russell D. Cohen, MD

Janice C. Colwell, MS, RN, CWOCN, FAAN

JoAnn Ermer-Seltun, MS, RN, ARNP, FNP-BC, CWOCN

Jane Fellows, MSN, RN, CWOCN

Alessandro Fichera, MD

Margaret T. Goldberg, MSN, RN, CWOCN

Barbara Hocevar, MSN, RN, CWOCN

Mary F. Mahoney, MSN, RN, CWON

Kimberly McIltrot, DNP, CPNP, CWOCN

Debra S. Netsch, DNP, APRN-CNP, FNP-BC, CWOCN

Denise Nix, MS, RN, CWOCN

Joseph J. Pariser, MD

Sanjay G. Patel, MD

Joyce Pittman, PhD, ANP-BC, FNP-BC, CWOCN

Michelle C. Rice, MSN, RN, CWOCN

Michele Rubin, APN, CNS, CGRN

Ginger Salvadalena, PhD, RN, CWOCN

Jody Scardillo, DNP, RN, ANP-BC, CWOCN

Adam C. Stein, MD

Gary D. Steinberg, MD

Linda Stricker, MSN, RN, CWOCN

The names and credentials are listed as they were printed during the time of the previous edition publication.

CONTRIBUTORS

Christine Baker, APRN, MSN, CWOCN
Advanced Practice Nurse
Section of Pediatric Surgery
University of Chicago Medicine Comer Children's
    Hospital

**Janice M. Beitz, PhD, RN, CS, CNOR, CWOCN-AP,
    CRNP, ANEF, FNAP, FAAN**
Professor of Nursing
Rutgers University Camden
Camden, New Jersey

Ruth A. Bryant, PhD, MS, RN, CWOCN
Director of Nursing Research
Nursing Research
Abbott Northwestern Hospital
Minneapolis, Minnesota

Jane Carmel, MSN, RN, CWOCN
Faculty, R.B. Turnbull, Jr., MD School of WOC Nursing
    Education Program
Cleveland Clinic
Cleveland, Ohio

Russell Cohen, MD
Professor of Medicine
Medicine
UChicago Medicine
Chicago, Illinois

Janice Colwell, APRN, CWOCN, FAAN
Advanced Practice Nurse
Surgery
UChicago Medicine
Chicago, Illinois

**JoAnn M. Ermer-Seltun, MS, RN, ARNP, FNP-BC,
    CWOCN, CFCN**
Co-Director, Family Nurse Practitioner
Vascular Wound Center and Continence Clinic
WEB WOC Nursing Education Programs
MercyOne North Iowa Medical Center
Mason City, Iowa

Jane Fellows, MSN, CWOCN-AP
Wound/Ostomy CNS
Oncology
Duke University Hospital
Durham, North Carolina

Linda Ferrari, MD
Colorectal and Pelvic Floor Surgeon
Colorectal Surgery
Guy's and Saint Thomas' NHS Foundation Trust
London, United Kingdom

Alessandro Fichera, MD
Division Chief, Colon and Rectal Surgery
Baylor University Medical Center at Dallas
Dallas, Texas

Margaret Goldberg, RN, MSN
Ostomy Consultant
Wound Center
Delray Medical Center
Delray Beach, Florida

**Virginia Hanchett, FNP, APRN-BC, DCNP, COCN,
    CWCN**
Program Director and Senior Nurse Practitioner
UR Medicine Ostomy Services
University of Rochester Medical Center
Rochester, New York

Barbara Hocevar, MSN, RN, CWOCN
WOCNEP Faculty
R.B.Turnbull, Jr., MD WOC Nursing Education Program
Cleveland Clinic
Cleveland, Ohio

Kathleen Hudson, BSN, RN, CWOCN
Clinical Nurse Educator, Wound and Ostomy Care
Nursing
University of Chicago Medicine
Chicago, Illinois

Kelly Jaszarowski, MSN, RN, CNS, CWOCN
Assistant Director WOC Program
R. B. Turnbull, Jr., MD WOC Nursing Education Program
Cleveland Clinic
Cleveland, Ohio

Mary F. Mahoney, MSN, RN, CWOCN, CFCN
UnityPoint at Home
West Des Moines, Iowa
Adjunct Faculty
WEB WOC Nursing Education Programs

Kimberly McIltrot, DNP, CPNP, CWOCN
DNP Program Director
John Hopkins School of Nursing
Baltimore, Maryland

Rose W. Murphree, DNP, RN, CWOCN, CFCN
Assistant Professor
General
Emory University Nell Hodgson Woodruff School of
    Nursing
Atlanta, Georgia

**Debra Netsch, DNP, APRN, FNP-BC, CNP,
    CWOCN-AP, CFCN**
Co-Director and Faculty/Advanced Practice WOC Nurse
    Practitioner
Ridgeview Wound & Hyperbaric Healing
    Center
WEB WOC Nursing Education Program/Ridgeview
    Medical Center
Minneapolis/Waconia, Minnesota

Denise Nix, MS, RN, CWOCN
Wound, Ostomy, Continence Nurse
WOC Nursing
M Health Fairview
Minneapolis, Minnesota

Vignesh T. Packiam, MD
Urologic Oncology Fellow
Urology Mayo Clinic
Rochester, Minnesota

Sanjay G. Patel, MD
Assistant Professor
Urology
Oklahoma State University Center for Health Sciences
Oklahoma City, Oklahoma

Laura Ann Phearman, BSN
Nurse Clinician Specialty
Nursing Children's and Women's Services
University of Iowa Children's Hospital
Iowa City, Iowa

**Joyce Pittman, PhD, RN, ANP-BC, FNP-BC, CWOCN,
    FAAN**
Associate Professor
College of Nursing
University of South Alabama
Mobile, Alabama

Michelle Rice, MSN, CWOCN
Wound/Ostomy CNS
Acute Care
Duke University Hospital
Durham, North Carolina

Michele Rubin, APRN, MSN, CNS, CGRN
IBD Colorectal APRN
IBD Colorectal Surgery
University of Chicago Medicine
Chicago, Illinois

Ginger Dawn Salvadalena, PhD, RN, CWOCN
Fellow, Clinical Research
Global Clinical Affairs
Hollister Incorporated
Libertyville, Illinois

Jody Scardillo, DNP, RN, ANP-BC, CWOCN
CNS Nurse Practitioner
CNS/NP
Albany Medical Center
Albany, New York

Sherief Shawki, MD
Colorectal Surgeon and Transplant Surgeon
Colorectal Surgery
Cleveland Clinic
Cleveland, Ohio

Adam C. Stein, MD
Assistant Professor in Medicine—Gastroenterology
Medicine
Northwestern Medical Center
Chicago, Illinois

Gary D. Steinberg, MD
Professor and Director
Urology
NYU Langone Health
New York, New York

Linda Jean Stricker, MSN, RN, CWOCN
Program Director, WOC School
R.B.Turnbull Jr.,MD WOC Nursing Education Program
Cleveland Clinic
Cleveland, Ohio

Ryan P. Werntz, MD
Assistant Professor
Urology
Prisma Health
Greenville, South Carolina

FOREWORD

I t is an honor to be invited to write the foreword to the *Wound, Ostomy, and Continence Nurses Society™ (WOCN®) Core Curriculum,* 2nd edition. Having served 22 years as a Wound, Ostomy, and Continence (WOC) Nursing Program Director, I can attest as to how valuable a resource these books will be to students, faculty, preceptors, and all clinicians caring for people with wounds, ostomies, and incontinence.

Terms currently popular in health care refer to patient-centered and patient-focused care. For those of you entering the wonderful WOC nursing specialty, know this: the patient has always been the focus of WOC nursing! In fact, our specialty grew from a need identified by patients themselves. As colorectal and urologic surgeries advanced, so did the number of people living with ostomies. In 1958, Akron, Ohio, native Norma N. Gill joined her surgeon, Rupert B. Turnbull Jr, MD, in founding what was then coined by Dr. Turnbull as enterostomal therapy (ET).

Beginning in 1948, when she was a 28-year-old mother of two young children, Norma began a long odyssey battling mucosal ulcerative colitis. She manifested all the gastrointestinal symptoms, including massive bouts of bloody diarrhea associated with this disease, along with many of the extraintestinal manifestations, such as uveitis, iritis, and extensive pyoderma gangrenosum on her face, chest, abdomen, and legs. During a brief remission in 1951, much to the amazement of Norma and her husband Ted, she became pregnant. The pregnancy was fraught with complications, the need for numerous blood transfusions, and fear for the lives of both mother and child throughout. Despite all of these life-threatening occurrences, in June 1952, Norma gave birth to a healthy baby girl. The complications continued after her baby's birth, and Norma's response to treatment was spotty at best. In October 1954, she was admitted to the Cleveland Clinic, and there her life was saved, and history forever changed. Dr. Turnbull operated to remove Norma's colon and create an ileostomy. Her postoperative course after ileostomy was rocky, and she had to undergo some additional operations to remove her rectum and have plastic surgery performed on her face.

Despite all of this, Norma began to feel better—incredibly better. As she was resuming her role as a wife and mother, she felt the need, as we now say, to "pay it forward." Norma wanted to help others who were facing the same challenges she had endured and emerged stronger than she had been before her illness. Her journey began with the Akron physicians and hospital she had come to know well during her illness. Norma started from scratch and cobbled together an inventory of the limited equipment available at the time. Soon she had many referrals from the surgeons and knew she had found her calling. In 1958, during an appointment with Dr. Turnbull, she told him what she was doing in Akron to help people with new ostomies and fistulae. He was impressed and called her a couple of months later to offer her a job at the Cleveland Clinic.

August 1958 is when the seeds for the modern specialty of WOC nursing were planted. It was not long before the word was out, and surgeons began requesting that their staff come to train with Norma and Dr. Turnbull. The R.B. Turnbull Jr., School of Enterostomal Therapy (now WOC Nursing) was established. After her long work day in Cleveland, Norma would return to Akron and see patients in hospitals there before heading home to her family and doing it all again the next day.

There was a child in an Akron hospital born with exstrophy of the bladder after years of urinary incontinence, reflux, and renal stones whose family made the lifesaving decision to have her undergo a urinary diversion. She always remembered her first encounter with Norma. Here was a woman who commanded respect. The surgeon, head nurse, and staff nurses, as well as the girl's mom, crowded around the bed as Norma taught the proper way to care for a new ileal conduit. The equipment at that time was very primitive. Heavy stoma plates, rubber pouches with complex assembly secured with cement and a belt and a prayer! Norma never gave up attempting to help her patients and along with Dr. Turnbull urged industry to develop better, more secure pouching systems. Thanks to a great family and the one and only Norma Gill, the child in that Akron hospital grew up well adjusted to her new stoma, that child grew up to be me! I knew I wanted to "pay it forward" just like Norma. The baby who was predicted never to be born to Norma and Ted is Sally Gill-Thompson—one of my best friends and a famous ET practitioner in her own right.

After establishment of the formal program in Cleveland, other ET schools soon opened, and graduates from the United States and abroad spread the word across the globe. Professional organizations were established, and admission criteria became more stringent as health care became more complex. ET nurses became well respected for their skills and experience caring for people with complex ostomies and fistulae. It was a natural extension of our practice to embrace wound and continence care. In the 1990s, we bid good-bye to our ET designation and became known as WOC nurses to better reflect our practice. After 38 years, I have retired from clinical practice but my passion for WOC nursing is not diminished. As you embark on your studies of WOC nursing, take time to reflect and appreciate the wonderful legacy you are continuing with your specialty practice. Your actions will have an immeasurable impact improving the lives of your patients through direct care and advocacy, educating your colleagues, expanding research to support our evidence-based practice. I know our future is in good hands.

Norma (and I) will be watching!

Paula Erwin-Toth, MSN, RN, FAAN

PREFACE

This text was developed for the student who will receive instruction in a Wound, Ostomy, and Continence Nursing Education Program (WOCNEP) specifically the ostomy educational program. The WOCNEP Directors have developed a curriculum blueprint that was approved by the Wound, Ostomy, and Continence Nurses Society™ (WOCN®) Accreditation Committee and Board of Directors. The curriculum objectives have been used to develop the content for this book. Each chapter begins with an outline and ends with review questions, answers and rationale that highlight the important issues in each chapter. The text has been written by experts in the field who provide care to patients undergoing ostomy surgery. As the editors, we have supported their work and edited this content to ensure it reflects the curriculum outline and current clinical practice.

The information in this book will help the future clinicians of ostomy services to provide a high level of care to their patients. We believe that the person with an ostomy should have the services of an educated nurse specialist and continued access to those services as they live their lives with a fecal and/or urinary diversion. Once educated in ostomy care, the specialty nurse has a unique role to contribute to the care of a person with an ostomy. It is our hope that this book will provide the foundation that helps deliver optimal care to all individuals with fecal and urinary diversions.

ACKNOWLEDGMENTS

The Wound, Ostomy, and Continence Nurses Society™ (WOCN®) wishes to thank all of the clinical experts who generously shared their time and expertise to create the second edition of this textbook. The Society would like to especially acknowledge the consulting editors, Jane Carmel, Janice Colwell, and Margaret Goldberg, for their inspiration, knowledge, and unwavering commitment to the development of this resource and to the field of wound, ostomy, and continence nursing.

The WOCN Society would like to acknowledge Hollister Incorporated for providing a commercially supported educational grant for the development of this textbook.

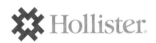

CONTENTS

Contributors   *vii*

Foreword   *ix*

Preface   *xi*

Acknowledgments   *xiii*

1   Professional Practice for Wound, Ostomy, and Continence Nursing   1
Rose W. Murphree and Kelly Jaszarowski

2   Anatomy and Physiology of the Gastrointestinal Tract   12
Debra Netsch

3   Anatomy and Physiology of the Urinary System   29
JoAnn M. Ermer-Seltun

4   Diseases That Lead to a Fecal Stoma: Colorectal Cancer   44
Linda Ferrari and Alessandro Fichera

5   Medical Management of Crohn's Disease and Ulcerative Colitis   59
Russell Cohen and Adam C. Stein

6   Surgical Management of Crohn's Disease and Ulcerative Colitis   71
Michele Rubin

7   Other Conditions That Lead to a Fecal Diversion   100
Janice M. Beitz

8   Urinary Diversions   117
Vignesh T. Packiam, Sanjay G. Patel, Ryan P. Werntz, and Gary D. Steinberg

9   Fecal and Urinary Stoma Construction   131
Linda Jean Stricker, Barbara Hocevar, and Sherief Shawki

10   Preoperative Preparation of Patients Undergoing a Fecal or Urinary Diversion   143
Margaret T. Goldberg and Mary F. Mahoney

11   Postoperative Nursing Assessment and Management   162
Janice Colwell and Kathleen Hudson

12   Selection of Pouching System   172
Janice Colwell and Kathleen Hudson

13   Postoperative Education for the Patient with a Fecal or Urinary Diversion   189
Jane Carmel and Margaret T. Goldberg

14   Adaptations, Rehabilitation, and Long-Term Care Management Issues   201
Jane Carmel and Jody Scardillo

15   Assessment and Management of the Pediatric Patient   223
Christine Baker, Laura Ann Phearman, and Kimberly McIltrot

16   Peristomal Skin Complications   250
Ginger Dawn Salvadalena and Virginia Hanchett

17   Stoma Complications   270
Joyce Pittman

18   Fistula Management   283
Denise Nix and Ruth A. Bryant

19   Nursing Management of the Patient with Percutaneous Tubes   304
Jane Fellows and Michelle Rice

Appendix A: Surgical Procedures   317

Appendix B: Selected Ostomy Support Resources   319

Appendix C: Selected Ostomy Product Suppliers and Manufacturers   321

Appendix D: Catheterization of an Ileal or Colon Conduit Stoma: Best Practice for Clinicians   322

Urostomy Urine Sample Collection Instruction Card   326

Appendix E: Colostomy and Ileostomy Products and Tips   327

Appendix F: WOCN Society and AUA Position Statement on Preoperative Stoma Site Marking for Patients Undergoing Urostomy Surgery   335

Appendix G: WOCN Society and ASCRS Position Statement on Preoperative Stoma Site Marking for Patients Undergoing Colostomy or Ileostomy Surgery   339

Appendix H: Urostomy Products and Tips   343

Appendix I: Care of Feeding Tubes   354

Appendix J: Ostomy Products HCPCS Codes (Healthcare Common Procedural Coding System)   361

Appendix K: Ostomy-Related Items   364

Appendix L: United Ostomy Associations of America: You Matter! Know What to Expect and Know Your Rights: Ostomy and Continent Diversion Patient Bill of Rights©   366

Appendix M: Pouching Infants/Children and Pediatric Pouches   367

Appendix N: Emergency Staff Procedure: Ileostomy Obstruction   369

Appendix O: Diagnosis and Management Algorithm for Acute Pouchitis   370

Glossary   371

Index   375

CHAPTER 1

PROFESSIONAL PRACTICE FOR WOUND, OSTOMY, AND CONTINENCE NURSING

Rose W. Murphree and Kelly Jaszarowski

OBJECTIVES

1. Define the nursing specialty of wound, ostomy, and continence nursing and describe the key role components.
2. Identify the WOC nurse's specific scope of practice based upon licensure
   a. WOC registered nurse
   b. WOC graduate registered nurse
   c. Advanced practice (APRN)
3. Describe the tri-specialty role of WOC nursing.
4. Name the various populations served by the WOC nurse.
5. List the WOC nurse practice settings.

TOPIC OUTLINE

Wound, Ostomy, and Continence Nursing Specialty 2

History and Evolution of WOC Nursing 2

Key Components of the WOC Nurse Role 2

Professional Practice Goals 3

Levels of the WOC Nursing Practice 3
WOC Registered Nurse 3
WOC Graduate Degree Registered Nurse 3
Advanced Practice WOC Registered Nurse 3

The Tri-specialty of WOC Nursing 4
Wound Specialty 4
Ostomy Specialty 4
Continence Specialty 4
Complex problems 4

WOC Nurse Roles 4
Clinician 4
Educator 4
Consultant 5
Researcher 5
Administrator 5
Preceptor 5
Dual/Multiple Roles 5

Populations Served by WOC Nurses 5
Pediatric Population 5
Older Adults 5
Palliative/Hospice Care 6

WOC Nurse Practice Settings 6
Acute Care 6
Outpatient Care 6
Home Health Care 6
Long-term/Extended Care 6
Rehabilitation 6
Industry 6
Academia 6
Research Consumer and Evidence-Based Practice 7

Care Coordination and Collaboration by WOC Nurse 7

Health Care Reimbursement 7
Continuous Professional Development 8
Certification 8

Ethics in WOC Nursing 8

Conclusion 9

WOUND, OSTOMY, AND CONTINENCE NURSING SPECIALTY

Wound, Ostomy, and Continence (WOC) nursing is a multifaceted, evidence-based practice that incorporates a unique body of knowledge to enable nurses to provide excellence in prevention of wound, ostomy, and/or continence problems and complications (WOCN, 2018). Also included in the scope of WOC nursing is health maintenance; therapeutic intervention; and rehabilitative and palliative nursing care to persons with select disorders of the gastrointestinal, genitourinary, and integumentary systems. The WOC nurse directs efforts at improving the quality of care, life, and health of health care consumers with wound, ostomy, and/or continence care needs. WOC nursing is a complex nursing specialty that encompasses the care of individuals of all ages, in all health care settings, and across the continuum of care.

HISTORY AND EVOLUTION OF WOC NURSING

WOC nursing originated as a lay practice to address the unmet needs of health care consumers with an ostomy. During the 1940s and 1950s, surgical techniques developed rapidly with an increase in ostomy surgeries (WOCN Society, 2010). Stoma construction was often poor, there were few pouching systems available and hospitals lacked support systems to help the affected individuals deal with the life-altering surgeries. To fill the gap in ostomy care, one particular individual with an ostomy began the quest to improve ostomy care and services (WOCN Society, 2010). In 1955, Norma Gill Thompson had surgery at Cleveland Clinic (Ohio) with Dr. Rupert Turnbull, which resulted in the creation of an ileostomy. During one of her postop follow-up visits, she spoke with Dr. Turnbull about her rehabilitation with her ostomy care. He was impressed with her adaptation, willingness to help others, and attitude toward life with an ostomy that he asked her to become an ostomy technician (the role became known as enterostomal therapist) for Cleveland Clinic. In 1961, they opened the first formal Enterostomal Therapy School to provide rehabilitative care and psychological support to individuals with ostomies. The following chronology highlights, adapted from the WOCN Scope and Standards (Wound, Ostomy and Continence Nurses Society™, 2018) documents some of the top defining moments in the history of WOC nursing.

- 1958: Norma Gill became the first "ostomy technician" at Cleveland Clinic.
- 1961: The first enterostomal therapy (ET) program was established at Cleveland Clinic.
- 1968: The first professional specialty organization was founded (American Association of Enterostomal Therapists), which later became known as the International Association for Enterostomal Therapy (IAET).
- 1976: Registered nurse licensure was required for entry into ET nursing education programs, which are now known as WOC nursing education programs.
- 1979: Certification in the specialty was first offered by the Enterostomal Therapy Nursing Certification Board, founded in 1978, which is a separate entity from the WOC nursing society, and is now known as the Wound, Ostomy and Continence Nursing Certification Board.
- 1982: The scope of practice was expanded to include the care of individuals with wounds and urinary and fecal continence disorders.
- 1985: A baccalaureate degree was implemented as the minimum educational requirement for admission to the WOC nursing education programs and eligibility for certification in the specialty.
- 1992: The International Association of Enterostomal Therapy evolved into the Wound, Ostomy and Continence Nurses Society: An Association of ET Nurses, which is now known as the Wound, Ostomy, and Continence Nurses Society™.
- 2010: Wound, ostomy, and continence nursing was recognized as a nursing specialty by the American Nurses Association.

KEY COMPONENTS OF THE WOC NURSE ROLE

Core values that guide the professional practice of the WOC nurse include integrity, leadership, and knowledge. These values are demonstrated by the following beliefs and behaviors (WOCN 2018):

- Integrity: WOC nurses are uncompromised in their dedication to being a trusted, unbiased, and credible source of evidence-based information, care, and expertise.
- Leadership: WOC nurses are stewards of excellence with a common passion for mutual respect, shared experiences, and lifelong learning.
- Knowledge: WOC nurses demonstrate a continued commitment to education and research to generate and disseminate knowledge that improves patient outcomes.

WOC nursing integrates art and science using creativity and innovation and assimilates evidenced-based practices to manage patients with wounds, abdominal stomas, fistulas, percutaneous tubes/drains, and continence problems. WOC nurses are often called on to create new products, modify therapies, use innovative approaches for topical therapies or products, and orchestrate interdisciplinary resources to provide treatment plans for individuals or groups of health care consumers to achieve optimum health and independence (WOCN, 2018). In addition to providing unique and creative clinical skills, WOC nurses address other problems that patients experience such as limited access to supplies, lack of support, and teaching family, caregivers and staff. Essential to the practice of WOC nursing is the establishment of a relationship with the patients and their families/caregivers to gain trust, to help set goals, and to move the patient toward an optimal state of health.

PROFESSIONAL PRACTICE GOALS

Throughout the process of care, key goals for WOC nurses are to promote safe, patient-centered, quality, effective, equitable, efficient, timely, evidence-based, and cost-effective care for health care consumers (WOCN, 2018). WOC nurses contribute to achieving these goals through a variety of activities including, but not limited to, the following (WOCN, 2018):

- Collaborating with the health care consumer, family members, and other health care providers to develop individualized care plans and outcomes
- Implementing and marketing the role
- Providing evidence-based care to promote quality, effective and safe care and practice, and optimal outcomes for health care consumers who are culturally, socioeconomically, and geographically diverse
- Preventing complications and reducing readmissions
- Using proactive risk management strategies to reduce health care–acquired injuries such as the following: surgical site and wound infections, catheter-associated urinary tract infections, medical adhesive–related skin injuries, pressure injuries, and medical device–related skin injuries, etc.
- Educating staff to improve the quality, effectiveness, and safety of care; and staff productivity, competency, and efficiency
- Using advanced technology for prevention, diagnosis, and treatment of wound, ostomy, and/or continence problems
- Coordinating care to promote continuity across health care settings
- Translating research into practice
- Developing metrics for quality outcomes
- Establishing standards for documentation and practice
- Developing formularies for supply management
- Developing protocols for cost-effective utilization of resources (e.g., pressure redistribution support surfaces, negative wound pressure therapy)
- Engaging in advocacy efforts for reimbursement of supplies and services
- Participating in/or conducting trials and evaluations of new products and treatments

LEVELS OF THE WOC NURSING PRACTICE

WOC REGISTERED NURSE

The WOC nurse is a registered nurse with a baccalaureate degree or higher, with at least 1 year of clinical nursing experience following RN licensure. To attend an accredited WOC Nursing Educational Program (WOCNEP), the applicant must have current clinical nursing experience within 5 years prior to applying to WOCNEP. Applicants can choose from several accredited WOCN Educational Programs, and the structure of each program is diverse. Programs follow the curriculum blueprint that is part of the WOCN accreditation of the educational program; all programs contain a didactic and clinical component. Upon completion of the educational program in wound, ostomy, and/or continence, the nurse is awarded a certificate designating WOC nurse or specialty status, and the graduate is qualified to take national board examinations to become board certified in wound ostomy and/or continence care.

Those nurses not attending a WOCNEP have advanced their knowledge through additional studying in the specialty area(s) as well as through clinical practical experience. It is the inclusion of a clinical practicum with an approved Certified Wound Ostomy Continence Nurse (CWOCN) preceptor, which sets the WOC nurse apart. Certification is through the WOC Nursing Certification Board (WOCNCB®), an organization that is separate and distinct from the WOCN® Society.

WOC GRADUATE DEGREE REGISTERED NURSE

The WOC graduate degree RN is licensed as an RN within the state of practice and has a masters or doctoral degree, but is not a graduate of an APRN educational program. They have attended an accredited WOCNEP or sought additional focused education and practical experience.

ADVANCED PRACTICE WOC REGISTERED NURSE

Advanced practice registered nurses (APRNs) have completed the educational requirements for licensure as an advanced practice nurse, either at the masters or doctoral level and are licensed in the state or states that they practice as APRNs. They have obtained education in one, two, or all three specialty areas through an accredited WOC Nursing Education Program (WOCNEP) or through additional study focused in the specialty or specialties including focused practical experience. Certification is through the WOC Nursing Certification Board (WOCNCB®). The WOC APRN may practice independently or in collaboration with a physician, which depends on the state board of nursing, where the nurse practices.

THE TRI-SPECIALTY OF WOC NURSING

WOUND SPECIALTY

WOC nurses provide care to health care consumers across the continuum of care with varied types of acute or chronic wounds due to pressure; venous, arterial, or diabetes/neuropathic disease; trauma; thermal injury; surgery; and/or other disease processes (e.g., cancer, infection, vasculitis, sickle cell disease, calciphylaxis, etc.). Wounds can have devastating effects on the health care consumer with increased morbidity and mortality due to complications. Pain, bleeding, odor, drainage, necrosis, infection, sepsis, and limb loss are some of the complications associated with wounds. Throughout the process of care, WOC nurses collaborate and coordinate with other health care providers in developing and implementing wound treatment plans.

OSTOMY SPECIALTY

Health care consumers undergoing ostomy surgery require intensive physical and emotional care and continued support to return to their normal lives. For health care consumers with fecal or urinary diversions, fistulas, or percutaneous tubes/drains, WOC nurses (regardless of the practice setting) provide specialized care to maximize the individual's independence in self-care and adaptation to the life-altering changes in their body image and function. According to the American Society of Colon and Rectal Surgeons, "... all patients who have ostomies should have access to an ostomy nurse for follow-up care, as needed and wherever possible" (Hendren et al., 2015).

After ostomy surgery, individuals are faced with life-altering changes that can be overwhelming and devastating without proper care and education. The selection and fitting of an ostomy pouching system requires a specially educated nurse who is qualified and skilled to assess and determine the unique medical and physical needs of each individual.

The need for specialized ostomy care continues well beyond the immediate surgical period. WOC nurses are needed to provide long-term support and follow-up care to health care consumers with ostomies.

CONTINENCE SPECIALTY

Living with fecal or urinary dysfunction and incontinence places a great burden on affected individuals and their families or caregivers. Loss of continence can cause skin and wound care complications and may contribute to individuals being prematurely placed in long-term care facilities (WOCN, 2013b). Unfortunately, many individuals, family/caregivers, and health care providers do not intervene in continence issues believing that loss of continence is a normal part of the aging process (WOCN, 2016). Successful outcomes for individuals with continence problems require specialized care, and WOC nurses play an important role in the management of fecal and urinary continence issues.

COMPLEX PROBLEMS

A fistula is an abnormal tract that develops between a body cavity or organ or an organ and the skin (Bryant & Best, 2016). Some of the most difficult fistulas that WOC nurses care for are enterocutaneous fistulas that develop an opening from the small intestine to the skin, enteroatmospheric fistulas that open into the base of a wound, and multiple fistulas (Bryant & Best, 2016). An interdisciplinary team is required to manage an individual with a fistula, and WOC nurses are essential members of the team. WOC nurses utilize a variety of creative and adaptive techniques for both pouching and nonpouching modalities to achieve the goals for topical management of fistulas: skin protection, containment and accurate measurement of drainage, odor control, comfort and mobility of the individual, and cost containment (Bryant & Best, 2016).

WOC nurses are also often consulted to assist in management of complications due to percutaneous tubes/drains (i.e., gastrostomy, jejunostomy, nephrostomy, biliary). Percutaneous tubes/drains are placed to provide drainage; relieve an obstruction and maintain an opening into an organ; and/or for administration of fluids, medications, or feedings. Multiple complications occur with enteral tubes/drains that include irritant dermatitis from leakage around the tube, device-related pressure ulcers/injuries from inappropriate stabilization of the tube, fungal infections, cellulitis, and hypertrophic granulation tissue (Fellows & Rice, 2016).

WOC NURSE ROLES

WOC nurses serve in a variety of roles including clinician, educator, consultant, researcher, and administrator, and they may engage in dual or multiple roles.

CLINICIAN

The WOC nurse provides care to individuals in multiple practice settings. The WOC nurse may also evaluate individuals and their care via telehealth services. To achieve optimal outcomes, the WOC nurse uses the nursing process when caring for health care consumers. Each plan of care is individualized to complement the developmental age of the health care consumer and their caregiver and achieve the best outcomes (ANA, 2010, 2015a).

EDUCATOR

Education is an integral component of every WOC nurse's role. The WOC nurse provides education directly to health care consumers, caregivers, nurses, clinical staff, and other health care providers. WOC nurses provide staff education through orientation, on the-job training, in-service education, and development of protocols and/or guidelines (WOCN, 2013a).

WOC nurses may also provide formal education in academia or other organized continuing education programs that focus on one or more aspects of wound, ostomy, or continence care (WOCN, 2013a). Educational webinars are examples of some of the numerous continuing education programs provided by WOC nurses and the WOCN® Society. These programs extend the reach of the WOC nurse and the WOCN® Society to areas and settings that lack a WOC nurse.

CONSULTANT

In a direct consultant role, the WOC nurse partners with the health care consumer and other members of the health care team (WOCN, 2013a). The WOC specialty nurse has unique skills to coordinate individualized care based on assessment of the needs of the health care consumer, knowledge of current best practices, and an ongoing evaluation of outcomes. Collaboration with other health care providers and groups is also an essential part of the WOC nurses consultant's role. Some WOC nurses serve as independent consultants with contractual arrangements for the delivery of wound, ostomy, and/or continence care services in various settings. WOC nurses may also utilize their expertise in other practice areas such as legal nurse consulting.

RESEARCHER

In the role of researcher, the WOC nurse advances the science and art of wound, ostomy, and/or continence care. Varied types of research are conducted using different methodologies (e.g., applied research/clinical trials, problem-focused research, exploratory research, etc.). WOC nurse researchers are active in all settings where WOC nurses practice including academia, industry, and direct patient care areas (WOCN, 2013a). At the clinical level, WOC nurses assist in the translation of research and evidence-based guidelines into practice to enhance the delivery of quality care.

ADMINISTRATOR

The WOC nurse may also assume the role of an administrator. As an administrator, the WOC nurse's duties and responsibilities include management and oversight of clinical staff and the delivery of services across a broad spectrum of care (WOCN, 2013a). Other activities involved in administration include program development and efforts to ensure quality outcomes. The WOC nurse manager may be responsible for developing and overseeing operating budget for their department/unit.

PRECEPTOR

A WOC nurse can assume the role of preceptor for students. The most common role of preceptor is for either graduate nursing students (if the WOC nurse is an advanced degree nurse) or for WOC nurse students.

The WOCNEP have a clinical component of 40 hours per specialty, and a WOC nurse who has completed the WOCNEP and is certified with an active practice can become a preceptor.

DUAL/MULTIPLE ROLES

Often WOC nurses assume dual or multiple roles, depending on their educational preparation and setting. In addition, WOC graduate-level prepared registered nurses and WOC advanced practice registered nurses contribute to the specialty and profession by delivering direct care as providers, examining systems, spearheading research, and providing clinical leadership in WOC nursing.

POPULATIONS SERVED BY WOC NURSES

Although the basic principles of wound, ostomy, and continence care are the same regardless of population or practice setting, certain populations may be at greater risk for wound, ostomy, and/or continence problems and complications. Also, they may require adaptation or modifications in their care to address their unique needs including, but not limited to, the following patient populations: pediatric patients (neonates, infants, children, adolescents), older adults, patients needing palliative or hospice care, and obese patients. WOC nurses have expertise in caring for individuals with wound, ostomy, and/or continence needs across the spectrum of ages and developmental stages, including those at end of life and others with unique or special needs.

PEDIATRIC POPULATION

Key concepts in effective management of the pediatric population include development of rapport with the patient, family, and caregivers; interdisciplinary collaboration and coordination of care; patient and family education; and ongoing follow-up, support, and positive reinforcement by the WOC nurse to promote cooperation and adherence to the treatment plan (Jinbo, 2016). Education must always be presented that is appropriate for the cognitive abilities of the child.

OLDER ADULTS

It is important for WOC nurses to collaborate and coordinate care with the patient, family and caregivers, and members of the interdisciplinary team to assess needs and provide appropriate, dignified care for the older adult with wound, ostomy, and/or continence needs. The assessment must include the preferences for care and personal goals of the older adult. Coordination of care with other disciplines (e.g., physical and occupational therapists, dieticians, social workers, etc.) is needed to provide comprehensive care to manage frail older adults and those with comorbid conditions.

PALLIATIVE/HOSPICE CARE

Increasing numbers of infants, children, adolescents, and adults are living with serious or critical illnesses or injuries (ANA & Hospice & Palliative Nurses Association [HPNA], 2017). Palliative care that includes hospice care is provided by an interdisciplinary team, and WOC nurses contribute in wound care (prevention or management of pressure injuries, malignant wounds), continence issues (fecal or urinary incontinence), and in management of fecal and urinary diversions.

 ## WOC NURSE PRACTICE SETTINGS

The majority of WOC nurses work in the acute care setting. In addition, WOC nurses have the opportunity to practice in other settings such as outpatient care, home health care, long-term care, nursing homes, industry, academia, private practice, etc. WOC nurses may practice in multiple clinical settings that are affiliated with/ or part of a large organization or health care system, or they may function as an independent consultant to several settings.

The following descriptions provide a brief overview of WOC nursing practice in some of the most common settings (WOCN, 2010).

ACUTE CARE

In the acute care setting, WOC nurses care for health care consumers with a wide variety of medical, surgical, and/or trauma diagnoses. The WOC nurse may provide services in one or more areas of the tri-specialty practice to health care consumers across the life span from newborns to the elderly. Health care consumers with wound, ostomy, and/or continence needs may be found in any level of care within the hospital setting including the emergency department, intensive/critical care units, operating room, and medical–surgical units.

OUTPATIENT CARE

WOC nurses may practice in outpatient care settings that include private practice settings, hospital-based outpatient clinics, and freestanding ambulatory care centers. WOC nurses may work in conjunction with physicians and surgeons (e.g., urologists, vascular specialists, colorectal surgeons) to optimize management of health care consumers with wound, ostomy, and/or continence disorders. WOC advanced practice registered nurses may also serve as providers within these practices.

HOME HEALTH CARE

In the home-care setting, WOC nurses provide direct care and consultation to health care consumers with wound, ostomy, and/or continence concerns. The prospective payment system in home care has fueled an increased demand for WOC nursing expertise to help streamline services, educate caregivers and staff, and contain costs.

WOC nurses can develop protocols for care and product formularies to reduce costs while maintaining quality care. In addition to serving as a direct care provider, the WOC nurse's responsibilities often include educating other home health nurses and clinical staff to promote quality, evidence-based care for management of health care consumers with wound, ostomy, and/or continence needs. WOC nurses are integral members of interdisciplinary teams and work closely with rehabilitation staff to facilitate self care and independence in the home environment. Additionally, the WOC nurse may serve as a case manager/care coordinator to facilitate care delivery.

LONG-TERM/EXTENDED CARE

In long-term care and extended care settings, WOC nurses may monitor, direct, or assist with care, and/or provide education to facilitate care by other registered and/or licensed practical/vocational nursing staff and nursing assistants. WOC nurses must be knowledgeable about the regulatory and risk management issues and assessment and documentation requirements that are unique to the setting. The WOC nurse may serve as an independent consultant or an employee of the facility.

REHABILITATION

Services in skilled nursing facilities focus on care that enables health care consumers to achieve maximum independence in self-care. WOC nurses, with their emphasis on optimizing self-care and strong educations skills, are able to meet the challenges posed by individuals who need rehabilitative services and have wound, ostomy, and/or continence issues. WOC advanced practice registered nurses who practice in this setting may be able to receive third-party reimbursement for their services.

INDUSTRY

WOC nurses may practice in one or more areas of the tri-specialty, depending on the industry's focus. The WOC nurse in this setting may function primarily as a researcher and/or educator to investigate and develop new products and teach the end users. The WOC nurse in industry may serve as a resource to direct care providers and provide research evidence about the clinical effectiveness of products for wound, ostomy, and/or continence care, and can offer guidance about the appropriate indications and use of products.

ACADEMIA

The WOC nurse in academia may function as an educator, researcher, administrator, or department head. The WOC nurse may provide formal education for one or more areas of the tri-specialty, or the content may be incorporated into other graduate or undergraduate courses. In addition to an academic appointment, a WOC nurse faculty member may have an active clinical practice as part of their role. Academic accreditation standards for nursing programs dictate faculty educational standards; therefore, the WOC nurse in this practice area will have an advanced degree.

RESEARCH CONSUMER AND EVIDENCE-BASED PRACTICE

Health care consumers and providers, including agencies such as the Centers for Medicare & Medicaid Services (CMS) and the health care insurance industry, expect care to be delivered based on the best available research and evidence. Many agencies and groups utilize and publish evidence-based clinical practice (EBP) guidelines, including the WOCN Society®. WOC nurses use all types of research and evidence to influence the quality of patient care that is provided while practicing in the full scope of WOC specialty nursing.

There are many roles for a WOC nurse in research and EBP, such as consumer and developer of EB guidelines and standards of care, investigator in a scientific research trial, as well as evaluator of products.

The WOC nurse can contribute to the development of evidence-based care in many ways without assuming the role (or responsibility) of a primary investigator such as by participating in the following activities:

Surveys or polls

Clinical trials or product evaluations (see section on product evaluation)

Data collection for pressure injury prevalence and incidence studies or continuous quality improvement projects/studies that relate to WOC care or foot and nail care

The components of EBP include a systematic search and appraisal of evidence to answer the clinical question(s), integration of the expertise and experience of the WOC nurse as well as consideration of the patient's preference, values, and concerns. As part of the critical appraisal process, it is necessary to be able to discern the level and quality of the evidence. There are levels and criteria for rating research evidence utilized by the WOCN® Society in developing clinical practice guidelines.

 ## CARE COORDINATION AND COLLABORATION BY WOC NURSE

The WOC nurse works collaboratively with other health care disciplines to provide comprehensive care. Successful collaboration between the WOC nurse, physicians, and other health care members increases member's awareness of each other's type of knowledge and skills that will lead to improvement in patients' treatment plan and successful outcome. In order to coordinate individualize patient care, the WOC nurse should partner with members of the health care team, patients' families/caregivers, and other health care providers across the continuum of care (WOCN, 2018). Collaboration and coordinating of care requires skill to ensure that the patient receives quality care.

The WOC nurse coordinates care for complex cases, utilizing their expertise, skills, and resources in various practice settings. The WOC APRN can provide additional services: order and interpret diagnostic and laboratory tests, prescribe pharmacological and nonpharmacological agents and treatments for wound, ostomy, and continence complications (WOCN, 2018).

 ## HEALTH CARE REIMBURSEMENT

Health care reimbursement has a direct effect on the amount and type of care provided to patients by all health care providers, including WOC nurses. Payment for health care in the United States involves several mechanisms, including self-pay by the consumers, insurance companies, and government agencies. The federal government is the single largest payer through Medicare, Medicaid, and the Department of Veterans Affairs (Sherman, 2012). Medicare is a federally provided health insurance program that is administered by the US Department of Health and Human Services through CMS. Medicare provides coverage for individuals over the age of 65, younger than 65 with disabilities, and with end-stage renal disease at any age.

Medicare Part A covers hospital and hospice visits, stays in skilled nursing facilities, and home health. Medicare Part B covers 80% of expenses incurred with outpatient visits/care, some home health, and durable medical equipment. Medicare Part C provides insurance coverage by private-run insurance companies. And Medicare Part D helps cover the cost of prescriptions. More information about Medicare can be found on the CMS Web site.

Medicaid is a joint state and federal health insurance program for low-income individuals. States establish and administer their own Medicaid programs and determine the type, amount, duration, and scope of services within broad federal guidelines. Medicaid provides health coverage to pregnant women, seniors and individuals with disabilities, and nonelderly, low-income parents or caretaker relatives and varies from state to state.

The Wound, Ostomy and Continence Nurses Society™ has developed two fact sheets about reimbursement for its members and are available on the Web site (http://www.wocn.org) in the Public Policy and Advocacy section. The fact sheet, *Reimbursement of Advanced Practice Registered Nurse Services*, provides information about reimbursement opportunities and challenges for the advanced practice RN (WOCN® Society, 2019a). In addition, the fact sheet, *Understanding Medicare Part B Incident to Billing*, provides some insight into cases where a nonadvanced practice WOC nurse might bill in the outpatient setting. "Incident to" is a billing mechanism for Medicare that allows services provided in an outpatient setting to be delivered by auxiliary personnel and billed under the provider's national provider identification (NPI). For example, under the incident to provision, a physician or APRN could develop the plan of care and a non-APRN could provide the care and bill under the provider's NPI (WOCN® Society, 2019b).

CONTINUOUS PROFESSIONAL DEVELOPMENT

Continued professional development is critical for the practicing WOC nurse. There are many opportunities through the WOCN® Society for the WOC nurse to maintain current, evidence-based practice. This can be accomplished by reading the *Journal of Wound Ostomy and Continence Nursing,* attending conferences, and working within the WOCN® Society as a volunteer. The WOCN offers an annual conference, which provides current research topics related to the wound, ostomy and continence practice. WOCN regions and affiliates offer on-site conferences. The WOCN® Society also provides live streaming/webcasts of sessions presented at the annual conference. Throughout the year, there are webinars available that provide continuing education credits. WOC nursing practice requires lifelong learning.

Involvement in professional activities can provide professional growth where opportunities are available to become a committee member to work on important projects, develop strategies to enhance care delivery as well as opportunities to develop relationships with other WOC nurse specialists. Examples of organizations that are within the scope of WOC practice include WOCN® Society, World Council of Enterostomal Therapists, and National Pressure Injury Advisory Panel.

Certification

Wound Ostomy Continence Nursing Certification Board (WOCNCB) is a national certified organization that provides credentials based on valid and reliable testing process. The WOCNCB is a separate and distinct organization from the WOC Nursing Society. WOCNCB validates the specialized knowledge, skills, and expertise of nurses who meet the requirements for certification. Certification is voluntary, however recommended as it provides assurance to patients and employers of a safe and competent practice. WOCN certification is granted for five years. Compliance must be demonstrated every five years by either reexamination or development of a professional growth program portfolio. Advance practice nursing certification in wound ostomy continence

TABLE 1-1 WOCNCB'S WOUND, OSTOMY AND CONTINENCE CERTIFICATION CREDENTIALS
CWOCN Certified Wound Ostomy Continence Nurse
CWCN Certified Wound Care Nurse
COCN Certified Ostomy Care Nurse
CCCN Certified Continence Care Nurse
CWON Certified Wound Ostomy Nurse
Advanced Practice Certifications Credentials
CWOCN-AP Certified Wound Ostomy Continence Nurse–Advanced Practice
CWCN-AP Certified Wound Care Nurse–Advanced Practice
COCN-AP Certified Ostomy Care Nurse–Advanced Practice
CCCN-AP Certified Continence Care Nurse–Advanced Practice
CWON-AP Certified Wound Ostomy Nurse–Advanced Practice

nursing is available through WOCNCB. (See **Table 1-1** on credentials.) For more information on WOCNCB and certification requirements, see their Web site: www.wocncb.org.

ETHICS IN WOC NURSING

WOC nursing as a specialty practice embraces the provisions of the *Code of Ethics for Nurses with Interpretive Statements* (ANA, 2015b). WOC nurses are obligated to "adhere to standards of ethical practice established by the WOCN Society and to conduct themselves in a manner that upholds the highest professional standards" (WOCN, 2018). The *Code of Ethics for Nurses:*

Provision 1. The nurse practices with compassion and respect for the inherent dignity, worth, and unique attributes of every person.

Provision 2. The nurse's primary commitment is to the patient, whether an individual, family, group, community, or population.

Provision 3. The nurse promotes, advocates for, and protects the rights, health, and safety of the patient.

Provision 4. The nurse has authority, accountability, and responsibility for nursing practice; makes decisions; and takes action consistent with the obligation to promote health and to provide optimal care.

Provision 5. The nurse owes the same duties to self as to others, including the responsibility to promote health and safety, preserve wholeness of character and integrity, maintain competence, and continue personal and professional growth.

Provision 6. The nurse, through individual and collective effort, establishes, maintains, and improves the ethical environment of the work setting and conditions of employment that are conducive to safe, quality health care.

Provision 7. The nurse in all roles and settings advances the profession through research and scholarly inquiry, professional standards development, and the generation of both nursing and health policy.

Provision 8. The nurse collaborates with other health professionals and the public to protect human rights, promote health diplomacy, and reduce health disparities.

Provision 9. The profession of nursing, collectively through its professional organizations, must articulate nursing values, maintain the integrity of the profession, and integrate principles of social justice into nursing and health policy.

For interpretive statements specific to WOC nursing are available in the full scope and standards document (WOCN, 2018).

CONCLUSION

WOC nurses are professionals dedicated to individuals with WOC care needs. It is the goal of the WOC nurse to enhance delivery of wound, ostomy, and continence care directly and indirectly to those persons in need of such care.

REFERENCES

American Nurses Association. (2010). *Nursing's social policy statement: The essence of the profession* (3rd ed.). Silver Spring, MD: Author.

American Nurses Association. (2015a). *Nursing: Scope and standards of practice* (3rd ed.). Silver Spring, MD: Author.

American Nurses Association. (2015b). Code of ethics for nurses with interpretive statements. Silver Spring, MD: Author.

American Nurses Association & Hospice and Palliative Nurses Association. (2017). Call for action: Nurses lead and transform palliative care. Retrieved August 21, 2017, from http://nursingworld. org/MainMenuCategories/ThePracticeofProfessionalNursing/PalliativeCare-Call-for-Action/Draft-PalliativeCare-ProfessionalIssuesPanel-CallforAction.pdf

Bryant, R., & Best, M. (2016). Management of draining wounds and fistulas. In R. Bryant & D. Nix (Eds.), *Acute & Chronic Wounds* (5th ed.). St. Louis, MO: Elsevier.

Fellows, J., & Rice, M. (2016). Nursing management of the patient with percutaneous tubes. In J. E. Carmel, J. C. Colwell, & M. T. Goldberg (Eds.), *Wound, Ostomy and Continence Nurses Society™ Core curriculum: Ostomy management* (pp. 220–230). Philadelphia, PA: Wolters Kluwer.

Hendren, S., Hammond, K., Glasgow, S. C., et al. (2015). Clinical practice guidelines for Ostomy surgery. *Diseases of the Colon and Rectum, 58*(4), 375–387. doi: 10.1097/DCR.0000000000000347.

Jinbo, A., & Bliss, D. (2016). Facilitators and barriers to adherence to prescribed bowel management programs by adolescents with neurogenic bowel conditions. Conference poster, WOCN 2016 Conference, Montreal, Canada.

Sherman, R., & Bishop, M. (2012). The business of caring: What every nurse should know about cutting costs. *American Nurse Today, 7*(11), 32–34.

WOCN Society. (2010). *Wound, ostomy, and continence nursing: Scope & standards of practice*. Mt. Laurel, NJ: Author.

Wound, Ostomy and Continence Nurses Society. (2013a). *Professional practice manual* (4th ed.). Philadelphia, PA: Wolters Kluwer/Lippincott Williams & Wilkins. Retrieved April 11, 2020, from the Lippincott Nursing Center at http://www.nursingcenter.com/journalarticle

Wound, Ostomy and Continence Nurses Society. (2013b). A quick reference guide for managing fecal incontinence. Retrieved April 3, 2017, from http://www.wocn.org/?page=QuickRefGuide

Wound, Ostomy and Continence Nurses Society. (2016). Reversible causes of acute/transient urinary incontinence: Clinical resource guide. Retrieved April 3, 2017, from http://www.wocn.org/?page=RevAcuteTransientUI

Wound, Ostomy and Continence Nurses Society. (2018). *Wound, ostomy and continence nursing scope & standards of practice* (2nd ed.). Mt. Laurel, NJ: Author.

Wound, Ostomy and Continence Nurses Society. (2019a). *Reimbursement of advanced practice registered nurse services: A fact sheet*. Mt. Laurel, NJ: Author.

Wound, Ostomy and Continence Nurses Society. (2019b). *Understanding Medicare Part B incident to billing: A fact sheet*. Mt. Laurel, NJ: Author.

QUESTIONS

1. Medicare Part B covers
  A. Hospice visits
  B. Durable medical equipment
  C. Prescriptions
  D. Hospital visits

2. When designing and implementing a WOC nurse role, it is important to
  A. Practice according to the WOCN® Scope and Standards
  B. Read the *Journal of WOC Nursing*
  C. Practice in all roles of the WOC nurse
  D. Provide annual reports to administration

3. Completion of an accredited WOCNEP to become a WOC nurse requires
  A. Didactic, special project, and passing final examination
  B. Didactic and 40 hours of clinical experience
  C. Didactic and acceptance of previous wound experience
  D. Didactic and 120 clinical hours with an approved CWOCN preceptor

4. As an educator, the WOC nurse is responsible for
  A. Providing staff nurse orientation
  B. Conducting clinical trials of products
  C. Developing protocols and guidelines
  D. Collecting data for quality improvement

5. Data collection for the WOC nurse should be
  A. Purposeful and outcome oriented
  B. Filled with everything the WOC nurse does
  C. Provided to administration annually
  D. Created by the WOC nurse only

6. As a research consumer, the role of the WOC nurse is
  A. Primary investigator for rigorous research studies
  B. Evaluator of WOC patient products
  C. Required to show proof of education in research
  D. Developer of evidence outside the scope of practice

7. The components of evidence-based practice include all of the following *except*
  A. Appraisal of evidence
  B. Systematic search of the literature
  C. Integration of the expertise of WOC nurse
  D. Work independently of others

8. Best practice documents provide which type of evidence?
  A. Randomized clinical trials
  B. Expert opinion
  C. Quasi-experimental studies
  D. Task force reviews

9. The first program for WOC nursing (previously enterostomal therapy) was located in
  A. Minneapolis
  B. New York City
  C. Cleveland
  D. Boston

10. Name two of the most common roles of the WOC nurse practices in acute care setting.
  A. Clinician and research
  B. Clinician and educator
  C. Educator and administrator
  D. Educator and preceptor

ANSWERS AND RATIONALES

1. B. Rationale: Medicare Part B covers durable medical equipment. Medicare Part A covers hospice and hospitals and Medicare Part D covers prescriptions.

2. A. Rationale: The WOCN® Scope and Standards is the foundation to incorporate into the WOC nursing practice.

3. D. Rationale: Requirements to complete a WOCNEP are didactic and 120 clinical hours (40 hours each specialty: in wound, ostomy, and continence) with an approved CWOCN preceptor.

4. A. Rationale: As an educator, the WOC nurse has the responsibility to provide orientation to staff nurses. Conducting clinical trials of products and developing guidelines is an example of the role in research. In the role of a clinician, the WOC nurse is responsible for quality improvement projects related to the specialty.

5. A. Rationale: Data collection is important to the WOC nurse's practice. It should be purposeful and outcome oriented to validate the role and position of the WOC nurse.

6. B. Rationale: The WOC nurse can contribute to research by evaluating WOC products.

7. D. Rationale: The components of evidence-based practice do not include work independently of others.

8. B. Rationale: Best practice documents' level of evidence is from expert opinion.

9. C. Rationale: Cleveland was the first site for an enterostomal therapy program (WOCN Program).

10. B. Rationale: Clinician and educator are the major roles of the WOC nurse in the acute care setting. The role of a consultant is also a major role for the WOC nurse.

CHAPTER 2

ANATOMY AND PHYSIOLOGY OF THE GASTROINTESTINAL TRACT

Debra Netsch

OBJECTIVE

Apply knowledge of normal anatomy and physiology of the GI system in nursing management and education of the patient with a fecal diversion.

TOPIC OUTLINE

Introduction **13**

Overview **13**

GI Tract (Alimentary Canal) **13**
    Histologic Characteristics 13
        Mucosa 13
        Submucosa 13
        Muscularis 14
        Serosa or Adventitia 14

Digestive Organs **15**
    Mouth 15
        Function 16
        Speech 16
        Ingestion 16
        Digestion 16
        Swallowing 16
    Esophagus 16
        Function 16

Abdominal Cavity Organs and Peritoneum **16**
    Stomach 17
        Function 18
        Digestion 18
        Secretion 18

        Absorption 18
        Elimination of Ingested Bacteria 18
Small Intestine 18
    Function 19
    Motility 19
    Secretion 20
    Absorption 20
Duodenum 20
Jejunum 20
Ileum 21
Ileocecal Valve 21
Large Intestine (Colon) 21
    Function 22
Colon Segments 22
Rectum 23
Anal Canal 23
Intestinal Bacteria 24
Accessory Organs 24
    Liver 25
    Gallbladder 25
    Exocrine Pancreas 25

Conclusions **26**

INTRODUCTION

The gastrointestinal (GI) system coordinates complex processes to prepare ingested food for cellular absorption and utilization, provides the body with water, and eliminates waste products. The physical state and chemical composition of the ingested food or liquid are changed through digestive, secretory, absorptive, and excretory functions to provide essential nutrition. This system is composed of the GI (alimentary) tract and accessory organs (salivary glands, liver, gallbladder, and exocrine pancreas; **Fig. 2-1**) (Patton & Thibodeau, 2014). It is through understanding of the normal anatomy and physiology of the GI system that pathological and surgical changes are more thoroughly appreciated. This chapter discusses the normal anatomy and physiology of the GI system.

 OVERVIEW

The digestive process begins in the mouth with chewing and continues in the stomach. In the stomach, food is mixed with enzymes, mucus, acid, and other secretions. The partially digested food and fluid pass from the stomach into the small intestine. The liver and exocrine pancreas secrete biochemicals and enzymes into the small intestine causing further breakdown into absorbable monosaccharides, amino acids, and fatty acids. These nutrients are transported through the small intestinal wall into blood vessels and lymphatics, which carry them to the liver for storage or further processing. The ingested food components not absorbed in the small intestine pass into the large intestine, which continues to absorb water. The fluid waste products are transported to the kidneys for elimination in the urine. Solid waste products pass into the rectum for elimination as stool through the anus.

The GI system functions with little conscious effort. The GI motility, other than chewing, swallowing, and defecation, is controlled by hormones and the autonomic nervous system (sympathetic and parasympathetic). The autonomic nervous system is controlled in the brain and by local stimuli mediated by intramural bundles of nerve fibers (plexuses) within the GI walls. The GI motility regulatory hormones particularly affect the small intestine. These are peptide and nonpeptide hormones. The peptide hormones including gastrin, cholecystokinin (CCK), secretin, insulin, and gastric inhibitory peptide (GIP) are produced and released throughout the GI tract to either stimulate or inhibit peristalsis and to facilitate digestion. Nonpeptide hormones include vitamin D, aldosterone, hydrocortisone, nitric oxide, and serotonin (Bryant, 2004; Doig & Huether, 2012; Reed & Wickham, 2009).

 GI TRACT (ALIMENTARY CANAL)

The GI tract is essentially a hollow muscular tube from the mouth to the anus. The length varies between individuals typically measuring during life around 7.62 m (25 feet) and after death closer to 10.67 m (35 feet) once smooth muscle tone is lost (OpenStax). It is composed of the mouth, esophagus, stomach, small intestine, large intestine, rectum, and anus. The digestive processes performed by the GI tract include (1) ingestion of food and fluids; (2) propulsion of food and waste products throughout the GI tract; (3) secretion of mucus, water, and digestive enzymes; (4) mechanical digestion of food particles; (5) chemical digestion of food particles; (6) absorption of nutrients; and (7) elimination of solid waste products by defecation (**Table 2-1**).

HISTOLOGIC CHARACTERISTICS

The alimentary canal has essentially the same four tissue layers from innermost to outermost: the mucosa, submucosa, muscularis, and serosa or adventitia (esophagus only; **Fig. 2-2**). These tissue layers vary in thickness and have sublayers.

Mucosa

The innermost tissue layer of the gut wall is the mucosal layer with sublayers of epithelium, lamina propria, and muscularis mucosa. The epithelium sublayer tissue is differentiated along the GI tract correlating with the regional-specific function. The mucosal epithelium is composed of protective stratified squamous epithelial cells at the beginning and end of the GI tract (mouth, esophagus, and anal canal). Simple columnar or glandular epithelial cells constitute the mucosal epithelium of the stomach, small intestine, and colon and secrete protective or digestive mucus, enzymes, and other biochemicals. This layer essentially provides lubrication and moisture, which facilitates the forward movement of food bolus while protecting the mucosa from abrasions. The mucosal lamina propria is the next sublayer outside the mucosal epithelium. It is primarily connective tissue containing blood vessels and lymphatics providing nutrients to the mucosal epithelium, transportation of hormones secreted by endocrine epithelium, and absorption of digestive end products from the lumen of the GI tract. The outermost mucosal sublayer is the muscularis mucosa. It is a thin layer of smooth muscle separating the mucosa and submucosa layers. Networks of widely distributed interstitial cells of Cajal (ICC) are considered the GI tract pacemaker cells. The ICC networks are present within the submucosal (ICC-SM), intramuscular (ICC-IM, ICC-DMP), and intermuscular layers (ICC-MY) of the GI tract from the esophagus to the internal anal sphincter.

Submucosa

The submucosa is the second tissue layer of the gut wall. It is a connective tissue layer containing blood vessels, lymphatics, submucosal glands, Meissner plexus (a submucosal nerve network affecting the muscularis smooth muscle), and a number of reticuloendothelial cells.

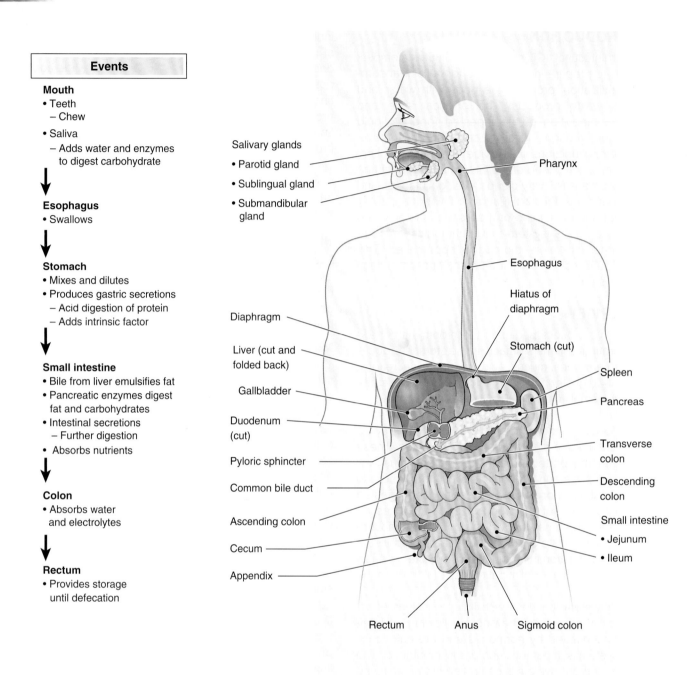

Events

Mouth
- Teeth
  - Chew
- Saliva
  - Adds water and enzymes to digest carbohydrate

↓

Esophagus
- Swallows

↓

Stomach
- Mixes and dilutes
- Produces gastric secretions
  - Acid digestion of protein
  - Adds intrinsic factor

↓

Small intestine
- Bile from liver emulsifies fat
- Pancreatic enzymes digest fat and carbohydrates
- Intestinal secretions
  - Further digestion
- Absorbs nutrients

↓

Colon
- Absorbs water and electrolytes

↓

Rectum
- Provides storage until defecation

Salivary glands
- Parotid gland
- Sublingual gland
- Submandibular gland

Pharynx

Esophagus

Hiatus of diaphragm

Diaphragm

Stomach (cut)

Liver (cut and folded back)

Spleen

Gallbladder

Pancreas

Duodenum (cut)

Pyloric sphincter

Transverse colon

Common bile duct

Descending colon

Ascending colon

Small intestine
- Jejunum
- Ileum

Cecum

Appendix

Rectum   Anus   Sigmoid colon

FIGURE 2-1. Normal Anatomy of the Digestive System. (From McConnell, T. H. (2007). *The nature of disease pathology for the health professions.* Philadelphia, PA: Wolters Kluwer.)

Muscularis

The muscularis is the third layer of the gut wall. It consists of two smooth muscle layers, a circular inner layer and longitudinal outer layer. The Auerbach (myenteric) plexus lies between these two muscle layers and coordinates rhythmic peristaltic contractions of the muscles resulting in the mixing and forward propulsion of the food bolus through the stomach and intestine.

Serosa or Adventitia

The outermost layer of the GI tract is a serous membrane. Structures within the peritoneal cavity are covered with serosa, which is connective tissue covered by the visceral peritoneum. This is continuous with the visceral peritoneum and is a factor in severe abdominal pain associated with transmural inflammatory bowel disease. If the serosa is exposed to air, it can lead to necrosis and sloughing of the serosal layer. Inflammation

TABLE 2-1 DIGESTIVE SECRETIONS

SOURCE	DAILY VOLUME (L)	pH	SODIUM (mmol)	POTASSIUM (mmol)	CHLORIDE (mmol)	BICARBONATE (mmol)	WATER (L)
Saliva	1.5	6.7–7.0	20–80	16–23	24–44	20–60	1
Gastric juice	2.0	1.0–3.5	20–100	4–12	52–124	0	2
Pancreatic	1.5	8.0–8.3	120–150	2–7	54–95	70–110	1.2
Bile	0.5	7.8	120–200	3–12	80–120	30–50	0.8
Intestinal juice	1.5	7.8–8.9	80–130	12–21	48–116	23–30	3.0

Modified from Bryant, R. (2004). Anatomy and physiology of the gastrointestinal tract. In J. Colwell, M. Goldberg, & J. Carmel (Eds.), *Fecal & urinary diversions: Management principles*. St. Louis, MO: Mosby-Elsevier; Ireland, A. P. (2004). Surgical fluids and electrolytes. Retrieved from http://surgstudent.org/lectures/flud/flud_centre_html.html

of the serosa (serositis) such as when stomas are not matured (everted) in surgery can result in partial or complete obstruction of the stoma. Structures outside the peritoneal cavity are surrounded with adventitia as the outermost layer instead of serosa. The adventitia is connective tissue that provides support to the organ it surrounds, such as the esophagus (Bryant, 2004; Doig & Huether, 2012; Patton & Thibodeau, 2014; Reed & Wickham, 2009; Takaki, 2003).

The continuity of the serosa with the visceral peritoneum is associated with pain of bowel inflammation despite the bowel not having pain receptors.

KEY POINT

One reason that stomas are typically matured at the time of surgery (primary matured or everted) is to avoid the complication of serositis.

KEY POINT

Stomas normally bleed a small amount when cleansed, due to the vascularity of the mucosa.

DIGESTIVE ORGANS

MOUTH

The mouth is the beginning or proximal end of the GI tract. The digestive process begins in the mouth through chewing and mixing of the food with saliva. This process is facilitated by the 32 teeth contained in the mouth. The tongue is muscular covered by moist squamous epithelium with the anterior surface covered by papillae containing thousands of taste buds. The taste buds or chemoreceptors differentiate between salty, sour, bitter, and sweet tastes. As the taste buds and olfactory nerves are stimulated, salivation is initiated and gastric juice is secreted in the stomach. Three pairs of salivary glands (submandibular,

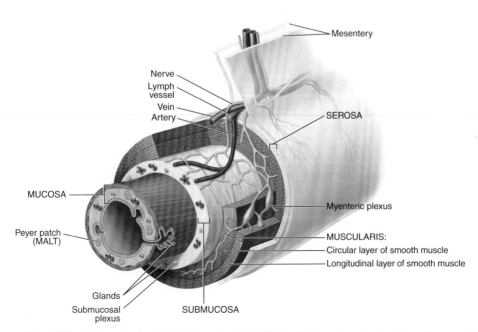

FIGURE 2-2. Layers of the GI Tract. (From Archer, P., & Nelson, L. A. (2012). *Applied anatomy & physiology for manual therapists.* Philadelphia, PA: Wolters Kluwer.)

sublingual, and parotid glands) are located in the mouth. The salivary glands produce approximately 1 to 1.5 L of saliva per day. Saliva consists primarily of water and a combination of mucus and sodium, bicarbonate, chloride, potassium, and salivary α-amylase (ptyalin), which is an enzyme that initiates carbohydrate digestion. It also contains immunoglobulin A and other antimicrobial substances, which prevent infection. Saliva sustains an alkaline pH around 7.4, which aids in neutralizing bacterial acids and preventing tooth decay.

Function
The functions performed by the structures of the mouth include speech, food ingestion, initiation of digestion, and swallowing.

Speech
The tongue and teeth are integral in the formation of words necessary for clear speech.

Ingestion
Nutrition is normally taken into the body through the mouth, which stimulates the taste buds and creates a pleasant sensation for future ingestion.

Digestion
Large food particles are broken into smaller particles through chewing or mastication of food. Thorough chewing of food increases the surface available for enzymatic or chemical digestion of carbohydrates, which reduce polysaccharides into maltose and isomaltose.

Swallowing
Swallowing is an important function of the propulsion of food into the digestive pathway requiring coordination of the mouth, palate, tongue, larynx, epiglottis, and esophagus. Ingested food is swallowed through the involuntary closing of the larynx opening, contraction of the pharyngeal muscles, inhibition of respiration, and relaxation of the upper esophageal sphincter allowing food to push through the pharynx and into the esophagus.

ESOPHAGUS
The esophagus is approximately 10 inches (25 cm) long connecting the oropharynx to the upper portion of the stomach traversing through the diaphragm. The esophagus is divided into three sections: the upper, middle, and lower. The upper third of the esophagus is composed of voluntary striated muscle. The lower two thirds contain involuntary smooth muscle innervated by preganglionic cholinergic fibers, with innervation of the entire esophagus originating from the vagus nerve. The vascular supply to the esophagus is from the esophageal branch of the thoracic aorta and the left gastric artery branching from the celiac trunk of the abdominal aorta. Each section of the esophagus has different venous return with the upper esophagus venous drainage through the superior vena cava, midesophagus

venous return by the azygos vein, and the lower esophagus venous drainage by the gastric veins, which empty into the portal system. Sphincters are present in the proximal and distal sections of the esophagus. The upper esophageal sphincter (cricopharyngeal muscle) prevents entry of air into the esophagus during respiration and prevents reflux from the esophagus into the oropharynx. The lower esophageal sphincter (cardiac sphincter) prevents reflux from the stomach with caustic injury to the esophagus. The esophagus is further protected from caustic injury by thick mucus produced in the submucosal layer delivered via ducts to coat the mucosal surface.

Function
The esophagus facilitates transport of food from the mouth and oropharynx into the stomach, completing swallowing. Swallowing starts in the oropharynx area, which was aforementioned. The esophageal phase of swallowing occurs when the bolus of food enters the esophagus and the esophagus relaxes preparing for the bolus to move. Peristalsis occurs through rhythmic waves of muscular contractions moving the food bolus forward causing relaxation of the lower esophageal sphincter and allowing the food bolus to enter into the stomach (Bryant, 2004; Doig & Huether, 2012; Hall & Guyton, 2011; Patton & Thibodeau, 2014; Reed & Wickham, 2009).

ABDOMINAL CAVITY ORGANS AND PERITONEUM
The abdominal cavity is located below the diaphragm and is continuous with the pelvic cavity. The majority of the GI tract organs are contained in the abdominal cavity, with portions of the colon being contained in the pelvic cavity. The peritoneum is a serous membrane lining much of the abdominal cavity (the parietal peritoneum) and covering most of the abdominal organs (visceral peritoneum). The parietal peritoneum nerve supply is adjacent to the body wall with sensitivity for pain. The visceral peritoneum is insensate. Retroperitoneal organs lie outside the peritoneum. A double layer of the peritoneum with a central layer of loose connective tissue constitutes the mesentery. It surrounds most of the small intestine, connecting it to the posterior abdominal wall. The mesentery is vital to the intestine providing blood supply to the bowel and nerve fibers for bowel innervation. The greater omentum is mesentery with a double fold that attaches the anterior stomach to the transverse colon and connects the stomach to the posterior abdominal wall (**Fig. 2-3A and B**). This is also known as the "fatty apron" since large amounts of fat are present between and among the double folds. Much of the lesser omentum lies posteriorly to the stomach extending among the liver, the stomach, and the duodenum (Bryant, 2004; O'Rahilly et al., 2008; Patton & Thibodeau, 2014).

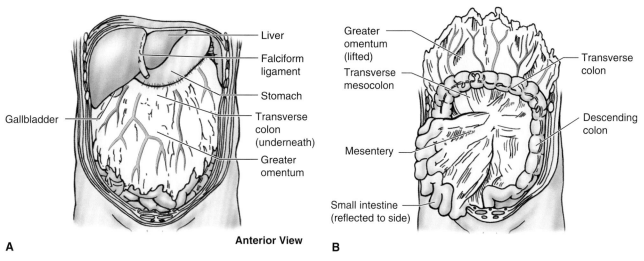

FIGURE 2-3. A. Omentum. **B.** Mesentery. (From Moore, K., & Dalley, A. F. (1999). *Clinically oriented anatomy* (4th ed.). Baltimore, MD: Wolters Kluwer.)

Stoma viability and function relies upon enough mesentery being kept with the bowel utilized to create a stoma since the mesentery is vital to providing blood supply to the bowel and nerve fibers for bowel innervation.

STOMACH

The stomach is a hollow, J-shaped muscular organ located just below the diaphragm (**Fig. 2-4**). The size and shape vary somewhat with a capacity of 1 to 1.5 L, measuring approximately 25 to 27.5 cm long and 10.25 cm wide. It consists of multiple anatomical areas with the cardia as a transitional narrow circular band surrounding the gastroesophageal junction (esophagus opening into the stomach). The fundus is the upper portion of the

stomach to the left of the cardia. The body is the middle portion, which curves to the right and is the largest portion containing numerous deep folds of the mucosal and submucosal layers, rugae. The rugae allow stretching of the stomach wall to accommodate filling. The antrum is the inferior or lower portion of the stomach and does not have rugae present, which are present in the rest of the stomach. The pylorus is the most distal stomach structure. The muscularis layer of the stomach has a circular muscle layer, oblique muscle layer, and a longitudinal muscle layer. The oblique muscle lies between the submucosa and the circular muscle layer. This is one more muscle layer than the rest of the GI tract, as a way to increase the ability to churn or mix the gastric contents.

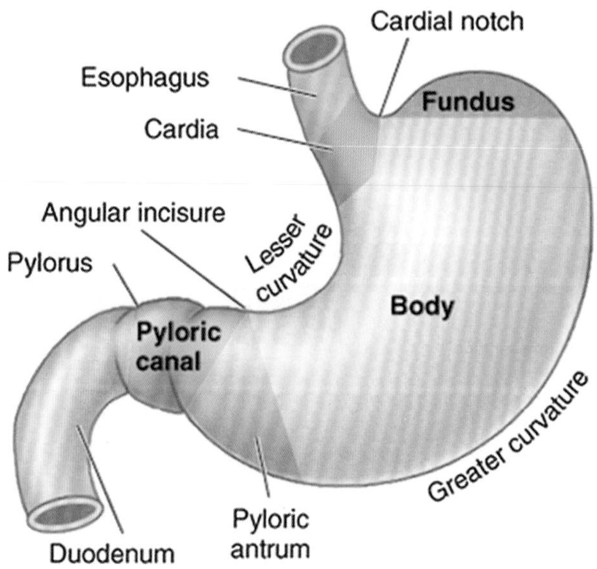

The muscular layer becomes progressively thicker in the body and antrum of the stomach. The blood supply is abundant to the stomach supplied by the branches of the celiac trunk. Venous drainage is from the splenic vein for the right side of the stomach and the gastric vein for the left side of the stomach both emptying into the portal vein. Innervation of the stomach is through the autonomic nervous system, with parasympathetic innervation provided by the vagus nerve and sympathetic innervation provided by the celiac plexus.

Columnar epithelial cells line the stomach and the gastric glands penetrating as gastric pits into the mucosal layer. The mucous cells secrete a protective viscous alkaline mucus. The mucus is approximately 1 to 1.5 mm thick blanketing the mucosa to neutralize acid with the mucosal bicarbonate, thus protecting the undisturbed innermost layer of mucus. The pH in the stomach itself is 2.0, while the innermost layer of mucus pH is 7.0. The gastric gland parietal cells produce hydrochloric acid (HCl), intrinsic factor, and TGF-α. The HCl creates the low pH, which inactivates salivary amylase and inhibits carbohydrate digestion. This also activates pepsin, a proteolytic enzyme, which initiates protein digestion and

FIGURE 2-4. The Stomach. (From Moore, K. L., Agur, A. M., & Dalley, A. F. (2014). *Essential clinical anatomy*. Philadelphia, PA: Wolters Kluwer.)

forms polypeptides in the stomach. The pepsin is inactivated when it enters the alkaline environment of the duodenum. The intrinsic factor binds with vitamin B_{12} and is key to the absorption of vitamin B_{12} in the terminal ileum (Bryant, 2004; Doig & Huether, 2012).

Function

The stomach receives food from the esophagus. As food reaches the end of the esophagus, it enters the stomach through a muscular valve called the lower esophageal sphincter.

The stomach secretes acid and enzymes that digest food.

Digestion

Swallowing relaxes the fundus (receptive relaxation) in preparation of a food bolus to be received from the esophagus. The food enters the stomach, which serves as a reservoir with controlled emptying into the duodenum. Peristaltic contractions mix the food with gastric secretions until it is chyme, a semifluid consistency. The mechanical mixing with chemical secretions in the stomach contributes to the digestive process. The more solid the food, the more mixing is required. The consistency of gastric contents, acidity, chyme fat content, vagal stimuli, osmolality, temperature, and emotional state all affect the rate of gastric emptying of the chyme into the duodenum through the pyloric sphincter.

Secretion

The stomach secretes 2 to 3 L/day of gastric juices and secretions (**Table 2-1**). These include mucus, acid enzymes, hormones, intrinsic factor, and gastroferrin. The gastric gland parietal cells produce HCl, intrinsic factor, and TGF-α. The HCl creates the low pH (high acidity), which inactivates salivary amylase and inhibits carbohydrate digestion. This also activates pepsin, which initiates protein digestion. The intrinsic factor binds with vitamin B_{12} (cyanocobalamin) and is key to the absorption of vitamin B_{12} in the terminal ileum. Lifelong injections of B_{12} will be necessary to prevent pernicious anemia if the stomach is removed. Gastroferrin facilitates iron absorption in the small intestine. Hormones secreted by the stomach also affect gastric secretion with secretin and gastric inhibitory polypeptides inhibiting stomach emptying through decreased gastric motor activity and gastric acid secretion. G cells make gastrin, which stimulates secretion of HCl promoting pepsinogen secretion and gastric motility. D cells secrete somatostatin, which inhibits secretion of gastric acid, gastrin, and intrinsic factor. Enterochromaffin (EC) cells produce serotonin. The zymogenic chief cells secrete lipase and pepsinogen, a precursor of pepsin. The amount of gastric secretions vary according to the time of day with the lowest volume and rate being in the morning, whereas the highest is in the afternoon and evening. The three phases of gastric secretion (cephalic, gastric, and intestinal phases) are influenced by multiple factors. The cephalic phase is stimulated by the thought, smell, and taste of food. The gastric phase is stimulated by food distention in the stomach. The intestinal phase is stimulated by chyme in the intestine. Gastric secretion is additionally stimulated by moderate amounts of alcohol and caffeine and interestingly by anger and hostility. Inversely, gastric secretion is inhibited by unpleasant odors, tastes, and the emotions of fear and depression.

Absorption

The role in nutrient absorption is limited in the stomach to include some partially chemically digested carbohydrates, alcohol, and some medications such as aspirin.

Elimination of Ingested Bacteria

The antibacterial effect of the stomach is provided by the extremely low pH, thus eliminating most of the ingested bacteria (Bryant, 2004; Doig & Huether, 2012; Hall & Guyton, 2011; Patton & Thibodeau, 2014; Reed & Wickham, 2009).

A patient with a large portion of the stomach resected may require lifelong vitamin B_{12} supplementation to avoid pernicious anemia since not enough intrinsic factor may be available to bind with vitamin B_{12} and facilitate absorption of vitamin B_{12}.

SMALL INTESTINE

The small intestine is divided into three functioning sections, the duodenum, jejunum, and ileum. Essentially, it stretches from the gastric pylorus to the ileocecal valve and is in total approximately 6.7 m (22 feet) varying from 5 to 8 m long. The duodenum starts at the pylorus and joins the jejunum at the ligament of Treitz, a suspension ligament. There is no line of separation to distinguish the jejunum from the ileum. The ileum ends at the ileocecal valve, which controls the flow of digested material from the small intestine into the large intestine and prevents reflux into the ileum. The duodenum lies retroperitoneal and attaches to the posterior abdominal wall. The jejunum and ileum are suspended from the posterior abdominal wall by the mesentery (**Fig. 2-5**). A branch of the celiac trunk provides the blood supply to the proximal (first portion) duodenum with the branches of the superior mesenteric artery supplying the majority of the

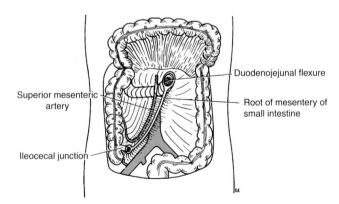

FIGURE 2-5. Attachment of the Root of the Mesentery of the Small Intestine to the Posterior Abdominal Wall. The ileocecal junction is identified. (From Snell, R. S. (2003). *Clinical anatomy* (7th ed.). Philadelphia, PA: Wolters Kluwer.)

small intestine, including the distal duodenum, jejunum, and ileum. The venous return is by the superior mesenteric vein, which joins the splenic vein and empties into the portal circulation. Both the parasympathetic and sympathetic components of the autonomic nervous system innervate the small intestine. The parasympathetic nerves mediate secretion, motility, pain sensation, and intestinal reflexes, that is, relaxation of sphincters. The sympathetic nerves inhibit motility and cause vasoconstriction. Intrinsic motor innervation is mediated by both the Auerbach plexus (myenteric plexus) and the Meissner plexus (submucosal plexus).

The submucosal and mucosal layers are unique in the small intestine being arranged in folds (plicae circulares), which increase the absorptive surface along with the villi (**Fig. 2-2**). The mucosal layer of the small intestine is lined with simple columnar epithelium. The epithelium contains enterocytes (absorptive cells) primarily with scattered goblet cells and occasional enteroendocrine cells. The lamina propria lies beneath the epithelial cell of the villi. This is a connective tissue layer of the mucous membrane and contains lymphocytes; plasma cells, which produce immunoglobulins; and macrophages. These numerous lymphoid cells of the small intestine produce more antibodies than does any other body site. This protects the mucosa from pathogens and ingested noxious substances. Peptides are also produced from the mucosal layer.

The villi are small intestinal structures of the mucosal layer, which are finger-like projections that cover the mucosal surface and increase the absorptive area of the small intestine, creating a velvety appearance of the lumen being 0.5 to 1 mm in length. Each villus contains a capillary network, lymph vessel, numerous white blood cells, and smooth muscle fibers. This protects the mucosa from pathogens and ingested noxious substances. Each villus has absorptive columnar cells and mucus-secreting goblet cells of the mucosal epithelium. Each villus is covered with absorptive cytoplasmic extensions (microvilli). Together, the villi and microvilli create the brush border, which, combined with the plicae circulares, increases the absorptive surface of the mucosa by 600 times what would be expected from a tube with the same diameter. The brush border has enzymes present including peptidases, disaccharidases, and nucleases. Between the villi are simple tubular glands (crypts of Lieberkühn). These crypts contain undifferentiated (stem) cells, mucus-secreting goblet cells, Paneth cells, and endocrine paracrine cells. Undifferentiated (stem) cells rise from the base of the crypts to the top of the villus, maturing as they rise reproducing mucosal cells on a continual basis with mucosal cell turnover between 48 and 72 hours and in entirety replaced every 4 to 7 days.

Interestingly, the villi are able to transform to some degree. They are able to elongate or become hypertrophied increasing the absorptive capacity, which helps to partially explain bowel adaptation after partial bowel resection. The villi may also temporarily atrophy with decreased absorptive capacity if food or fluids are not ingested. Beneath the epithelial cell of the villi of the small intestine lies the lamina propria. This is a connective tissue layer of the mucous membrane and contains lymphocytes; plasma cells, which produce immunoglobulins; and macrophages. These numerous lymphoid cells of the small intestine produce more antibodies than does any other body site (Bryant, 2004; Doig & Huether, 2012; Dyer, 2014; Hall & Guyton, 2011; Patton & Thibodeau, 2014; Reed & Wickham, 2009).

Because the villi are able to transform to some degree and elongate or become hypertrophied, they are able to increase the absorptive capacity taking on some of the function of the colon when the colon is surgically removed.

As the villi atrophy and flatten, decreased absorption occurs. Additionally, as gut atrophy progresses, there is increased risk of bacterial translocation and the immune functions of the GI tract are impaired.

Function

The small intestine is the organ responsible for much of the digestive process, absorption of nutrients, electrolytes, vitamins, minerals, and miscellaneous substances. It is a major contributor to maintaining fluid and electrolyte balance. The specific functions contributing to the digestive process include intestinal motility, secretion, and absorption.

Motility

The motility of the small intestine facilitates both digestion and absorption. Chyme arriving in the duodenum from the stomach stimulates intestinal mixing of secretions from the liver, pancreas, and intestinal glands containing enzymes as well as bile salts. The luminal contents are brought into contact with the absorbing villi through a churning motion (short segmental contractions). The plicae or mucosal folds slow the motility of the chyme allowing for more time for digestion and absorption. The chyme is pushed further through the small intestine toward the large intestine by propulsive movements (peristaltic waves). Distention of the intestinal wall by the luminal contents stimulates the peristalsis. The myenteric plexus (Auerbach plexus) lies between the longitudinal and circular muscle layers and is primarily responsible for control of peristalsis and segmentation. Food entering into the stomach causes the ileum to empty into the large intestine (gastroileal reflex). The average normal transit time from the mouth to the colon is 4 to 9 hours with 3 to 5 hours of that time spent continually mixing the chyme in the small intestine (Bryant, 2004; Doig & Huether, 2012; Hall & Guyton, 2011; Reed & Wickham, 2009).

Secretion

Extensive amounts of mucus are secreted within only the first few centimeters of the duodenum by the Brunner glands (compound mucous glands). These glands secrete mucus to protect the duodenal wall from being digested by the highly acidic chyme emptying into the duodenum from the stomach. The mucus neutralizes the HCl contained in the chyme as the mucus contains a large amount of bicarbonate ions, which combine with the bicarbonate ions from pancreatic secretion and liver bile. The epithelium covering villi and Lieberkühn crypts contains secretory cells of two types, goblet cells and enterocytes. Large amounts of mucus are secreted by goblet cells, which serve to lubricate and protect the intestinal surfaces. The enterocytes secrete approximately 3 L of extracellular fluid into the small bowel lumen each day. The pH of this fluid is slightly alkaline 7.5 to 8 (**Table 2-1**). This watery intestinal fluid is almost all extracellular fluid and contains no enzymes. It promotes the absorptive process by providing a flow of fluid from the crypts into the villi for osmotic absorption of substances from the chyme as it contacts the villi.

The enterocytes of the villi contain digestive enzymes that digest food substances while they are being absorbed through the epithelium. These digestive enzymes include (1) peptidases, which split small peptides into amino acids; (2) four enzymes, sucrase, maltase, isomaltase, and lactase, which split disaccharides into monosaccharides; and (3) intestinal lipase in small amounts, which split neutral fats into glycerol and fatty acids (Bryant, 2004; Doig & Huether, 2012; Hall & Guyton, 2011; O'Rahilly et al., 2008; Patton & Thibodeau, 2014; Reed & Wickham, 2009).

Absorption

The digestive processes break down complex molecules into substances that are more easily absorbed into the bloodstream. The vast amount of absorption occurs in the proximal small intestine (duodenum and jejunum) where the villi and brush border are ample. The ileum can absorb a substantial amount if necessary. The amount of bowel necessary to absorb enough nutrition to sustain life is difficult to determine due to variations in measurement techniques. However, digestion and absorption of nutrients is more than 90% completed within the first 100 cm of the small intestine. The absorption of intraluminal fluid is significant with as much as 5 to 6 L/day received by the proximal small bowel, an additional 3 L/day produced (**Table 2-1**). Of this total 8 to 9 L, 7 to 8 L is reabsorbed back into the small intestine. Only 1 to 2 L of fluid per day is passed through the ileocecal valve (Bryant, 2004; Hall & Guyton, 2011; Patton & Thibodeau, 2014).

DUODENUM

The duodenum is the first section of the small intestine; being C shaped, the concavity encloses the head of the pancreas. It is the shortest segment of the small intestine being 25.4 cm (10 inches) long extending from the pylorus to the duodenojejunal flexure. It lies retroperitoneally in close proximity to the stomach, the accessory organs (liver, gallbladder, and pancreas), and the transverse colon. The common bile duct and pancreatic duct empty into the duodenum at Vater ampulla. The flow of secretions through Vater ampulla into the duodenum is controlled by the sphincter of Oddi. The ligament of Treitz separates the duodenum and the jejunum. This ligament suspends the duodenum at an angle facilitating passage of the contents.

The major function of the duodenum is to neutralize acidic gastric contents as they enter the duodenum. The acidic chyme is partially neutralized by alkaline mucus secreted by Brunner glands located in the submucosal layer of the duodenum, as previously discussed. Additionally, secretin is released as the acid chyme enters the duodenum. The secretin stimulates the pancreas to secrete high concentrations of bicarbonate ions draining through the pancreatic duct and emptying into the duodenum at Vater ampulla helping to neutralize the chyme. The presence of fats in the duodenum stimulates delivery of alkaline bile, which further neutralizes gastric acids.

The second function of the duodenum is to continue the digestive processes. The presence of fatty acids and amino acids in the duodenum stimulates CCK release, which in turn contracts the gallbladder, and secretion of pancreatic enzymatic juices. Bile is delivered to the duodenum to emulsify the fats, making them more susceptible to enzymatic breakdown. The pancreatic juice contains many digestive enzymes: amylase, to continue carbohydrate digestion; lipases, to continue lipid digestion; and the trypsin precursor of proteolytic enzymes, which is activated in the duodenum by enterokinase. Once trypsin is activated, it then activates the other proteolytic enzymes: chymotrypsin and carboxypeptidase.

Absorption is also another function of the duodenum. Substances absorbed include carbohydrates and minerals including iron, calcium, and magnesium. The villi are flatter with less frequent plicae in the duodenum compared to the jejunum (Bryant, 2004; O'Rahilly et al., 2008; Patton & Thibodeau, 2014).

JEJUNUM

The jejunum is the middle section of the small intestine. The ligament of Treitz is considered the division of the duodenum and jejunum, though it is difficult to distinguish between the distal part of the jejunum and the ileum. It is approximately 2.7 m (9 feet) long with a diameter of 2.5 to 3.8 cm. The jejunum is the primary organ of nutritional absorption of most fats, proteins, vitamins, and the remaining carbohydrates. Digestion is finalized by the enzymes of the ample villi brush border. Absorption is through the carrier systems and the large volume of intestinal secretions. Additionally, absorption is facilitated through prominent villi and frequent plicae circulares (Bryant, 2004; O'Rahilly et al., 2008; Patton & Thibodeau, 2014).

ILEUM

The third and most distal section of the small intestine is the ileum. It is almost 4 m (12 feet) in length extending from the ligament of Treitz to the ileocecal valve. The width of the ileum is approximately 2.5 cm. The ileum has proportionately the most goblet cells of the small bowel. Increased amounts of mucosal lymphoid tissue are also present in the ileum with conspicuous cluster called Peyer patches. The Peyer patches together with the tonsils, appendix, and other diffuse lymphoid tissue constitute gut-associated lymphoid tissues (GALTs). The ileum is narrower than the jejunum with less prominent villi and no plicae circulares. The ileum absorbs nutrients not absorbed previously by the duodenum or jejunum. The terminal ileum contains the only receptors to absorb the intrinsic factor–vitamin B_{12} complex and bile salts. Patients who have had significant lengths of the terminal ileum resected may require lifelong vitamin B_{12} replacement to prevent pernicious anemia, improve fat intolerance, and reduce weight loss. Fat intolerance occurs when the bile salts in the terminal are not reabsorbed, which reduces bile production in the liver. Bile is produced in the liver and stored concentrated in the gallbladder until CCK stimulates the gallbladder to contract and deliver bile into the duodenum. Fats are emulsified by the bile, and the residual bile salts continue to pass further through the bowel until they are reabsorbed in the terminal ileum. Recycling of bile salts is known as the enterohepatic circulation, which promotes bile production and thus fat absorption (Bryant, 2004; Doig & Huether, 2012; Hall & Guyton, 2011; O'Rahilly et al., 2008; Patton & Thibodeau, 2014).

> **KEY POINT**
>
> Patients who have had significant lengths of the terminal ileum resected may require lifelong vitamin B_{12} replacement to prevent pernicious anemia, improve fat intolerance, and reduce weight loss.

ILEOCECAL VALVE

The ileocecal valve is a one-way valve separating the ileum and the cecum (separates the small intestine from the large intestine; **Fig. 2-5**). The ileocecal valve (sphincter) is 2 to 3 cm of smooth muscle intrinsically regulated. It typically remains closed until peristaltic waves occur in the last few centimeters relaxing or opening the ileocecal valve and allows controlled amounts of chyme to pass through to the large intestine. Distention of the cecum causes increased contractions and constriction

of the ileocecal valve, which protects the small bowel from distention and reflux (Bryant, 2004; Doig & Huether, 2012; O'Rahilly et al., 2008; Patton & Thibodeau, 2014).

As a native one-way valve, the ileocecal valve is used at times as a continence mechanism for continent diversions.

> **KEY POINT**
>
> Ostomies of the small intestine are smaller in diameter than those of the large intestine due to the relatively smaller diameter of the small intestine compared with the large intestine.

LARGE INTESTINE (COLON)

The large intestine consists of the cecum with appendix appendage, ascending colon, transverse colon, descending colon, sigmoid colon, rectum, and anal canal. It is approximately 1.2 to 1.5 m (4 to 5 feet) long and is somewhat horseshoe shaped. The diameter is 2.5 to 5.5 cm, the largest at the cecum with the caliber decreasing distally (further down the colon).

Unique to the colon are several features of the tissue layers from the rest of the GI tract. The outer layer (serosa) forms peritoneal sacs, which enclose fat and hang from the bowel (epiploic appendices). The longitudinal muscle of the colon unlike that of the small intestine is gathered into three muscular bands or taeniae. The taeniae coli extend from the appendix to the rectosigmoid junction where the taeniae fuse into one continuous, circumferential longitudinal muscle. The taeniae are shorter than the colon, which causes a sacculated or gathered appearance (haustra). Colonic contractions and relaxation of the circular muscle make the haustra more or less prominent. The mucosa of the colon has many features different from the mucosa of the small intestine. The mucosa has folds (rugae) between the haustra. Villi are not present in the large intestine (colon). Lieberkühn crypts are deeper extending into the muscularis mucosae. Paneth cells are scattered throughout the cecum and ascending colon but absent in the rest of the colon.

The Lieberkühn crypts along with goblet cells produce colonic secretions of water, mucus, potassium, and bicarbonate. The bicarbonate secretion creates alkaline fecal matter with a pH of 7.8. Mucus produced by the goblet cells provides (1) lubrication to facilitate transportation of the fecal bolus and (2) protection from mucosal injury and (3) serves as a binding agent for the fecal material. Mucous production is stimulated by colonic irritants (bacterial, mechanical, or chemical) and the parasympathetic nervous system. Mucous secretion is decreased with anxiety and tension. The superior mesenteric artery provides the blood supply to the cecum, the right colon, and the transverse colon to the splenic flexure (**Fig. 2-6**). The inferior mesenteric artery provides the blood supply to

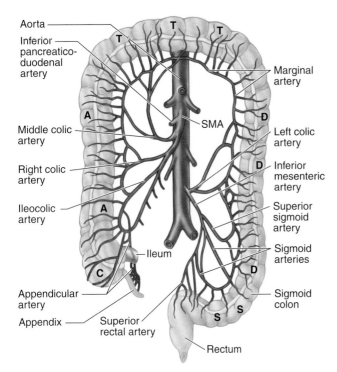

FIGURE 2-6. Blood Supply to the Large Intestine, Cecum, and Appendix. A, ascending colon; C, cecum; D, descending colon; S, sigmoid colon; SMA, superior mesenteric artery; T, transverse colon. (From Moore, K. L., Agur, A. M., & Dalley, A. F. (2014). *Essential clinical anatomy.* Philadelphia, PA: Wolters Kluwer.)

the descending colon, the sigmoid colon, and the proximal portion of the rectum. The middle and inferior hemorrhoidal arteries, arising from the internal iliac arteries, supply the remainder of the rectum. The venous return is from the veins corresponding to the arteries supplying the colon. The superior mesenteric vein provides venous drainage for the cecum, the right colon, and the transverse colon to the splenic flexure. The inferior mesenteric vein provides venous drainage to the descending colon, the sigmoid colon, and the proximal portion of the rectum. The blood from these veins is delivered to the liver as part of the portal vein system. The middle and inferior hemorrhoidal veins drain the remainder of the rectum and drains into the iliac veins as part of the systemic circulation (Bryant, 2004; Doig & Huether, 2012).

Function
The functions of the colon are collection, concentration, transportation, and elimination of fecal waste materials. The proximal half of the colon concerns essentially absorption, and the distal half of the colon concerns primarily storage. The intestinal materials pass into the cecum through the ileocecal valve totaling 1 to 1.5 L/day. Water, electrolytes (sodium and chloride), glucose, and urea are absorbed from this material. As the intestinal matter progresses through the colon, more fluid is absorbed from the fecal material and the consistency

thickens from being fluid (in the ascending colon) to semifluid or soft (in the transverse colon) to solid (in the descending colon). Once the intestinal content reaches the sigmoid colon, it becomes feces, a collection of solid fecal waste products.

Transportation of the fecal material is through synchronous longitudinal and circular muscle movements that propel the fecal material forward primarily not only through segmentation (kneading) but also through several types of peristalsis. Historically, this was referred to gastrocolic reflex and is stimulated when chyme enters from the ileum (most commonly during or immediately after eating). This reflex stimulates propulsion of the fecal material rapidly into the sigmoid colon and rectum, stimulating elimination. Relaxation of the colon is important to moving fecal material through the colon. The cecum fills with receptive relaxation, the fecal material accumulates and is stored with adaptive relaxation, pendulum movements (continuous back and forth movement) aid in absorption, and mass movement (en masse contraction of the left colon) propels the fecal bolus into the rectum to be evacuated. In summary, the cecum, ascending colon, transverse colon, and descending colon provide absorption and epithelial transport. When the fecal material mass reaches the sigmoid colon, it is entirely composed of waste products (undigested food residue, unabsorbed GI secretions, epithelial cells, and bacteria) and is considered feces or stool. The rectosigmoid section serves essentially as storage until it is time to defecate (Bryant, 2004; Doig & Huether, 2012).

The colon's main functions of fluid absorption, fecal material transportation and storage, and elimination of feces lend the colon to be considered by some as an "organ of convenience" and not necessary to sustain life.

COLON SEGMENTS
The *cecum* is the first section of the colon essentially forming a pouch below the ileocecal valve. It measures 6 to 7.6 cm in length containing the ileocecal valve. The *ileocecal valve* lies between the terminal ileum and the cecum preventing reflux of colonic material and bacteria into the small intestine. The *appendix* is a finger-like appendage of the cecum lying 1 to 2 cm below the ileum. The mucosa of the appendix is laden with lymphoid tissue. The *ascending colon* extends from the cecum to the right hepatic flexure, being the segment that is in a vertical position on the right side of the colon. It is 15 cm long and slightly smaller in diameter than is the cecum. The ascending colon is covered with peritoneum on the front and sides. The *hepatic flexure* is a sharp 90-degree left turn in the colon as it continues as the transverse colon. The *transverse colon* lies horizontally across the upper portion of the abdomen and is approximately 45 to 50 cm in length.

At the distal or furthest end, the transverse colon makes an extremely sharp (almost 180-degree) downward turn, which is the *splenic flexure*. The transverse colon is only fixed at two points (hepatic and splenic flexures), so it is quite mobile and may sag downward. In front of the transverse colon lies the greater omentum. The splenic flexure lies higher than the hepatic flexure. The *descending colon* is the next segment, extending from the splenic flexure to the true pelvic brim measuring around 22 cm. The descending colon lies vertically on the left side of the abdomen. The front and both sides of the descending colon are covered with the peritoneum. As the descending colon passes over the psoas muscle, the *sigmoid colon* starts and continues in an S-shaped curve to the left and continues to the upper end of the rectum. The length of the sigmoid colon is varied on average 40 cm. The sigmoid colon is covered with the peritoneum on the front, posterior, and sides. The remaining portions include the *rectum* and *anal canal*, which follow (Bryant, 2004; Doig & Huether, 2012; Hall & Guyton, 2011; O'Rahilly et al., 2008).

The S-shaped curve to the left of the sigmoid colon is the reason why patients are positioned on their left side for endoscopic examinations or enemas.

RECTUM

The rectum is distensible as an angulated hollow structure 12 to 15 cm (6 inches) in length (**Fig. 2-7**). It is slightly wider or the same in diameter than the preceding sig-moid colon segment and is similar anatomically. The rectum begins where the sigmoid colon terminates and is marked by the third sacral vertebra following the curve of the sacrum and coccyx. It angles sharply downward and backward in a straight manner. The rectum does not have haustra or epiploic appendices. It is normally collapsed being surrounded by strong muscular longitudinal fibers of the merging of the taeniae coli.

The rectal mucosa creates three transverse folds, which are the valves of Houston (two on the left and one on the right). The valves of Houston are composed of mucosa, muscularis mucosa, submucosa, and circular muscle, which help support the weight of the fecal matter and reduce the frequency of the urge to defecate. Rectal compliance (resistance of the rectal wall to stretch or the amount of stiffness of the rectal wall) is related to rectal capacity (volume). Together, they are integral components of continence. In clinical practice, stool frequency and rectal compliance are correlated in patients with an ileal pouch. Poor outcomes are found when compliance of the ileal pouch fails to increase postoperatively.

The rectum becomes the anal canal as it passes through the levator ani muscle (Bryant, 2004; Doig & Huether, 2012; Fox et al., 2006; Hall & Guyton, 2011; O'Rahilly et al., 2008).

ANAL CANAL

The anal canal is a short canal approximately 3 to 4 cm in length and is the last portion of the colon positioned from the anorectal junction to the anal verge (typically the portion visible at skin level). A distinction in tissue types occurs at the midpoint of the anal canal known as the dentate line (also known as the pectinate line). Proximal (above) the dentate line, the mucosa has a pleated appearance referred to as the columns of Morgagni. These longitudinal folds occur as the rectum narrows into the anal canal. The anal canal is lined with columnar epithelium above the dentate line. Below the dentate line, to the anal verge, the anal canal is lined with modified squamous epithelium. The transition of tissue types from columnar epithelium to the squamous epithelium occurs gradually, approximately 6 to 12 mm proximal to the dentate line, and is known as the transition (cloacogenic) zone. Above the dentate line, the epithelium changes to a purple hue from the internal hemorrhoidal plexus. Above the dentate line, the epithelium is innervated with autonomic nerves, whereas the submucosa distal to the dentate line contains numerous encapsulated and free sensory nerve endings allowing high sensitivity to pain, touch, and other sensations.

The anoderm (area below the dentate line) resembles skin minus the accessory skin structures (i.e., hair, sebaceous glands, and sweat glands). The anal canal is surrounded by two sphincters, the internal anal sphincter and the external anal sphincter. The internal anal

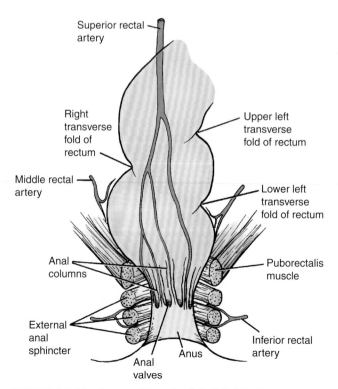

FIGURE 2-7. The Rectum. (From Snell, R. S. (2011). *Clinical anatomy by regions*. Philadelphia, PA: Wolters Kluwer.)

sphincter is formed by thick circular smooth muscle (involuntary sphincter) surrounding the anal canal to 1.5 cm distal of the dentate line. It is tonically contracted. Overlapping it distally, surrounding the anal canal is the striated muscle of the external anal sphincter (voluntary sphincter). The deep portion of the external sphincter is not attached posteriorly while it is continuous with the puborectalis muscle (one of four divisions of the levator ani pelvic floor muscle) in the proximal portion. It is innervated by the pudendal nerve. The external sphincter is also tonically contracted. These sphincters along with coordination of the pelvic floor muscles and voluntary efforts maintain continence and allow voluntary defecation. The anal verge is the level where the anal canal walls make contact in their normal resting state and have a puckered appearance. The perianal skin is considered the 5-cm radius of skin around the anal verge.

A mass movement of feces is delivered to the rectum, causing distention. Rectosigmoid distention causes stimulation of the mechanoreceptors, which elicit a reflex causing internal sphincter relaxation (rectoanal inhibitory reflex) while simultaneously the external anal sphincter contracts. The sensitive anal canal epithelium "samples" the contents to determine if the composition is air, liquid, or solid (sampling reflex). If defecation is desired and straining occurs to push the fecal mass into the rectum, intrarectal pressures increase. The increased pressure is sufficient to overcome the external sphincter contraction except at times of micturition or voluntary contraction of the external sphincter. Simultaneously, the external sphincter and pelvic floor muscles relax, causing straightening of the rectum and eliminating resistance by Houston valves or rectal angles. The squatting position also reduces rectal angles. Fecal mass stimulation of the anal canal mucosa allows continued relaxation of the external sphincter (Bryant, 2004; Doig & Huether, 2012; Hall & Guyton, 2011; Heitkemper, 2006; Reed & Wickham, 2009).

The cell type differences lining above and below the dentate line in the anal canal are associated with common types of cancer above and below the dentate line (adenocarcinoma above the dentate line associated with colorectal cancer and squamous cell carcinoma below the dentate line associated with anal cancer).

INTESTINAL BACTERIA

The presence of bacteria in the GI tract increases from the stomach to the distal colon. The stomach is rather sterile due to the high acidity that obliterates ingested pathogens or inhibits bacterial growth. The duodenum and jejunum have a relatively low aerobic bacterial concentration (10^{-1} to 10^{-4}) since in the duodenum, bile acid secretion, intestinal motility, and antibody production reduce bacterial growth. The aerobic bacteria that are present include streptococci, lactobacilli, staphylococci,

and enterobacteria. Anaerobic bacteria are not found proximal to the ileocecal valve but are found distal of the ileocecal valve in the colon. Bacteria are quite prevalent in the colon and are vital to many functions. The anaerobes found from the ileocecal valve to the cecum include *Bacteroides*, clostridia, anaerobic lactobacilli, and coliforms.

Anaerobic bacteria decompose remaining proteins and indigestible residue; synthesize folic acid, vitamin K, nicotinic acid, riboflavin, and some B vitamins; and convert urea salts into ammonium salts and ammonia absorption into the portal circulation. *Escherichia coli*, *Enterobacter aerogenes*, *Clostridium perfringens*, and *Lactobacillus bifidus* are common colonic bacteria. The bacteria become more concentrated the further or more distal in the colon. Anaerobic bacteria compose approximately 95% of colonic fecal flora and contribute one third of the solid bulk of feces. Together, these bacteria are responsible to some degree for fecal odor and intestinal gas production.

The normal intestinal bacteria flora is not virulent or pathogenic. Endogenous infections of the GI tract occur through three major methods: bacterial overgrowth, intestinal perforation, and contamination of nearby structures. Prebiotics are plant fibers that promote healthy bowel flora growth. Probiotics are probiotic bacteria that arrive to the bowel in an active state. They interact with epithelial and immune cells boosting systemic immune activity and epithelial function. Synbiotics are synergistic combinations of both probiotics and prebiotics. The use of probiotics decreases bacterial overgrowth and reestablishes a healthy bowel flora. They are clinically used mainstream as therapeutic treatment of many GI disorders and disease processes, that is, irritable bowel syndrome, inflammatory bowel disease, antibiotic-associated diarrhea, and *Clostridium difficile* colitis and diarrhea (Beisner et al., 2010; Bryant, 2004; Doig & Huether, 2012; Fedorak & Madsen, 2004).

Bacterial concentration increases distally in the bowel. This is the reason why there is more gas and odor for a sigmoid colostomy compared to an ileostomy.

The ability of probiotics and symbiotics to promote healthy bowel flora, facilitate epithelial transport, and boost the immune system is the rationale behind the accepted therapeutic use to treat pouchitis of continent diversions.

ACCESSORY ORGANS

The accessory organs of digestion include the liver, gallbladder, and exocrine pancreas, all of which secrete substances that are necessary for the digestion of chyme. The secretions are delivered in the duodenum. The liver provides bile for the digestion and absorption of fats. The bile produced by the liver is stored in the gallbladder when food is not being digested. The exocrine pancreas provides enzymes necessary for digestion of three main types of food: carbohydrates, proteins, and fats. The exocrine pancreas produces an alkaline fluid that contains large amounts of bicarbonate ions helping to neutralize acidic chyme leaving the stomach as it empties into the duodenum.

The liver metabolizes or synthesizes nutrients absorbed by the small intestine into forms that can be more readily absorbed by the body's cells. These nutrients are then either released into the bloodstream or stored for later use (Bryant, 2004; Doig & Huether, 2012; Hall & Guyton, 2011; Patton & Thibodeau, 2014; Reed & Wickham, 2009).

Liver

The liver is the largest internal organ of the body and weighs between 1,200 and 1,600 g. It lies under the right diaphragm. The liver is divided into right and left lobes, with the larger right lobe subdivided into the caudate and quadrate lobes. The liver is suspended from the anterior abdominal wall, the inferior diaphragmatic surface by the falciform ligament, the coronary ligament, and the round ligament. The liver is unique in having a blood supply of both arterial and venous sources (the hepatic artery and the portal vein). The hepatic artery is a branch of the abdominal aorta and provides the liver with oxygenated blood at the rate of 400 to 500 mL/min or 25% to 33% of the cardiac output.

The portal vein receives nutrient-rich, deoxygenated blood from the splenic, inferior, and superior mesenteric veins (blood from the intestines, pancreas, spleen, stomach, and mesentery) at the rate of 1,000 to 1,200 mL/min or 70% to 75% of the liver's blood supply. The portal vein branches into the sinusoids supplying each of the lobules. The sinusoids empty the venous blood into the intralobular vein, which eventually empties into the hepatic vein and the inferior vena cava. The volume of the liver's blood supply and proximity to the cells individually is thought to allow for the liver's ability to regenerate. On average, regeneration is believed to occur within 3 weeks functioning normally within 4 weeks.

Blood vessels, lymphatics, and nerves are supplied to the liver by the Glisson capsule, which covers the liver. If the liver is diseased or swollen, the distention of this capsule causes pain and the lymphatics may ooze fluid into the peritoneal space.

The lobules are the functional units of the liver that are formed from hepatocytes. The plates of hepatocytes contain capillaries or sinusoids and small channels (bile canaliculi) that are adjacent to the hepatocytes. Hepatocytes secrete electrolytes, lipids, lecithin, bile acids, and cholesterol into the small channels (bile canaliculi). Bile is also secreted via the hepatocytes and contains these substances as well as bilirubin (a by-product of destroyed red blood cells), which provides the bile pigment. The alkaline bile (7.5 pH) flows through the canaliculi channels to bile ducts that drain into the common bile duct and empties into the duodenum through the sphincter of Oddi (the major duodenal papilla). Bile salts are conjugated bile acids required for intestinal fat emulsification and absorption. Most bile salts are absorbed in the terminal ileum and returned to the liver via the portal circulation with this recycling of bile salts termed the enterohepatic circulation. Vitamin B_{12} is likewise absorbed in the terminal ileum and returned to the liver for storage.

The liver lobules sinusoids are lined with highly permeable endothelium. This allows the transport of nutrients into the hepatocytes for metabolism. The liver lobules sinusoids are also lined with phagocytic Kupffer cells (tissue macrophages), which destroy foreign substances, kill bacteria from the blood, and play a role in bilirubin production. Interstitial fluid is drained into the hepatic lymphatic system by Disse space (the endothelial lining of the sinusoid and hepatocyte) (Bryant, 2004; Doig & Huether, 2012; Hall & Guyton, 2011; Patton & Thibodeau, 2014; Reed & Wickham, 2009). The liver's ability to regenerate is significant allowing for up to 70% liver destruction before becoming symptomatic.

Gallbladder

The gallbladder is sac-like and pear shaped and is located on the inferior aspect of the liver. Bile flows through the cystic duct into the gallbladder from the liver. The bile is stored in the gallbladder and concentrated until it is needed for digestion. The bile concentrates as it is stored through absorption of water and electrolytes through the gallbladder wall, which creates a highly concentrated mixture of bile salts, bile pigments, and cholesterol, changing the pH of the bile to 7. Bile flows from the liver and gallbladder into the duodenum through the major duodenal papilla (sphincter of Oddi) into the duodenum as chyme enters the duodenum. After the duodenum empties, the major duodenal papilla closes, causing the gallbladder to fill with bile until the cycle begins again (Bryant, 2004; Doig & Huether, 2012; Hall & Guyton, 2011; Patton & Thibodeau, 2014; Reed & Wickham, 2009).

Exocrine Pancreas

The pancreas is fish shaped weighing approximately 85 g and approximately 20 cm long by 5 cm wide with four sections (head, neck, body, and tail). Its head is tucked into the C-shaped curve of the duodenum near the pyloric valve, the body is behind the stomach, and the tail touches the spleen at the level of the first and second lumbar vertebrae. The blood supply to the pancreas is supplied from branches of the celiac, splenic, and superior mesenteric arteries. The venous return is through the splenic and superior mesenteric veins, which drain blood into the portal circulation. The pancreas is innervated by sympathetic and parasympathetic fibers.

The pancreas uniquely has both exocrine and endocrine functions. Endocrine pancreatic cells are located within the islets of Langerhans and directly secrete hormones into the bloodstream. The hormones are insulin (secreted by beta cells), glucagon (alpha cells elucidate), somatostatin (produced by delta cells), and pancreatic polypeptide (produced by PP cells).

The exocrine (digestive) pancreas is composed of acinar cells and networks of ducts lined with columnar epithelial cells that secrete enzymes and aqueous bicarbonate fluids important to digestive functions secreting 700 to 1,000 mL daily. The clusters of the acinar cells for an acinus will form lobules. Connective tissue joins each lobule together forming the pancreas. Each acinus contains small ducts that empty into lobules where the secretions from the acinar cells are received and empty into the Wirsung duct. The Wirsung duct runs the entire length of the pancreas and connects to the duodenum through the Vater ampulla being surrounded by the sphincter of Oddi. The alkaline pancreatic juice (pH of 8.3) neutralizes the acidic chyme as it enters the duodenum and creates an optimal environment to active digestive enzymes (Bryant, 2004; Doig & Huether, 2012; Hall & Guyton, 2011; Patton & Thibodeau, 2014; Reed & Wickham, 2009).

CONCLUSIONS

This chapter has covered the normal anatomy and physiology of the GI tract including the structures, functions, blood supply, and innervation of the different organs involved throughout the entire process. The GI tract is complex with many interrelated functions and structures. It is through a better understanding of normal anatomy and physiology that more thorough comprehension of physiologic or surgical changes can occur.

REFERENCES

Beisner, J., Stange, E., & Wehkamp, J. (2010). Innate antimicrobial immunity in inflammatory bowel diseases. *Expert Review of Clinical Immunology, 6*(5), 809–818.

Bryant, R. (2004). Anatomy and physiology of the gastrointestinal tract. In J. Colwell, M. Goldberg, & J. Carmel (Eds.), *Fecal & urinary diversions: Management principles*. St. Louis, MO: Mosby-Elsevier.

Doig, A., & Huether, S. (2012). Structure and function of the digestive system. In S. Huether & K. McCance (Eds.), *Understanding pathophysiology* (5th ed.). St Louis, MO: Mosby-Elsevier.

Dyer, J., (2014). *Anatomy & physiology made incredibly visual* (2nd ed.). Philadelphia, PA: Wolters Kluwer.

Fedorak, R., & Madsen, M. (2004). Probiotics and prebiotics in gastrointestinal disorders. *Current Opinion in Gastroenterology, 20*, 146–155.

Fox, M., Thumshirn, M., & Fried, M. (2006). Barostat measurement of rectal compliance and capacity. *Diseases of the Colon & Rectum, 49*, 360–370.

Hall, J., & Guyton, A. (2011). *Guyton and hall textbook of medical physiology* (12th ed.). St Louis, MO: Elsevier.

Heitkemper, M. (2006). Physiology of bowel function. In D. Doughty (Ed.), *Urinary & fecal incontinence: Current management concepts* (3rd ed.). St Louis, MO: Mosby-Elsevier.

Ireland, A. P. (2004). Surgical fluids and electrolytes. Retrieved from http://surgstudent.org/lectures/flud/flud_centre_html.html

OpenStax. (February 26, 2016). Anatomy & Physiology. OpenStax CNX. Retrieved from http://cnx.org/contents/14fb4ad7-39a1-4eee-ab6e-3ef2482e3e22@8.24

O'Rahilly, R., Muller, F., Carpenter, S., et al. (2008). Basic human anatomy: A regional study of human structure. Online version developed at: Dartmouth Medical School. Retrieved from http://www.dartmouth.edu/~humananatomy/index.html. Accessed initially on September 1, 2014.

Patton, K., & Thibodeau, G. (2014). *Mosby's handbook of anatomy & physiology* (2nd ed.). St. Louis, MO: Mosby.

Reed, K., & Wickham, R. (2009). Review of the gastrointestinal tract: From macro to micro. *Seminars in Oncology Nursing, 25*(1), 3–14.

Takaki, M. (2003). Gut pacemaker cells: the interstitial cells of Cajal (ICC). *Journal of Smooth Muscle Research, 39*(5), 137–161.

QUESTIONS

1. The GI tract is essentially a hollow muscular tube from the mouth to the anus. The length varies between individuals typically measuring
   A. 15 feet
   B. 25 feet
   C. 45 feet
   D. 100 feet

2. Which tissue layer of the alimentary canal coordinates rhythmic peristaltic contractions of the muscles, which results in the mixing and forward propulsion of the food bolus through the stomach and intestine?
   A. Mucosa
   B. Submucosa
   C. Muscularis
   D. Serosa

3. Which tissue layer of the alimentary canal is involved when a patient is experiencing the pain of bowel inflammation?
   A. Mucosa
   B. Submucosa
   C. Muscularis
   D. Serosa

4. What complication may be avoided when stomas are matured (everted) at the time of surgery?
   A. Serositis
   B. Bowel perforation
   C. Prolapse
   D. Stoma prolapse

5. Which postsurgical patient would the WOC nurse monitor for pernicious anemia due to impaired absorption of vitamin B$_{12}$?
   A. A patient with an ileostomy
   B. A patient with a large part of the stomach resected
   C. A patient with a bowel resection
   D. A patient with a colostomy

6. Which structure of the small intestine may take on some of the functions of the colon when the colon is surgically removed?
   A. Crypts of Lieberkühn
   B. Villi
   C. Paneth cell
   D. Epithelium

7. A patient is undergoing surgery for a continent diversion. Which structure of the small intestine may be used as a continence mechanism for this patient?
   A. Terminal ileum
   B. Ligament of Treitz
   C. Ileocecal valve
   D. Duodenojejunal flexure

8. Of all the organs of the digestive tract, which one is considered by some to be an "organ of convenience" and is not necessary to sustain life?
   A. Ileum
   B. Jejunum
   C. Duodenum
   D. Colon

9. Patient should be positioned on the left side for a colonoscopy because of an S-shaped curve to the
   A. Sigmoid colon
   B. Rectum
   C. Anal canal
   D. Duodenum

10. Which organ has the ability to regenerate for up to 70% destruction before becoming symptomatic?
    A. Liver
    B. Pancreas
    C. Gallbladder
    D. Appendix

ANSWERS AND RATIONALES

1. **B. Rationale:** The GI tract is essentially a hollow muscular tube from the mouth to the anus. The length varies between individuals typically measuring during life around 7.62 m (25 feet) and after death closer to 10.67 m (35 feet).

2. **C. Rationale:** The muscularis consists of two smooth muscle layers, a circular inner layer and longitudinal outer layer, and coordinates rhythmic peristaltic contractions of the muscles resulting in the mixing and forward propulsion of the food bolus through the stomach and intestine.

3. **D. Rationale:** The serosa, which covers the structures within the peritoneal cavity, is in continuity with the visceral peritoneum and is associated with pain of bowel inflammation.

4. **A. Rationale:** The outer layer of the bowel is serosa and if exposed to air, it can lead to necrosis and sloughing called serositis (inflammation of the serosa). If a stoma is not everted at the time of creation, the serositis can cause a partial or complete obstruction of the nonmatured stoma.

5. **A. Rationale:** A patient with an ileostomy will have had significant lengths of the terminal ileum resected and may require lifelong vitamin B12 replacement to prevent pernicious anemia, improve fat intolerance, and reduce weight loss.

6. **B. Rationale:** Villi are able to transform to some degree, elongate, or become hypertrophied and thus are able to increase the absorptive capacity taking on some of the function of the colon when the colon is surgically removed.

7. C. Rationale: The ileocecal valve is smooth muscle that can function to prevent stoma output from a continent diversion.

8. D. Rationale: The colon function (fluid absorption, transportation of the fecal material, and storage) is not necessary to sustain life. The small intestine villi are able to transform to some degree and are able to increase the absorptive capacity taking on some of the colon function when the colon is surgically removed.

9. A. Rationale: The sigmoid colon is on the left side of the abdomen, and the endoscopist will be able to move the scope into the S-shaped sigmoid colon if the patient is laying on the left side.

10. A. Rationale: It is thought that the liver's blood supply and proximity to individual cells allows the liver to regenerate.

CHAPTER 3

ANATOMY AND PHYSIOLOGY OF THE URINARY SYSTEM

JoAnn M. Ermer-Seltun

OBJECTIVE

Apply knowledge of anatomy and physiology of the renal and urologic system in nursing management and education of the patient with a urinary diversion.

TOPIC OUTLINE

Introduction   30

Kidney Location and Structure   30

Elimination of Urine   31
Ureters   31
Ureter Function   32
Ureter Clinical and Surgical Implications   33

Structure and Function of the Lower Urinary Tract   33
Urinary Bladder   33
Urethra   34
Pelvis   35
Pelvic Floor   35
Female Pelvic Floor   35
Levator Ani   36
Endopelvic Fascia   36
Perineal Membrane, Perineal Body, and Anal Sphincter   36
Male Pelvic Floor   36
Adrenal Glands and Adjacent Organs   36

Function of the Kidneys   36
Urine Formation   36
Urine Concentration and Volume   37
Urine pH   37

Fluid and Electrolyte Balance   37
Water Regulation   38

Electrolyte Balance and Renin–Angiotensin–Aldosterone System   38
Potassium Regulation   38
Calcium, Phosphate, and Magnesium Regulation   39
Vitamin D   39
Calcitonin   39
Magnesium   39
Summary of Calcium, Phosphate, and Magnesium Regulation   39
Acid–Base Balance   39
Endocrine Function   40
Erythropoietin   40
Renin–Angiotensin–Aldosterone System   40
Vitamin D$_3$ 40

Conclusions   40

INTRODUCTION

A fundamental understanding of the urinary system and the changes in urine filling, storage, and elimination associated with urinary reconstruction is essential in providing care for a person with a urinary diversion. This complex system provides homeostasis or equilibrium to maintain a stabilized internal environment for optimal cell and tissue metabolism. This arduous task is accomplished through excretion of water and waste; fluid and electrolyte balance; regulation of acid–base balance and endocrine function by secreting hormones: erythropoietin (EPO) to promote red blood cell production and renin–angiotensin–aldosterone to regulate blood volume and pressure; and activation of vitamin D to promote ossification of bones and teeth. The urinary system consists of the upper urinary tract, which is responsible for urine formation and transportation (pair of kidneys, renal pelves, and ureters), and lower urinary tract (urinary bladder, urethra, and support structures), which provides urine storage and elimination (**Fig. 3-1**). This chapter concentrates on the normal structure and function of the urinary system.

KIDNEY LOCATION AND STRUCTURE

The kidneys are a pair of reddish brown, bean-shaped organs situated near the twelfth thoracic (T12) and third lumbar (L3) vertebrae, lying on either side of the vertebral column. They are located against the deep muscles of the back in the retroperitoneal space. The right kidney is lower than the left to accommodate the liver. The lateral aspect of the kidney is convex, while the medial surface is quite concave. The hilum is located at the resulting medial depression that leads into a hollow chamber called the renal sinus, which contains blood vessels, nerves, lymphatic vessels, and the proximal ureter. The renal pelvis is a funnel-shaped sac, which is the superior end of the expanded ureter that is created by the convergence of two or three tubes called major calyces (Huether, 2019).

A bisected kidney discloses two distinct regions: an inner medulla and outer cortex, which is often referred as the parenchyma or "meat of the kidney" (**Fig. 3-2**). The inner medulla is made up of conical masses of tissue called renal pyramids. The base of the pyramids orientates toward the convex surface, whereas their apices form the renal papillae, which arise from the calyces approaching the hilum. The renal papilla is a valvular-like system that promotes outward (antegrade) flow from the nephron (functional unit of the kidney) into the renal pelvis to prevent reflux (retrograde flow) into the renal cortex. The renal cortex is granular in nature and forms a shell around the medulla. It dips into the medulla to fill the space between the pyramids forming renal columns and lobules. The cortex is protected by a dense adherent covering (renal capsule) and embedded in a mass of fat tissue. In addition, a double layer of renal fascia (Gerota fascia) over the perinephric fat, and other fibrous tissue helps protect and anchor the kidneys to the posterior abdominal wall. Therefore, the renal capsule, fat cushion, and perirenal and Gerota fascia, as well as the abdominal muscles, diaphragm, quadratus lumborum muscles, and ribs, offer protection and absorb shock if a blow occurs from the abdomen or flank region (Huether, 2019; Shier et al., 2019a; Weinberg et al., 2018).

The functional unit of the kidney is the nephron (**Fig. 3-3**). Its primary function is to remove waste and toxic products from the plasma and control the composition of

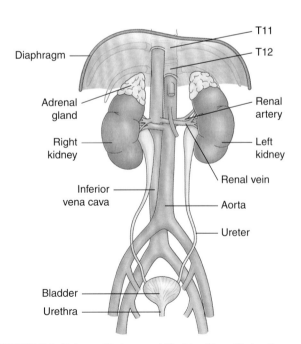

FIGURE 3-1. Kidneys, Ureters, and Bladder. (From Timby, B. K., & Smith, N. E. (2013). *Introductory medical-surgical nursing.* Philadelphia, PA: Wolters Kluwer.)

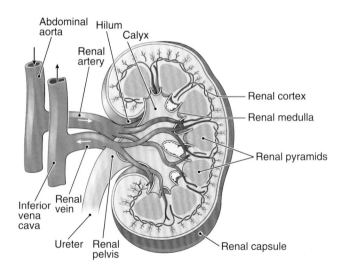

FIGURE 3-2. Structure of the Kidney. (From Cohen, B. J. (2012). *Memmler's structure and function of the human body.* Philadelphia, PA: Wolters Kluwer.)

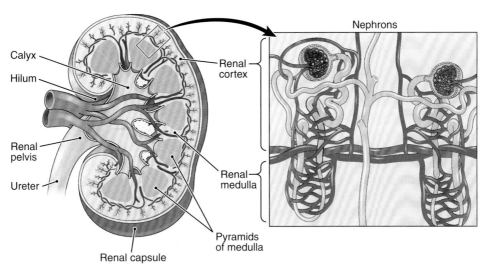

FIGURE 3-3. Kidney (*Left*) with Nephron (Enlarged to Show Detail, *Right*). (From Cohen, B. J. (2012). *Medical terminology*. Philadelphia, PA: Wolters Kluwer.)

body fluids. There are about 1.2 million nephrons in each renal parenchyma, so one can envision how tiny and condensed each unit must be. The nephron is a tube-like structure subdivided into the renal corpuscle (glomerulus and Bowman capsule) and a renal tubule. The glomerulus begins as a complex filtering unit composed of a tangled collection of blood capillaries that is surrounded by a thin-walled, cup-like structure called a Bowman capsule. It continues with a proximal convoluted (highly coiled) tubule, loop of Henle, and ends with the distal convoluted tubule, which empties into a collecting duct where multiple distal convoluted tubules merge. The fluid (glomerular filtrate) then drains into the top of the renal pyramid and then to the renal papillae (prevents retrograde flow) where it joins the minor calyx and major calyx and lastly empties into the renal pelvis, which connects to the proximal portion of the ureter (Weinberg et al., 2018). Of interest, epithelial and smooth muscle cells line the walls of the minor and major calyx, renal pelvis, and ureter and contract to propel urine to the bladder (Huether, 2019).

Blood supply to the nephron enters by an afferent arteriole, which gives rise to the glomerulus's tangled capillaries and exits the glomerulus via the efferent arteriole. It continues through the peritubular and vasa recta capillary system near the nephron loop where it joins blood from other peritubular capillary systems and ultimately unites with the kidney's venous system. The intricate adjacent capillary system of the nephron is crucial for renal filtration and urine formation (Weinberg et al., 2018).

There are three types of nephrons, superficial cortical (majority of all nephrons), midcortical, and juxtamedullary. The kidney is a highly vascular organ. Although the kidneys account for only 1% of a person's body weight, it receives over 15% to 30% (1,000 to 1,200 mL/min) of the total cardiac output when a person is at rest (Shier et al., 2019a). Blood is supplied to the kidney from usually

a single (pairing can occur) renal artery, which directly branches off from the abdominal aorta. The position of the artery may vary in individuals; therefore, best surgical approach may need to be determined by the urologist prior to reconstruction. As the renal artery enters the hilum, it splits into the interlobar arteries, which pass through the renal pyramids and then branch to form a series of incomplete arches at the junction between the medulla and cortex called arcuate arteries. These arteries in turn branch into cortical radiate arteries, which finally give rise to the afferent arterioles that lead to the functional kidney units called nephrons. Venous return follows the same flow series as does the arterial return (Huether, 2019; Shier et al., 2019a).

ELIMINATION OF URINE

Urine forms as the result of glomerular filtration of the blood plasma, tubular reabsorption, and minus tubular secretion. Once the glomerular filtrate passes through the collecting ducts, the urine remains unchanged. It exits the collecting ducts, drains into the minor and major renal calyces, and enters the renal pelvis, which is formed from the convergence of two to three major calyces. The renal pelvis is the funnel-shaped portion of the proximal ureter. The urine is transported from the kidney and ureters to a sac-like muscle (bladder) in an antegrade fashion (efflux) while avoiding retrograde (reflux) movement of the urine through peristalsis. The bladder serves as a reservoir for urine and exits the body through a tubular structure called the urethra (Huether, 2019; Weinberg et al., 2018).

URETERS

The ureter is a long, tubular organ with an approximate length of 22 to 30 cm, with the left ureter slightly longer due to the inferior location of the right kidney

(Huether, 2019; Shier et al., 2019a). The superior aspect of the ureter consists of the funnel-shaped renal pelvis, which holds approximately 15 to 20 mL of urine and tapers to 2 mm where it becomes officially the ureter, known as the ureteropelvic junction (UPJ). The UPJ is a common site for congenital or acquired obstruction, that is, stones. The ureter continues in an inverted "S" shape in a downward and medial fashion until it terminates into the posterior base of the bladder (trigone) called the ureterovesical junction (UVJ).

A variety of sources supply arterial blood to the ureters, and these vary among people. Branches of the renal, gonadal, or adrenal arteries supply the upper ureters, while branches of the obturator artery, deferential artery in men, or uterine artery in women supply the lower (pelvic) ureter region. Venous return parallels the arterial supply as well as lymphatic drainage channels.

KEY POINT

The ureteropelvic junction (UPJ) obstruction is a common congenital or acquired condition.

URETER FUNCTION

The main function of the ureter is to transport urine to the bladder in a fashion that promotes emptying without reflux. Several mechanisms promote antegrade urine flow: peristalsis through mechanical distention; neurologic, endocrine, and pharmacologic stimulation; as well as the UVJ structure. The renal pelvis holds about 15 to 20 mL of urine, and this distension initiates muscular peristaltic waves at a rate consistent with amount of urine present in the renal pelvis. For instance, if urine is formed quickly (i.e., diuretic therapy), then the peristaltic wave may occur every few seconds; in contrast, if glomerular filtration rate (GFR) is slow (i.e., dehydration), the peristalsis may occur every few minutes (Shier et al., 2019a). In recent research, it appears that interstitial cells of Cajal (ICC) are more likely the modulators of smooth muscle activity involved in ureteral peristalsis (Hurtado et al., 2014; Iskander et al., 2018).

Resting intraluminal pressure is elevated with each peristaltic contraction, which pushes the bolus of urine before it is at relatively low pressure. Because urine transport is at low pressure, any disorder that increases bladder pressure (i.e., low bladder wall compliance or bladder outlet obstruction) can elevate the risk of upper tract damage such as hydroureteronephrosis, recurrent urinary tract infections (UTIs), vesicoureteral reflux, and potentially irreversible renal damage. Gap junctions (electrochemical communication between ureteral muscle cells) allow the ureter to function as a single unit to propel urine forward through the entire ureter to the bladder in one single peristaltic contraction, even if innervation to the ureter is compromised or the ureter is transplanted. In addition to mechanical distention, neu-

rologic, endocrine, and pharmacologic factors aid in ureteral peristaltic action. Sympathetic stimulation within the ureteral wall of the alpha-adrenergic receptors causes increase strength and number of contractions, while beta-adrenergic stimulation causes relaxation of the ureter. Parasympathetic stimulation of cholinergic receptors with medications such as epinephrine (catecholamine) creates strong peristaltic action.

Since urine transport is at low pressure, any disorder that increases bladder pressure (i.e., low bladder wall compliance or bladder outlet obstruction) can elevate the risk of upper tract damage such as hydroureteronephrosis, recurrent UTIs, vesicoureteral reflux, and potentially irreversible renal damage.

The UVJ plays a pivotal role in promoting antegrade urine flow from the kidney into the bladder and preventing reflux (retrograde movement) from the bladder to the upper tracts. It consists of the distal ureter, the adjoining bladder wall, and the trigone of the bladder, which acts together as a unit to prevent retrograde urine movement by three methods (Gray & Moore, 2009). First, the terminal ureter tunnels the adjacent bladder wall and trigone at a gentle angle for about 1.5 cm. This layout promotes sealing of the ureter when the bladder or trigone contract. The outer layer (adventitia) of the intramural (tunneled) ureter contains three sheaths known as Waldeyer sheath, to provide limited mobility and solid attachment to the bladder. Second, the smooth muscle bundles arranged in a circular and longitudinal manner within the bladder offer additional support as well as promotion of UVJ closure during urination. Lastly, the trigone is a triangular-shaped smooth muscle at the base of the bladder with the apex extending into the bladder neck in women and the verumontanum (an elevation in the floor of the prostrate where seminal ducts enter) in men. The trigone is divided into two distinct segments, superficial and deep (Gray & Moore, 2009).

Urine is expelled into the bladder following a peristaltic contraction through a flap-like fold of the mucous membrane. This fold acts like a valve at the UVJ in that it allows urine to enter the bladder but prevents backing up of urine from the bladder to the ureter even during coughing, sneezing, and physical exertion (Shier et al., 2019a). As the bladder fills with urine, both the detrusor and trigone regions are relaxed due to sympathetic nerve stimulation to allow urine to pass through the UVJ. Beta-adrenergic receptors in the bladder cause smooth muscle relaxation, while alpha-adrenergic receptors in the bladder neck cause the smooth muscle to contract to prevent urine leakage while filling and storage.

In contrast, during micturition, the bladder contracts due to parasympathetic stimulation of the cholinergic receptors and indirectly inhibits sympathetic stimulation of the bladder neck (causes relaxation of the bladder neck) to promote urine elimination. The contraction of the bladder and trigone raises the closing pressure of the intramural ureter (UVJ) to prevent reflux. Moreover, the trigone contracts an additional approximately 20 seconds after micturition to further lessen the risk of reflux (Huether, 2019; Kurz & Guzzo, 2017).

URETER CLINICAL AND SURGICAL IMPLICATIONS

Due to the narrowing along the ureter at three sites (1) upper ureter at UPJ; (2) middle ureter as it enters the brim of the pelvis, crossing the iliac vessels; and (3) distal ureter at UVJ), stone formation is common (Lescay & Tuma, 2019). The UVJ was the most common site reported of ureteral calculi in an ER setting (Eisner et al., 2009). In addition, injuries to the ureter are usually iatrogenic (Lescay & Tuma, 2019), specifically the result of hysterectomies or colorectal surgeries (Barbic et al., 2018; Douissard et al., 2018). Strategies to prevent ureter injures during surgical interventions is preoperative ureteral stenting, which in itself may lead to an iatrogenic ureter injury (Douissard et al., 2018). Signs or symptoms of ureteral injuries may include flank pain, ileus, hematuria, elevated and prolonged drain production, as well as BUN and creatinine elevations (Matsumura et al., 2018). Significant narrowing of the ureter from either strictures or stone formation that lead to partial or complete obstruction may necessitate nephrostomy tube placement (Siddiqi & Schwartz, 2017), as well as laparoscopic stents or ureteroureterostomy due iatrogenic injuries to facilitate urine drainage (Gild et al., 2018).

 ## STRUCTURE AND FUNCTION OF THE LOWER URINARY TRACT

The lower urinary tract consists of the bladder, urethra, and pelvic floor muscles. These structures work together as a unit to maintain continence through storage and elimination of urine at a desirable time.

URINARY BLADDER (**FIG. 3-4**)

The urinary bladder is a hollow, muscular organ that has a fixed base and quite a distensible body designed to fill with urine at low pressures, stores approximately 300 to 600 mL urine in the healthy adult, and eliminates urine. The bladder lies within the pelvic cavity and is located posterior to the symphysis pubis and inferior to the parietal peritoneum. In females, the anterior uterine wall and vagina come in contact with the bladder, while in males, the posterior bladder neighbors the rectum (Shier et al., 2019a). The pressure of surrounding organs modifies the spherical shape of the bladder, but the size and shape of the bladder are dependent upon the amount of urine being stored. Often, anatomic drawings inaccurately depict an air bubble in the bladder; however, as the bladder empties, the walls collapse down upon the fixed base creating a tetrahedron (triangular pyramid)-like shape.

As the bladder fills, the superior surface expands upward into a dome; it pushes above the pubic crest if distended and near the umbilicus if greatly distended (Shier et al., 2019a). The trigone is the anterior floor of the bladder with an inlet at each of the angles, the UVJ orifices as described above, and a funnel-shaped extension into the apex of the trigone is called the bladder neck or UVJ. There are four histological layers in the wall of the bladder: mucosa, lamina propria or submucosa, muscularis, and serous coat or adventitia (Kurz & Guzzo, 2017; Shier et al., 2019a). The mucosa coat is composed of several thicknesses of the transitional epithelial cells or uroepithelium that are similar to the lining of the renal pelvis and ureters as well as the upper portion of the urethra. The thickness of this layer becomes reduced (only one to two cells deep) as the bladder fills and distends and returns to five to seven cells deep with urine elimination.

The uroepithelium is impermeable to the contents of the urine and manufactures a very thick, mucoid-like substance called glycosaminoglycans (GAG layer) to protect the mucosa from irritants in the urine. The second layer, lamina propria, is loosely connected to the uroepithelium but firmly attached to the third layer, muscularis. It contains connective tissue, nerves, blood vessels, as well as interstitial cells that communicate considerably by gap junctions. The third layer consists of a complex meshwork of smooth muscle bundles (unlike the organized circular and longitudinal layers of the intestine) known as the detrusor muscle. The muscle layer contains collagen and elastin to provide structural integrity to the bladder.

Unfortunately, some lower urinary tract disorders such as seen in specific types of denervation and obstruction result in excessive collagen deposition. This consequence creates trabeculation (thickening or hypertrophy of bladder muscle) and ineffective contractility of the bladder leading to elevated urine residuals, elevated risk for UTIs, and compromised upper tract urine production and drainage (Kurz & Guzzo, 2017). The muscularis also contains interstitial cells connected by gap junctions to provide communication and coordination of detrusor activity.

The fourth layer is the serosal coat or adventitia. It covers most of the bladder with fibroelastic connective

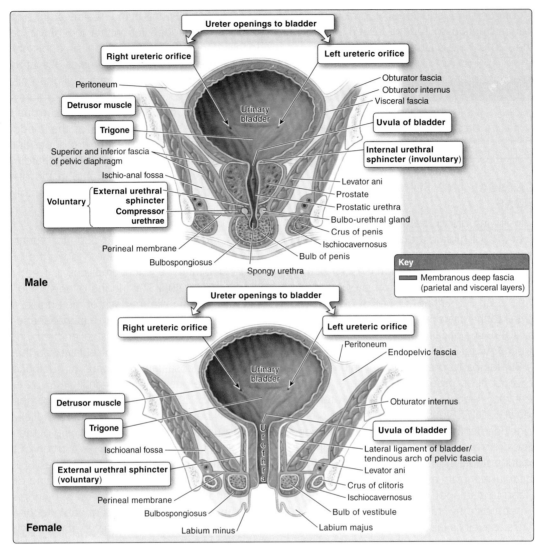

FIGURE 3-4. Bladder and Urethra, Male and Female. (Used with permission from Leeper-Woodford, S. K. (2016). *Sistemas Integrados.* Wolters Kluwer.)

tissue except the upper portion of the bladder where simple squamous epithelium covers the area along with a small amount of connective tissue. Perivesical fat covers beyond the serosa/adventitia. The bladder receives its arterial blood supply via the superior, inferior, and medial vesical arteries, in addition to branches of the obturator, inferior gluteal, or internal iliac arteries. Females also receive arterial blood to the bladder from uterine and vaginal arteries. This profuse blood supply to the bladder accounts for blood in the urine (hematuria) that easily arises with UTIs, trauma, or surgery (Huether, 2019).

KEY POINT

The urinary bladder is also known as the detrusor muscle. The detrusor smooth muscle contains collagen and elastin as well as a rich blood supply.

URETHRA

Urine is expelled from the bladder through a collapsible tube called the urethra. Like the upper urinary tract and bladder, the urethra is composed of the same four histological layers (urothelium, lamina propria, muscularis, and serosa or adventitia) but differs in that it is composed of both smooth and specialized striated muscle that aids in maintaining continence. The urethra has specialized striated muscle that contains both fast-twitch and short-twitch muscle fibers that aid in tone of the urethra during periods of sudden increase in abdominal pressure (i.e., cough) and prolong periods needed for continence between voids. In females, the urethra is about 4 cm in length, which begins at the bladder neck and terminates at the urethral meatus between the vagina and clitoris (Kurz & Guzzo, 2017).

To promote female continence, the anterior vaginal wall is fused with the distal two thirds of the urethra and shares vascular components, muscular and endopelvic fascial support (Pradidarcheep et al., 2011; Sampselle & DeLancey, 1998; Siccardi & Valle, 2019). The female urethra is short compared to the male urethra but acts as a continence mechanism almost the entire length. In contrast, the male urethra is approximately 18 to 20 cm in length and acts as a passageway to transport not only urine but cells and secretions from the reproductive organs. It can be divided into three sections: prostatic urethra approximately 3 cm, membranous urethra approximately 2.5 cm, and penile urethra approximately 15 cm (Kurz & Guzzo, 2017; Shier et al., 2019a).

The male urethra is composed of uroepithelium, lamina propria, muscularis, and adventitia but devoid of the muscularis layer in the distal portion. The proximal urethra wall contains both smooth and striated muscle that contributes to the continence sphincter mechanism. Females receive their urethral arterial blood supply from the vaginal artery, while males receive theirs from the pudendal artery. Venous return occurs from the venous pelvic plexus in females; in males, venous return occurs through the deep dorsal vein. Lymphatic drainage takes place through the superficial and deep inguinal nodes, hypogastric, obturator, as well as internal and external iliac nodes (Kurz & Guzzo, 2017).

PELVIS

The pelvis is a ring of bones composed of the sacrum and fusion of paired bones of the iliac, ischial, and pubic bones. The female pelvis accommodates both locomotion and childbirth by being larger and broader than that of a male (tall, narrow, and compact) as well as having an ovoid-shaped inlet in contrast to the male heart-shaped inlet.

PELVIC FLOOR

The pelvic floor consists of several muscle groups and ligaments that help support the pelvic viscera and deliver sphincter-like action in the anal canal and vagina (Ashton-Miller & DeLancey, 2007; Perucchini & DeLancey, 2008; Sampselle & DeLancey, 1998). The lower urinary tract is also supported by the perineal membrane, perineal body (PB), and anal sphincter.

Female Pelvic Floor

Female functional continence mechanism is complex and depends on the integrity of the pelvic floor. The pelvic floor is made of three primary layers: (1) superficial perineum, (2) urogenital diaphragm or deep perineum, and (3) pelvic floor diaphragm (**Fig. 3-5**). Key support structures within these layers provide vital support to the pelvic soft organs (viscera) and the urethral continence

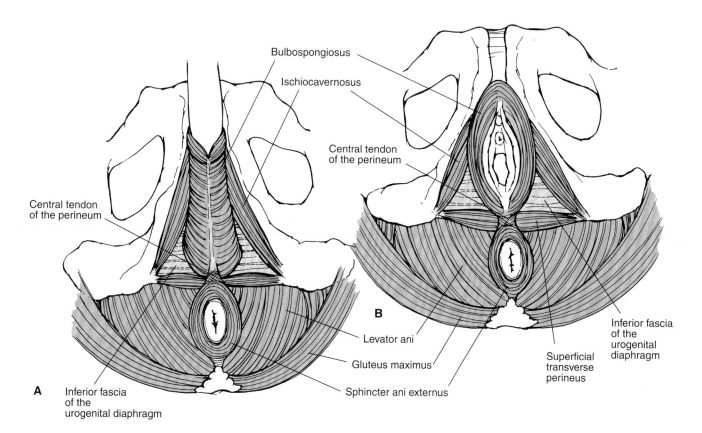

FIGURE 3-5. Pelvic Floor Muscles, Male **(A)** and Female **(B)**. (Used with permission from Oatis, C. A. (2016). *Kinesiology—The mechanics and pathomechanics of human movement* (3rd ed.). Wolters Kluwer.)

mechanism: endopelvic fascia, levator ani muscle, perineal membrane, PB, and external anal sphincter (Bordoni et al., 2019).

Levator Ani

Within the third layer (pelvic floor diaphragm) resides the principal source of support of the pelvic floor, the levator ani, which consists of the pubovisceral (pubococcygeus, pubourethralis, pubovaginalis, and puborectalis) and iliococcygeus muscles that function as a single unit (Pradidarcheep et al., 2011; Sampselle & DeLancey, 1998). The primary function of the levator ani is to lift the anus, vagina, and urethra and to pull them forward; this anterior pull creates a compressive force against the lumen of these organs that promotes closure through increased intraurethral, intravaginal, and intra-anal pressures (Bordoni et al., 2019; Sampselle & DeLancey, 1998).

Endopelvic Fascia

The pelvic floor layers and viscera must anchor to the bony structures of the pelvis in order to provide optimal support. The endopelvic fascia is complex internal system made of dense connective tissue composed of collagen, elastin, and smooth muscle. It provides suspensory support by encapsulating the pelvic viscera (urethra, vagina, bladder, uterus) as well as the levator ani and connecting them to the boney pelvis as well to each other. In general, endopelvic fascia serves to compartmentalize organs and muscles to maintain form and function, assists in sliding yet limits friction during motion, responds to stretch and distention, and serves as a shock absorber (Siccardi & Valle, 2019).

Perineal Membrane, Perineal Body, and Anal Sphincter

The perineal membrane, PB, and anal sphincter comprise an inferior supportive layer of the pelvic floor. The perineal membrane is a triangular fibrous structure that spans the anterior pelvis; the vagina and urethra pass through a central hole in this supportive membrane. The primary function of the perineal membrane is to limit descent of the pelvic organs by attaching the PB to the pubic bones. The perineal membrane provides secondary support by limiting descent of the PB and vagina when the levator ani is relaxed during the processes of defecation, urination, and birth (Sampselle & DeLancey, 1998).

Male Pelvic Floor

The pelvic floor of the male is also made up of three primary layers with key support structures within the layers: endopelvic fascia, levator ani, and perineal membrane, PB, and anal sphincter. The endopelvic fascia is analogous to that of the female, but condensations of the fascia provide specific support to the prostate gland, bladder base, and urethra. The levator ani is separated into two muscles as seen in females (pubovisceral and iliococcygeus) but is a thicker and larger U-shaped muscle as well as the primary support structure for the bladder and urethra. The perineal membrane, PB, and anal sphincter also provide secondary support (Pradidarcheep et al., 2011).

KEY POINT

The primary support for the pelvic organs is the levator ani, which is actually a group of smaller muscles that function as a single unit.

ADRENAL GLANDS AND ADJACENT ORGANS

The adrenal glands are pyramid shaped, superior to each kidney, and entrenched in adipose tissue as well as Gerota fascia that encompasses the kidney. Although the adrenal glands are closest in proximity to the kidneys, they are functionally and anatomically distinct. They consist of two parts that secrete different hormones: adrenal medulla (central portion) and adrenal cortex (the outer portion).

The other organs adjacent to the kidneys include the duodenum, pancreas tail, hepatic flexure of the large intestine, ascending colon, and descending and sigmoid colon. Therefore, identification and protection of these adjacent organs by the surgeon during urinary reconstruction surgery are crucial to prevent life-threatening inter- and postoperative complications.

FUNCTION OF THE KIDNEYS

The function of the renal system is to maintain homeostasis of the body's internal environment through the regulation of body fluid volume, pH, and composition. This vital task is accomplished through (1) excretion of water and waste through urine production, (2) fluid and electrolyte balance, (3) regulation of acid–base balance, and (4) endocrine function by secreting hormones such as EPO to promote red blood cell production and renin and aldosterone to regulate blood volume and pressure and activation of vitamin D to promote bone growth and preservation (Huether, 2019; Shier et al., 2019b).

URINE FORMATION

Urine is an end product of glomerular filtration plus tubular secretion minus tubular reabsorption. Urine is composed of wastes, excess water, and electrolytes and is excreted from the body by the lower urinary tract. The nephrons are responsible for filtering 180 L of fluid every 24 hours with a formation of 1 to 2 L of urine per day, depending upon health, hydration, activity, and environmental factors. Excessive or poor urine production requires further medical evaluation.

GFR is the amount of filtrate through the nephron system per minute and often used as a marker reflecting kidney health. Filtration begins as the glomerular capillaries that filter the water dissolve molecules and ions out of the capillary plasma and into the glomerular capsules. The resulting glomerular filtrate composition is mostly water, glucose, amino acids, urea, uric acid, creatine, creatinine, sodium, chloride, potassium, calcium, bicarbonate, phosphate, and sulfate ions. Three forces affect the GFR favorably or negatively: hydrostatic pressure, filtration pressure, and plasma oncotic pressure. The sum of these three forces is net filtration pressure and normally is positive, causing filtration. The GFR is directly proportional to the net filtration pressure. Therefore, anything affecting hydrostatic pressure of the glomerulus capillaries or Bowman capsule, and capillary oncotic pressure will also affect the GFR. Examples of GFR alterations include obstruction as seen in strictures, renal calculi, tumors of urinary system which increases pressure in Bowman capsule, vomiting, diarrhea, or excessive sweating modifies protein levels consequently reducing GFR, in contrast, changes in protein plasma levels in blood may increase GFR as seen in severe malnutrition or liver disease (Huether, 2019).

KEY POINT

The greatest factor that drives net filtration and GFR is the glomerular hydrostatic pressure.

URINE CONCENTRATION AND VOLUME

The average GFR for a healthy adult is 125 mL/min, which translates into 45 gallons of protein-free filtrate in a 24-hour period (Shier et al., 2019a,b). GFR is the most reliable measure of kidney function (Huether, 2019). Obviously, to maintain homeostasis, only 1 to 2 L of filtrate is excreted as urine, and the remaining filtrate (99%) is reabsorbed by the renal tubular system. Once the filtrate reaches the loop of Henle, over 60% to 70% of filtered water and sodium have been reabsorbed. In addition, over half of the urea and more than 90% of the potassium, glucose, bicarbonate, calcium, and phosphate have been reabsorbed as well (Huether, 2019). Glomerular filtrate may be hypotonic, isotonic, or hypertonic when it reaches the loop of Henle; thus, concentration or dilution is the responsibility of the loop of Henle, distal tubules, and collecting ducts (Huether, 2019). Of interest, an abundant protein in urine called uromodulin is manufactured by the thick ascending loop of Henle to bind uropathogens to prevent UTIs, as well as protects against injury to the uroepithelium, and renal calculi formation; it is also linked with chronic kidney disease (Scolari et al., 2015).

KEY POINT

The primary purpose of the loop of Henle is to determine urine concentration and hydration needs by the body. It also produces a protein uromodulin that is protective against UTI and kidney stone formation.

URINE pH

Urine pH is approximately 4.6 to 8.0. Under normal conditions, the urine is more acidic but can vary depending upon dietary intake and acid–base balance mechanism. A higher pH may be due to large intake of citrus fruits, legumes, and vegetables, and an acidic pH may be due to a robust diet of meat or cranberry. Upon rising in the morning, urine is more acidic due to a slower respiratory rate (more CO_2 [acid] retained) during sleep. Urea is a by-product of protein metabolism, and the amount eliminated in the urine reflects the amount of ingested dietary protein. Urine is primarily made up of urea and water with 50% of the filtered urea reabsorbed by the renal tubules. Uric acid is a by-product of purine and guanine metabolism from the intake of meat and seafood. Only 10% is excreted in the urine. If in excess, uric acid may precipitate in the blood and cause painful deposits in joints called gout (Huether, 2019).

Some species of bacteria (especially *Proteus* strains, *Klebsiella*, *Staphylococcus*, and *Pseudomonas*) produce an enzyme called urease. Urease converts urea into ammonia and carbon dioxide, which leads to a significant rise in urine pH. Unfortunately, phosphate will precipitate in an alkaline urine environment and create struvite crystals made of magnesium–phosphate–ammonium leading to kidney stones as well as peristomal encrustations in a person with a urinary diversion. Struvite stones account for about 10% to 15% of the renal calculi, often called the "infection stone" and affect mostly women and those prone to UTIs, that is, patients with indwelling catheters, stents, or foreign bodies (Flagg & Joiner, 2017). Stone formation can occur in both high alkaline (calcium phosphate, calcium carbonate, magnesium phosphate stones) and acidic urine environments (uric acid, cystine, and calcium oxalate stones). However, under general circumstances, it is thought that an acidic urine pH is beneficial, imparting a hostile environment for bacterial growth (Huether, 2019). Any conditions that alter the H^+ balance (vomiting, diarrhea, uncontrolled diabetes, COPD, dehydration, diet, some medications, etc.) will alter urine pH values to compensate and bring about homeostasis in acid–base balance as described below (Hacker, 2019).

KEY POINT

High urine pH in a urinary diversion can cause peristomal lesions. Acidic urine creates a hostile environment for bacterial growth in urine.

FLUID AND ELECTROLYTE BALANCE

The second function of the renal system is to balance the body's fluid volume and electrolytes to maintain homeostasis since they are interdependent. Four key points to remember when discussing fluid and electrolyte balance are as follows: (1) aldosterone causes reabsorption of sodium (Na^+) and secretion of potassium (K^+); (2) antidiuretic hormone (ADH) causes water reabsorption; (3) Na^+ is the main ion outside the cell (interstitial and vascular), while K^+ is the main ion within the actual cell; and (4) water easily diffuses through a membrane readily from low to high solute concentration, while other ions need active or passive transport to cross membranes.

WATER REGULATION

The distribution of body fluids is not uniform and occupies different compartments in varying compositions. The body has approximately 40 L of water with 63% (25 L) of this total body water volume occupying the intracellular fluid compartment, while 37% (15 L) is in the extracellular fluid compartment. A seemingly simplistic yet complex equilibrium must exist; water intake must equal water output. The average oral intake is approximately 2,500 mL with approximately 60% (1,500 mL) lost in urine and 6% (150 mL) in feces and sweat (150 mL), while 28% (700 mL) will be lost in evaporation from the skin and lungs (Shier et al., 2019a,b).

Life-sustaining measures of water balance are primarily regulated through the renal system and urine production since the other avenues (feces, sweat, skin, lungs) of water output are less in volume and variability. The primary effectors for the regulation of water output in the urine are the renal distal convoluted tubules and collecting ducts, although water reabsorption starts in the proximal renal tubules (Shier et al., 2019a,b). The renal convoluted tubules and collecting ducts are impermeable to water unless ADH is present. ADH stimulates the cells in these structures to become greatly permeable to water, so water rapidly leaves the tubules/ducts through osmosis into the pericapillary system and the hypertonic medulla. This process creates a more concentrated urine, and water is conserved in the internal environment.

Dehydration is the epitome of excess water loss via sweat, water deprivation, and illnesses that cause prolonged vomiting and/or diarrhea. Infants and the elderly are at higher risk for water imbalance. Infants have less efficient water conservation by the kidneys, while the elderly have a reduced thirst mechanism, possible immobility issues, and lack of autonomy to obtain adequate fluid intake. In contrast, water intoxication can occur with excessive oral intake of fluids that leads to low serum sodium levels and intravascular water diffusion into the cells by osmosis leading to cellular swelling that can increase intracranial pressure, central nervous system (CNS) symptoms, and death in rare cases.

ELECTROLYTE BALANCE AND RENIN–ANGIOTENSIN–ALDOSTERONE SYSTEM

Electrolyte balance, like water equilibrium, occurs when ionic gains equal losses. The kidneys regulate important electrolytes (sodium, chloride, potassium, calcium, phosphate, magnesium, bicarbonate, and hydrogen) that are essential in cell membrane permeability, impulse conduction along an axon, muscle fiber contraction, and pH balance. The intake and regulation of intake of electrolytes usually is satisfied by ingestion of foods and beverages in response to thirst and hunger as well as existing as by-products of metabolic reactions.

Electrolyte loss or output is reflected in perspiration and feces, but the greatest output arises from the end result of kidney function and urine production. Remember, sodium ions represent 90% of the positively charged ions in the extracellular fluid. In contrast, potassium positively charged ions predominate in the intracellular fluid. In review, most of the Na^+ (60% to 70%) and 90% of K^+ and other electrolytes are reabsorbed by the proximal convoluted tubule and loop of Henle. In addition, aldosterone regulates both Na^+ and K^+. Low serum Na^+ and low renal artery pressure and $beta_1$ adrenergic receptor stimulation (within the juxtaglomerular apparatus) incite the juxtaglomerular cells to secrete the enzyme renin (Hacker, 2019; Shier et al., 2019b).

The renin–angiotensin–aldosterone system (RAAS) plays a critical role in influencing cardiac output and arterial pressure by regulating blood volume and systemic vascular resistance (Klabunde, 2014). Renin reacts with angiotensinogen (a blood protein), which releases angiotensin I. This reacts with angiotensin-converting enzyme (ACE) that is supplied from lung endothelial blood vessels, which in turn changes angiotensin I into angiotensin II.

Angiotensin II (a potent vasoconstrictor) travels in the bloodstream to stimulate the adrenal gland to release aldosterone (in the presence of adrenocorticotropic hormone [ACTH] as well as ADH [also called vasopressin for its mild vascular constricting properties]) from the posterior pituitary to conserve water. Aldosterone then stimulates the distal convoluted tubules and collecting ducts to reabsorb Na^+ and water and secrete K^+. Angiotensin II also stimulates the thirst centers in the brain to help increase fluid volume and facilitates norepinephrine release from adrenergic receptor sites to promote sympathetic function. Renin secretion is inhibited by normalization of blood pressure and plasma sodium concentration. Another hormone, atrial natriuretic peptide (ANP), is secreted by the atrial heart cells in response to stretching from increased blood volume. ANP inhibits renin secretion from the juxtaglomerular cells and aldosterone from the adrenal gland resulting in lower blood volume and pressure through Na^+ and water excretion. In summary, Na^+, water, and blood volume regulation is primarily controlled by renal tubule system in response to fluid and Na^+ concentrations, the RAAS, and ANP (Hacker, 2019; Huether, 2019; Shier et al., 2019b).

POTASSIUM REGULATION

In addition to previous content discussing potassium regulation, an elevated K^+ level is a powerful stimulus for the adrenal gland to secrete aldosterone to reduce

K^+ concentrations by distal tubular secretion (as well as reabsorption of Na^+ and water). Diuretic therapy (K^+ sparing or loop), presence of aldosterone, dietary intake, and hydrogen ion concentration for acid–base balance are primarily controlled by potassium balance (Huether, 2019; Shier et al., 2019a,b).

CALCIUM, PHOSPHATE, AND MAGNESIUM REGULATION

Minerals account for about 4% of the total body weight and are primarily located in bone and teeth. Calcium and phosphorus contribute up to 75% of that weight (Huether, 2019; Shier et al., 2019b). As in Na^+ and K^+ reabsorption, calcium, phosphate, and magnesium are resorbed mostly by the proximal convoluted tubules and loop of Henle (approximately 85%), while the distal convoluted tubule actively makes the final adjustments in concentration through the effect of parathyroid hormone (PTH), calcitonin, and glucagon (Hacker, 2019). In addition, dietary intake, H^+ ion concentration (regulated by acid–base balance), and vitamin D may influence homeostasis of these minerals. Noteworthy, Ca-sparing diuretics (thiazides) promote reabsorption of calcium thereby reducing urinary excretion, while loop diuretics promote calcium urinary excretion to reduce serum calcium.

Vitamin D

Vitamin D is obtained through the diet or made in the skin but must be converted to a metabolic active form by the liver and then kidneys (Huether, 2019; Shier et al., 2019b). In addition to enhancing absorption of calcium and phosphate from the gut, vitamin D increases bone reabsorption, which releases calcium and phosphate into the blood and augments phosphate reabsorption in the kidneys.

Calcitonin

The C cells of the thyroid secrete calcitonin in response to elevated calcium serum levels. It acts as an antagonist compared to vitamin D and PTH by decreasing serum Ca through promotion of bone development and reduction of renal reabsorption of calcium. Calcitonin plays a lesser role in calcium metabolism than do PTH and vitamin D (Hacker, 2019).

Magnesium

Often labeled the forgotten cation, magnesium plays a critical role in intracellular and extracellular function, which prevents cardiac arrhythmias, hypertension, possible CAD, neuromuscular and neuropsychiatric disturbances, and osteoporosis (van de Wal-Visscher et al., 2018). Some emerging studies report that low levels of magnesium may be a central factor in the development of type 2 diabetes, asthma, migraines, and nephrolithiasis (van de Wal-Visscher et al., 2018). Balancing levels of Mg is dependent upon intestinal uptake, amount in bone and skeletal storage, and renal elimination with the kidney as the main regulator in maintaining Mg homeostasis. Noteworthy, calcium and magnesium antagonize each other's gut absorption; high calcium intake reduces magnesium absorption, while low magnesium intake promotes calcium absorption. Mainly poor renal function as seen in chronic kidney disease; alteration in PTH, calcium, and possible vitamin D levels; as well as gut malabsorption and poor intake may alter magnesium balance (Hacker, 2019).

Summary of Calcium, Phosphate, and Magnesium Regulation

In summary, PTH and vitamin D increase serum calcium, while calcitonin reduces serum calcium. PTH promotes excretion of phosphate, while vitamin D promotes reabsorption. Presence of calcium in the gut reduces magnesium absorption in contrast to the presence of PTH and vitamin D, which promote magnesium absorption. Diseases that affect the bone, kidney, and parathyroid gland, as well as altered vitamin D levels may lead to hypo or hyper conditions of calcium, phosphate, and magnesium.

ACID–BASE BALANCE

An acid is an electrolyte that releases hydrogen ions (H^+) in water; in contrast, an electrolyte that releases ions that combine with a hydrogen ion is called a base. Buffers are substances that assist in normalizing pH change by donating a hydrogen ion when depleted or combining with a hydrogen ion when in excess. Normal blood pH is 7.35 to 7.45, whereas acidosis is 7.0 to 7.3, and alkalosis is 7.5 to 7.8. Homeostatic mechanisms to maintain this narrow pH range is primarily done by the kidneys and lungs to maintain hydrogen (H^+) balance. Bicarbonate (HCO_3—base) is regulated by the kidneys and normally reabsorbed by the proximal tubules and a small amount in the distal tubules, while carbon dioxide (CO_2—acid) is blown off by the lungs as a by-product of respiratory metabolic processes. Both of these systems help maintain H^+ balance to regulate or buffer the pH when acid–base disturbances occur that cannot be compensated (Hacker, 2019).

In urinary diversions where a segment of intestine is used as a conduit or reservoir, electrolyte and acid–base balance may occur because the intestinal segment continues to perform its physiological function of secretion and reabsorption as well as mucous production. In a urinary diversion, the bowel will secrete sodium and bicarbonate and reabsorb ammonia, hydrogen (acid), and chloride from urine. Depending upon the patient's comorbid conditions (i.e., baseline renal function, age), length and type of intestinal segment used will determine the risk and extent of an acid–base problem. Typically, a respiratory-compensated metabolic acidosis with hyperchloremia is a complication of ileal or colonic segments when interposed into urinary system (Vasdev et al., 2013).

KEY POINT

Metabolic acidosis with hyperchloremia can occur with urinary diversions.

ENDOCRINE FUNCTION

The kidneys possess endocrine-like function by secreting hormones: EPO to promote red blood cell production and renin–angiotensin–aldosterone to regulate blood volume and pressure, and activation of vitamin D to promote ossification of bones and teeth.

Erythropoietin

EPO is a glycoprotein hormone that stimulates the bone marrow through cytokine properties to create red blood cells in response to hypoxia due to reduced renal blood flow (bleeding) or exposure to high altitudes (reduced oxygen levels). EPO is created mainly by fibroblast cells lining the peritubular capillary system near the renal tubules and minimally by the liver except during fetal gestation. Chronic kidney disease can drastically reduce EPO production and may lead to anemia and reduced hematocrit. Recumbent human EPO is often used to treat anemia produced by renal failure, inflammatory bowel disease, and myelodysplasia occurring from cancer treatment involving chemotherapy or radiation (Huether, 2019; Shier et al., 2019a,b).

Renin–Angiotensin–Aldosterone System

As previously discussed, the kidneys monitor blood pressure and take a corrective action by producing renin in response to low afferent arteriole pressure caused by either systemic hypotension or renal artery stenosis. In short, renin acts upon angiotensinogen, which creates angiotensin I. Angiotensin I is cleaved by a peptidase (ACE) generated by blood vessels in the lung to create angiotensin II. Angiotensin II causes multiple reactions to help elevate low blood pressure and volume including constriction of arterioles to reduce capillary bed flow, thereby enhancing vascular resistance; stimulation of the proximal tubules to reabsorb sodium (thus water); stimulation of the adrenal gland to produce aldosterone, which promotes Na^+ reabsorption and K^+ secretion at the distal convoluted tubes; excitation of the posterior pituitary gland to release ADH (vasopressin) to promote water reabsorption at the collecting ducts; and increase in the strength of the heartbeat (Huether, 2019; Klabunde, 2014; Shier et al., 2019b).

Vitamin D₃

The inactive form of vitamin D_3 (calciferol) is synthesized in the skin when ultraviolet rays trigger the conversion of dehydrocholesterol into calciferol or is supplied through diet or supplementation. It is then changed into an active form of vitamin D_3 through a two-step process that occurs first in the liver then in the kidneys. Vitamin D_3 plays a vital role in intestinal calcium and phosphate absorption from food and promotes healthy bones and teeth through ossification (Huether, 2019; Shier et al., 2019a,b).

 ## CONCLUSIONS

The role of the renal system is to provide homeostasis to maintain a stabilized internal environment for optimal cell and tissue metabolism. It accomplishes this vital task through filtration of toxins from the blood and excretion of water and waste. Moreover, it provides homeostasis through fluid, electrolyte, and acid–base balance as well as hormonal secretion. The created filtrate (urine) leaves the kidneys through the renal pelves and ureters and is then transported to the bladder where it is stored and eliminated depending upon physiologic, psychological, and social influences that create a desire to urinate. The renal and urologic system is multifaceted where essential knowledge of the anatomy and physiology is imperative for optimal care of a patient who is a candidate for a urinary diversion due to a urological disorder. Depending upon the type of urinary diversion, alteration in the functions of the kidney may occur such as fluid and electrolyte and acid–base imbalances, urinary reflux, hydronephrosis, and renal failure. The primary goal when creating a urinary diversion is to preserve the function of the upper urinary tract.

REFERENCES

Ashton-Miller, J. A., & DeLancey, J. O. (2007). Functional anatomy of the female pelvic floor. *The Annals of the New York Academy of Sciences, 1101*, 266–296.

Barbic, M., Telenta, K., Noventa, M., et al. (2018). Ureteral injuries during different types of hysterectomy: A 7-year series at a single university center. *European Journal of Obstetrics & Gynecology and Reproductive Biology, 225*, 1–4.

Bordoni, B., Sugumar, K., & Leslie, S. W. (2019). Anatomy, abdomen and pelvis, pelvic floor. [Updated April 25, 2019]. *StatPearls* [Internet]. Treasure Island, FL: StatPearls Publishing. Retrieved from https://www.ncbi.nlm.nih.gov/books/NBK482200/

Douissard, J., Ris, F., Morel, P., et al. (2018). Current strategies to prevent iatrogenic ureteral injury during colorectal surgery. *Surgical Technology International, 32*, 119–124.

Eisner, B. H., Reese, A., Sheth, S., et al. (2009). Ureteral stone location at emergency room presentation with colic. *The Journal of Urology, 182*(1), 165–168.

Flagg, L., & Joiner, C. M. (2017). Urinary stone disease. In D. K. Newman, J. F. Wyman, & V. W. Welch (Eds.), *SUNA core curriculum for urologic nursing* (1st ed., pp. 375–443). Pitman, NJ: SUNA.

Gild, P., Kluth, L. A., Vetterlein, M. W., et al. (2018). Adult iatrogenic ureteral injury and stricture-incidence and treatment strategies. *Asian Journal of Urology, 5*(2), 101–106.

Gray, M., & Moore, K. N. (2009). Atlas of genitourinary anatomy and physiology. In M. Gray, & K. N. Moore (Eds.), *Urologic disorders: Adult and pediatric care* (pp. 12–43). St. Louis, MO: Mosby.

Hacker, C. (2019). Renal system. In C. R. Rebar, N. M. Heimgartner, & C. J. Gersch (Eds.), *Pathophysiology made incredible easy!* (6th ed., pp. 285–320). Philadelphia, PA: Wolters Kluwer.

Huether, S. E. (2019). Structure and function of the renal and urologic system. In S. E. Huether, & K. L. McCance (Eds.), *Understanding pathophysiology* (8th ed.). St. Louis, MO: Elsevier.

Hurtado, R., Bub, G., & Herzlinger, D. (2014). A molecular signature of tissues with pacemaker activity in the heart and upper urinary tract involves coexpressed hyperpolarization-activated cation and T-type Ca^{2+} channels. *FASEB Journal, 28*(2), 730–739.

Iskander, S. M., Feeney, M. M., Yee, K., et al. (2018). Protein kinase 2β is expressed in neural crest-derived urinary pacemaker cells and required for pyeloureteric contraction. *Journal of the American Society of Nephrology*, 29(4), 1198–1209. doi: 10.1681/ASN.2017090951.

Klabunde, R. (2014). Cardiovascular physiology concepts: Renin-angiotensin-aldosterone system. Retrieved from http://cvphysiology.com/Blood%20Pressure/BP015.htm

Kurz, D. A., & Guzzo, T. J. (2017). Genitourinary anatomy and physiology. In D. K. Newman, J. F. Wyman, & V. W. Welch (Eds.), *SUNA core curriculum for urologic nursing* (1st ed., pp. 375–443). Pitman, NJ: SUNA.

Lescay, H. A., & Tuma, F. (2019). Anatomy, abdomen and pelvis, ureter. [Updated November 13, 2018]. In *StatPearls* [Internet]. Treasure Island, FL: StatPearls Publishing. Retrieved from https://www.ncbi.nlm.nih.gov/books/NBK532980/

Matsumura Y, Iemura Y, Fukui S, et al. (2018). [Iatrogenic injuries of urinary tract: Outcomes of surgical repairs]. *Hinyokika Kiyo*, 64(3), 95–99.

Perucchini, D., & DeLancey, J. (2008). Functional anatomy of the pelvic floor and lower urinary tract. In K. Baessler, et al. (Eds.), *Pelvic floor re-education* (2nd ed.). London, UK: Springer Verlag.

Pradidarcheep, W., Wallner, C., Dabhoiwala, N. F., et al. (2011). Anatomy and histology of the lower urinary tract. In K. E. Andersson & M. C. Michel (Eds.), *Urinary tract, handbook of experimental pharmacology* (pp. 117–148). Berlin/Heidelberg, Germany: Springer-Verlag.

Sampselle, C. A., & DeLancey, O. L. (1998). Anatomy of female continence. *Journal of Wound, Ostomy, and Continence Nursing*, 25(2), 63–74.

Scolari, F., Izzi, C., & Ghiggeri, G. M. (2015). Uromodulin: From monogenic to multifactorial diseases. *Nephrology, Dialysis, Transplantation*, 30(8), 1250–1256.

Shier, D., Butler, J., & Lewis, R. (2019a). Urinary system. In D. Shier, J. Butler, & R. Lewis (Eds.), *Hole's human anatomy & physiology* (15th ed., pp. 767–802). New York, NY: McGraw-Hill.

Shier, D., Butler, J., & Lewis, R. (2019b). Water, electrolyte, and acid–base balance. In D. Shier, J. Butler, & R. Lewis (Eds.), *Hole's human anatomy & physiology* (15th ed., pp. 804–823). New York, NY: McGraw-Hill.

Siccardi, M. A., & Valle, C. (2019). Anatomy, bony pelvis and lower limb, pelvic fascia. [Updated January 24, 2019]. In *StatPearls* [Internet]. Treasure Island, FL: StatPearls Publishing. Retrieved from https://www.ncbi.nlm.nih.gov/books/NBK518984/

Siddiqi, N. H., & Schwartz, B. F. (2017). Percutaneous nephrostomy. Retrieved November 2, 2019, from https://emedicine.medscape.com/article/1821504-overview

van de Wal-Visscher, E. R., Kooman, J. P., & van der Sande, F. M. (2018): Magnesium in chronic kidney disease: Should we care? *Blood Purification*, 45, 173–178. doi: 10.1159/000485212.

Vasdev, N., Moon, A., & Thorpe. (2013). Metabolic complications of urinary intestinal diversion. *Indian Journal of Urology*, 29(4), 310–315.

Weinberg, K., Telegrafi, S., & Kozirovsky, M. (2018). Urinary system. In S. Hagen-Ansert (Ed.), *Textbook of diagnostic sonography* (8th ed., pp. 375–443). St. Louis, MO: Elsevier.

QUESTIONS

1. The functional unit of the kidney is the nephron. What is the primary function of this structure?
   A. Removing waste and toxic products from the plasma
   B. Secreting mucus, water, and enzymes
   C. Forming urine
   D. Absorbing nutrients

2. Which structure of the urinary system assists with urine storage and elimination?
   A. Kidneys
   B. Renal pelves
   C. Ureters
   D. Bladder

3. Which structure of the urinary system is a common site for congenital or acquired obstruction, such as stones?
   A. Kidney
   B. Urinary bladder
   C. Ureteropelvic junction (UPJ)
   D. Urethra

4. The urethra is composed of both smooth and specialized striated muscle. What is the important function of this structure?
   A. Maintaining homeostasis
   B. Maintaining continence
   C. Storing excess urine
   D. Providing perfusion

5. Which of the organs adjacent to the kidneys needs to be protected by the surgeon during urinary reconstruction?
   A. Ascending large intestine
   B. Abdominal aorta
   C. Liver
   D. Gallbladder

6. Which of the following statements accurately describes a function of the renal system when maintaining homeostasis of the body's internal environment?
   A. The kidneys secrete renin–angiotensin–aldosterone to regulate blood volume and pressure.
   B. Erythropoietin (EPO) causes multiple reactions to help elevate low blood pressure and volume.
   C. Carbon dioxide (CO_2—acid) is regulated by the kidneys and normally reabsorbed by the proximal tubules and a small amount in the distal tubules.
   D. Vitamin K plays a vital role in intestinal calcium and phosphate absorption from food and promotes healthy bones and teeth through ossification.

7. What condition might occur when an excess of uric acid is precipitated in the blood?
   A. Hypertension
   B. Diabetes mellitus
   C. Diabetes insipidus
   D. Gout

8. What important point should be emphasized when explaining how the renal system works to regulate the body's fluid and electrolyte balance?
   A. Aldosterone causes secretion of sodium (Na^+) and reabsorption of potassium (K^+).
   B. Antidiuretic hormone (ADH) causes water reabsorption.
   C. Potassium (K^+) is the main ion outside the cell, while sodium (Na^+) is the main ion within the actual cell.
   D. Water needs active or passive transport to cross membranes.

9. What is the primary goal when creating a urinary diversion?
   A. Preserve the function of the upper urinary tract.
   B. Preserve the function of the lower urinary tract.
   C. Maintain acid–base balance.
   D. Prevent damage to the kidneys.

10. What condition might occur when erythropoietin (EPO) production is suppressed by chronic kidney disease?
   A. Elevated hematocrit
   B. Anemia
   C. Urinary incontinence
   D. Acid–base imbalances

ANSWERS AND RATIONALES

1. A. Rationale: The functional unit of the kidney is the nephron. Its primary function is to remove waste and toxic products from the plasma and control the composition of body fluids.

2. D. Rationale: The urinary bladder is a hollow, muscular organ designed to fill with urine at low pressures, stores approximately 300 to 600 mL urine in the healthy adult, and eliminates urine.

3. C. Rationale: The UPJ is a common site for congenital or acquired obstruction, that is, stones.

4. B. Rationale: The urethra has specialized striated muscle that contains both fast-twitch and short-twitch muscle fibers that aid in tone of the urethra during periods of sudden increase in abdominal pressure to prevent urinary incontinence.

5. A. Rationale: Organs adjacent to the kidneys include the duodenum, pancreas tail, hepatic flexure of the large intestine, ascending colon, and descending and sigmoid colon. Identification and protection by the surgeon during urinary reconstruction surgery are crucial to prevent life-threatening inter- and postoperative complications.

6. A. Rationale: The kidneys possess endocrine-like function by secreting hormones: EPO (erythropoietin) to promote red blood cell production and renin–angiotensin–aldosterone to regulate blood volume and pressure. Homeostatic mechanisms to maintain narrow blood pH range is primarily done by the kidneys and lungs to maintain hydrogen (H^+) balance. Bicarbonate (HCO_3—base) is regulated by the kidneys.

7. D. Rationale: Uric acid is a by-product of purine and guanine metabolism from the intake of meat and seafood. Only 10% is excreted in the urine. If in excess, uric acid may precipitate in the blood and cause painful deposits in joints called gout.

8. B. Rationale: Four key points to remember when discussing fluid and electrolyte balance are as follows: (1) aldosterone causes reabsorption of sodium (Na^+) and secretion of potassium (K^+); (2) antidiuretic hormone (ADH) causes water reabsorption; (3) Na^+ is the main ion outside the cell (interstitial and vascular), while K^+ is the main ion within the actual cell; and (4) water easily diffuses through a membrane readily from low to high solute concentration.

9. A. Rationale: Depending upon the type of urinary diversion, alteration in the functions of the kidney may occur such as fluid and electrolyte and acid–base imbalances, urinary reflux, hydronephrosis, and renal failure. The primary goal when creating a urinary diversion is to preserve the function of the upper urinary tract.

10. B. Rationale: EPO is created mainly by fibroblast cells lining the peritubular capillary system near the renal tubules. Chronic kidney disease can drastically reduce EPO production and may lead to anemia and reduced hematocrit.

CHAPTER 4

DISEASES THAT LEAD TO A FECAL STOMA: COLORECTAL CANCER

Linda Ferrari and Alessandro Fichera

OBJECTIVE

Describe the disease states that lead to creation of a fecal stoma: colorectal cancer.

TOPIC OUTLINE

- **Introduction 44**
- **Colorectal Adenocarcinoma 44**
  - Etiology 44
  - Risk Factors 45
  - Primary Prevention 45
  - Risk Assessment and Patient Stratification 45
  - Secondary Prevention: Colorectal Cancer Screening 45
  - Presentation/Workup 46
  - Treatment Algorithms 47
  - Colon Cancer Management: Surgical Resection 47
  - Rectal Cancer Treatment: Neoadjuvant Therapy and Surgical Resection 49
  - Adjuvant Treatment 51
    - Advanced Disease 51

- **Other Cancers of the Colon and Rectum 51**
  - Carcinoid Tumors 52
  - Melanoma: Primary and Metastatic 52
  - Gastrointestinal Stromal Tumor 52
  - Sarcoma 52
  - Lymphoma 52
- **Indications for Stoma Formation for Colorectal Neoplasia 52**
  - Temporary Stoma 52
  - Timing to Reverse Temporary Stoma 53
  - Permanent Stoma 53
  - Quality of Life With or Without Stoma After Low Anterior Resection 54
    - Surveillance 54
- **Conclusions 55**

INTRODUCTION

In the United States, colorectal cancer (CRC) is the fourth most common malignancy and second most common cause of cancer-related death (National Cancer Institute, 2019). Fortunately, due to significant efforts in both screening and treatment, those rates are decreasing on the order of approximately 3% and 2.8% yearly for CRC incidence and deaths, respectively (National Cancer Institute, 2019). Despite these promising trends, there have been an estimated 145,600 new cases of colon cancer in 2019, making care of the CRC patient in need of either temporary or permanent stoma a very common occurrence in clinical practice.

COLORECTAL ADENOCARCINOMA

ETIOLOGY

Adenocarcinoma accounts for the majority of cancers in the colon and rectum. CRC is the second most common cancer diagnosed in women and the third most in men. In the United States, the incidence of CRC per 100,000 people decreased from 60.5 in 1976 to 46.4 in 2005 (Cheng et al., 2011), with the exception in patients younger than 50 years, for whom the incidence has been increasing (Bailey et al., 2014). In 2019, the estimated new cases are 145,600, with estimated death of 51,020, they respectively represent 8.3% of all new cancer cases and 8.4% of all cancer deaths (National Cancer Institute, 2019). The origin of these tumors is believed to be a single transformed cell that undergoes abnormal growth and division leading to formation of an adenoma and ultimately adenocarcinoma. In order to progress to carcinoma, the cell must undergo a series of genetic mutations causing inactivation of tumor suppressor genes such as *APC*, *DDC*, and *p53* or activation of proto-oncogenes like *K-ras*, which is associated with poor prognosis (Conlin et al., 2005).

RISK FACTORS

There are both modifiable and nonmodifiable risk factors for CRC development. Modifiable risk factors include high-fat and/or low-fiber diet, decreased physical activity, smoking, excessive alcohol intake, increased bodyweight, and red and processed meat consumption (Dekker et al., 2019). Nonmodifiable risk factors include age >50 years, patient disease, family history of polyps or CRC, and genetic predisposition. Positive family history plays an important role in 10% to 20% of all patients with CRC, with different risk depending on number and degree of affected relatives and age of CRC diagnosis (Henrikson et al., 2015). Patients suffering from long-standing inflammatory bowel disease (i.e., Crohn's disease or ulcerative colitis) are at an increased risk of developing CRC with a lifetime risk of 3.7% to 5.4% (Eaden et al., 2001). Their risk is proportional to the duration of inflammation, extent of colonic involvement, and age of onset. Personal history of neoplastic polyps (i.e., adenomas) carries a two- to fivefold increased risk of carcinoma, which is not surprising given the natural history of CRC development. A family history of adenoma or CRC yields a two- to fourfold increased risk of CRC, with greater risk for CRC over adenoma, family age of diagnosis at <50 years, and multiple affected family members (Johns & Houlston, 2001).

While the majority of CRCs are sporadic, approximately 15% are associated with an inherited colon cancer predisposition via a germ-line genetic mutation. Hereditary CRC syndromes can be divided as nonpolyposis, such as hereditary nonpolyposis colon cancer (HNPCC), and familial polyposis, such as familial adenomatous polyposis (FAP) syndrome. FAP is caused by mutations in the oncogene *APC* and is inherited in an autosomal dominant pattern with a 100% risk of developing colon cancer by age 40 years. Individuals with FAP develop hundreds to thousands of adenomatous polyps in the colon and in the duodenum and stomach. Each of these is at risk for malignant transformation. Individuals with FAP should undergo total colectomy or proctocolectomy (removal of the colon and rectum) for treatment and risk reduction rather than segmental resection alone. There is a high risk of recurrence in the rectum if proctectomy is not performed, and therefore, these individuals must continue rectal screening postoperatively.

HNPCC (Lynch syndrome) is inherited by mutations in one of several mismatch repair genes (*MLH1*, *MSH2*, *MSH6*, and *PMS2*) leading to microsatellite instability. It is estimated that HNPCC accounts for 5% of CRCs. The lifetime CRC risk is slightly lower than with FAP at a rate of 70% to 90%. These individuals do not develop diffuse adenomatous disease as with FAP, and the cancers are typically flat and difficult to detect by colonoscopy. These tumors have a predilection for the right colon and can be treated with total colectomy alone without proctectomy as with FAP. Additionally, they are at risk for extracolonic cancers such as endometrial, ovarian, stomach, small bowel, and bladder. Women with HNPCC are counseled to undergo surveillance if premenopausal or consider prophylactic total abdominal hysterectomy and bilateral salpingo-oophorectomy if finished with childbearing.

KEY POINT

People with a history of colorectal cancer in one or more first-degree relatives (parents, sibling, or children) are at increased risk to develop colorectal cancer.

PRIMARY PREVENTION

Recommendations to reduce the risk of development for CRC include smoking cessation, regular physical activity for at least 30 minutes, and healthy diet comprehensive of fresh fruits, vegetables, whole grains, fiber, and calcium (Song et al., 2015). In addition, regular use of vitamin supplements and hormone replacement therapy seem to reduce the risk of CRC. In 2016, the US Preventive Task force recommended the use of low-dose aspirin for primary prevention of cardiovascular disease and CRC in adults between 50 and 69 years (Bibbins-Domingo, 2016). However, possible beneficial effects should be balanced against possible side effects, such as gastrointestinal bleeding.

RISK ASSESSMENT AND PATIENT STRATIFICATION

Depending on their risk of developing CRC, the National Comprehensive Cancer Network (NCCN) guidelines for CRC screening stratify patients into three groups, average group, increased risk group, and patients with high-risk syndrome. Risks assessment in people without family history should be considered by 40 years of age, with the aim to understand when to start the screening program.

SECONDARY PREVENTION: COLORECTAL CANCER SCREENING

CRC screening programs vary among different countries, based on the local health system. The two most commonly used choices are endoscopic evaluation and fecal-based screening tests. Endoscopic evaluation of the colon is the primary means of CRC screening, through either sigmoidoscopy or colonoscopy. Endoscopic tests, especially colonoscopy, have high sensitivity and specificity but are invasive studies and carry a risk of iatrogenic perforation and bleeding. Main advantage is that they offer the possibility to remove precursor lesions and early cancers. General consensus for a complete colonoscopy to the cecum is that 10-year interval is appropriate for the majority average-risk population.

Stools tests aim to detect possible markers that might indicate the presence of CRC. The two primary fecal-based screening tests are the fecal occult blood test (FOBT) and fecal immunochemical test (FIT). The advantage of these techniques are that they are not invasive and have high compliance. Patients with positive tests should have a colonoscopy and complete a two-step screening program. It has been demonstrated that screening with FOB reduced CRC mortality by 16% (Hewitson et al., 2008), while screening with FIT reduces cancer mortality of 22% compared to prescreening period (Zorzi et al., 2015). FIT is the most common screening tool in Europe, with high rate of participation.

CT colonography is an additional screening modality that has the advantage of improved visualization of the colonic mucosa without the risks of an invasive procedure. However, positive findings require a colonoscopy, and the issue about radiation exposure needs to be considered. At present, it might be used for patients suspected of CRC too frail for full bowel preparation prior colonoscopy.

Current NCCN guidelines recommend colonoscopy every 10 years, annual FOBT or FIT tests every 3 years, flexible sigmoidoscopy every 5 to 10 years, or CT-colonography every 5 years starting at age 50 for average-risk individuals, until 76 years (National Comprehensive Cancer Network, Version 2.2019, 2019). Screening between 76 and 85 years needs to be assessed based on individual conditions, based on weighting risks and benefits, and based on frailty and life expectation as well.

> **KEY POINT**
>
> The National Comprehensive Cancer Network has Colon Cancer Guidelines for Patients (http://www.nccn.org/patients/guidelines/colon/index.html#1).

PRESENTATION/WORKUP

If not diagnosed through a screening modality, patients with CRC may present with a variety of symptoms including blood per rectum, decreased stool caliber, nonspecific abdominal pain, weight loss, and fatigue. Initial evaluation includes endoscopy if not previously performed, to assess tumor location and obtain biopsies to confirm suspected diagnosis of CRC. Once the diagnosis is confirmed, further studies are used to evaluate extent of tumor invasion and tumor spread including CT chest, abdomen and pelvis, CEA, and MRI or endoscopic ultrasound for rectal cancers. Based on this information, the cancer is staged using tumor invasion, spread to lymph nodes, and distant metastatic spread (TNM classification, **Table 4-1**) (Amin et al., 2017).

TABLE 4-1 TNM CLASSIFICATION

AJCC STAGE	TNM CLASSIFICATION	DEFINITION
0	Tis (carcinoma in situ)	Tis: tumor involves mucosa only
I	T1, N0, T2, N0, M0	T1: tumor invades submucosa T2: tumor invades muscularis propria
IIA	T3, N0, M0	T3: tumor invades through muscularis propria to subserosa (colon) or perirectal tissues (rectal)
IIB	T4a, N0, M0	T4a: tumor invades surface of visceral peritoneum
IIC	T4b, N0, M0	T4b: tumor directly invades adjacent structures
IIIA	T1–T2, N1/N1C, M0 T1, N2a, M0	N1: metastasis to 1–3 regional lymph nodes N2a: metastasis to 4–6 regional lymph nodes
IIIB	T3–T4, N1/N1C, M0 T2–T3, N2a, M0 T1–T2, N2b, M0	N2b: metastases to ≥7 regional lymph nodes
IIIC	T4a, N2a, M0 T3–T4a, N2b, M0 T4b, N1–N2, M0	N3: any node along major named vascular trunk
IVA	Any T, any N, M1a	M1a: distant metastasis confined to one organ
IVB	Any T, any N, M1b	M1b: distant metastases in more than one organ/site
IVC	Any T, any N, M1c	M1c: peritoneal metastases with or without metastases of other organs

Adapted from Amin, M. B., Edge, S. B., Greene, F. L., et al. (Eds.). (2017). *AJCC cancer staging manual* (8th ed.). New York, NY: Springer.

TREATMENT ALGORITHMS

Based on staging information, specifically local tumor invasion and metastatic disease, patients may be treated with preoperative neoadjuvant therapy or go directly to surgical resection, followed by adjuvant therapy if indicated.

COLON CANCER MANAGEMENT: SURGICAL RESECTION

Surgical resection is commonly a first step in the treatment of CRC depending on stage and location (colon vs. rectal) (**Figs. 4-1 and 4-2**) (National Comprehensive Cancer Network, Version 4.2019, 2019). It is estimated that over 200,000 colectomies are performed yearly in the United States, making it one of the most commonly performed procedures (Bal, 1992; Etzioni et al., 2009). A preoperative evaluation must be performed to determine the patient's fitness for the planned operation.

The steps of resection include ligation of the feeding blood supply with en bloc resection of tumor and involved adjacent structures and inclusion of the draining lymph nodes, followed by primary anastomosis (**Fig. 4-3A and B**). Originally it was believed that 5-cm proximal and distal margins were required; however, mural spread rarely extends past 2 cm from the palpable tumor (Quirke et al., 1986). This is often not measured in practice as oncologic principles and blood supply necessitate resection proximally and distally to the next named feeding vessel. Specifically, with right colon resections, there is not a set distance of terminal ileum required for adequate resection.

KEY POINT

Surgical resection is the first step in the treatment of CRC depending upon the stage.

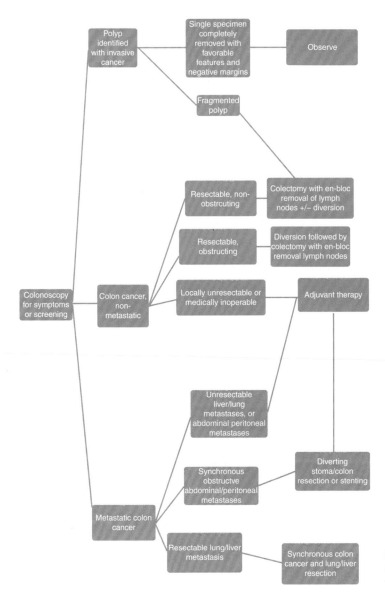

FIGURE 4-1. Treatment Algorithm for Colon Cancer. (Adapted from NCCN Guidelines. Colon cancer. Version 4.2019.)

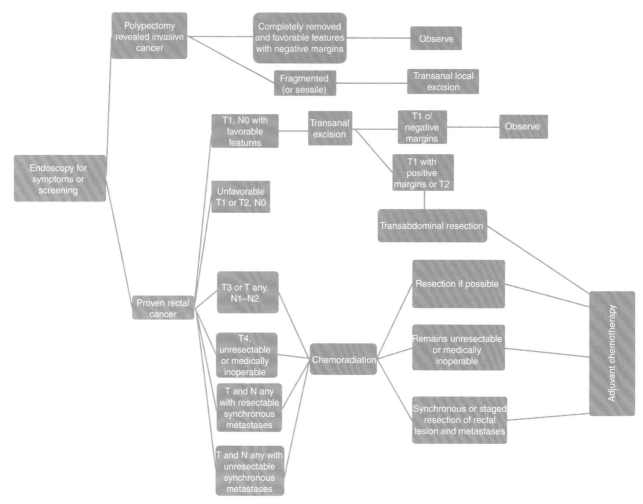

FIGURE 4-2. Treatment Algorithm for Rectal Cancer. (Adapted from NCCN Guidelines. Rectal cancer. Version 3.2019.)

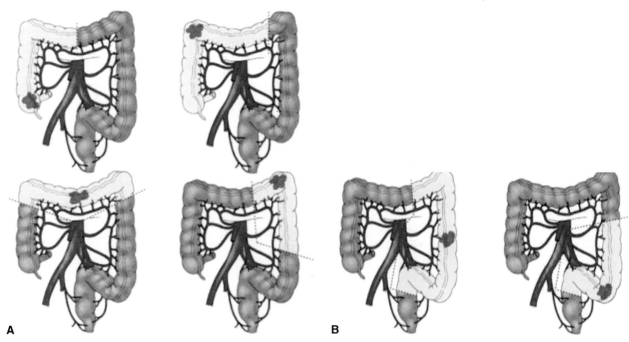

FIGURE 4-3. A. Segmental colon resection for colon cancer based on tumor location. **B.** LAR for distal colon or mid/upper rectal cancers. (From Fisher, S. M. (2010). *ABSITE review*. Philadelphia, PA: Wolters Kluwer.)

Over the past two decades, laparoscopic colectomy has become a valid option for patient with resectable disease. According to COLOR (Deijen et al., 2017) and CLASSIC (Jayne et al., 2007) trials, laparoscopy is not inferior to open approach and has similar rates of disease-free survival, overall survival, and recurrence rate. In the COST trial, 872 patients have been randomly assigned to undergo open or laparoscopic colectomy for colon cancer. After a median follow-up of 7 years, they have observed similar 5-year overall survival and recurrence rate. Perioperative care and prehabilitation programs have significantly reduced the length of hospital stay and complication rates after procedures. The EnROL trial (Kennedy et al., 2014) has shown same outcome between open and laparoscopy, with a significant reduction in terms of hospital stay in favor of the laparoscopic group (5 vs. 7 days, p = 0.033).

RECTAL CANCER TREATMENT: NEOADJUVANT THERAPY AND SURGICAL RESECTION

Rectal cancer management differs from colon cancer due to the absence of a serosa surrounding the rectum, which is the reason for the higher risk of local recurrence. To minimize these risks, radiation therapy is recommended for rectal cancers with advanced local disease or lymph node involvement (stage II or stage III) (**Figs. 4-4 and 4-5**). For these tumors, the incidence of local recurrence is decreased from 30% to 65% to 5% to 10% with adjuvant radiation (Colorectal Cancer Collaborative Group, 2001).

Rectal cancers are treated by one of three operations depending on extent of local disease and tumor location:

transanal local excision/transanal endoscopic microsurgery (TEM), low anterior resection (LAR) (**Fig. 4-3B**), transanal total mesorectal excision (TaTME), or abdominoperineal resection (APR) (**Fig. 4-6**).

Low-grade, node-negative tumors (T1N0) may be treated with TEM with curative intent. It involves a full-thickness excision performed through the rectal wall into the perirectal fat and requires 3-mm deep mucosal margins to be considered an oncologic resection. Local excision has the advantages of minimal morbidity and mortality and rapid postoperative recovery (Baxter & Garcia-Aguilar, 2007). On the other hand, local lymphs are not sampled, potentially leaving micro-metastatic disease that is typically not identified by preoperative images.

Advanced cancers in the upper and middle third of the rectum are treated with LAR (**Fig. 4-3B**), while low rectal cancers may require APR (**Fig. 4-6**) due to sphincter involvement or inability to obtain clear distal margin. LAR encompasses the sigmoid and involved rectum while leaving distal rectum and sphincter complex intact (usually with a temporary loop ileostomy) (**Fig. 4-7**), whereas resection of the entire rectum and anus and creation of an end colostomy is required with an APR (with a permanent colostomy) (**Fig. 4-6**). Both LAR and APR require total meso-rectal excision (TME) for adequate oncologic resection, entailing complete resection of mesorectum and other surrounding perirectal tissues. Pathologic specimens are evaluated for adequacy of TME as well as involvement of circumferential radial margin (CRM). Laparoscopic approach for rectal cancer resection has been investigated in

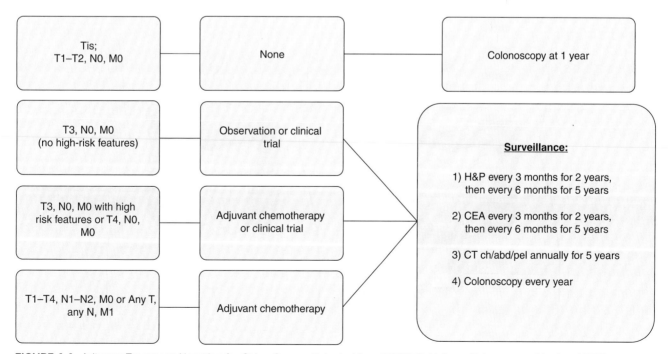

FIGURE 4-4. Adjuvant Treatment Algorithm for Colon Cancer. (Adapted from NCCN Guidelines. Colon cancer. Version 4.2019.

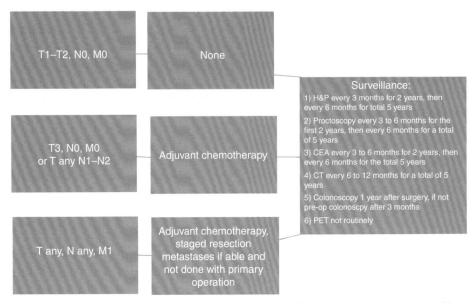

FIGURE 4-5. Adjuvant Treatment Algorithm for Rectal Cancer. (Adapted from NCCN Guidelines. Rectal cancer. Version 3.2019.)

randomized trials where it has been compared to open approach (Jayne et al., 2010; van der Pas et al., 2013) with the results that laparoscopic resections are noninferior to open approach in disease-free survival and overall survival. Pathologic outcomes have been reported in the ACOSOG Z6051 trial (Fleshman et al., 2015), which has the primary end point to achieve clear resection margin (CRM) >1 mm, negative distal margin, and completeness of TME. Criteria of noninferiority of laparoscopic approach were not reached, and nearly complete TME was achieved in 92.1% in the laparoscopic arm and 95.1% in the open resection arm, for a difference of −3.0 (95% CI, −7.4 to 1.5; p = 0.20). Similar results have been obtained from ALaCaRT trail (Stevenson et al., 2015), where successful resections were achieved in 82% of the laparoscopic group and 89% of the open resection ones, for a difference of −7 (95% CI, −12.4% to infinity). Two-year disease-free survival and local recurrence rate haven't been found to be different between patients treated with laparoscopic and open resection for stage II and III rectal cancer enrolled in the ACOSOG Z6051 randomized trial (Fleshman et al., 2019). From this recent published results, we can consider laparoscopy noninferior to open technique

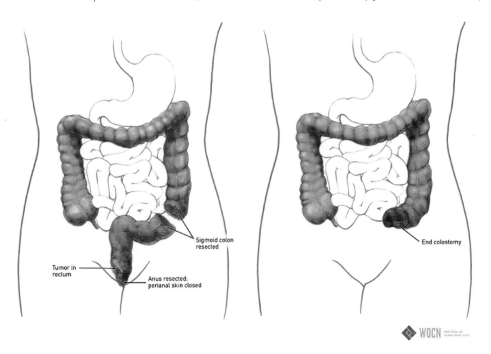

FIGURE 4-6. Abdominal Perineal Resection.

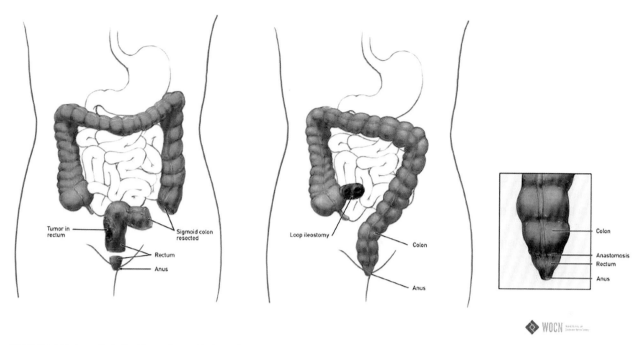

FIGURE 4-7. Low Anterior Resection with Loop Ileostomy.

for rectal cancer resections. Disease-free survival is negatively impacted by positive circumferential margins, low position of the tumor in the rectum, rectal perforation during resection, but not by laparoscopic approach. TaTME is a relatively new technique (Sylla et al., 2010) developed to overcome the difficulties to conduct a laparoscopic TME in obese patients with narrow pelvis. With this approach, the laparoscopy is used simultaneously (two-team) or sequentially (one-team). Potential advantage is to allow precise identification of the distal margin under direct vision through the trans-anal approach. Disadvantages are the increased risk of urethral injury and pelvic autonomic nerves. There are controversial results in terms of oncologic outcomes, with a study conducted in The Netherlands (Hol et al., 2019), in high volume centers reporting local recurrence rate of 2% and 4% at 3 and 5 years, respectively (which are in line with COLOR II trial), and a study from Norway (Larsen et al., 2019), conducted in 4 hospitals, reporting local recurrence rate of 9.5% at 11 months. Randomized control trials in high volume centers and further training are necessary before drawing appropriate conclusion about the use of this technique in colorectal surgical oncology.

KEY POINT

When an APR is performed, the left colon is used to create the colostomy, and generally the stoma will be located on the left side of the abdomen.

ADJUVANT TREATMENT

Systemic treatment with chemotherapy is beneficial for patients with locally advanced tumors (T3 with high risk of recurrence or T4) as well as those metastasized to lymph nodes or distant sites (**Fig. 4-5**). Based on the results of the MOSAIC trial and the National Surgical Adjuvant Breast and Bowel Project (NSABP) C-07, the current adjuvant regimen consists of 5-FU, leucovorin, and oxaliplatin (FOLFOX) (André et al., 2009; Kuebler et al., 2007). Both overall survival and disease-free survival were improved on the order of 5% on the FOLFOX regimen.

In addition to the regimen, timing of adjuvant therapy after surgical resection is important. An important meta-analysis has showed that every 4-week delay in delivery chemotherapy results in a 14% decreased in overall survival, so adjuvant therapy should be administered as soon as the patient is available after surgery (Biagi et al., 2011).

Advanced Disease

The most common site of metastases for colon or rectal cancer is the liver. CRC may also spread to the lungs, bones, brain, or spinal cord. Options for treatment may include surgery, chemo or radiation therapy, and/or immunotherapy.

OTHER CANCERS OF THE COLON AND RECTUM

Although adenocarcinoma is the predominant colorectal neoplasm, there are several other tumors of the colon and rectum that occur with less frequency but may require surgical management and possible stoma formation.

CARCINOID TUMORS

Carcinoid tumors are a type of neuroendocrine tumor originating from the crypts of Lieberkühn. Approximately 65% of carcinoid tumors arise within the gastrointestinal tract, 30% of which arise in the colon, and 20% in the rectum (Kulke & Mayer, 1999). These tumors are twice as common in individuals of African American descent and occur primarily in the fifth or sixth decades of life. Carcinoid syndrome is present in 10% to 18% of patients with symptoms including flushing, watery diarrhea, abdominal pain, wheezing, and right-sided heart failure. Unfortunately, 90% of symptomatic patients already have advanced or metastatic disease. Colorectal carcinoids are more commonly asymptomatic and identified on screening colonoscopy. Small (<2 cm) rectal carcinoids may be treated with transanal local excision alone. Rectal tumors >2 cm and all colon carcinoid tumors are treated with standard oncologic colorectal resection. Patients with carcinoid syndrome may be treated with somatostatin analogs for symptomatic control.

MELANOMA: PRIMARY AND METASTATIC

Melanoma of the gastrointestinal tract is most commonly metastatic from a different primary site and occurs in the small intestine. Approximately only 15% of melanoma metastatic to the GI tract occurs in the colon (Allen & Cott, 2002; Rengtgen et al., 1984). Primary GI melanoma may occur in the rectum or anus with only case reports of primary colonic melanoma (Avital et al., 2004; Miliaras et al., 2018). Unfortunately, GI melanoma carries a worse prognosis than cutaneous melanoma, which may be attributed to a later stage at diagnosis and pathways of metastatic spread. Patients are often asymptomatic but may present with bleeding, obstruction, or pain. The only curative treatment modality is wide surgical excision; however, there is no survival benefit with radical excision with an APR, and therefore, this is reserved for those with intractable pain.

GASTROINTESTINAL STROMAL TUMOR

Gastrointestinal stromal tumors (GISTs) can occur anywhere in the GI tract and arise from the interstitial cells of Cajal. They are most commonly diagnosed in men in their fifth or sixth decades of life (Tryggvason et al., 2005). GISTs are slow growing and can grow to a very large size before causing symptoms. Median size at diagnosis for symptomatic patients was found to be 8.9 cm as compared to 2.7 cm in asymptomatic patients (Kingham & DeMatteo, 2009). They occur most commonly in the small intestine and may occur in the rectum but are rarely present in the colon. These tumors spread hematogenously to the liver or peritoneum, and lymphatic spread

is rare. These tumors are unfortunately not responsive to chemotherapy or radiation and are treated with surgical resection alone. A grossly negative margin of 1 cm is recommended in order to obtain a microscopically negative margin. These tumors have a high rate of local recurrence, and therefore, all patients should be considered for adjuvant therapy with a tyrosine kinase inhibitor, such as imatinib or sunitinib. Recurrence is decreased for rectal GISTs with APR or LAR as compared to wide local excision (Yeh et al., 2000). If the tumor is deemed unresectable, consider neoadjuvant therapy to potentially decrease tumor burden and allow resection in the future.

SARCOMA

Sarcomas may involve the lower intestine either as a primary colorectal sarcoma or as direct extension from a surrounding sarcoma such as a retroperitoneal sarcoma. Primary colorectal sarcomas are rare and are usually of the subtype leiomyosarcoma. As with all sarcomas, tumor grade is the most significant prognostic indicator, and treatment includes radical en bloc resection of all tumors including adjacent structures if able.

LYMPHOMA

The gastrointestinal tract is the most common site of extra-nodal lymphoma with colorectal lymphoma accounting for 15% to 20% of GI lymphomas (Koch et al., 2001; Quayle & Lowney, 2006). Due to the increased concentration of lymphatic tissue, approximately 70% of colorectal lymphomas are located in the cecum and ascending colon. Patients most often present in the fifth to seventh decades of life with symptoms of abdominal pain or palpable abdominal mass. Colorectal lymphomas are generally considered to be a widespread systemic process and therefore are most often treated with radiation for locoregional control and systemic chemotherapy for intermediate- or high-grade disease. Surgery may be considered for truly localized disease but is generally reserved for diagnostic purposes or to treat lymphoma-related complications such as perforation, bleeding, and obstruction.

 ## INDICATIONS FOR STOMA FORMATION FOR COLORECTAL NEOPLASIA

Patients with colorectal tumors may require a stoma that can be categorized as permanent or temporary.

TEMPORARY STOMA

Temporary stomas provide diversion of the fecal stream to either decompress proximal to an obstructing mass or protect a distal anastomosis. These are generally loop colostomies or loop ileostomies (**Fig. 4-8**) depending on the patient's anatomy, tumor location, and indication for diversion. Patients with obstructing CRC who are not

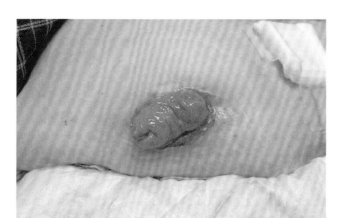

FIGURE 4-8. Diverting Loop Ileostomy in a Patient with a Distal Rectal Cancer and a Low Anastomosis.

candidates for immediate resection may benefit from a diverting stoma. This allows for continued GI function, while the patient completes the workup or undergoes neoadjuvant treatment to reduce tumor burden, or for palliative intent for unresectable and/or metastatic disease.

A temporary stoma may be created at the time of surgical resection to "defunctionalize" or "protect" a distal anastomosis. Surgical management of colon and upper third rectal cancers includes resection of tumor with adequate proximal and distal margins including lymph nodes and blood supply, segmental colon resection (**Fig. 4-3A**), and LAR (**Fig. 4-3B**), respectively. Both are followed by primary anastomoses of the remaining segments. Anastomoses must be made with adequately perfused healthy tissue without tension and without evidence of leak. Anastomotic leakage is a severe complication related to colorectal surgery, and it can increase not only postoperative morbidity and mortality but also local recurrence rate (Mirnezami et al., 2011) and poor bowel function long term (Emmertsen et al., 2013). Several factors have been analyzed to assess the risk for anastomotic leakage and the most relevant seems to be male gender, preoperative radiotherapy, smoking habit (Richards et al., 2012), need for blood transfusion, and anastomotic distance from anal verge (Arezzo et al., 2019). Loop diverting stomas may be created at this time to protect anastomoses that do not meet one or more of these criteria and are therefore at risk for future breakdown, for example, low anastomosis in male patients with history of smoking who previously received adjuvant chemoradiotherapy and who are at increased risk of anastomotic leak.

When marking a stoma site for the patient with CRC, consult the surgeon to determine if marking both sides of the abdomen might be prudent as the surgical procedure may depend upon intraoperative findings.

KEY POINT

When undergoing a low anterior resection (LAR), a temporary diverting loop ileostomy (see **Fig. 4-7**) may be created to divert stool from the anastomosis. This is especially true for the patient who may be at risk for anastomotic breakdown such as patients who had adjuvant chemoradiotherapy or have a history of smoking.

TIMING TO REVERSE TEMPORARY STOMA

Patients with a temporary protective ileostomy (diverting stoma) are at lower risk of developing clinical anastomotic leak, peritonitis and concomitant-associated morbidity, resulting in poor quality of life and function. The appropriate time to close the loop ileostomy after pelvic surgery has not been established, and it ranges between 2 months after surgery until the end of chemotherapy, with a percentage of patients who will never have the stoma reversed. Early closure of protective ileostomy (within 2 months) is a safe procedure but can negatively influence completion of chemotherapy due to anastomotic issues. On the other hand, a late closure, which means having an ileostomy during adjuvant chemotherapy, might increase the risk of high stoma output, electrolytes impairment, dehydration, and renal failure (Oliphant et al., 2015). A recent meta-analysis has demonstrated that loop ileostomy closure during adjuvant chemotherapy following rectal cancer resection might be associated with comparable results to the closure of ileostomy after completion of chemotherapy (Hajibandeh et al., 2019). Further research is needed to determine impact in quality of life and completeness of chemotherapy protocol to determine the right timing to closure.

PERMANENT STOMA

Permanent stomas generally take the form of an end colostomy (**Fig. 4-9**) or ileostomy. These may be created when reestablishment of intestinal continuity will not be achieved or when the disease process necessitates resection of the anal sphincter complex. Such opera-

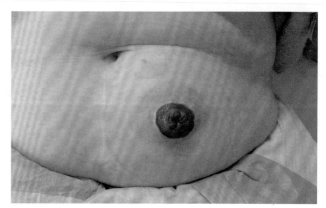

FIGURE 4-9. End Colostomy After APR.

tions include APR (**Fig. 4-6**) and pelvic exenteration. Indications for APR include cancers of the distal rectum in which distal negative margins cannot be achieved, those with direct extension into levator muscles, or patients with preoperative fecal incontinence. APR includes resection of the sigmoid colon, rectum, and anus; closure of the perineum; and creation of end colostomy. Total pelvic exenteration includes resection of other pelvic structures including the uterus, vagina, bladder, urethra, and rectum. This is indicated for rectal tumors with invasion to adjacent pelvic structures or gynecologic or urinary malignancies with involvement of the rectum. Depending on cancer location and extent of local invasion, patients may require an anterior, posterior, or total pelvic exenteration. Anterior exenteration includes only genitourinary and gynecologic structures, while posterior exenteration includes only GI and gynecologic structures. Given resection of both GI and GU structures with total pelvic exenteration, patients will have both a permanent colostomy and urostomy (**Fig. 4-10**). Both operations, APR and pelvic exenteration, are highly morbid and should be performed primarily for curative intent in patients fit to tolerate the operation as well as its possible complications.

Preoperative stoma site marking is essential for those either with a planned stoma creation or at high risk for requiring a stoma (Salvadalena et al., 2015). Special attention must be taken for patients in whom an intraoperative decision will be made regarding type of stoma and for those needing both a colostomy and urostomy (see Chapter 10). This becomes more of an issue in patients who have already had a stoma reversed and now need a second diversion.

QUALITY OF LIFE WITH OR WITHOUT STOMA AFTER LOW ANTERIOR RESECTION

After restoration of bowel function and closure of diverting stoma, more than 40% of patients develop a combination of increased stool frequency, urgency, clustering,

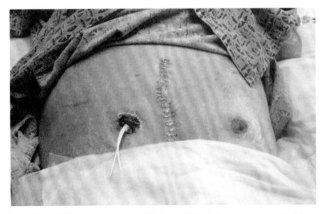

FIGURE 4-10. Urostomy on *Right* and End Colostomy on *Left* in a Patient with Pelvic Exenteration. (Courtesy of Mary Arnold Long, MSN, RN, CRN, CWOCN-AP, ACNS-BC.)

and incontinence, which is defined as low anterior resection syndrome (LARS) which could have important repercussion in patients' quality of life (Bregendahl et al., 2013). These symptoms often appear after temporary stoma closure, decrease after few months, and reach plateau within the first 2 years (Hallbook & Sjodahl, 2000). Quality of life and bowel function have been assessed in patients who have undergone restorative anterior resection as part of a multicentric study (Battersby et al., 2016) among 462 patients. Overall, 85% of patients reported a various degree of bowel-related quality of life impairment and over 40% considered that bowel dysfunction had a major effect on their quality of life at a median 5 years after surgery. Determinants for bowel-related quality of life (BQoL) impairment were preoperative radiotherapy and low tumor location; when both risks factors are present, 93% of patients have major BQoL impairment. These findings are important during preoperative discussion with patients and might help to manage long-term patients' expectations after surgery.

In a recent study from Denmark, 898 patients were assessed for quality of life after rectal cancer surgery (Feddern et al., 2019). Patients with tumor <10 cm from the anal verge had worse quality of life than patients with an end colostomy. Tumor location and preoperative radiation should be factored in when having preoperative discussions with patients centered on quality of life. Preoperative planning should educate the patients about risks of developing LARS, using the recently published POLARS (preoperative LARS) score (Battersby et al., 2018). POLARS score estimates patients' postoperative bowel function as it pertains to LARS. This can potentially help in individualizing care during preoperative patients' discussion and multidisciplinary meeting. Variables considered are age at diagnosis, gender, tumor height from anal verge, preoperative radiotherapy, surgical procedure such as partial meso-rectal excision or total meso-rectal excision, and presence of a temporary stoma. Patients at increased risk for LARS are young female undergoing preoperative radiotherapy followed by TME for a low rectal cancer and having a temporary stoma. LARS patients are divided into no LARS for score between 16 and 20, minor LARS for score between 20 and 30, and major LARS for score above 30 (4.9). The score can be calculated using the nomogram (**Fig. 4-11**), alternatively the online calculator may be used via https://www.pelicancancer.org/our-research/bowel-cancer-research/polars/. Predicting bowel function before rectal cancer treatment is important as it has been demonstrated that preoperative patients' education and counseling reduce the impact of symptoms and improve postoperative quality of life (Fink et al., 2013).

Surveillance
The goal for follow-up care for the patient with colon or rectal cancer is early detection of a cancer that has

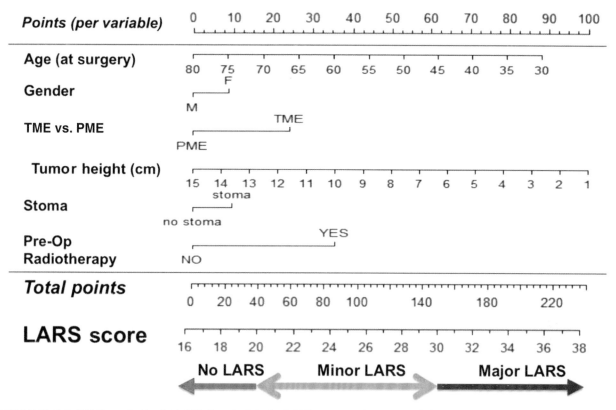

FIGURE 4-11. POLARS Score to Predict LARS. To calculate the LARS category draw a straight line down to find the patients predicted LARS value. The LARS categories are No LARS, score <20; minor LARS, 20 ≤ score < 30; and major LARS, score ≥30. PME, partial mesorectal excision; TME, total mesorectal excision; LARS, low anterior resection syndrome. (Used with permission from Battersby, N. J., Bouliotis, G., Emmertsen, K. J., et al.; UK and Danish LARS Study Groups. (2018). Development and external validation of a nomogram and online tool to predict bowel dysfunction following restorative rectal cancer resection: The POLARS score. *Gut, 67*(4), 688–696.)

returned. Treatment will depend upon the stage of the cancer and location of the cancer; see **Figures 4-4** and **4-5** for surveillance guidelines.

 CONCLUSIONS

CRC remains a very common diagnosis in the United States, and these patients are frequently managed with surgery as a component of a multidisciplinary approach. The majority of patients will have restoration of intestinal continuity; however, colostomies and ileostomies are often necessary for the reasons previously mentioned. Preoperative planning with site marking, patient counseling, precise operative technique, and postoperative patient follow-up and education are hallmarks of optimal outcomes.

REFERENCES

Allen, P. J., & Cott, D. G. (2002). The surgical management of metastatic melanoma. *Annals of Surgical Oncology, 9*(8), 762–770.

Amin, M. B., Edge, S. B., Greene, F. L., et al. (Eds.). (2017). *AJCC cancer staging manual* (8th ed.). New York, NY: Springer.

André, T., Boni, C., Navarro, M., et al. (2009). Improved overall survival with oxaliplatin, fluorouracil, and leucovorin as adjuvant treatment in stage II or III colon cancer in the MOSAIC trial. *Journal of Clinical Oncology, 27*, 3109–3116.

Arezzo, A., Migliore, M., Chiaro, P., et al. (2019). The REAL (Rectal anastomotic Leak) score for prediction of anastomotic leak after rectal cancer surgery. *Techniques in Coloproctology, 23*, 649–663.

Avital, S., Romaguera, R. L., Sands, L., et al. (2004) Primary malignant melanoma of the right colon. *The American Surgeon, 70*, 649–651.

Bailey, C. E., Hu, C. Y., You, Y. N., et al. (2014). Increasing disparities in the age-related incidences of colon and rectal cancers in the United States, 1975–2010. *JAMA Surgery*, 1–6.

Bal, D. G. (1992). Cancer in African Americans. *CA: A Cancer Journal for Clinicians, 42*, 5–6.

Battersby, N. J., Bouliotis, G., Emmertsen, K. J., et al.; UK and Danish LARS Study Groups. (2018). Development and external validation of a nomogram and online tool to predict bowel dysfunction following restorative rectal cancer resection: The POLARS score. *Gut, 67*(4), 688–696.

Battersby, N. J., Juul, T., Christensen, P., et al.; United Kingdom Low Anterior Resection Syndrome Study Group. (2016). Predicting the risk of bowel-related quality-of-life impairment after restorative resection for rectal cancer: A multicenter cross-sectional study. *Diseases of the Colon & Rectum, 59*(4), 270–280.

Baxter, N. N., & Garcia-Aguilar, J. (2007). Organ preservation for rectal cancer. *Journal of Clinical Oncology, 25*, 1014–1020.

Biagi, J. J., Raphael, M. J., Mackillop, W. J., et al. (2011). Association between time to initiation of adjuvant chemotherapy and survival in colorectal cancer: A systematic review and meta-analysis. *JAMA, 305*(22), 2335–2342.

Bibbins-Domingo, K. (2016). Aspirin use for the primary prevention of cardiovascular disease and colorectal cancer. U.S. Preventive services Task Force recommendation statement. *Annals of Internal Medicine, 64*, 836–845.

Bregendahl, S., Emmertsen, K. J., Lous, J., et al. (2013). Bowel dysfunction after low anterior resection with and without neoadjuvant therapy for rectal cancer: A population-based cross-sectional study. *Colorectal Disease*, 15(9), 1130–1139.

Cheng, L., Eng, C., Nieman, L. Z., et al. (2011). Trends in colorectal cancer incidence by anatomic site and disease stage in the United States from 1976 to 2005. *American Journal of Clinical Oncology*, 34(6), 573–580.

Colorectal Cancer Collaborative Group. (2001). Adjuvant radiotherapy for rectal cancer: A systematic overview of 8,507 patients from 22 randomized trials. *Lancet*, 358(9290), 1291–1304.

Conlin, A., Smith, G., Carey, F. A., et al. (2005) The prognostic significance of K-ras, p53 and APC mutations in colorectal carcinoma. *Gut*, 54(9), 1283–1286.

Deijen, C. L.,Vasmel, J. E., de Lange-de Klerk, E. S. M., et al. (2017). Ten-year outcomes of a randomised trial of laparoscopic versus open surgery for colon cancer. *Surgical Endoscopy*, 31, 2607–2615.

Dekker, E., Tanis, P. J., Vleugels, J. L. A., et al. (2019). Colorectal cancer. *Lancet*, 394(10207), 1467–1480.

Eaden, J. A., Abrams, K. R., & Mayberry, J. F. (2001). The risk of colorectal cancer in ulcerative colitis: A meta-analysis. *Gut*, 48(4), 526–535.

Emmertsen, K. J., Laurberg, S.; Rectal Cancer Function Study Group. (2013). Impact of bowel dysfunction on quality of life after sphincter preserving resection for rectal cancer. *British Journal of Surgery*, 100, 1377–1387.

Etzioni, D. A., Beart, R. W. Jr., Madoff, R. D., et al. (2009). Impact of the aging population on the demand for colorectal procedures. *Diseases of the Colon and Rectum, 52*, 583–590; discussion 590–591.

Feddern, M. L., Emmertsen, K. J., & Laurberg, S. (2019). Quality of life with or without sphincter preservation for rectal cancer. *Colorectal Disease*, 21(9), 1051–1057.

Fink, C., Diener, M. K., Bruckner, T., et al. (2013). Impact of preoperative patient education on prevention of postoperative complications after major visceral surgery: Study protocol for a randomized controlled trial (PEDUCAT trial). *Trials*, 14,271.

Fleshman, J., Branda, M. E., Sargent, D. J., et al. (2019). Disease-free survival and local recurrence for laparoscopic resection compared with open resection of stage II to III rectal cancer: Follow-up results of the ACOSOG Z6051 randomized controlled trial. *Annals of Surgery*, 269(4), 589–595.

Fleshman, J., Sargent, D. J., Green, E., et al. (2007). Laparoscopic colectomy for cancer is not inferior to open surgery based on 5-year data from the COST Study Group trial. *Annals of Surgery, 246*, 655–662.

Hajibandeh, S., Hajibandeh, S., Sarma, D. R., et al. (2019). Meta-analysis of temporary loop ileostomy closure during or after adjuvant chemotherapy following rectal cancer resection: The dilemma remains. *International Journal of Colorectal Disease*, 34(7), 1151–1159.

Hallbook, O., & Sjodahl, R. (2000). Surgical approaches to obtaining optimal bowel function. *Seminars in Surgical Oncology*, 18, 249–258.

Henrikson, N. B., Webber, E. M., Goddard, K. A., et al. (2015). Family history and the natural history of colorectal cancer: Systematic review. *Genetics in Medicine*, 17(9), 702–712.

Hewitson, P., Glasziou, P., & Watson, E. (2008). Cochrane systematic review of colorectal cancer screening using the fecal occult blood test (hemoccult): An update. *American Journal of Gastroenterology, 103*, 1541–1549.

Hol, J. C., van Oostendorp, S. E., Tuynman, J. B., et al. (2019). Long-term oncological results after transanal total mesorectal excision for rectal carcinoma. *Techniques in Coloproctology*, 23(9), 903–911.

Jayne, D. G., Guillou, P. J., Thorpe, H., et al. (2007). Randomized trial of laparoscopic-assisted resection of colorectal carcinoma: 3-year results of the UK MRC CLASICC Trial Group. *Journal of Clinical Oncology*, 25, 3061–3068.

Jayne, D. G., Thorpe, H. C., Copeland, J., et al. (2010). Five-year follow-up of the Medical Research Council CLASICC trial of laparoscopically assisted versus open surgery for colorectal cancer. *British Journal of Surgery*, 97(11), 1638–1645.

Johns, L. E., & Houlston, R. S. (2001). A systematic review and meta-analysis of familial colorectal cancer risk. *The American Journal of Gastroenterology, 96*(10), 2992–3003.

Kennedy, R. H., Francis, E. A., Wharton, R., et al. (2014). Multicenter randomized controlled trial of conventional versus laparoscopic surgery for colorectal cancer within an enhanced recovery programme: EnROL. *Journal of Clinical Oncology*, 32, 1804–1811.

Kingham, T. P., & DeMatteo, R. P. (2009). Multidisciplinary treatment of gastrointestinal stromal tumors. *Surgical Clinics of North America*, 89, 217–233.

Koch, P., del Valle, F., Berdel, W. E., et al. (2001). Primary gastrointestinal non-Hodgkin's lymphoma: I. Anatomic and histologic distribution, clinical features, and survival data of 371 patients registered in the German Multicenter Study GIT NHL 01/92. *Journal of Clinical Oncology*, 19(18), 3861–3873.

Kuebler, J. P., Wieand, H. S., O'Connell, M. J., et al. (2007). Oxaliplatin combined with weekly bolus fluorouracil and leucovorin as surgical adjuvant chemotherapy for stage II and III colon cancer: Results from NSABP C-07. *Journal of Clinical Oncology*, 25, 2198–2204.

Kulke, M. H., & Mayer, R. J. (1999). Carcinoid tumours. *New England Journal of Medicine, 340*, 858–868.

Larsen, S. G., Pfeffer, F., Kørner, H.; Norwegian Colorectal Cancer Group. (2019). Norwegian moratorium on transanal total mesorectal excision. *British Journal of Surgery*, 106(9), 1120–1121.

Miliaras, S., Ziogas, I. A., Mylonas, K. S., et al. (2018). Primary malignant melanoma of the ascending colon. *Case Reports, 2018*, bcr-2017-223282.

Mirnezami, A., Mirnezami, R., Chandrakumaran, K. et al. (2011). Increased local recurrence and reduced survival from colorectal cancer following anastomotic leak: Systematic review and meta-analysis. *Annals of Surgery*, 259, 930–938.

National Cancer Institute. (2019). Surveillance, epidemiology, and end results program; SEER Stat Fact Sheets: Colon and rectum cancer. Retrieved from http://seer.cancer.gov/statfacts/html/colorect.html

National Comprehensive Cancer Network, Version 2.2019. (2019). Clinical practice guidelines in oncology: Colorectal cancer screening. Retrieved November 21, 2019, from https://www.nccn.org/professionals/physician_gls/pdf/colorectal_screening.pdf

National Comprehensive cancer Network, Version 4.2019. (November 9, 2019). Clinical practice guidelines in oncology: Colon cancer. Retrieved from https://www.nccn.org/professionals/physician_gls/pdf/colon.pdf

Oliphant, R., Czerniewski, A., Robertson, I., et al. (2015). The effect of adjuvant chemotherapy on stoma-related complications after surgery for colorectal cancer: A retrospective analysis. *Journal of Wound, Ostomy, and Continence Nursing*, 42(5), 494–498.

Quayle, F. J., & Lowney, J. K. (2006). Colorectal lymphoma. *Clinics in Colon and Rectal Surgery*, 19, 49–53.

Quirke, P., Dixon, M. F., Dundey, P., et al. (1986). Local recurrence of rectal adenocarcinoma due to inadequate surgical resection: Histopathologic study of lateral tumor spread and surgical excision. *Lancet, 2*, 996–998.

Rengtgen, D. S., Thompson, W., Garbutt, J., et al. (1984). Radiologic, endoscopic and surgical considerations of melanoma metastatic to the GI tract. *Surgery, 95*, 635–639.

Richards, C. H., Campbell, V., Ho, C., et al. (2012). Smoking is a major risk factor for anastomotic leak in patients undergoing low anterior resection. *Colorectal Disease*, 14(5), 628–633.

Salvadalena, G., Hendren, S., McKenna, L., et al. (2015). WOCN Society and ASCRS position statement on preoperative stoma site marking for patients undergoing colostomy or ileostomy surgery. *Journal of Wound Ostomy & Continence Nursing*, 42(3), 249–252.

Song, M., Garrett, W. S., & Chan, A. T. (2015). Nutrients, foods, and colorectal cancer prevention. *Gastroenterology*, 148(6), 1244–1260.

Stevenson, A. R., Solomon, M. J., Lumley, J. W., et al. (2015). Effect of laparoscopic-assisted resection vs open resection on pathological outcomes in rectal cancer: The ALaCaRT randomized clinical trial. *JAMA, 314*, 1356–1363.

Sylla, P., Rattner, D. W., Delgado, S., et al. (2010). NOTES Transanal rectal cancer resection using transanal endoscopic microsurgery and laparoscopic assistance. *Surgical Endoscopy, 24*, 1205–1210.

Tryggvason, G., Gisalason, H. G., Magnusson, M. K., et al. (2005). Gastrointestinal stromal tumors in Iceland, 1990–2003: The Icelandic GIST study, a population based incidence and pathologic risk stratification study. *International Journal of Cancer, 117*, 289–293.

Van der Pas, M. H., Haglind, E., Cuesta, M. A., et al.; COlorectal cancer laparoscopic or open resection II (COLOR II) Study Group. (2013). Laparoscopic versus open surgery for rectal cancer (COLOR II): Short-term outcomes of a randomised, phase 3 trial. *The Lancet Oncology, 14*(3), 210–218.

Yeh, C., Chen, H., Tang, R., et al. (2000). Surgical outcome after surgical resection of rectal leiomyosarcoma. *Diseases of the Colon and Rectum, 43*, 1517–1521.

Zorzi, M., Fedeli, U., Schievano, E., et al. (2015) Impact on colorectal cancer mortality of screening programmes based on the faecal immunochemical test. *Gut, 64*, 784–790.

QUESTIONS

1. Which intervention by a WOC nurse is directed at reducing a nonmodifiable risk factor for colorectal cancer development?
   A. Planning a diet for the patient that is high in fiber
   B. Instructing the patient to eat foods that are low in fat
   C. Investigating a family history of polyps
   D. Developing an exercise plan for the patient

2. The WOC nurse is providing teaching to a patient diagnosed with familial adenomatous polyposis (FAP). What information accurately describes this condition?
   A. FAP is inherited in an autosomal dominant pattern with a 100% risk of developing colon cancer by age 40 years.
   B. It is recommended that individuals with FAP undergo segmental resection rather than total colectomy or proctocolectomy for treatment.
   C. FAP is inherited by mutations in one of several mismatch repair genes leading to microsatellite instability.
   D. People with FAP are at risk for extracolonic cancers such as endometrial, ovarian, stomach, small bowel, and bladder.

3. A 55-year-old patient visits a gastroenterologist with complaints of anal bleeding upon defecation. Which test would most likely be ordered for this patient to perform diagnostic biopsies and/or therapeutic procedures?
   A. FOBT
   B. Sigmoidoscopy or colonoscopy
   C. CT colonography
   D. Virtual colonoscopy

4. Which symptom is *not* characteristic of colorectal cancer?
   A. Nonspecific abdominal pain
   B. Weight loss
   C. Fatigue
   D. Increased stool caliber

5. A patient is diagnosed with colon cancer manifested by a tumor that invades to the submucosa. What stage of cancer would be documented?
   A. Stage 0
   B. Stage I
   C. Stage II
   D. Stage III

6. A patient with a TNM stage IVa rectal cancer would need to meet which diagnostic requirement for this staging?
   A. Tumor invading surface of visceral peritoneum
   B. Metastasis to one to three regional lymph nodes
   C. Distant metastasis confined to one organ or site
   D. Distant metastases in more than one organ/site or the peritoneum

7. A patient undergoing a colonoscopy is diagnosed with nonmetastatic, obstructing colon cancer that is resectable. What is the recommended treatment for this patient?
   A. Diversion followed by colectomy with en bloc removal of lymph nodes
   B. Colectomy with en bloc removal of lymph nodes +/– diversion
   C. Adjuvant therapy alone
   D. Diversion with adjuvant therapy

8. A patient diagnosed with colon cancer is scheduled for synchronous colon cancer and lung/liver resection. This treatment is recommended for which type of colon cancer?
   A. Polyp identified with invasive cancer
   B. Nonmetastatic colon cancer that is resectable/obstructing
   C. Nonmetastatic colon cancer that is resectable/nonobstructing
   D. Metastatic colon cancer with resectable lung/liver metastases

9. A patient who is diagnosed with rectal cancer by endoscopy presents with the following findings: T1, N0 with favorable features. A transanal excision shows T1/negative margins. What is the recommended treatment for this patient?
   A. Observation
   B. Chemoradiation alone
   C. Chemoradiation and resection if possible
   D. Synchronous or staged resection of rectal lesion and metastases

10. A patient is diagnosed with a very low rectal cancer. For what type of resection would the WOC nurse prepare the patient?
   A. Low anterior resection
   B. Abdominoperineal resection
   C. Segmental colectomy
   D. Total mesorectal excision

ANSWERS AND RATIONALES

1. C. Rationale: While other risk factors such as dietary (reduction of red meats and low fiber) and exercise and weight loss are modifiable (dietary consultation, initiation of an exercise program), the risk factor of a family history is not modifiable and an important assessment that should be considered in a patient work up for risk of colorectal cancer development. Positive family history plays an important role in 10% to 20% of all patients with colorectal cancer.

2. A. Rationale: FAP is inherited in an autosomal dominant pattern with a 100% risk of developing colon cancer by age 40 years. Individuals with FAP should undergo total colectomy or proctocolectomy for treatment and risk reduction rather than segmental resection alone. There is a high risk of recurrence in the rectum if proctectomy is not performed.

3. B. Rationale: Initial evaluation includes endoscopy if not previously performed, to assess if a tumor is present and to determine tumor location and obtain biopsies to confirm suspected diagnosis of CRC. Endoscopic tests, especially colonoscopy, have high sensitivity and specificity.

4. D. Rationale: Nonspecific abdominal pain, weight loss, and fatigue maybe presenting symptoms for the patient with suspected colorectal cancer. However, the stool caliber maybe *reduced* in the patient presenting with CRC because the tumor may decrease the lumen of the colon, presenting a partial obstruction or narrower channel.

5. B. Rationale: The tumor has grown into the submucosa, which is the layer of tissue underneath the mucosa or lining of the colon making this a Stage I cancer.

6. C. Rationale: Stage IVa describes distant metastasis that has spread to one other body location. The "a" after Stage IV means one other body part, stage IV that the cancer has spread.

7. A. Rationale: A fecal diversion should be done to divert the stool from the obstruction, followed by a colectomy (removal of the area with the colon cancer) and removal of lymph nodes. The tumor can then be staged and treatment prescribed.

8. D. Rationale: The most common site of metastases for colon or rectal cancer is the liver. Colorectal cancer may also spread to the lungs, bones, brain, or spinal cord. Options for treatment may include surgery, chemo or radiation therapy, and/or immunotherapy.

9. A. Rationale: The treatment was the excision of the tumor, a full-thickness excision through the anus. Since there was no extension of the disease and the tumor only invaded the submucosa observation with surveillance (see Figure 4-5) would be the treatment plan.

10. B. Rationale: A low rectal cancer may involve the sphincter or there may be an inability to obtain a clear distal margin necessitating an abdominal perineal resection (removal of the rectum).

CHAPTER 5

MEDICAL MANAGEMENT OF CROHN'S DISEASE AND ULCERATIVE COLITIS

Russell Cohen and Adam C. Stein

OBJECTIVES

1. Understand the epidemiology and differential diagnosis of Crohn's disease and ulcerative colitis.

2. Describe the modern medical treatment of Crohn's disease and ulcerative colitis.

3. Identify important supportive measurements and the role of diet in patients with Crohn's disease and ulcerative colitis.

TOPIC OUTLINE

- Introduction **60**
- Etiology **60**
- Presentation **60**
   - Epidemiology 60
   - Overview and Differential Diagnosis 61
   - Ulcerative Colitis 61
   - Crohn's Disease 62
- Medical Management **63**
   - Ulcerative Colitis 63
      - Mild to Moderate Disease 63
      - Moderate to Severe Disease 64
   - Crohn's Disease 64
      - Fistulizing Disease 64
      - Strictures 65

- Extraintestinal Manifestations **65**
- Cancer Risk **65**
- Diet in IBD **65**
- Nutrition in IBD **65**
   - Protein and Caloric Malnutrition 66
   - Micronutrient Deficiencies 66
   - Wound Healing 66
   - Supportive Care 66
- Conclusions **66**

INTRODUCTION

Crohn's disease (CD) and ulcerative colitis (UC) are chronic inflammatory bowel diseases (IBD) characterized by relapsing and remitting inflammation in the gastrointestinal (GI) tract. Clinical presentation typically mirrors the location and severity of disease, which can range from bloody, loose stools due to rectal inflammation to obstructive-type symptoms caused by stricturing in the small bowel. The underlying etiology of these disorders remains elusive, and as such, traditional treatments such as steroids target the inflammatory cascade rather than the actual disease process. These treatments often fail to control the disease, leading to surgery and consequences of bowel resection including the chance of having a permanent ostomy. Recent advances in medical therapy, along with a paradigm shift in treatment goals, have led to glimpses of improved outcomes and potentially decreasing surgical rates (Bouguen et al., 2015; Laharie et al., 2013). This section focuses on the presentation and medical management of IBD, and the following Chapter 6 discusses surgical management.

 ETIOLOGY

Accounts of IBD in the scientific literature date back to the 17th century, yet it was not until 1932 that a cohort of patients with "regional enteritis" was rigorously characterized and published in the medical literature, a disease later named Crohn's disease after the first author of the paper (Crohn et al., 1932). Efforts since have characterized many different clinical presentations of IBD, grouped into the two major types of IBD, CD and UC. Despite careful phenotypic characterization and rigorous scientific research, the mechanisms leading to disease onset and progression remain largely unknown.

Leading concepts regarding the pathogenesis of both CD and UC involve a multifactorial process where genetically predisposed individuals have a dysregulated, inappropriate immune response to one or more of a variety of environmental insults, leading to bowel inflammation (Knights et al., 2013). Multiple genes have been identified in various populations with IBD; the best studied has been the *Nod-2* gene, which is important in immune-mediated events, such as stimulation of the release of inflammatory cell signals (cytokines), the creation of proteins directed against microorganisms, as well as intracellular trafficking and killing of intracellular microbes (Abraham & Cho, 2006). Postulated environmental factors include but are not limited to infection, antibiotic use, tobacco use, tobacco cessation, and overall hygiene (Berg et al., 2013). Evidence suggests that environmental insults lead to alterations in the GI microbiota, which play a role in triggering or furthering this aberrant immune response (Kostic et al., 2014). As a result, virtually all of the prior and current therapies target the immune system, inflammatory cascade, and/or the microbes themselves.

Overall, however, the etiology remains a mystery. This impacts therapeutic approaches, as it is not clear what target(s) are the ultimate causes of disease in most patients. As a result, therapies to date have focused on curbing the immune system, rather than eliminating or arresting the actual cause of disease. Currently, no medical therapy has been found to be definitively disease modifying to the point of creating a reliable, long-term, disease-free state. Medications instead target the inflammatory cascade, which mechanistically is well characterized. Newer classes of drugs utilize antibodies targeted to biological targets such as proteins or cellular receptors. These have proven to be effective, yet less than half of patients achieved a disease-free state, and long-term safety and efficacy data are limited for the newest therapies (Allen & Peyrin-Biroulet, 2013).

 PRESENTATION

EPIDEMIOLOGY

Once thought to be a disease of the "westernized" nations, IBD is now considered to be a worldwide disease, with patients increasingly diagnosed in developing countries that are becoming more industrialized (Duricova et al., 2014). This highlights the role of environmental influences on the development of IBD, including the hygiene hypothesis. Nonetheless, the highest annual incidence rates continue to be seen in Europe, North America, and Australia. The incidence is continuing to rise throughout the world, regardless of industrialization. In the United States, the incidence of UC and CD has been reported to be 8.8 and 7.9 per 100,000; the prevalence was 214 and 174 per 100,000 (figures are adjusted using data from Olmstead County, Minnesota) (Shivashankar et al., 2017). The highest annual incidence rates in the world have been reported for UC as 24.3 per 100,000 (Iceland) and for CD as 29.3 per 100,000 (Australia) (Duricova et al., 2014). While patients can present at any age, both for CD and UC, the vast majority will present within the second to fourth decades of life (Duricova et al., 2014). For unknown reasons, patients with CD on average tend to be diagnosed earlier than do those with UC. A "second peak" of new UC cases in the fifth and sixth decades has been reported in many series and is attributed to individuals who have stopped smoking cigarettes (Regueiro et al., 2005). In fact, smoking seems to "protect against" developing UC; unfortunately, it is strongly linked to CD (especially aggressive disease) (Nunes et al., 2013). As these are chronic conditions that often require hospitalization and even surgery, these diseases especially at a young age can lead to significant emotional and financial burden.

KEY POINT

Smokers with Crohn's disease are more refractory to medical treatment, as are ex-smokers who develop ulcerative colitis.

OVERVIEW AND DIFFERENTIAL DIAGNOSIS

CD and UC are chronic, relapsing, and remitting diseases, with periods of time without significant symptoms, called "remission," and times where they have symptoms of inflammation, called "active disease" or "flaring." Clinical presentations can vary widely and for the most part are dependent on the pathophysiologic inflammatory process, including the severity and histologic depth of inflammation as well as the location of disease (**Table 5-1**). Patients may often exhibit signs and symptoms for years prior to diagnosis; many patients ignore or overlook symptoms until they interfere with their life or persist without resolution.

An initial step in patients who present with diarrhea, hematochezia (bloody stools), or other similar symptoms is to first rule out an infectious cause. Adequate patient history should be taken and stools tested for *Clostridium difficile* (*C. difficile*), other bacterial agents, *Giardia*, other parasites, and pathogens specific to the location or setting that the patient presents or visited.

It is important to differentiate IBD from other diseases and disorders of the GI tract. Symptoms of either UC or CD often overlap with other etiologies, including other inflammatory conditions such as celiac disease or autoimmune enteritis as well as noninflammatory or functional disorders such as irritable bowel syndrome ("IBS"). Symptoms of functional bowel disorders can be difficult to distinguish from those related to IBD, yet treatments differ substantially between the two. Additionally, functional bowel disorders are often present in patients with

IBD, and distinguishing the etiology of symptoms will prevent overaggressive treatment of inflammation that may not be present. Workup including imaging, stool studies assessing inflammation (fecal calprotectin or fecal leukocytes), and/or endoscopic assessment can help define causality and guide further evaluation.

Patients who are already diagnosed with IBD that subsequently present with active inflammatory symptoms should prompt workup into the trigger of their symptoms. Concurrent infection may worsen inflammation and prevent traditional treatments from optimally working. Patients should be assessed for more common enteric infections such as *C. difficile*, *Giardia*, and *Cytomegalovirus* (*CMV*) and promptly treated if these are found. Many patients may flare due to noncompliance with their treatment regimens or major stressors (i.e., death, divorce, employment change, etc.).

> **KEY POINT**
>
> The clinical distinction between ulcerative colitis and Crohn's disease is vital, since the type of inflammatory bowel disease will direct the therapeutic approach.

ULCERATIVE COLITIS

Inflammation in UC follows a characteristic pattern: the rectum is always involved, and it extends proximally to include part or all of the colon. Classically, the pattern of inflammation is broken down into three major categories: (1) proctitis (involving only the rectum), (2) left-sided colitis (involving the area of the colon distal to the splenic flexure, or 60 cm as measured from the anal verge on colonoscopy), and (3) extensive colitis (involving the colon proximal to the splenic flexure as well as the areas distal). Within this last category, the term "pancolitis" refers to the entire colon being involved. The additional category "proctosigmoiditis" is also used in some settings to describe disease involving the rectum and sigmoid colon (**Table 5-2**).

The pattern of inflammation is continuous and circumferential, which often differentiates UC from the often patchy and discontinuous inflammation seen in CD. Histologically, inflammation is limited to the superficial mucosal lining of the bowel but does not extend deeper into the submucosa, muscularis, or serosal surface of the colon (**Table 5-1**). Symptoms consist of frequent, bloody stools associated with urgency to defecate, sometimes waking patients up from sleep to have a bowel movement. There may or may not be abdominal cramping, particularly around times of bowel movements. Otherwise, constant abdominal pain is not commonly seen because inflammation is limited to the mucosa lining where there is little nervous innervation. As the severity increases, patients may have fevers, night sweats,

TABLE 5-1	DISTINGUISHING FEATURES OF ULCERATIVE COLITIS COMPARED TO CROHN'S DISEASE	
	ULCERATIVE COLITIS	**CROHN'S DISEASE**
Location	Colon only	Anywhere in the GI tract
Endoscopic appearance	Continuous	Patchy; skip areas
Mucosal penetration	Superficial	Full thickness
Histological inflammation	Continuous	Patchy
Granulomas	No	Yes
Extraintestinal manifestations	Yes	Yes
Fistulas	No	Yes
Perianal disease	No	Yes
Strictures	No	Yes
Smoking association	Nonsmokers or ex-smokers	Commonly smokers
Bleeding	Yes	Yes
Pain	Minimal (crampy)	Yes

TABLE 5-2 MAJOR CLASSIFICATIONS OF ULCERATIVE COLITIS

DISEASE TYPE	DISEASE LOCATION	DISTANCE MEASURED FROM ANAL VERGE
Proctitis	Rectum only	20 cm
Proctosigmoiditis	Rectum and sigmoid colon	~35–40 cm
Left-sided ulcerative colitis	From rectum extending up to the splenic flexure	60 cm
Extensive ulcerative colitis	From rectum extending beyond the splenic flexure	>60 cm
Pancolitis	Entire colon	Entire colon

weight loss, and fatigue. Additionally, patients may have other symptoms outside of the colon; these extraintestinal manifestations include the joints (arthritis), skin (erythema nodosum, pyoderma gangrenosum), and eyes (iritis, uveitis, episcleritis).

Patients suspected of having UC typically undergo assessment of their colon via colonoscopy or flexible sigmoidoscopy. There is a characteristic inflammatory pattern on endoscopy, with inflammation starting in the rectum and extending proximally in a circumferential, continuous pattern. Inflammation may be limited to the rectum or extend the entire length of the colon. In rare cases, inflammation may continue into the last portion of the small bowel, the terminal ileum, but characteristically, the small bowel is not affected. Histologically, only the superficial layer of the colon, the mucosa, is involved.

KEY POINT

The person with ulcerative colitis will present with chronic persistent or intermittent diarrhea and/or rectal bleeding. The inflammation usually spares the small bowel, except in severe extensive disease when the terminal ileum may display inflammation called backwash ileitis.

CROHN'S DISEASE

CD differs from UC in that inflammation may occur anywhere within the GI tract, from the mouth to the anus, and may be continuous or patchy, and symptoms are based on the area or areas of involvement. The most commonly affected area is the terminal ileum, and many of those patients have cecal and/or right colonic involvement as well. About 20% of patients have disease limited to the colon, and 5% have involvement of the mouth, esophagus, stomach, or upper small bowel. Symptoms of patients with distal colonic involvement, including the rectum and sigmoid, often include bloody, frequent

stools, similar to UC. Isolated small bowel involvement usually presents as abdominal pain, loose but less frequent stools usually with minimal or no blood, and weight loss. Inflammation in the small bowel can lead to narrowing and even obstruction, and patients can present with obstructive symptoms. Upper GI involvement is variable, presenting as painful oral ulcerations, dysphagia, odynophagia, or upper abdominal pain. Regardless of location, patients may have weight loss and sometimes require parenteral nutrition (PN) depending on the severity of malnutrition and treatment plan.

CD differs also from UC in that inflammation can extend beyond the mucosal layer, penetrating deep into the submucosa, even extending the full thickness of the bowel wall. As inflammation progresses deep into the bowel, fluid collections outside of the bowel can form, known as abscesses. Additionally, inappropriate connections between the bowel and other organs, called fistulas, may form. Fistulas can occur between the bowel and adjacent organs, including other parts of the bowel, the bladder, the vagina, and the skin. When this involves the rectum or anal canal, characteristic abscess formation and even drainage can occur in the perianal area, commonly referred to as the phenotypic CD with perianal disease.

Ongoing deep bowel inflammation in CD can also lead to scar formation, causing narrowing, or stricturing of the bowel. This mostly occurs in the small bowel. Over time, strictures can lead to blockages, and surgery is required for treatment.

CD, like UC, can have extraintestinal manifestations. These are similar in nature to UC and often parallel underlying bowel inflammation. This is discussed later in the chapter.

Workup of CD should focus on characterizing the location and extent of inflammation, as well as fistulizing or perianal disease. This usually requires both endoscopic and radiologic assessments. The colon and terminal ileum are usually assessed by colonoscopy, which allows not only for assessment of disease activity but also for biopsy. The small bowel can be assessed either radiologically or endoscopically depending on the resources available. Classically, dynamic barium studies under x-ray were utilized; however, now, both computerized tomography (CT) and magnetic resonance (MR) enterography can be used to get detailed images of the small bowel and also evaluate for fistulas or perianal disease. Recent advances in endoscopy now allow imaging of the small bowel via either video capsule endoscopy (VCE) or deep enteroscopy. For VCE, the patient swallows a camera, the shape and size of a large pill, which takes several thousand pictures over a period of time and transmits them for viewing. A number of different techniques for deep enteroscopy allow for endoscopic assessment of the small bowel, with capability of visualization of the entire small bowel around 50% of the time.

The danger of VCE in CD is capsule retention at an area of stricturing, which may require deep enteroscopy or surgery to remove (Collins, 2016).

 MEDICAL MANAGEMENT

Management of IBD is unique in that most patients are diagnosed at an early age and are otherwise healthy, yet despite medical therapy, many will require surgery at some point during their lifetime. Additionally, many of the medications, while for the most part are safe and well tolerated, have potential serious complications. As such, the decision regarding treatment, either medical or surgical, needs to be done in partnership with the patient.

In principle, management for all patients with IBD is based on location of inflammation as well as disease severity. The basic tenets of treatment for UC and CD are the same: get patients well ("induction") and keep them well ("maintenance"). Medications used for induction therapy often overlap with maintenance therapy, with some notable exceptions. Fortunately, the armamentarium of medical options for both UC and CD has substantially increased over the past several years (**Table 5-3**). Now, more than ever, patients have several reasonably effective medications to choose from. This is paramount as patients often lose response or fail to respond to medications; having alternate medications can often prevent surgery or needing to be on more toxic, induction-only medications as maintenance therapy. Additionally, based on disease severity, consideration for early, aggressive treatment that may potentially be disease modifying must be weighed against the more traditional approach of adding systemically acting medications as less potent medications fail to control inflammation.

Disease severity dictates not only treatment options but also if treatment can safely be provided at home or if hospitalization is required. This decision is primarily based on symptomatic severity, need for expedited workup, urgent surgical consultation, and ability to meet nutritional and hydration needs.

ULCERATIVE COLITIS

Mild to Moderate Disease

Both induction and maintenance involve medications that act directly on the colonic mucosa with limited systemic absorption, including 5-aminosalicylic acid (5-ASA) and topical steroids such as budesonide and hydrocortisone (Marshall & Irvine, 1995; Marshall et al., 2010, 2012; Ruddell et al., 1980). Systemically acting medications such as prednisone are usually not needed but may be reserved for induction therapy only. The route of medication depends on the extent of inflammation as well as patient preference. Disease limited to the rectum responds well to topical therapy delivered per rectum, while disease extending beyond the distal sigmoid colon will respond to oral medication plus rectal topical therapy. Topical therapy includes hydrocortisone, budesonide, and 5-ASA and can be delivered via suppository, foam, or enema. Typically, patients with active rectal inflammation may have difficulty initially retaining rectal therapy, so they are often started on topical budesonide or hydrocortisone foam or enema twice a day as a fast-acting agent, with transition to 5-ASA therapy with improvement in inflammatory symptoms as well as ability to retain medication. As the extent of disease moves further into the colon, the addition of oral therapy is warranted. Oral therapy options include 5-ASA, sulfasalazine, and extended-release budesonide (Cohen et al., 2000; Rubin et al., 2017; Travis et al., 2014). If using 5-ASA, combination of oral and topical rectal therapy is superior to oral therapy alone; however, patient preference can often dictate if rectal therapy is given (Safdi et al., 1997). Sulfasalazine, 5-ASA, and extended-release budesonide may be given as oral therapy alone.

TABLE 5-3 MEDICATIONS COMMONLY USED IN ULCERATIVE COLITIS AND CROHN'S DISEASE		
MEDICATION CLASS	**ULCERATIVE COLITIS**	**CROHN'S DISEASE**
Aminosalicylate	Balsalazide, mesalamine, olsalazine, sulfasalazine	Balsalazide, mesalamine, olsalazine, sulfasalazine
Traditional corticosteroids	Hydrocortisone, prednisolone, prednisone	Hydrocortisone, prednisolone, prednisone
Corticosteroids with minimal systemic impact	Budesonide	Budesonide
Immunosuppressants	Azathioprine, 6-mercaptopurine, cyclosporine, tacrolimus	Azathioprine, 6-mercaptopurine, methotrexate
Anti-TNF	Adalimumab, infliximab, golimumab	Adalimumab, certolizumab, infliximab
Antiadhesion molecule	Vedolizumab	Natalizumab, vedolizumab
Anti-IL12/23	Ustekinumab	Ustekinumab
Janus kinase inhibitor	Tofacitinib	—

Anti-TNF, anti–tumor necrosis factor antibodies; Anti-IL 12/23, anti-interleukin 12/23 antibodies.

Moderate to Severe Disease

With increasing disease burden, systemic therapy is required. New treatment paradigms have positioned the biological therapies earlier in management, with the goal of limiting or even eliminating corticosteroids from the algorithm (Cohen & Stein, 2019; Dassopoulos et al., 2015; Rubin et al., 2019). For sick patients who require an immediate therapeutic intervention, corticosteroids are often initially started, either oral or intravenous (IV); IV therapy is typically reserved for patients who are failing oral steroids or require hospitalization. Glucocorticoids have several short- and long-term side effects and should only be given for a limited period of time. As such, a treatment strategy allowing successful tapering of steroids is necessary and should be implemented as early as possible. Multiple non–steroid-containing medical options are available as induction therapy: anti–tumor necrosis factor (anti-TNF) antibodies including infliximab (Rutgeerts et al., 2005), adalimumab (Sandborn et al., 2012), and golimumab (Sandborn et al., 2014); anti-integrin antibodies (vedolizumab) (Feagan et al., 2013); anti-IL 12/23 antibodies (ustekinumab) (Sands et al., 2019), as well as the very potent calcineurin inhibitors cyclosporine (Lichtiger et al., 1994) and tacrolimus (Ogata et al., 2006).

Anti-TNFs, vedolizumab, and ustekinumab carry the benefit of being effective for both induction and maintenance of remission. Cyclosporine and tacrolimus are only used as an induction agent, and a separate strategy is required for maintenance. If symptoms persist despite maximal medical therapy including steroids, or steroids are unable to be weaned, surgery should be considered. With symptomatic improvement, maintenance strategies beyond anti-TNF or vedolizumab include the immunomodulators azathioprine (AZA) (Jewell & Truelove, 1974) and 6-mercaptopurine (6MP) (George et al., 1996) as well as 5-ASA (Miner et al., 1995). Of note, immunomodulators are often added to anti-TNF or anti-integrin therapy, as evidence suggests that the combination of a monoclonal antibody and an immunomodulator is more efficacious than is either medication alone (Panaccione et al., 2014).

Tofacitinib is the first of potentially many oral small molecule agents that has shown efficacy in the treatment of UC. Working through the inhibition of the janus kinase (i.e., "JAK") pathway, tofacitinib has proven efficacy in the induction and maintenance of remission in patients with UC (Sandborn et al., 2017), although safety concerns over potentially higher risk of venous thromboses have currently delegated this agent to be used only after failure or intolerance of an anti-TNF agent with specific caution in people 50 years or older with at least one cardiovascular risk factor (Sandborn et al., 2019). While the clinical trials for tofacitinib in CD were disappointing, other experimental JAK inhibitors are under study for both UC and Crohn's.

CROHN'S DISEASE

In general, most treatment options for CD are in line with that of UC. The role of sulfasalazine and 5-ASA is limited to mild disease. The immunomodulator methotrexate has been proven effective in CD (Feagan et al., 2000), and it is an important part of the treatment regimen. The current anti-TNF agents approved by the FDA for use in CD are infliximab (Hanauer et al., 2002; Rutgeerts et al., 1999; Targan et al., 1997), adalimumab (Colombel et al., 2007; Hanauer et al., 2006; Sandborn et al., 2007), and certolizumab (Schreiber et al., 2007). In the anti-integrin antibody category, both vedolizumab (Sandborn et al., 2013) and natalizumab (Targan et al., 2007) are effective in CD. Ustekinumab is the first approved agent in the IL12/23 pathway that has shown efficacy in the induction and maintenance or remission in CD (Feagan et al., 2016).

The addition of the immunomodulators azathioprine or 6-mercaptopurine to anti-TNF agents has shown superior efficacy and decreased antidrug antibody levels (Colombel et al., 2010; Lichtenstein et al., 2018). The role of the cyclosporine and tacrolimus are less clear, as studies did not show as promising results as in UC. Due to the full-thickness and penetrating characteristics of CD, there are some other notable differences in treatment than for UC, which are discussed in detail below. Recent treatment guidelines have been updated to reflect these changes (Lichtenstein et al., 2018).

Unlike UC, in which surgical intervention typically removes the entire colon and rectum, CD surgery often only removes the affected area, and the disease returns at the site of resection unless effective medications are started (or restarted) after surgery to prophylaxis against recurrence (Rutgeerts et al., 1990).

KEY POINT

Patients undergoing biologic therapy must be tested for tuberculosis because the drugs can increase the risk of reactivating TB for those who have been exposed. Similarly, testing for hepatitis B is required due to potential worsening of disease upon exposure to the anti-TNF agents.

Fistulizing Disease

Medical options for fistulizing disease are limited, and surgery is often required for drainage of abscesses or removal of the fistulous tract. The treatment approach is dictated by the location of the fistulas and the presence of infection. For patients with perianal disease, it is important to assess for the presence of an abscess. If there is concern for abscess, antibiotics with coverage of enteric flora (typically ciprofloxacin [side effect tendonitis, Achilles tendon rupture] and metronidazole) should be initiated with surgical drainage and set on placement to prevent recurrence (Van Assche et al., 2010). Additionally, systemic anti-inflammatory medication should be initiated after active infection is treated. Thiopurines and the anti-TNFs infliximab (Present et al., 1999; Sands et al., 2004) and adalimumab have the most supporting evidence for efficacy in fistulizing disease (Van Assche et al., 2010).

For perianal fistulas without abscess, or fistulas outside the perianal area without associated infection, anti-inflammatory treatment with thiopurines or anti-TNFs should be utilized. Consideration should be placed on bowel rest with parenteral nutritional support to limit flow through the fistula. Surgical treatment should be considered if medical therapy fails or complex fistulizing disease is present. For management of enterocutaneous fistulas, see Chapter 18.

Strictures

Prolonged inflammation can lead to scarring and over time luminal narrowing. This may lead to obstructive-type symptoms, which, depending on the location of the narrowing and grade of obstruction, can present as abdominal pain, distention, nausea, and vomiting. Treatment depends on the grade of obstruction, with complete obstruction often requiring prompt surgical resection, and lower-grade obstructions with carefully observed conservative nonoperative management in the hospital setting. There should be evaluation for an inflammatory component; inflammation in the area of a prior stricture may lead to worsening luminal narrowing causing symptoms. In this situation, treating inflammation can lead to symptomatic improvement, as can the implementation of antibiotics (classically ciprofloxacin or metronidazole) to decrease bacterial overgrowth, as well as other possible functions. Ultimately, surgery is usually needed to remove the narrowed area or areas.

 ## EXTRAINTESTINAL MANIFESTATIONS

Patients with UC or CD can develop inflammatory-type involvement of areas outside of the GI tract (Vegh et al., 2014). These extraintestinal manifestations can involve a number of different areas, including joints, skin, eyes, and the liver. For the most part, these extraintestinal manifestations parallel the course of intestinal inflammation; patients with active extraintestinal manifestations are likely to also have active bowel inflammation.

For wound, ostomy, and continence nurses, a less common but serious extraintestinal manifestation of the skin is pyoderma gangrenosum. This is an ulcerating, inflammatory disorder of the skin, characterized by the progression of a single papule or pustule on the skin that turns into painful ulcerated, purulent wounds. It often is precipitated by mild trauma, including peristomal appliance maintenance. Peristomal pyoderma gangrenosum can be difficult to manage and requires close follow-up with the patient to ensure progress.

Once recognized, the initial treatment for peristomal pyoderma gangrenosum is a combination of wound care and medical therapy. Topical or systemic corticosteroids are normally used as first line to help decrease inflammation. The challenge is to manage an open moist wound in the area where the pouch adhesive must make a seal. Hydrocolloid and foam dressings can be considered for use to cover the open areas and provide a dry surface for the pouch seal. If these measures fail to produce wound healing, the medical management is usually escalated by adding either an anti-TNF agent or a T-cell inhibitor (cyclosporine or tacrolimus) (see Chapter 16).

 ## CANCER RISK

In patients with IBD, chronic intestinal inflammation is one of the primary risk factors for the development of GI malignancy. Cancers as a result of chronic intestinal inflammation include colorectal cancer, small bowel adenocarcinoma, intestinal lymphoma, anal cancer, and cholangiocarcinoma (Alexrad et al., 2016). The risk and pathogenesis of inflammation-associated cancer has chiefly been described in colitis-associated colorectal cancer. In a meta-analysis, quantitative estimates of colorectal cancer risk in UC have been reported to be 2% after 10 years, 8% after 20 years, and 18% after 30 years of disease (Eaden et al., 2001).

 ## DIET IN IBD

The link between diet and IBD remains an area of relative speculation and uncertainty. Given the increased incidence of IBD in more socioeconomically developed populations, the environment likely has some role in the pathogenesis of inflammation. Speculation exists that a more "westernized" diet influences the development of IBD, perhaps by changing the gut microbiota, or the increased fat content; however, this has yet to be fully elucidated (Wu et al., 2013).

Mixed evidence suggests that dietary modification may provide some limited benefit to symptomatic improvement, especially in CD. However, there is a paucity of evidence regarding dietary manipulation as an effective treatment of IBD. This is not surprising given both the uncertain role in the etiology of IBD and the difficulty in rigorously controlling the day-to-day food and drink consumption needed to produce scientifically sound results. There is some evidence in the pediatric population that a severely restrictive elemental diet with or without PN leads to some improvement in CD; however, this remains controversial and not universally accepted (Sigall-Boneh et al., 2014; Zachos et al., 2007). Overall, there is a lack of evidence at this time to suggest dietary modification as first-line therapy for IBD, especially in the adult population.

 ## NUTRITION IN IBD

Malnutrition is common among patients with IBD, with manifestations based on severity and location of bowel inflammation. The most evident signs of malnutrition are loss of weight and muscle mass, and common symptoms include fatigue and decreased energy. Even in the absence of more obvious physical attributes of malnutrition, more subtle examination findings such as hair loss, rash, visual changes, and neuropathic-type symptoms such as numbness, tingling, and balance problems indicate the presence of micronutrient deficiencies. As such, nutritional assessments including measuring micronutrients should be performed periodically throughout the disease course, especially during periods of time with active disease. Abnormalities should be addressed promptly and interventions performed as appropriate. Specific recommendations for treatment are outside the scope of this chapter.

PROTEIN AND CALORIC MALNUTRITION

There are a multitude of factors that lead to deficiencies in protein and calories in patients with IBD. The overall state of inflammation leads to a hypermetabolic rate, which given abdominal symptoms is nearly impossible to match via dietary intake. This caloric deficit leads to weight loss, which in turn is exacerbated by protein loss in the stool from luminal inflammation along with decreased protein intake. Prolonged inflammation leads to loss of weight and muscle mass. In the pediatric and young adult population, this can lead to major consequences with decreased growth and development, delayed puberty, and decreased peak bone mass.

MICRONUTRIENT DEFICIENCIES

The source of most vitamins and minerals, at least in part, is dietary. Patients with IBD are at risk for deficiencies due to a multitude of potential processes, including decreased availability from poor oral intake and absorptive capacity, and losses coming from diarrhea and bleeding (Hwang et al., 2012). The specific types of deficiencies patients are at risk for depend on the nature and location of inflammation. Clinically, there are often subtle findings suggesting possible micronutrient deficiencies, with nonspecific skin changes and oral lesions that indicate a potential underlying problem (Kaminski & Drinane, 2014).

For the most part, vitamins and minerals are absorbed in the small bowel. Patients with CD who have either small bowel inflammation or small bowel resections are at risk for specific deficiencies based on involvement. At-risk patients should have levels routinely monitored and deficiencies repleted, and often taking a proactive approach of supplementation even prior to low levels is appropriate and encouraged. In CD, the most common location of inflammation and surgical resection is the terminal ileum, which is primarily responsible for vitamin B_{12} absorption.

Typically, patients at risk for vitamin B_{12} deficiency are given supplementation even prior to onset of deficiency. Aggressive repletion should be done if a deficiency is identified. Surgery to remove the terminal ileum often involves resecting the ileocecal valve and cecum. This can lead to loose stools even without inflammation due to rapid transit, bile salt wasting, or fat malabsorption. In this setting, deficiencies include fat-soluble vitamins and zinc. Repletion involves improvement in diarrhea by addressing the underlying cause and oral repletion. The use of bile acid sequestrants such as cholestyramine, colestipol, and colesevelam before meals can dramatically decrease diarrhea in many cases. Patients who have lost too much small bowel to surgery, disease, or both may end up with inadequate absorptive surface area and require PN.

While patients with UC do not have small bowel disease, they are still at risk for iron deficiency due to blood loss and other vitamin/mineral deficiencies from decreased nutritional intake.

WOUND HEALING

A common belief is that malnutrition, including micronutrient deficiencies, contributes to both the potential for developing wounds and the degree and success of overall wound healing. The evidence is mixed, however. These divergent results are likely multifactorial, including running the risk of relative undertreatment or overtreatment of nutritional deficiencies, with many micronutrients having deleterious effects on wound healing both at deficient and toxic levels. Despite the mixed evidence regarding wound healing, we recommend nutritional optimization for both prevention and promotion of wound healing as well as treatment of any other abnormal physiologic processes contributing to impaired wound healing such as elevated blood glucose levels and infection.

SUPPORTIVE CARE

If malnutrition is suspected, it is important that a comprehensive nutritional assessment be performed and any vitamin/mineral deficiencies be addressed. Certain situations make oral nutrition difficult or contraindicated, such as obstructive disease, fistulizing disease, or pending surgical treatment. In these situations, there should be consideration for PN (Nguyen et al., 2016).

CONCLUSIONS

CD and UC are the two common categories of IBD. These chronic relapsing disorders possibly result from a misguided immune response stimulated by an environmental factor in a genetically susceptible host. Often striking the young, therapeutic approaches have centered on therapies with anti-inflammatory or immunosuppressive properties. Newer biological and novel small molecule therapies have supplanted corticosteroids and traditional immunosuppressants for patients with moderate to severe disease. CD can occur anywhere in the GI tract, often with skip areas, transmural inflammation, and sometimes with fistulas or other perianal disease. UC is limited to the mucosal layer of the colon, with a continuous pattern of inflammation from the rectum, extending proximally. Extraintestinal manifestations can be seen with both conditions; dietary implications are often more of an issue with CD, as the small intestine is important for maintaining proper nutritional state. Future breakthroughs in determining more predictably the epidemiology, disease course, and selection of therapeutic regimens are anticipated in the coming years.

REFERENCES

Abraham, C., & Cho, J. H. (2006). Functional consequences of NOD_2 ($CARD_{15}$) mutations. *Inflammatory Bowel Diseases, 12*(7), 641–650.

Alexrad, J. R., Lichtiger, S., & Yajnik, V. (2016). Inflammatory bowel disease and cancer: The role of inflammation, immunosuppression, and cancer treatment. *World Journal of Gastroenterology, 22*, 4794–4801.

Allen, P. B., & Peyrin-Biroulet, L. (2013). Moving towards disease modification in inflammatory bowel disease therapy. *Current Opinion in Gastroenterology, 29*(4), 397–404. doi: 10.1097/MOG.0b013e3283622914.

Berg, A. M., Dam, A. N., & Farraye, F. A. (2013). Environmental influences on the onset and clinical course of Crohn's disease—part 2: Infections and medication use. *Gastroenterology & Hepatology, 9*(12), 803–810.

Bouguen, G., Levesque, B. G., Feagan, B. G., et al. (2015). Treat to target: A proposed new paradigm for the management of Crohn's disease. *Clinical Gastroenterology and Hepatology, 13*(6), 1042–1050. e1042. doi: 10.1016/j.cgh.2013.09.006.

Cohen, R. D., & Stein, A. C. (2019). Management of moderate to severe ulcerative colitis in adults. In D. Basow (Ed.), *UpToDate*. Waltham, MA: UpToDate.

Cohen, R. D., Woseth, D. M., Thisted, R. A., et al. (2000). A meta-analysis and overview of the literature on treatment options for left-sided ulcerative colitis and ulcerative proctitis. *The American Journal of Gastroenterology, 95*(5), 1263–1276. doi: 10.1111/j.1572-0241.2000.01940.x.

Collins, P. D. (2016). Video capsule endoscopy in inflammatory bowel disease. *World J Gastrointest Endosc, 8*(14), 477–488.

Colombel, J. F., Sandborn, W. J., Reinisch, W., et al. (2010). Infliximab, azathioprine, or combination therapy for Crohn's disease. *New England Journal of Medicine, 362*(15), 1383–1395. doi: 10.1056/NEJMoa0904492.

Colombel, J. F., Sandborn, W. J., Rutgeerts, P., et al. (2007). Adalimumab for maintenance of clinical response and remission in patients with Crohn's disease: The CHARM trial. *Gastroenterology, 132*(1), 52–65.

Crohn, B. B., Ginzburg, L., & Oppenheimer, G. D. (1932). Regional ileitis: A pathologic and clinical entity. *JAMA, 99*, 1323–1329.

Dassopoulos, T., Cohen, R. D., Scherl, E. J., et al. (2015). Ulcerative colitis care pathway. *Gastroenterology, 149*(1), 238–245.

Duricova, D., Burisch, J., Jess, T., et al. (2014). Age-related differences in presentation and course of inflammatory bowel disease: An update on the population-based literature. *Journal of Crohn's & Colitis, 8*(11), 1351–1361. doi: 10.1016/j.crohns.2014.05.006.

Eaden, J. A., Abrams, K. R., Mayberry, J. F. (2001). The risk of colorectal cancer in ulcerative colitis: A meta-analysis. *Gut, 48*(4), 526–535.

Feagan, B. G., Fedorak, R. N., Irvine, E. J., et al. (2000). A comparison of methotrexate with placebo for the maintenance of remission in Crohn's disease. North American Crohn's Study Group Investigators. *New England Journal of Medicine, 342*(22), 1627–1632. doi: 10.1056/NEJM200006013422202.

Feagan, B. G., Rutgeerts, P., Sands, B. E., et al. (2013). Vedolizumab as induction and maintenance therapy for ulcerative colitis. *New England Journal of Medicine, 369*(8), 699–710.

Feagan, B. G., Sandborn, W. J., Gasink, C., et al.; for the UNITI–IM-UNITI Study Group. (2016). Ustekinumab as induction and maintenance therapy for Crohn's disease. *New England Journal of Medicine, 375*(20), 1946–1960. doi: 10.1056/NEJMoa1602773.

George, J., Present, D. H., Pou, R., et al. (1996). The long-term outcome of ulcerative colitis treated with 6-mercaptopurine. *American Journal of Gastroenterology, 91*(9), 1711–1714.

Hanauer, S. B., Feagan, B. G., Lichtenstein, G. R., et al. (2002). Maintenance infliximab for Crohn's disease: The ACCENT I randomised trial. *Lancet, 359*(9317), 1541–1549.

Hanauer, S. B., Sandborn, W. J., Rutgeerts, P., et al. (2006). Human anti-tumor necrosis factor monoclonal antibody (adalimumab) in Crohn's disease: The CLASSIC-I trial. *Gastroenterology, 130*(2), 323–333; quiz 591.

Hwang, C., Ross, V., & Mahadevan, U. (2012). Micronutrient deficiencies in inflammatory bowel disease: From A to zinc. *Inflammatory Bowel Diseases, 18*(10), 1961–1981. doi: 10.1002/ibd.22906.

Jewell, D. P., & Truelove, S. C. (1974). Azathioprine in ulcerative colitis: Final report on controlled therapeutic trial. *British Medical Journal, 4*(5945), 627–630.

Kaminski, M. V., Jr., & Drinane, J. J. (2014). Learning the oral and cutaneous signs of micronutrient deficiencies. *Journal of Wound, Ostomy, and Continence Nursing, 41*(2), 127–135; quiz E121–E122. doi: 10.1097/WON.0000000000000012.

Knights, D., Lassen, K. G., & Xavier, R. J. (2013). Advances in inflammatory bowel disease pathogenesis: Linking host genetics and the microbiome. *Gut, 62*(10), 1505–1510. doi: 10.1136/gutjnl-2012-303954.

Kostic, A. D., Xavier, R. J., & Gevers, D. (2014). The microbiome in inflammatory bowel disease: Current status and the future ahead. *Gastroenterology, 146*(6), 1489–1499. doi: 10.1053/j.gastro.2014.02.009.

Laharie, D., Filippi, J., Roblin, X., et al. (2013). Impact of mucosal healing on long-term outcomes in ulcerative colitis treated with infliximab: A multicenter experience. *Alimentary Pharmacology & Therapeutics, 37*(10), 998–1004. doi: 10.1111/apt.12289.

Lichtenstein, G. R., Loftus, E. V., Isaacs, K. L., et al. (2018). ACG clinical guideline: Management of Crohn's disease in adults. *The American Journal of Gastroenterology, 113*(4), 481–517. doi: 10.1038/ajg.2018.27.

Lichtiger, S., Present, D. H., Kornbluth, A., et al. (1994). Cyclosporine in severe ulcerative colitis refractory to steroid therapy. *New England Journal of Medicine, 330*(26), 1841–1845.

Marshall, J. K., & Irvine, E. J. (1995). Rectal aminosalicylate therapy for distal ulcerative colitis: A meta-analysis. *Alimentary Pharmacology & Therapeutics, 9*(3), 293–300. doi: 10.1111/j.1365-2036.1995.tb00384.x.

Marshall, J. K., Thabane, M., & Steinhart, A. H. (2010). Rectal 5-aminosalicylic acid for induction of remission in ulcerative colitis. *Cochrane Database of Systematic Reviews*, (1), CD004115.

Marshall, J. K., Thabane, M., & Steinhart, A. H. (2012). Rectal 5-aminosalicylic acid for maintenance of remission in ulcerative colitis. *Cochrane Database of Systematic Reviews, 11*, CD004118.

Miner, P., Hanauer, S., Robinson, M., et al. (1995). Safety and efficacy of controlled-release mesalamine for maintenance of remission in ulcerative colitis. Pentasa UC Maintenance Study Group. *Digestive Diseases and Sciences, 40*(2), 296–304.

Nguyen, D. L., Parekh, N., Bechtold, M. L., et al. (2016). National trends and in-hospital outcomes of adult patients with inflammatory bowel disease receiving parenteral nutrition support. *Journal of Parenteral and Enteral Nutrition, 40*(3), 412–416. doi: 10.1177/0148607114528715.

Nunes, T., Etchevers, M. J., Domenech, E., et al.; Tobacco-Eneida Study Group of GETECCU. (2013). Smoking does influence disease behaviour and impacts the need for therapy in Crohn's disease in the biologic era. *Alimentary Pharmacology & Therapeutics, 38*(7), 752–760. doi: 10.1111/apt.12440.

Ogata, H., Matsui, T., Nakamura, M., et al. (2006). A randomised dose finding study of oral tacrolimus (FK506) therapy in refractory ulcerative colitis. *Gut, 55*(9), 1255–1262.

Panaccione, R., Ghosh, S., Middleton, S., et al. (2014). Combination therapy with infliximab and azathioprine is superior to monotherapy with either agent in ulcerative colitis. *Gastroenterology, 146*(2), 392–400.e393.

Paul, D., & Collins, P. D. (2016). Video capsule endoscopy in inflammatory bowel disease. *World Journal of Gastrointestinal Endoscopy, 8*(14), 477–488.

Present, D. H., Rutgeerts, P., Targan, S., et al. (1999). Infliximab for the treatment of fistulas in patients with Crohn's disease. *New England Journal of Medicine, 340*(18), 1398–1405. doi: 10.1056/NEJM199905063401804.

Regueiro, M., Kip, K. E., Cheung, O., et al. (2005). Cigarette smoking and age at diagnosis of inflammatory bowel disease. *Inflammatory Bowel Diseases, 11*(1), 42–47. doi: 10.1097/00054725-200501000-00006.

Rubin, D. T., Ananthakrishnan, A. N., Siegel, C. A., et al. (2019). ACG clinical guideline: Ulcerative colitis in adults. *The American Journal of Gastroenterology, 114*(3), 384–413. doi: 10.14309/ajg.0000000000000152.

Rubin, D. T., Cohen, R. D., Sandborn, W. J., et al. (2017). Budesonide multimatrix is efficacious for mesalamine-refractory, mild to moderate ulcerative colitis: A randomised, Placebo-controlled trial. *Journal of Crohn's & Colitis, 11*(7), 785–791. doi: 10.1093/ecco-jcc/jjx032.

Ruddell, W. S., Dickinson, R. J., Dixon, M. F., et al. (1980). Treatment of distal ulcerative colitis (proctosigmoiditis) in relapse: Comparison of hydrocortisone enemas and rectal hydrocortisone foam. *Gut, 21*(10), 885–889.

Rutgeerts, P., D'Haens, G., Targan, S., et al. (1999). Efficacy and safety of retreatment with anti-tumor necrosis factor antibody (infliximab) to maintain remission in Crohn's disease. *Gastroenterology, 117*(4), 761–769.

Rutgeerts, P., Geboes, K., Vantrappen, G., et al. (1990). Predictability of the postoperative course of Crohn's disease. *Gastroenterology, 99*(4), 956–963.

Rutgeerts, P., Sandborn, W. J., Feagan, B. G., et al. (2005). Infliximab for induction and maintenance therapy for ulcerative colitis. *New England Journal of Medicine, 353*(23), 2462–2476.

Safdi, M., DeMicco, M., Sninsky, C., et al. (1997). A double-blind comparison of oral versus rectal mesalamine versus combination therapy in the treatment of distal ulcerative colitis. *American Journal of Gastroenterology, 92*(10), 1867–1871.

Sandborn, W. J., Feagan, B. G., Marano, C., et al. (2014). Subcutaneous golimumab induces clinical response and remission in patients with moderate-to-severe ulcerative colitis. *Gastroenterology, 146*(1), 85–95; quiz e14–e85. doi: 10.1053/j.gastro.2013.05.048.

Sandborn, W. J., Feagan, B. G., Rutgeerts, P., et al. (2013). Vedolizumab as induction and maintenance therapy for Crohn's disease. *New England Journal of Medicine, 369*(8), 711–721.

Sandborn, W. J., Hanauer, S. B., Rutgeerts, P., et al. (2007). Adalimumab for maintenance treatment of Crohn's disease: Results of the CLASSIC II trial. *Gut, 56*(9), 1232–1239.

Sandborn, W. J., Panes, J., Sands, B. E., et al. (2019). Venous thromboembolic events in the tofacitinib ulcerative colitis clinical development programme. *Alimentary Pharmacology & Therapeutics, 50*(10), 1068–1076. doi: 10.1111/apt.15514.

Sandborn, W. J., Su, C., Sands, B. E., et al.; OCTAVE Sustain Investigators. (2017). Tofacitinib as induction and maintenance therapy for ulcerative colitis. *New England Journal of Medicine, 376*(18), 1723–1736. doi: 10.1056/NEJMoa1606910.

Sandborn, W. J., van Assche, G., Reinisch, W., et al. (2012). Adalimumab induces and maintains clinical remission in patients with moderate-to-severe ulcerative colitis. *Gastroenterology, 142*(2), 257–265.e251–e253. doi: 10.1053/j.gastro.2011.10.032.

Sands, B. E., Anderson, F. H., Bernstein, C. N., et al. (2004). Infliximab maintenance therapy for fistulizing Crohn's disease. *New England Journal of Medicine, 350*(9), 876–885. doi: 10.1056/NEJMoa030815.

Sands, B. E., Sandborn, W. J., Panaccione, R., et al.; for the UNIFI Study Group. (2019). Ustekinumab as induction and maintenance therapy for ulcerative colitis. *New England Journal of Medicine, 381*(13), 1201–1214. doi: 10.1056/NEJMoa1900750.

Schreiber, S., Khaliq-Kareemi, M., Lawrance, I. C., et al. (2007). Maintenance therapy with certolizumab pegol for Crohn's disease. *New England Journal of Medicine, 357*(3), 239–250.

Shivashankar, R., Tremaine, W. J., Harmsen, W. S., et al. (2017). Incidence and prevalence of Crohn's disease and ulcerative colitis in Olmsted County, Minnesota from 1970 through 2010. *Clinical Gastroenterology and Hepatology, 15*(6), 857–863. doi: 10.1016/j.cgh.2016.10.039.

Sigall-Boneh, R., Pfeffer-Gik, T., Segal, I., et al. (2014). Partial enteral nutrition with a Crohn's disease exclusion diet is effective for induction of remission in children and young adults with Crohn's disease. *Inflammatory Bowel Diseases, 20*(8), 1353–1360. doi: 10.1097/MIB.0000000000000110.

Targan, S. R., Feagan, B. G., Fedorak, R. N., et al. (2007). Natalizumab for the treatment of active Crohn's disease: Results of the ENCORE Trial. *Gastroenterology, 132*(5), 1672–1683.

Targan, S. R., Hanauer, S. B., van Deventer, S. J., et al. (1997). A short-term study of chimeric monoclonal antibody cA2 to tumor necrosis factor alpha for Crohn's disease. Crohn's Disease cA2 Study Group. *New England Journal of Medicine, 337*(15), 1029–1035. doi: 10.1056/NEJM199710093371502.

Travis, S. P., Danese, S., Kupcinskas, L., et al. (2014). Once-daily budesonide MMX in active, mild-to-moderate ulcerative colitis: Results from the randomised CORE II study. *Gut, 63*(3), 433–441.

Van Assche, G., Dignass, A., Reinisch, W., et al. (2010). The second European evidence-based Consensus on the diagnosis and management of Crohn's disease: Special situations. *Journal of Crohn's & Colitis, 4*(1), 63–101. doi: 10.1016/j.crohns.2009.09.009.

Vegh, Z., Burisch, J., Pedersen, N., et al.; EpiCom-Group. (2014). Incidence and initial disease course of inflammatory bowel diseases in 2011 in Europe and Australia: Results of the 2011 ECCO-EpiCom inception cohort. *Journal of Crohn's & Colitis, 8*(11), 1506–1515. doi: 10.1016/j.crohns.2014.06.004.

Wu, G. D., Bushmanc, F. D., & Lewis, J. D. (2013). Diet, the human gut microbiota, and IBD. *Anaerobe, 24*, 117–120. doi: 10.1016/j.anaerobe.2013.03.011.

Zachos, M., Tondeur, M., & Griffiths, A. M. (2007). Enteral nutritional therapy for induction of remission in Crohn's disease. *Cochrane Database of Systematic Reviews,* (1), CD000542. doi: 10.1002/14651858.CD000542.pub2.

QUESTIONS

1. Which of the following environmental factor is often present in Crohn's disease but *not* in ulcerative colitis?
A. Gluten allergy
B. Cigarette smoking
C. Exposure to household pets as a child
D. Breast-fed as an infant

2. Which is true regarding the worldwide incidence rates of Crohn's disease and ulcerative colitis?
A. Rates are lowering in both.
B. Rates are lowering in Crohn's but increasing in ulcerative colitis.
C. Rates are lowering in ulcerative colitis but increasing in Crohn's.
D. Rates are increasing in both.

3. Which is true of colonic inflammation typically seen in patients with ulcerative colitis?
A. Often appears in both the small bowel (ileum) and colon
B. Often appears in the right colon, rarely in the rectum
C. Always appears in the rectum, occasionally in the right colon
D. May skip around in the colon with areas of normal mucosa interspersed between areas of colitis

4. All of the following are considered to be "Crohn's defining" in patients with IBD *except for*
A. Inflammation limited to the mucosal lining of the colon
B. Perianal fistula
C. Granulomas seen under the microscope
D. Midsmall intestinal inflammation

5. Which medication would *not* be used for maintenance therapy for patients with ulcerative colitis?
A. Corticosteroids
B. Mesalamine
C. Infliximab
D. Vedolizumab

6. Which of the following statements is true regarding Crohn's perianal fistulas?
A. Always require surgery
B. Never require surgery
C. Indicate that the patient really has ulcerative colitis
D. May require combined medical and surgical treatments

7. Which of the following is true regarding peristomal pyoderma gangrenosum?
A. Often precipitated by an injury or trauma to the area
B. Not seen in patients with Crohn's disease
C. Best treated by keeping the stoma uncovered to allow to heal
D. Many regress with initiation of cigarette smoking

8. Which of the following is true regarding diet and IBD?
A. Diet can help control inflammation.
B. A gluten-free diet has been proved effective in ulcerative colitis.
C. Mixed evidence suggests that dietary modification may provide some limited benefit to symptomatic improvement.
D. A specific carbohydrate diet has been proven effective in Crohn's disease.

9. Which vitamin is often deficient in patients with Crohn's disease who have had the end of the small intestine removed surgically?
A. Thiamine (B_1)
B. Riboflavin (B_2)
C. Pyridoxine (B_6)
D. Cyanocobalamin (B_{12})

10. Which disease may include a fistula between the anorectum and vagina?
A. Crohn's disease
B. Ulcerative colitis
C. Can occur in both Crohn's disease or ulcerative colitis
D. Vaginal fistulas only occur following birth canal tears at delivery

ANSWERS AND RATIONALES

1. B. Rationale: Active cigarette smoking is present in many Crohn's disease patients and is linked to more refractory disease, fistulous disease, and quicker relapse following bowel resection. The opposite is true in ulcerative colitis; this is a condition of nonsmokers; smokers typically only get ulcerative colitis when they stop smoking.

2. D. Rationale: Rates of ulcerative colitis and Crohn's disease are both increasing worldwide. This is particularly true in parts of the world that are becoming "westernized" (i.e., Southeast Asia) and in populations that have migrated to Western countries.

3. C. Rationale: Ulcerative colitis always appears in the rectum; the inflammation is circumferential, continuous, without skip areas. Less than one third of patients have inflammation that extends to the right colon.

4. A. Rationale: Inflammation limited to the mucosal lining of the colon is only seen in ulcerative colitis. Crohn's disease is a full-thickness inflammation, extending deeper than just the mucosal lining, into the muscular layers of the colon and often all the way to the serosal surface. The other options are not seen in ulcerative colitis and are considered to be "Crohn's defining."

5. A. Rationale: Corticosteroids are never used for maintenance therapy in either Crohn's disease or ulcerative colitis due to their side effect profile and lack of efficacy. The other options are all effective in both inducing and maintaining a disease response in ulcerative colitis.

6. D. Rationale: Perianal fistulas are Crohn's defining in patients with IBD. Some patients can be treated entirely with medical therapies (antibiotics, immunosuppressants, biologics), while others may require surgical treatment if the medical therapy fails.

7. A. Rationale: Pyoderma gangrenosum is often precipitated by trauma or injury to the area, including stoma formation or repeated trauma to the peristomal area. It is treated by both topical wound care and medical therapy. It can be seen in either Crohn's disease, ulcerative colitis, or in patients who never had IBD.

8. C. Rationale: While diet manipulations may be effective in decreasing symptoms, no diet to date has been shown to actually decrease inflammation in either Crohn's disease or ulcerative colitis.

9. D. Rationale: While the B vitamins are typically well absorbed even in patients who have had intestinal resections, cyanocobalamin (B_{12}) is absorbed primarily at the end of the ileum, which is often diseased or resected in patients with Crohn's disease. It is important to verify normal vitamin B_{12} levels in these patients.

10. A. Rationale: Up to one third of Crohn's disease patients may develop a fistula, and in many cases, these start at the anorectum junction (the dentate line) and tunnel to surrounding organs such as the vagina, scrotum, or perineum. These fistulas do not occur in patients with ulcerative colitis.

OBJECTIVE

Describe the surgical management of inflammatory bowel disease.

TOPIC OUTLINE

Crohn's Disease   72
  Indications for Surgery   72

Preoperative Preparation   72
  Medical Optimization   72
  Immunosuppressive or Biologic
    Therapy   72
  Abdominal imaging   73
  Ostomy Site Selection/Patient Education   73
  Mechanical Bowel Preparation Combined with
    Antibiotics   73
  Venous Thromboembolism Prophylaxis   73
  Laparoscopic Versus Open Approach   73
  Bowel Resection   73
    Subtotal Colectomy   76
    Proctocolectomy with Ileostomy   77
  Potential Complications   77
    Nonhealing Perineal Wound, Urinary and
      Sexual Function   77
    Stricturoplasty   78

Ulcerative Colitis   79
  Indications for Surgery   80
  Operative Management   80
    Proctocolectomy with Ileostomy   81
    Ileal Pouch–Anal Anastomosis   82

Minimally Invasive Surgery: Laparoscopic and
    Robotic   85
  Laparoscopic Surgery   85
  Robotic Surgery   85

Management of the Patient with IPAA   85
  Between Stages with a Diverting Loop
    Ileostomy   85
  Measures to Reduce Stool Frequency and
    Perianal Skin Irritation with an IPAA   86
  Ileal Pouch–Anal Function and Expected
    Outcomes   87
  Potential IPAA Complications   87
    Pouchitis Management   88
  Continent Ileostomy   90
    Indications   90
    Contraindications   91
    Surgical Procedure   91
    Complications with the Continent Ileostomy   92
    Management of a Continent Ileostomy
      Catheter Care   92
    Diet   93
    Stoma Care   93
    Pregnancy and Childbirth   93

Conclusions   94

CROHN'S DISEASE

Crohn's disease (CD) is a chronic, unremitting, panintestinal disease that may affect any part of the GI tract but is most often located at the terminal ileum (Strong et al., 2015). Although medical management is effective, surgical therapy will be required in at least one half of patients during their disease course. Operative management is reserved for patients who develop complications or have disease refractory to medical therapy, and undergoing surgery can alleviate symptoms, manage serious complications, or improve quality of life. If the disease is diagnosed and medically treated early, then the need for surgical intervention within the first 2 years of diagnosis has decreased in some settings (Takayuki et al., 2020). It remains to be seen whether more aggressive and newer personalized medical therapies with a treat-to-target targeting approach (treat to target: to achieve disease remission by adjusting therapy according to the achievement [or not] of predefined treatment response target) and early postoperative management will decrease the need for surgical intervention in the future (Bernstein et al., 2012). However, the need for surgery should not be perceived as a failure of medical management, rather that surgery is another treatment modality in addition to medical therapy and each is required at different times. In the surgical treatment of CD, a fecal stoma may be indicated either as a permanent or as a temporizing procedure until inflammation subsides or the healing of diseased tissue occurs.

INDICATIONS FOR SURGERY

Because of the high rate of disease recurrence after segmental bowel resection, the guiding principle of surgical management of CD is preservation of intestinal length and function (Kornbluth et al., 1998). In some clinical settings, surgical resection may be the most efficient means to restore health and improve quality of life. Approximately 85% to 90% of patients develop disease recurrence within the first postoperative year (Rutgeerts et al., 1990). Therefore, every attempt at conserving the small bowel should be made in the surgical approach to CD. The recommended indications for surgical treatment of CD are outlined in **Box 6-1**.

 ## PREOPERATIVE PREPARATION

MEDICAL OPTIMIZATION

Although the majority of patients requiring operative intervention for Crohn's disease are young, those who present acutely (e.g., with sepsis or perforation) could be seriously ill, and those who present with chronic symptoms (e.g., with strictures) could be malnourished. The patient's medical condition should be optimized by correcting anemia, fluid depletion, electrolyte imbalance, and malnutrition prior to surgery if possible. Although

---

> **BOX 6-1   INDICATIONS FOR SURGICAL TREATMENT IN CROHN'S DISEASE**
>
> - Unresponsive to medical management
> - Perforation—may require diverting stoma, surgical drainage with or without resection
> - Obstruction due to fibrotic stricture not amendable to medical treatments or that cannot be surveyed
> - Hemorrhage that cannot or fails to be managed
> - Cancer/neoplasia
> - Growth retardation or extraintestinal manifestations with the presence of significant growth retardation in perpetual patients despite appropriate medical treatment, presence of symptomatic dermatologic, oral, ophthalmologic, or joint disorders refractory to medical management

---

some patients may require total parenteral nutrition (TPN) due to prolonged intolerance of oral nutrition, long-term preoperative TPN should be avoided as it can increase the risk of infectious complications. In patients with fistulizing disease, the exclusive use of enteral nutrition has been shown to reduce postoperative septic complications (Li et al., 2014).

IMMUNOSUPPRESSIVE OR BIOLOGIC THERAPY

Most patients with Crohn's disease who require surgery are on one or more immunosuppressive drugs or biologic agents (i.e., infliximab). Most immunosuppressive drugs can be discontinued just before surgery without negative sequelae. In patients who can tolerate it, early discontinuation of immunosuppressive drugs should be considered as this may allow time for the serum levels to decrease, which might improve surgical outcomes. Glucocorticoids need to be continued but at the lowest dose to maintain remission and tapered after surgery.

The impact of preoperative biologic agents upon surgical outcomes is controversial (Kotze & Coy, 2014). In some studies, preoperative use of infliximab did not increase postoperative complication rates (Colombel et al., 2004; Gaertner et al., 2007; Marchal et al., 2004; Myrelid et al., 2014; Nasir et al., 2010; Subramanian et al., 2006). Other studies have suggested negative effects of newer biologic agents such as vedolizumab (Lightner et al., 2018); however, no negative effects were found with ustekinumab (Lightner et al., 2018). A recent study found no overall infection or surgical site infection risk from exposed and unexposed tumor necrosis factor (TNF) inhibitor patients. In contrast, factors that were associated with increased risk for postoperative infection included higher burden of comorbidities, active smoking, and use of TPN. For surgical site infections, risk factors included comorbidities, revision of a previous bowel resection, urgent surgery, and use of preoperative steroids. More studies are needed to evaluate the effect of duration of anti-TNF exposure, including the interval between last dose and surgery and to compare the infection risks among the different types of procedures, such as creation of an anastomosis. Surgeons have different preferences as to the timing of stopping the immunosuppressants and biologic therapies. Thus, whenever possible, stopping biologics a week or 2 prior to surgery or in situations where surgery is more urgent, diverting stomas may be considered to avoid catastrophic anastomotic complications.

ABDOMINAL IMAGING

Abdominal imaging studies are essential in determining the anatomical distribution and complexities of Crohn's disease. Both computed tomography enterography (CTE) and magnetic resonance enterography (MRE) are highly accurate in assessing lesions and complications (e.g., abscess, fistula) of Crohn's disease (Lee et al., 2009; Malgras et al., 2012). MRE has the added benefit of not requiring radiation (Qui et al., 2014).

OSTOMY SITE SELECTION/PATIENT EDUCATION

In nonemergency situations, the potential sites for an ileostomy or colostomy placement should be marked by the WOC nurse before surgery to ensure proper placement for the patient's body habitus and to optimize better function and overall outcomes (Salvadalena et al., 2015). At the same time, education on living with the stoma should be provided (see Chapter 10).

MECHANICAL BOWEL PREPARATION COMBINED WITH ANTIBIOTICS

A mechanical bowel preparation (MBP) with oral antibiotics is generally recommended prior to any elective colorectal surgery to decrease the colonic bacteria in the bowel with intent to decrease postoperative infections. MBP combined with preoperative oral antibiotics is typically recommended for elective colorectal resections (Migaly et al., 2019). The mechanical bowel prep is left to the discretion of the operating surgeon; however, the suggestion is to use an MBP combined with oral antibiotics:

- MBP is usually accomplished with polyethylene glycol solution.
- Oral antibiotics should follow MBP in the afternoon or evening before surgery. Three repeated doses of one of the following combinations of antibiotics are given orally over a period of approximately 10 hours (Bratzler et al., 2013):
  - Neomycin sulfate 1 g and erythromycin base 1 g
  - Neomycin sulfate 1 g and metronidazole 1 g

This suggestion is consistent with surgical site infection guidelines issued by the American College of Surgeons and Surgical Infection Society (Ban et al., 2017).

VENOUS THROMBOEMBOLISM PROPHYLAXIS

Patients who undergo abdominal surgery for inflammatory bowel disease are at a moderate to high risk for developing a deep venous thrombosis (DVT) and should receive primary prophylaxis when hospitalized. The American Society of Colorectal Surgeons Clinical Practice Guideline for the Prevention of Venous Thromboembolic Disease in Colorectal Surgery (Fleming et al., 2018) states: pharmacological thromboprophylaxis with either low molecular weight heparin or low-dose unfractionated heparin should typically be given to patients undergoing colorectal operations who are deemed to be at moderate or high risk for VTE, who are not identified as high risk for bleeding complications.

The optimal duration is not known, but in high risk patients such as those who undergo major abdominal and/or pelvic surgery for cancer, compromised mobility concerns, etc., longer duration is recommended and may extend up to 3 to 4 weeks (Nguyen et al., 2014a,b).

LAPAROSCOPIC VERSUS OPEN APPROACH

CD is an ideal indication for the laparoscopic approach especially given the recurrent nature of the disease. The laparoscopic approach to CD has been shown to be feasible as well as safe (Liu et al., 1995; Sardini & Wexner, 1998), including those who develop recurrent disease after open surgery (Aytac et al., 2012). Studies have found that the need for conversion to an open procedure was predicted by the severity of disease; independent predictors of conversion included a history of recurrent medical episodes of CD and the presence of intra-abdominal abscesses or fistula at the time of laparoscopy (Bergamaschi et al., 2003; Maartense et al., 2006). In a long-term follow-up study, the recurrence rates in laparoscopic ileocolic resection compared favorably with those in conventional surgery (Chaudhary et al., 2011). The laparoscopic approach has been found to shorten the duration of postoperative ileus, decrease morbidity, shorten length of hospital stay, and reduce costs while decreasing the incidence of small bowel obstruction and incisional hernias due to fewer developments of adhesions and reduced incision size (Maartense et al., 2006; Tan & Tjandra, 2007; Young-Fadok et al., 2001). Patients who undergo laparoscopic abdominal surgery tend to experience a better quality of life than do those with an equivalent open approach. In addition, patients who undergo laparoscopic resection report that they are more satisfied with the physical appearance of their scars (Eshuis et al., 2008). Thus, the laparoscopic approach to bowel resection in Crohn's disease is preferred when the appropriate expertise is available.

BOWEL RESECTION

Resection of the diseased bowel is the most common surgical procedure performed for CD, especially ileal or ileocolonic disease. An ileocecectomy (**Fig. 6-1**) with removal

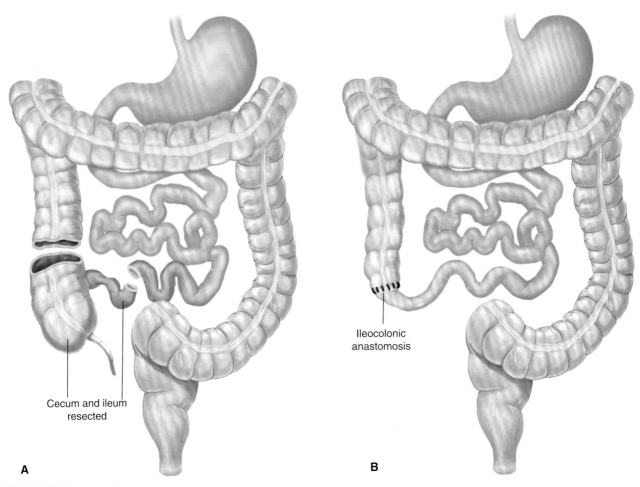

A

B

Cecum and ileum
resected

Ileocolonic
anastomosis

FIGURE 6-1. Ileocecectomy.

of the terminal ileum and the cecum is the most common operation performed, as this is the most common site for the development of CD. Given the risk of recurrent disease after intestinal resection, surgical resection of diseased bowel should be conservative, resecting only sections causing symptomatic complications, such as obstruction, bleeding, or perforation. The two ends of bowel are brought together in a side-to-side or side-to-end anastomosis per surgeon preference as one type of anastomosis has not been conclusively shown to be superior to another based on available data (Michelassi, 2014). With an ileocolonic resection, a side-to-side anastomosis is preferred by some surgeons as it is thought that the large width at the anastomosis leads to less fecal stasis, thereby impeding the development of symptomatic recurrence. A meta-analysis of eight comparative studies found that a side-to-side anastomosis was associated with fewer anastomotic leaks and postoperative complications, that is, need for a stoma, a shorter hospital stay, and lower perianastomotic recurrence rates compared with end-to-end anastomosis (Similus et al., 2007).

The Kono-S anastomosis, a novel functional end-to-end anastomosis, resulted in fewer surgical recurrences

(recurrences requiring reoperations) than conventional side-to-side anastomosis (Kono et al., 2011). In one study, none of 69 patients who underwent small bowel or colonic resection for Crohn's disease followed by Kono-S anastomosis developed a surgical recurrence in the 5 years of follow-up (Kono et al., 2011).

In a Kono-S anastomosis, the bowel stumps are first reinforced with absorbable sutures, then sutured together to create a common support column, a unique feature of this technique. Bowels on both sides of the center support column are then opened longitudinally at the antimesenteric border starting at 1 cm from the support column. The longitudinal incisions are then hand-sewn closed transversely using absorbable sutures in a single-layer manner to complete the anastomosis. In the completed anastomosis, the support column is positioned between the anastomosis and the mesentery (**Fig. 6-2**). The potential advantage of this anastomotic configuration is the ability to maintain intestinal diameter and thus prevent distortion or stenosis associated with recurrent strictures, which usually start from the mesenteric side of the lumen (Kono et al., 2011).

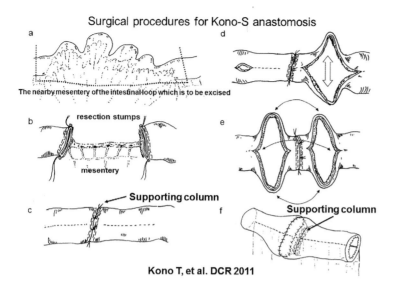

Surgical procedures for Kono-S anastomosis

Kono T, et al. DCR 2011

FIGURE 6-2. Kono S Anastomosis. (Used with permission from Kono, T., Maeda, K., Sakai, Y., et al. (2015). Surgical prophylaxis of anastomotic recurrence by Kono-S anastomosis in luminal Crohn's disease: a multicenter long-term study in Japan: 1823. *American Journal of Gastroenterology, 110*, S775–S776.)

Decisions as to whether primary anastomosis should be performed will depend on whether the procedure is performed electively or as an emergency, the status of the patient including the nutritional status, whether the patient is on high doses of steroids and/or biologics and immunosuppressive agents, and the local condition of the bowel if obstructed or if there is presence of an abscess. The optimal procedure depends upon the extent of disease and the clinical setting.

A segmental colectomy (partial removal of the colon) **(Fig. 6-3)** may be adequate for isolated areas of colonic involvement, and an ileorectal (small intestine to the rectum) anastomosis can be performed if the rectum has no disease involvement; however, one half of such cases

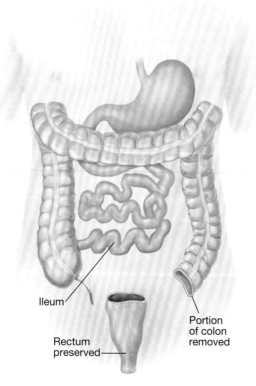

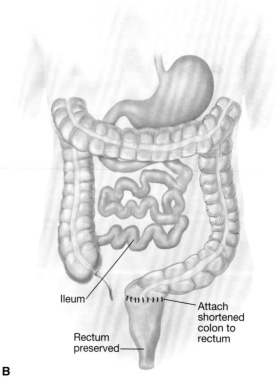

A

B

FIGURE 6-3. Segmental Colectomy with Ileorectal Anastomosis.

require a subsequent proctectomy with removal of the rectum and anus with an end ileostomy due to disease recurrence (Horgan & Dozois, 1999). Although the probability of clinical recurrence after undergoing an ileorectal anastomosis is 58% and 83% at 5 and 10 years, respectively, the probability of rectal preservation at 10 years was as high as 86% (Leinicke & Dietz, 2019). About one half of patients who had an end ileostomy and a defunctionalized rectum after a total colectomy because of rectal disease required a secondary proctectomy in 6 to 10 years (Yamamoto & Watanabe, 2014). In suboptimal conditions, it may be safest to perform a subtotal colectomy and bring out the proximal end of the bowel as an ileostomy or to perform an anastomosis and a diverting ileostomy with the plan to re-anastomose the bowel at a later date. If surgery is performed in an emergency because of a free perforation, abscess, or obstruction, it may be too risky to perform an anastomosis because of the risk of developing an anastomotic leak. In this situation, the proximal end can be brought out as an ileostomy or colostomy with a Hartmann's pouch (see below) or the anastomosis can be performed with a proximal diverting ileostomy.

KEY POINT

The terminal ileum and the cecum are the most common site for the development of CD.

Subtotal Colectomy

In patients with severe perianal disease and associated sepsis of the rectum and anus, it is recommended to initially perform a subtotal colectomy and ileostomy with a Hartmann's pouch. A Hartmann's pouch, named after the surgeon Hartmann who developed the procedure, consists of the anus and rectum that remain in place with the top of the rectum sewn closed as a defunctionalized segment (**Fig. 6-4**). If initially a completion proctectomy is planned, a low short Hartmann's procedure is considered in the presence of severe anorectal disease and ongoing sepsis. Once the disease and sepsis subsides, the proctectomy can be performed using a perineal approach without going back through the abdomen, thereby reducing postoperative hospitalization and recovery time (Sher et al., 1992).

KEY POINT

It is important to remind patients with a Hartmann's pouch that they will have a discharge from the rectum and feel the urge to pass it like a bowel movement. This is normal, and it is a mucus discharge they pass once a day or even less frequently. These patients, however, can develop a recurrent flare of the disease or a diversion proctitis of the retained rectum with increased urgency, tenesmus, and frequent watery or bloody discharge requiring medical management with rectal topical therapies.

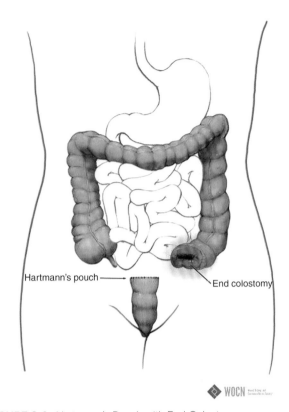

FIGURE 6-4. Hartmann's Pouch with End Colostomy.

A diverting stoma is often indicated in patients who have severe perianal disease that is unresponsive to more conservative surgical therapy with drains, setons (silastic bands placed through a fistula tract from the anus/rectum to the outside perianal skin [**Fig. 6-5**]), and medical therapy. The stoma allows the fecal stream to be diverted from the diseased portion of bowel in order to allow the perianal disease to go into remission. Placement of drains into an abscess cavity or setons into fistula tracts to decrease inflammation, in addition to a diverting stoma, is a frequently temporizing procedure to an eventual need for a permanent end stoma in perianal CD.

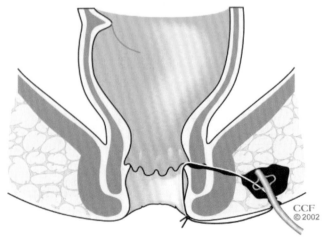

FIGURE 6-5. Seton Placement for Fistula Drainage. (Used with permission from Cleveland Clinic Foundation.)

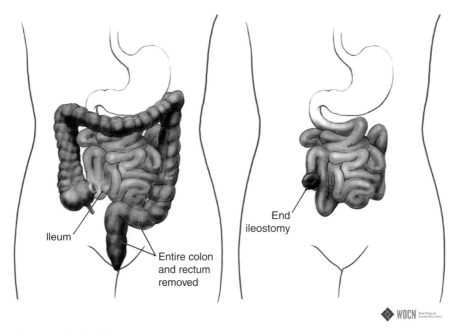

FIGURE 6-6. Proctocolectomy with End Ileostomy.

Often, it is not possible to take down the stoma in the future because of the risk of CD recurring once the fecal stream is returned. However, the diverting stoma often reduces the risk of perianal sepsis such that a proctectomy can be safely performed at a later time when the infection has subsided (Bauer et al., 1986). Initially, these patients may not be willing to have a permanent stoma but may be more accepting knowing that there is a remote possibility of it being temporary (Smith et al., 2009; Thorpe et al., 2009). When severe perianal CD patients experience an improved quality of life with the diverting stoma and decreased perineal sepsis without pain, constant fistula drainage, and inability to sit or walk, many are much more accepting of having the completion of proctectomy for a permanent stoma.

Proctocolectomy with Ileostomy

Proctocolectomy with permanent end ileostomy is the procedure of choice for patients with pancolitis, extensive colorectal CD, or have malignant/premalignant lesions in either the colon or the rectum. The entire colon, rectum, and anus are removed and an end ileostomy performed (**Fig. 6-6**). Total proctocolectomy in properly selected patients has been associated with low morbidity, low risk of recurrence, and a long interval to recurrence (Fichera et al., 2005).

KEY POINT

An important factor in the initial acceptance of a permanent ileostomy is that the decision needs to be the patient's decision of choice and he or she needs to own it. This means that the patient needs to have all the information necessary to make an informed choice and understand that a permanent ileostomy is the best option given his or her medical condition.

Often, this procedure is initially difficult for patients to accept, as they do not want to wear a pouching system and have body image, quality of life, activity, relationship, and sexual concerns. However, with time, once patients begin to feel better, learn how to live with and manage the ileostomy, as well as regain an improved quality of life, most patients are very happy living with an ileostomy (Recalla et al., 2013).

It is also noted that patients with colonic CD who have had a proctocolectomy with end ileostomy have a decreased risk of a recurrence of CD in the small bowel (Leal-Valdivesio et al., 2012). However, when disease does recur, it occurs usually at the stoma site with complications of a stricture or fistulae or as a localized skin manifestation around the stoma such as pyoderma gangrenosum.

KEY POINT

A restorative procedure, such as the ileal pouch–anal anastomosis (IPAA), should generally **not** be performed in patients with CD because of a high risk of pouch failure and disease recurrence in the pouch.

POTENTIAL COMPLICATIONS

Nonhealing Perineal Wound, Urinary and Sexual Function

An intersphincteric proctectomy (the resection of the rectum with a distal dissection in the space between the internal and external anal sphincter) is recommended to minimize the risk of a nonhealing wound and sexual or urinary dysfunction. The major complication of any proctectomy, however, is the risk of a nonhealing perineal wound with a small sinus tract, which has been reported to occur in 20% of patients (Bauer et al., 1986). Six months of healing time is given for the perianal wound or sinus tract to fully heal. If needed, an examination under anesthesia with curettage and debridement of the wound is performed to stimulate granulation tissue to close the wound (Bauer et al., 1986).

Often, warm sitz baths help promote wound drainage and cleanliness, and if indicated by the presence of drainage and or odor, topical antibiotic such as silver sulfadiazine can be applied to the open wound to decrease surface bacteria. In addition, use of silver nitrate applied to the nonhealing hypergranular tissue to stimulate the healing cycle can be attempted prior to the need for additional surgery. Clipping the hair around the perineal wound can also help decrease bacteria in the wound and prevent the hair from curling into the open wound.

Patient education on the use of a pressure redistribution seat pad while sitting is important in order to decrease pressure on the perineal wound. Sitting from side to side from one buttock to the other may also help to relieve the pressure from sitting and the pulling tension put on the incisional wound. Patients need to be reminded not to use a donut cushion as it causes a pulling or spreading of the incisional wound and applies pressure on the outer buttocks, which impedes the blood flow to the area. In addition, very warm sitz baths or shower water concentrated in the perineum will help to cleanse and soothe the area as well as allow any excess serosanguinous fluid to drain so the wound can heal. If drainage from the perineal wound causes skin irritation, moisture barrier ointments and the use of an anal leakage pad may wick away and absorb the drainage (**Box 6-2**).

The nerves related to urinary and sexual function lie close to the rectum in the pelvis, and if disturbed or irritated during the removal of the rectum, their function may be suboptimal or delayed until complete healing occurs. Pelvic nerve injury is rare but an important complication in which male patients may develop decreased erections or retrograde ejaculation. In female patients, dyspareunia (pain with intercourse) may occur due

to scar tissue, which lessens over time as scar tissue softens and becomes more pliable. The ability to conceive may be compromised due to adhesions causing a blockage of the fallopian tubes (Cornish et al., 2007). Use of laparoscopic and robotic-assisted technique may cause less manipulation of tissue and scar tissue formation, decreasing the risk of nerve damage related to urinary and sexual function (Miller et al., 2012).

Stricturoplasty

Stricturoplasty is a surgical procedure performed to alleviate bowel narrowing due to scar tissue that has built up in the intestinal wall and is used for the treatment of fibrotic strictures (scarring and thickening of bowel due to periods of inflammation) in CD. Stricturoplasty is an alternative to bowel resection for Crohn's patients who have multiple skip lesions of the small bowel or especially those who have lost significant length of small bowel to previous resections (Fichera et al., 2005). Stricturoplasty should not be performed in an acutely inflamed bowel or if there is an associated fistula. Stricturoplasty can relieve an obstruction and can be performed with or without a synchronous small bowel resection. It involves the creation of a longitudinal incision through the narrowed area while closing the incision transversely, which widens the intestinal lumen. The Heineke-Mikulicz is performed for short strictures up to 10 cm (**Fig. 6-7**), and the Finney stricturoplasty is performed for longer strictures up to 15 cm (**Fig. 6-8**). For extensive and/or strictures occurring sequentially

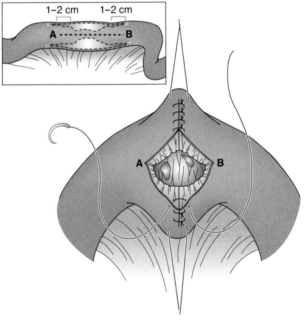

FIGURE 6-7. Heineke-Mikulicz Stricturoplasty. This technique is limited to patient with short segment disease in close proximity. (Adapted from Milsom, J. W. (1999). Stricturplasty and mechanical dilation in strictured Crohn's disease. In F. Michelassi, & J. W. Milsom (Eds.), *Operative strategies in inflammatory bowel disease* (pp. 259–267). New York, NY: Springer-Verlag.)

BOX 6-2   PERINEAL WOUND CARE

Use a pressure redistribution pad; do not use a donut-shaped pad.

Take warm sitz baths or concentrate the shower water daily to cleanse and soothe the wound; pat dry.

Alternate sitting from one buttock cheek to the other to avoid pressure directly on the incision.

Wear an anal leakage pad or butterfly pad to absorb any seepage from the wound.

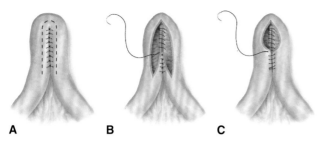

FIGURE 6-8. Finney Stricturoplasty. **A.** After a row of interrupted sutures is placed between the two loops of bowel, a longitudinal enterotomy is created along the antimesenteric border of the strictured segment. **B.** The enterotomy is then closed using a running suture from the posterior wall of the stricturoplasty and then (**C**) on the anterior wall of the stricturoplasty. (From Wexner, S. D., & Fleshman, J. W. (2011). *Colon and rectal surgery: Abdominal operations*. Philadelphia, PA: Wolters Kluwer.)

over long intestinal segments, a Michelassi side-to-side isoperistaltic stricturoplasty (SSIS) is safe and effective (**Fig. 6-9**). With this procedure, the portion of long segment of strictured bowel is divided in half and then overlapped with a side-to-side anastomosis, thereby avoiding a resection, a blind loop, or a bypassed segment of bowel (Campbell et al., 2012; Michelassi et al., 2000; Michelassi & Upadhyay, 2004).

Stricturoplasty has been associated with excellent results, including relief of obstruction, ability to withdraw steroids, and improvement in symptoms. The risk of fistula or recurrent stricture formation is low and comparable to resection (Ambe et al., 2012; Bellolio et al., 2012; Campbell et al., 2012). Whether preservation of diseased bowel increases the long-term risk of malignancy is unknown, although case reports have documented adenocarcinoma arising in sites of previous

stricturoplasty after many years of disease (Menon et al., 2007). The SSIS is a safe, effective, and durable bowel-sparing procedure in patients with extensive fibrostenosing Crohn's disease of the small bowel, and the majority of patients maintain the original SSIS after a median follow-up of 11 years. Postoperative iron deficiency is frequent and may require supplementation (Michelassi et al., 2000).

⬤ ULCERATIVE COLITIS

Ulcerative colitis (UC) is a chronic disease of the colon and rectum characterized by relapsing and remitting episodes of inflammation. Although ulcerative colitis is primarily treated medically, surgery may be required in patients who become refractory to medical therapy or develop severe complications. Surgery is viewed as definitive therapy for UC with removal of the entire colon and rectum with end ileostomy. Total proctocolectomy (removal of the colon and rectum) with a permanent ileostomy is often curative, alleviating symptoms and removing the risk of colonic adenocarcinoma (**Fig. 6-6**). Prior to 1980, total proctocolectomy was the mainstay of therapy. However, since the late 1970s, continence-preserving procedures involving the ileal pouch–anal anastomosis (IPAA) have been refined and the IPAA has become the procedure of choice for patients with UC who wish to maintain continence and not have a permanent ileostomy. However, a temporary ileostomy is indicated between procedures in the IPAA, as the procedure is often performed in multiple steps. It is estimated that approximately 20% to 30% of patients with UC will eventually require surgery (Langholz, 2010).

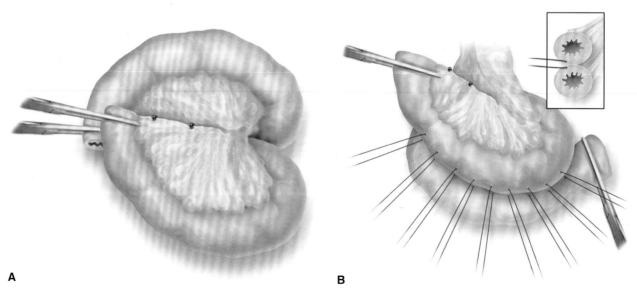

FIGURE 6-9. A. Michelassi stricturoplasty: the mesentery and bowel wall are transected at the midpoint. **B.** The loops of the small intestine are overlaid with dilated segments of the proximal loop aligned with stenotic segments of the distal segment.

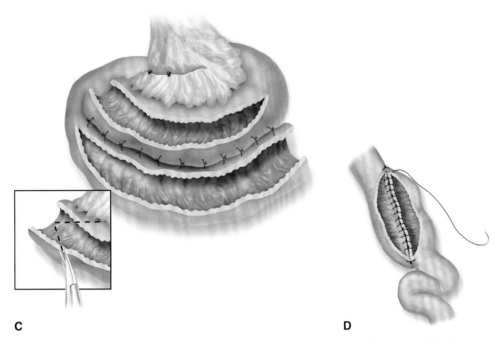

C   **D**

FIGURE 6-9 (*Continued*) **C.** The inner layer is completed on the back wall and runs medially from the end of the stricturoplasty. **D.** The completed side-to-side isoperistaltic stricturoplasty. (From Wexner, S. D., & Fleshman, J. W. (2011). *Colon and rectal surgery: Abdominal operations*. Philadelphia, PA: Wolters Kluwer.)

INDICATIONS FOR SURGERY

Indications for surgery in UC can be either urgent or elective (**Table 6-1**). Failure of medical management is the most common indication for surgery. An acute attack of UC that fails to respond to IV steroid therapy within 10 days warrants surgical intervention. Steroid dependency is a predictor for the need for surgery and is a marker for more severe disease (Becker & Stucchi, 2009). Advances in medical therapy, including the use of infliximab, have made it less likely that patients with toxic megacolon or fulminant colitis will

require emergent colectomy (Cohen, 2009; Halverson & Jarnerot, 2009). However, a long duration of inhospital medical therapy that is ineffective delays surgical therapy in patients with acute severe UC and thereby increases the risk of complications (Windsor et al., 2013).

Lifesaving operative management should not be delayed in hope of saving the colon (Randall et al., 2010). In addition, the use of chromoendoscopy (dye used to detect tissue type or pathology) to identify surveillance dysplastic lesions has reduced the need for surgery given that dysplastic lesions can be detected and removed more successfully (Efthymicu et al., 2013). In children, the presence of pancolitis is the strongest predictor of the need for surgery, and more than 80% of patients who require surgery have total colonic involvement (Falcone et al., 2000). One major goal of management in children is the avoidance of growth retardation caused by long-term steroid use.

OPERATIVE MANAGEMENT

The choice of procedure is dependent on a number of factors that must be individualized to the patients' clinical condition. Three operative approaches in which a temporary or permanent stoma is often required are the proctocolectomy with end ileostomy, a staged restorative proctocolectomy with IPAA with an ileostomy between steps, and the proctocolectomy with continent ileostomy. These three surgical procedures can be performed either in a single stage or in multiple stages for patients with UC. Each technique can improve the quality of life and reduce the risk of colonic malignancy, and each has its own advantages and disadvantages (Hulten, 1998; McCLeod, 1999) (**Table 6-2**).

TABLE 6-1 INDICATIONS FOR SURGERY IN THE MANAGEMENT OF THE PATIENT WITH ULCERATIVE COLITIS	
Indications for urgent surgery	Toxic megacolon refractory to medical management
	Fulminant attack refractory to medical management
	Uncontrolled colonic bleeding
	Perforation (free or walled off)
	Obstruction and stricture with suspicion for cancer
Indications for elective surgery	Refractory disease with failure of medical management
	Chronic steroid dependency
	Dysplasia or adenocarcinoma found on screening biopsy
	Disease present for 7–10 y
	Systemic complications from medicine, particularly steroids
	Failure to thrive in children

TABLE 6-2 CHOICE OF OPERATIONS, ADVANTAGES, AND DISADVANTAGES IN THE MANAGEMENT OF THE PATIENT WITH ULCERATIVE COLITIS

OPERATION	ADVANTAGES	DISADVANTAGES
Proctocolectomy with permanent ileostomy	Complete excision of large intestinal disease—curative One operation	Stoma Need for pouching system Risk of parastomal hernia
Ileal pouch anastomosis	**Hand-Sewn Anal Anastomosis**	
	Transanal defecation and fecal continence preserved Complete excision of large intestinal disease with decreased risk of rectal cancer—curative No permanent ileostomy	Staged multiple operations often required with ileostomy between stages Possible nighttime fecal incontinence up to around 9 mo Risk of pouchitis or other pouch complications
	Stapled Rectal Anastomosis	
	Transanal defecation and fecal continence preserved Better nighttime fecal continence right away No permanent ileostomy Technically easier to perform	Staged multiple operations often required with ileostomy between stages Excision of large intestinal disease except 1–3 cm of rectal mucosa remains at risk for rectal cancer or cuffitis Risk of pouchitis or other pouch complications

Optimal surgical outcomes depend on surgical expertise, the clinical setting, and careful patient selection. The patient's age, previous intestinal or anal surgery, previous vaginal deliveries or history of anal incontinence, obesity, patient occupation, liver disease, and cancer risk should be considered. In general, the choice of operative procedure is dictated by the presentation of disease as urgent or nonurgent (**Table 6-3**). In the acute setting, a total abdominal colectomy (colon removed) is the operation of choice for management of acute fulminant UC with or without toxic megacolon or those patients who are in poor medical condition and on combination immunosuppressive therapy that includes IV or high-dose steroids, cyclosporin, and/or infliximab (Gaetano et al., 2018; Selvaseker et al., 2007; Windsor et al., 2013).

Typically, in urgent clinical settings, the rectum is not removed but is managed as a mucous fistula or Hartmann's pouch and a temporary ileostomy is constructed. This approach is the safest procedure with less operative risk for the patient (Windsor et al., 2013). In the case of indeterminate colitis, when a definitive diagnosis of UC versus CD is not possible prior to surgery, an abdominal colectomy can be performed so that pathological review of the entire colectomy specimen may provide a more definitive diagnosis. Once the patient has recovered from the colectomy, the next choice of the surgical procedure can be made electively as to either an IPAA or a completion proctectomy.

TABLE 6-3 CHOICE OF OPERATIVE PROCEDURE IN THE MANAGEMENT OF THE PATIENT WITH ULCERATIVE COLITIS: URGENT VERSUS NONURGENT

PATIENT PRESENTATION	PREFERRED PROCEDURE
Urgent	
Fulminate UC, toxic megacolon, perforation, hemorrhage, indeterminate colitis	Total abdominal colectomy, Hartmann's pouch with subsequent surgery
Nonurgent	
Chronic UC, nonemergent circumstances	Restorative proctocolectomy with IPAA and diverting ileostomy for patients in good health, continent, and <65 y of age Total proctocolectomy with end ileostomy or continent ileostomy in older patients or patients with poor continence
Chronic UC malignancy	Procedures same as above but oncologic considerations dictate operation selected For rectal cancers, mucosectomy is recommended with IPAA

UC, ulcerative colitis.

KEY POINT

By leaving the rectum in as a placeholder, the option remains available for the patient to later undergo an IPAA procedure or a completion proctectomy, if the patient so desires.

Proctocolectomy with Ileostomy

Proctocolectomy with ileostomy involves removing the entire colon, rectum, and anus with a permanent end ileostomy (**Fig. 6-6**). The procedure is curative for UC and can be performed laparoscopically as hand-assisted or robotic-assisted technique with removal of the rectum (Fichera et al., 2011; Miller et al., 2012). The indications for a total proctocolectomy with a permanent ileostomy include the following:

- Patient preference for one operation
- Medically unable to tolerate multiple operations (e.g., comorbidities, advanced age)
- Very low or ultralow rectal cancer, not amenable to sphincter-sparing procedures
- Poor anal sphincter function associated with fecal incontinence

An important factor in the acceptance of a permanent ileostomy is that the decision needs to be the patients' decision of choice and he or she needs to own it. This means that the patient needs to have all the information necessary to make an informed choice and understand that a permanent stoma is the best option given his or her medical condition.

Telling a patient he or she needs a proctocolectomy with permanent ileostomy is often difficult, as most patients would prefer not to have a permanent ileostomy. The concerns are often related to body image, embarrassment related to accidental leaks of stool and smell, interpersonal relationships and their acceptance, and sexual relationships. These patients need a coordinated team approach with the gastroenterologist, surgeon, nurse, and WOC nurse all working together to assist the patient in understanding and accepting the need for an ileostomy, its benefit to their overall health and quality of life, as well as education on stoma management and lifestyle concerns (Bass et al., 1997). Early discussions and providing the time needed for the patient and family to ask questions, express feelings, and verbalize their concerns in a supportive environment is the key to overall acceptance.

Ileal Pouch–Anal Anastomosis

A restorative proctocolectomy with an IPAA removes the entire colon and rectum while preserving the anal sphincter and hence normal bowel function and fecal continence (**Fig. 6-10**). The ileal pouch serves as an internal pelvic reservoir or "new rectum" for intestinal contents (Parks & Nicholls, 1978). Confirming a diagnosis of UC versus CD both clinically and by pathological review of tissue slides is important. The IPAA procedure is not routinely recommended in patients with CD due to the high incidence of pouch failure and pouch-related fistulas (Reese et al., 2007). However, with an indeterminate diagnosis without terminal ileal inflammation or perianal manifestations of abscess or fistulas, the IPAA may be considered but the potential risk of developing CD in the pouch needs to be clearly understood as these patients are at a higher risk. In addition, a preoperative history of *Clostridium difficile* has been found to be associated with pouch failure after reconstruction, and vigilant postoperative monitoring in patients who have had previous *C. difficile* infection is recommended (Skowron et al., 2016).

The procedure can be performed in one, two, or three steps, with approximately 3 months between surgeries to allow the scar tissue to heal; however, most are done in two or three steps (**Fig. 6-10**).

- A one-step IPAA procedure includes the following: removal of colon and rectum, creation of the IPAA with connection to the anus, and no fecal diversion. If at the time of surgery, the ileal pouch reaches down to the anus with minimal to no tension; the procedure can be performed without a diverting ileostomy as one step. This is predicated on the overall condition of the patient (see below).
- A two-step IPAA procedure includes the following:
  - *Step 1*—removal of the colon and rectum, creation of the IPAA with connection to the anus, and the creation of a diverting loop ileostomy to allow the anastomosis of the pouch to the rectum to heal (**Fig. 6-10B**).
  - *Step 2*—after approximately 3 months of healing and radiologic confirmation that the pouch has healed, the diverting ileostomy can then be taken down as the second step, and bowel continuity is restored (**Fig. 6-10C**).
- A three-step IPAA procedure includes the following:
  - *Step 1*—removal of the colon, creation of an end ileostomy and Hartmann's pouch. This allows the patient to get off all medications, recover nutritionally, and reduce the risk of infectious complications before moving forward to the second step (**Fig. 6-10A**).
  - *Step 2*—takedown of the stoma, removal of the rectum, creation of the ileal pouch from distal segment of ileum with attachment to the anus, and the creation of a loop ileostomy (**Fig. 6-10B**).
  - *Step 3*—approximately 3 months of healing and radiologic confirmation that the pouch has healed, the diverting ileostomy can then be taken down as the third step, and bowel continuity is restored (**Fig. 6-10C**).

There are several considerations for which procedure is the best for patients undergoing an IPAA. A one- or two-step procedure can be performed electively on a thin patient, who is not on immune suppressants, high-dose steroids, or anti-TNF medications and who has relatively quiescent disease. On the other hand, if the ileal pouch reaches down to the anus with considerable tension and there is risk for an anastomotic dehiscence, then a diverting ileostomy would be required as the first step.

A three-step procedure is often indicated in clinical settings, such as pregnancy, acute fulminant colitis that is refractory to medical therapy, need for emergent operative management, obesity, narrow pelvis, and indeterminate colitis, or if a patient is in poor medical condition with immunosuppression and/or malnourished. These are all conditions of high risk for an ileal–anal anastomotic

**Total abdominal colectomy with
end ileostomy and rectum retained
(Hartmann's pouch)**

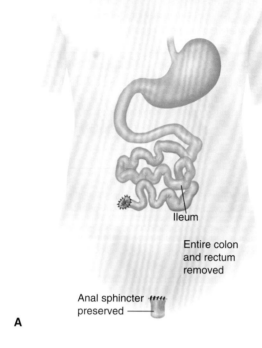

Ileum

Entire colon
and rectum
removed

Anal sphincter
preserved

A

**Rectum removed J pouch created
with diverting ileostomy**

**Ileostomy closed, bowel
continuity restored**

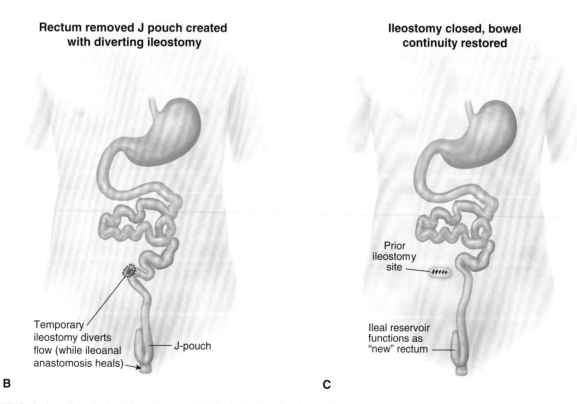

Temporary
ileostomy diverts
flow (while ileoanal
anastomosis heals)

J-pouch

Prior
ileostomy
site

Ileal reservoir
functions as
"new" rectum

B   **C**

FIGURE 6-10. Ileal Pouch–Anal Anastomosis (IPAA). **A.** Total abdominal colectomy with end ileostomy. **B.** Rectum removed, J-pouch created, and diverting loop ileostomy created. **C.** Takedown of loop ileostomy.

TABLE 6-4 ILEAL POUCH–ANAL ANASTOMOSIS: THREE STAGES WITH MANAGEMENT CONSIDERATIONS

STAGE ONE	MANAGEMENT CONSIDERATIONS
Removal of the colon Creation of end ileostomy and Hartmann's pouch	The patient has end ileostomy Disease still present in retained rectum but usually goes into remission with no stool flow Expect a clear grayish mucous drainage per rectum, can be bloody while coming off anti-inflammatories Allows the patient to get off all medications Recovers nutritionally
STAGE TWO	**MANAGEMENT CONSIDERATIONS**
Removal of the rectum Formation of ileal pouch from distal segment of the ileum with pouch–anal anastomosis Diverting loop ileostomy	Approximately 2 feet of small bowel is bypassed, and the patient can experience high stoma output and dehydration Loop stomas can be a management challenge due to lack of adequate protrusion High stoma output that is very liquid and frequent may at times pass into the blind loop, and patients may report passing stool through the anus
STAGE THREE	**MANAGEMENT CONSIDERATIONS**
Ileostomy takedown, bowel continuity restored	Initially may have multiple loose stools Nighttime minor seepage of stool/wetness may occur initially Perianal dermatitis is common when stools are frequent, loose, or due to frequent wiping after bowel movements Annusitis (frequent bloody stools, urgency and tenesmus in the retained 1–2 cm of rectal cuff) could occur Pouchitis symptoms usually do not occur before 5–6 mo after takedown and only occur in 50% of all patients

leak and pouch failure (Pandey et al., 2011). Because of the trend toward suspected more frequent postoperative complications associated with corticosteroids and anti-TNF medications, a three-staged procedure has been typically advocated (Selvaseker et al., 2007; Windsor et al., 2013). However, recent studies and a meta-analysis have found no increased risk for postoperative complications or advantage to the three-stage IPAA in such patients (Hicks et al., 2013; Skowron et al., 2016; Yang et al., 2012). The choice of right operation for the right patient will depend upon a thorough assessment of the patient and the surgeon's judgment (**Table 6-4**).

The IPAA is performed using the stapled or hand-sewn technique (**Fig. 6-11**). Generally, a hand-sewn anastomosis removes all the rectal mucosa and is used in patients with biopsy-proven dysplasia or a colon cancer in the anal transition zone (ATZ). A hand-sewn anastomosis may be performed to decrease the risk of dysplastic tissue developing in the retained cuff (Holder-Murray & Fichera, 2009; Remzi et al., 2003) (**Fig. 6-11A**).

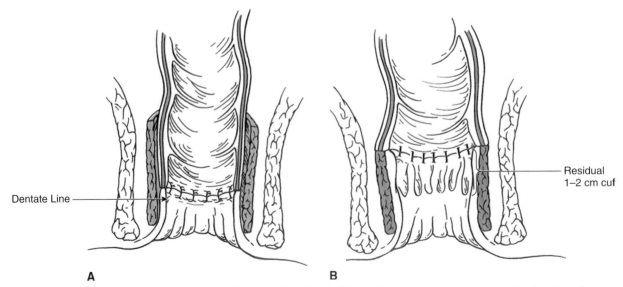

FIGURE 6-11. Ileal Pouch–Anal Anastomosis Hand-Sewn and Stapled. **A.** Sutured (hand-sewn) anastomosis at dentate line after mucosectomy. **B.** Stapled anastomosis. There is a residual 1- to 2-cm cuff of rectal mucosa. (From Dimick, J. B., Upchurch, G. R., & Sonnenday, C. J. (2012). *Clinical scenarios in surgery*. Philadelphia, PA: Wolters Kluwer.)

A discussion with the patient on potential risk for leakage of stool, at least initially and for up to 9 months after take-down of the ileostomy, is important (Fichera et al., 2007).

A stapled anastomosis leaves 2 to 3 cm of rectal mucosa and is used when there is no evidence of dysplasia or a colon cancer in the ATZ. The stapled anastomosis is technically easier to perform and preserves the ATZ, which is the area where the anal and rectal mucosa meets (**Fig. 6-11B**). This 2 to 3 cm of ATZ is the area where sensations of passing gas or stool and the signals to the sphincter muscles to squeeze to hold stool and maintain stool continence (Fichera et al., 2007; Holder-Murray & Fichera, 2009). Dysplasia of the ATZ occurring after a stapled IPAA is infrequent. ATZ preservation has not led to the development of cancer with a minimum of 10 years of follow-up. There is speculation that if the patient has had UC for >10 years, the risk for developing a dysplasia or cancer may increase and long-term follow-up is recommended (Holder-Murray & Fichera, 2009).

The best data comparing the two anastomotic techniques came from a nonrandomized, prospective study of 3,382 patients undergoing IPAA. Compared with a stapled anastomosis, a hand-sewn anastomosis was associated with a higher frequency of anastomotic stricture, septic complications, bowel obstruction, and pouch failure. Patients who had the hand-sewn anastomosis reported more incontinence, seepage, and pad usage, as well as dietary, social, and work restrictions (Hiroaki et al., 2015).

KEY POINT

A permanent ileostomy will be required if an IPAA is not technically possible.

In a large series of 1,789 patients undergoing proctocolectomy, IPAA was attempted but abandoned intraoperatively in 4.1% (Browning & Nivatvongs, 1998). An ileostomy may also be required if the pouch fails postoperatively due to anastomotic complications, infection, fistulization, development of Crohn's disease, disease recurrence, or poor function.

Minimally Invasive Surgery: Laparoscopic and Robotic

Minimally invasive surgery (laparoscopic and robotic) is done using small incisions through which surgical instruments are place. Minimally invasive surgery may cause less pain, scarring, and damage to healthy tissue, and the patient may have a faster recovery than traditional surgery.

Laparoscopic Surgery

Laparoscopic surgery refers to a technique where the surgeon makes several small incisions about ½ inch in size, instead of a single large incision. For most colon and rectal operations, three to five incisions are needed. Small tubes, called "trocars," are placed through these incisions and into the abdomen. Carbon dioxide gas is used to inflate the abdomen in order to give the surgeon room to work. This allows the surgeon to use a camera attached to a thin metal telescope (called a laparoscope) to watch a magnified view of the inside the abdomen on operating room monitors (ASCRS, 2019). Laparoscopic-assisted restorative proctocolectomy has a positive impact on body image and cosmesis, particularly for women, and the laparoscopic approach is a safe and effective approach with short-term advantages in most clinical settings with fewer wound infections, lower rate of intra-abdominal abscesses, and shorter hospital stays (Dunkar et al., 2001; Larson et al., 2005; Polie et al., 2007). As experience with laparoscopic colorectal surgery increases, there are no absolute contraindications to laparoscopy, and the decision is based upon surgeon judgment, skills, and experience. Laparoscopy can be performed electively as well as in the emergent setting of acute fulminant colitis. The laparoscopic approach is associated with significantly fewer incisional, abdominal, and pelvic adhesions (Indar et al., 2009).

Robotic Surgery

Robotic surgery or "robotic-assisted surgery" is very similar to standard laparoscopic surgery in that instruments are passed into the abdomen through trocars. Rather than manipulate the instruments manually, the surgeon sits at a console, or special computer desk, and manipulates small controllers while observing the inside of the abdomen with a 3-D monitor. The computer system translates the movements of the surgeon's hands to the robot, which then moves the surgical instruments (ASCRS, 2019).

Technical advances have allowed skilled laparoscopists to perform single-port and robotic-assisted proctocolectomy with IPAA (Fichera et al., 2011). In addition, laparoscopic and robotic IPAA have equivalent postoperative morbidity related to superficial surgical site infection, peripouch abscess, pelvic sepsis, readmission, or reoperation underscoring the safety of the continued expansion of the robotic platform for pouch surgery (Lightner et al., 2019).

MANAGEMENT OF THE PATIENT WITH IPAA

BETWEEN STAGES WITH A DIVERTING LOOP ILEOSTOMY

With the formation of the ileal pouch (in a two- and three-step procedure), a loop ileostomy is created so that the final step to take down the stoma and reconnect the two ends of bowel is easily performed at the stoma site. The patient with an end ileostomy that was performed in the initial step (a three-step procedure) with removal of the colon and formation of Hartmann's pouch will need to be educated on the differences of an end stoma versus a temporary diverting loop stoma. It is important that the patient understands that the loop stoma will most probably be in the same location on the abdomen as the end stoma and that it may not protrude above the skin as the end stoma but instead may be flush with the skin. In that setting, difficulty in managing a good seal to prevent leakage of stool may be more challenging and may require a convex pouching system to bring out the stoma and close management surveillance by the WOC nurse.

Dehydration is more common with a loop ileostomy than an end ileostomy in the patient with an IPAA, as several inches to feet are below the stoma and no longer absorbing fluid. High output of 1,500 to 2,000 mL/24 hours is common with a loop ileostomy since it is more proximal in the small bowel and bypasses 20% or more of distal small bowel, which can lead to dehydration (Williams et al., 2007). Signs and symptoms of dehydration include fatigue, decreased energy, light-headedness and dizziness on standing, thirst, dark-colored urine, decrease in urination, and a high liquid ostomy output. Patients are advised to drink liquids with meals and snacks but not on an empty stomach. Foods that will act like a sponge to soak up the liquids include starch-based products such as bread, pasta, crackers, pretzels or applesauce, and bananas.

KEY POINT

Education on the signs and symptoms of dehydration as well as measures to maintain hydration and a thickened output are key principles in patient education with a loop ileostomy (Recalla et al., 2013).

In addition, the use of antidiarrheal medications such as loperamide hydrochloride (Imodium©) or diphenoxylate/atropine (Lomotil©) (prescriptive) before meals and at bedtime can thicken stool output and slow down the number of times the pouch needs to be emptied. Remind the patient to take the antidiarrheal medication on a consistent basis 30 minutes before meals and at bedtime, as needed. It is recommended to start out with one dose before breakfast and dinner and then increase doses as needed before lunch and bedtime until a thickened output is achieved at least 75% to 80% of the times the pouch is emptied in 24 hours. Maximum dosage is eight tablets of loperamide hydrochloride (Imodium©) or diphenoxylate/atropine (Lomotil©) per day.

Patients best understand the concept of balancing liquid and solid intake by using the following example: by eating and then drinking, the foods eaten will soak up the liquids you drink, thereby slowing down the transit time of both through your intestines so the fluids and nutrients have time to be absorbed. Drinking liquids without food often causes fluids to move rapidly through the intestines with minimal absorption, resulting in dehydration over time.

Assessing sexual and urinary function after the IPAA procedure is particularly important as most of the surgery is performed in the pelvis with removal of the rectum and placement of the ileal pouch (Zulkowski, 2012). IPAA has been associated with a small risk of sexual dysfunction; the risk is greatest in patients who require reoperative pelvic surgery. Postoperative impotence and retrograde ejaculation have been observed in approximately 1.5% and 4% of men, respectively. Transient dyspareunia occurs in about 7% of women, although coital frequency and the ability to experience orgasm remain unchanged (Cornish et al., 2007; Wax et al., 2003). The nerves related to urinary and sexual function may be manipulated or affected by swelling of tissues during the operation, and in males, the erections may initially be weak. The ability to urinate may also be affected where the urine stream is not as strong or difficulty in getting the urine flow started. Often, with time and healing of the pouch and pelvic tissues, these symptoms resolve (Cornish et al., 2007). If these problems continue after healing has occurred, the patient should be referred to an urologist for medical evaluation of urinary or sexual performance issues.

MEASURES TO REDUCE STOOL FREQUENCY AND PERIANAL SKIN IRRITATION WITH AN IPAA

In the early postoperative phase when bowel continuity has been restored, patient's daily assessment of dietary intake, bowel function, and condition of the perianal skin is an important component to understanding and achieving successful outcomes with the ileal–anal pouch (Michelassi et al., 2003; Perry-Woodford & McLaughlin, 2008). Initially, patients may experience a high number (8 to 10) of loose bowel movements per day with some minor leaks of stool until they get into a pattern of eating foods to thicken their stool and to drink the bulk of liquids with meals.

KEY POINT

Keeping a diet and stool diary is most helpful in the beginning as patients quickly learn how dietary intake can influence their bowel function.

Use of antidiarrheal medications before meals and at bedtime and/or bulk-forming agents can be most helpful in decreasing the number of stools or leaks per day and night as well as increasing the stool consistency to pasty at least 75% to 80% per day. Patients often state that high-roughage foods such as raw vegetables or fruit, popcorn, or nuts as well as foods that are high in acid such as tomato sauce or fruit juices cause an increased number of stools and/or burning discomfort just inside the anus and near the anal opening. The burning discomfort may be due to bile salt diarrhea and can be treated with bile salt binding agents such as colestipol (Colestid©) or cholestyramine (Questran©) (Young & Vanderhoof, 2012). Patients either avoid these types of food or limit the frequency as to when and how often they include them in their diet. Eating a large meal late at night or after 7 PM can increase a patient's chance of having bowel movements at nighttime. One bowel movement during the night is often normal (Fichera et al., 2007; Michelassi et al., 2003).

It is important to note that most patients eventually do not avoid any foods and that each person is individually unique and what bothers one person may not bother another. Each person needs to try food items one at a time to determine which foods increase symptoms and if symptoms are tolerable.

When a patient experiences 10 or more loose to watery stools per day, he or she is at risk for developing perianal skin irritation and breakdown and burning discomfort. Frequent wiping with toilet paper that can be rough and harsh also contributes to perianal skin irritation (Zulkowski, 2012). Use of moisturized cleansing pads as well as moisture barrier skin ointments is recommended to protect the skin, especially when stools are loose, with leakage of stool, or when experiencing an increased number of stools with frequent wiping. Moisture barrier ointments should be used when the patient is experiencing frequent, loose bowel movements or leakage of stool, as stool contains digestive enzymes that are irritating to the skin. In addition, use of fecal incontinent pads or butterfly absorbing pads wick away the wetness or seepage of stool to protect the skin.

It is important to instruct the patient to be sure the skin is dry before applying the barrier ointment in order to not trap wetness on the skin. Skin that is exposed to continual wetness can appear denuded and has the potential for developing infections such as candidiasis (Gray, 2007; Zulkowski, 2012). Use of antifungal powder or an ointment is recommended after each bowel movement and at nighttime as needed until the rash subsides. Patients should carry wet wipes, a moisture barrier ointment, and an antifungal barrier cream with them whenever they have issues with bowel frequency or leaks of stool or when traveling distances from home. It is important to understand the cause of the skin irritation or breakdown of tissue such as high number of loose stools, leakage of stool, types of foods eaten which irritate, etc., so that steps can then be taken to minimize or eliminate the causes while treating the skin condition.

ILEAL POUCH–ANAL FUNCTION AND EXPECTED OUTCOMES

Ileal–anal pouch function continues to improve incrementally every 3 months the first year, and patients may see improvements for up to 2 years following

TABLE 6-5 ASSESSMENT OF FUNCTION IN THE PATIENT WITH AN ILEAL–ANAL POUCH

Bowel movements	Number per day, number during the night, percentage of consistency as watery, loose, pasty, or formed
Leakage of stool	Episodes during the day and night, actual stool or a wetness, requires wearing a pad to absorb stool day/night
Perianal skin integrity	Skin loss, erythema, denuded skin, fungal infection
Ileal–anal anastomosis	Digital examination to assess patency or a stenosis, squeeze tone
Quality of life	Interferes with work, daily routines, sleep, diet, exercise, relationships
Sexual function	In women—dyspareunia, ability to reach orgasm, ability to get pregnant In men—erectile function, ability to reach orgasm, ejaculate present
Medications	Use of antidiarrheal medication, fiber preparations, and bile salt inhibitors Antibiotic use for pouchitis

restoration of bowel continuity. It is important to assess these patients every 3 months the first year as this is the adjustment phase in which pouch function improves as the pouch heals and the patient learns to live with an ileal pouch (Michelassi et al., 2003; Perry-Woodford & McLaughlin, 2008). The important factors to assess at each IPAA patient encounter in patients with an IPAA are outlined in **Table 6-5**.

Frequent assessment and monitoring the first year and then yearly thereafter, unless issues arise, will ensure that the patient has a successful outcome and keeps the patient focused on what good functional results can be expected and measures to maintain good results. Often, these patients develop a "new normal" and may revert back to losing their perspective over time if not followed, as to what good functional results are with a pouch. They may forget to use stool-bulking agents or to call and speak to their health care provider as symptoms change with increased stools, perianal skin irritations, and breakdown or they develop pouchitis symptoms. Like when UC patients develop a "new normal" with increased UC symptoms over time, so do patients with an IPAA develop a "new normal" with increased symptoms over time. Overall expected functional outcomes for patients after an IPAA are listed in **Box 6-3**.

POTENTIAL IPAA COMPLICATIONS

Complications of mechanical, inflammatory, functional, neoplastic, and metabolic conditions related to the pouch can occur postoperatively (Shen et al., 2008). Early and late complications include bowel obstruction, anastomotic dehiscence, pelvic abscess, wound infection, urinary tract infection, anastomotic stenosis requiring mechanical dilation, impotence, retrograde ejaculation, and dyspareunia (Farouk et al., 2000; Michelassi et al., 2003; Shen et al., 2008). Acute and chronic complications can lead to pouch failure such as recurrent pelvic sepsis, CD of the pouch with fistulas, chronic unrelenting pouchitis, or poor pouch function. CD of the pouch has inflammatory, fibrostenotic, and fistulizing phenotype, paralleling to the nonpouch CD findings. Patients with CD of the pouch usually have segmental inflammation of the pouch body and/or afferent limb. Pelvic sepsis is a common early complication of IPAA and occurs in 6% to 16% of patients, and postoperative anastomotic leak with pelvic sepsis is associated with poor pouch function as well.

IPAA surgery in patients with medically refractory UC was linked to high morbidity, according to an analysis of the American College of Surgeons National Quality Improvement Program (ACS-NSQIP) database. Among 1,882 patients who underwent IPAA surgery, the most common reasons for readmission were surgical site infection ($n = 88$), dehydration ($n = 77$), small bowel obstruction ($n = 38/18$), and abdominal pain ($n = 28$). This study brings the possibility and considerations for national health care initiatives in surgical management undergoing IPAA surgery and efforts to improve outcomes on surgical site infection and postoperative dehydration (Aydinli et al., 2017).

Pelvic contrast MRI or a dynamic proctography has proven to be invaluable for the diagnostic assessment of patients with clinically suspected pouch-related complications including leaks and fistulas. Pelvic sepsis is treated with antibiotics, and in some cases, a fluid collection may require drainage with interventional radiology drain placement. ATZ inflammation or cuffitis is an acute and chronic inflammation of the 1 to 2 cm of retained rectal mucosa in a stapled anastomosis (Andersson et al., 2011; Shen et al., 2008). Symptoms are severe tenesmus, urgency, bleeding, and frequent number of bowel movements with small amounts of stool. This can occur in a small number of patients and is treated with 5-ASA or steroid suppository or enema preparations. It is important to note that pouchitis and cuffitis can coexist. Based on the response to topical medical therapy, cuffitis can be classified into steroid/mesalamine-responsive, steroid/mesalamine-dependent, and steroid/mesalamine-refractory types. The development of dysplasia in the ATZ is infrequent and has not led to the development of cancer in a minimum of up to 10 years of follow-up. Biopsy of the ATZ is recommended every 3 to 5 years after an IPAA procedure, but if a patient experiences multiple episodes of pouchitis or ongoing inflammation, then surveillance of the pouch should occur yearly (Fichera et al., 2007; Holder-Murray & Fichera, 2009; Remzi et al., 2003). An ileostomy may be required if the pouch fails due to anastomotic complications, infection, fistulization, development of Crohn's disease, disease recurrence, or poor function. See **Table 6-6** for symptoms of ileal pouch disorders and complications.

Pouchitis Management

The most common late complication is inflammation of the IPAA called pouchitis. It is an acute inflammatory process of the pouch that occurs in 25% to 40% of patients, which in a minority can become chronic (Hurst et al., 1996, 1998; Pardi et al., 2009; Shen et al., 2008). Potential risk factors include extraintestinal manifestations such as primary sclerosing cholangitis (PSC), backwash ileitis, and extensive UC; use of nonsteroidal anti-inflammatory drugs (NSAIDs) over an extended period of days; and being a nonsmoker (Pardi et al., 2009; Shen et al., 2008). Pouchitis should be expected in any patients who experience abdominal cramps, increased stool frequency, watery diarrhea, urgency, and fatigue. Patients may or may not report blood in the stool, fever, leakage of stool, or a flare of joint or body aches. Patients commonly state "It feels like UC all over again or flu-like symptoms."

The exact cause of pouchitis is unclear, but it is often successfully treated with a 2-week course of antibiotics, particularly metronidazole or ciprofloxacin. If intolerant, other antibiotics such as augmentin, levofloxacin, or sulfamethoxazole and trimethoprim can also be considered. Symptoms of pouchitis usually resolve within 24 to 48 hours after the start of the antibiotic, but the patient needs to complete the full 2 weeks dosage. Around 30% of pouchitis patients develop a single episode, 60% develop two or more episodes, and about 10% develop chronic pouchitis (Hurst et al., 1996; Pardi et al., 2009; Shen et al., 2008). In chronic pouchitis, if the patient develops a prompt recurrence of symptoms within a week or 2 after stopping the antibiotic, then he or she needs to go back on a chronic antibiotic regimen

TABLE 6-6 SYMPTOMS OF ILEAL POUCH DISORDERS AND COMPLICATIONS

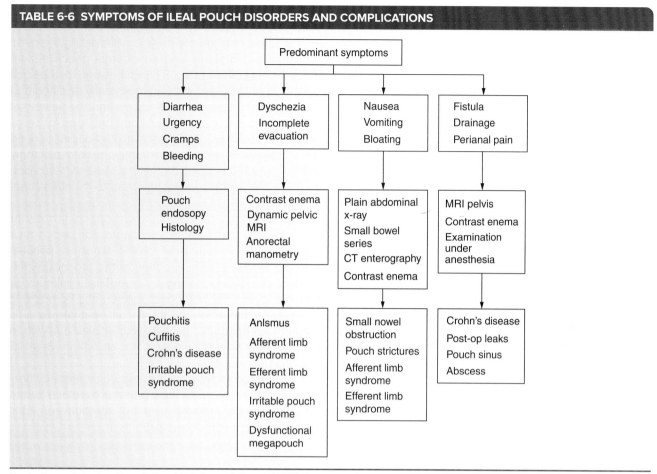

Used with permission from Shen, B., Remzi, F. H., Lavery, I. C., et al. (2008). A proposed classification of ileal pouch disorders and associated complications after restorative proctocolectomy. *Clin Gastroenterol Hepatol, 6,* 145.

and possibly a maintenance probiotic (VSL#3), which has been researched with conflicting and yet some positive results in the treatment of pouchitis prevention (Singh et al., 2015).

Attempts should be made to taper off the antibiotics when possible. VSL#3 is most effective in mild pouchitis symptoms but is not usually as effective for acute pouchitis and is often used as maintenance treatment (Pardi et al., 2009). Sometimes, a combination of antibiotics or cycling antibiotics may be effective when loss of response occurs.

When antibiotics are no longer effective, topical steroids, 5-ASA enemas, budesonide, and immunomodulators may be utilized. In patients with concurrent pouchitis and enteritis, oral budesonide may be effective (Neva-neethan et al., 2012; Sambuelli et al., 2002). Chronic treatment of pouchitis involves induction therapy as well as maintenance therapy, similar to the management of IBD. Chronic pouchitis may eventually develop into CD. In patients with underlying Crohn's disease or concurrent autoimmune disorders (e.g., rheumatoid arthritis, psoriasis), anti-TNF agents (e.g., infliximab, adalimumab) are given (Barreiro-de Acosta et al., 2012; Kelly et al., 2016). Patients with chronic antibiotic-resistant pouchitis

or Crohn's disease of the pouch may benefit from induction therapy as well as maintenance therapy from infliximab (Kelly et al., 2016) or adalimumab. Other agents have been used for treating chronic antibiotic refractory pouchitis, although data are limited. Vedolizumab, an anti-integrin antibody (Bar et al., 2018; Peter et al., 2018; Philpott et al., 2017), and ustekinumab, an anti-interleukin 12/23 antibody (Peter et al., 2018; Tran-Minh et al., 2018), appear to be effective in some cases.

In patients with PSC or IgG4-associated pouchitis, oral budesonide or budesonide enema is used (Neva-neethan et al., 2012; Sambuelli et al., 2002). The use of low-dose mercaptopurine (50 mg daily) or methotrexate (7.5 to 12.5 mg daily, oral or intramuscular) may be used in patients who fail to respond to budesonide and in patients with multiple extraintestinal manifestations of autoimmune pouchitis.

Patients who develop chronic antibiotic-resistant pouchitis or Crohn's disease of the pouch have a high risk for needing pouch excision. Patients who fail immunomodulator and/or biologic therapy after the exclusion of secondary causes should be referred to a colorectal surgeon for consideration of pouch excision and permanent ileostomy. These patients have a high risk of pouch excision. Many patients, however, are treated on the presence of clinical symptoms, but an accurate diagnosis requires endoscopic visualization of the pouch and histologic evaluation (Pardi et al., 2009; Shen et al., 2008).

IPAA may have long-term effects on female productive health. Some women experience increased dyspareunia, although the ability to experience orgasm and coital frequency remain unchanged. Female fertility and fecundity may be decreased due to pelvic adhesions, although successful pregnancies happen regularly (Cornish et al., 2007; Pardi et al., 2009; Wax et al., 2003). It is still not clear whether use of laparoscopic and/or robotic-assisted techniques may improve these outcomes.

Pregnancy and delivery are safe in women with an IPAA. Women may experience a transient increase in stool frequency and incontinence during pregnancy as the fetus grows in size next to the pelvic pouch. Women should not be discouraged from childbearing because of the pouch. Whether vaginal or cesarean delivery is better for women remains controversial. The type of delivery should be influenced by obstetric considerations as well as the potential risk of sphincter injury (Cornish et al., 2007).

Long-term functional results and quality of life with an IPAA are typically superior to that of patients with a Brooke ileostomy, continent Kock ileostomy, or medically treated colitis (Andersson et al., 2011; Pemberton et al., 1989; Wasmuth et al., 2009). However, it is still unclear whether this complex procedure results in an improved quality of life because the disease was removed or because they could control their stools. Other authors have shown that the quality of life improves no matter what procedure is performed and is due to eradication of the disease (Andersson et al., 2011; Jimmo & Hyman, 1998). In one study on ranking the impact of altered bowel emptying on quality of life and disability, the patients with pelvic pouches were found to rank altered bowel emptying as a significantly worse area than did those with stomas (O'Bichere et al., 2000). Although it is generally accepted that avoiding an abdominal stoma will improve quality of life by maintaining body image, it is unclear if the relative change in bowel emptying with a pouch causes enhanced quality of life relative to a stoma.

CONTINENT ILEOSTOMY

Continent ileostomy (Oxford Radcliff Hospitals, 2013) is an alternative to an end ileostomy for patients who have undergone total proctocolectomy (**Fig. 6-6**). The continent (permanent) ileostomy is performed by surgeons who specialize in this type of procedure. An internal pouch is created from the small intestine using a limb of small bowel to create a valve that prevent stool from draining from the stoma. The stoma and ileal reservoir are intubated by the patient on a regular basis to

provide elimination of reservoir contents. The continent ileostomy introduced by Kock has been demonstrated to improved patients' quality of life by eliminating the need for a protruding stoma and an external pouch system (Kock, 1969a,b; Kock et al., 1977). Enthusiasm for the Kock pouch was initially strong but subsequently declined due to complexity of pouch construction and the valve that is associated with complications and the need for reoperation is high. In addition, Parks and Nicholls introduced an alternative in 1978, the restorative proctocolectomy or IPAA, which preserves the natural route of defecation by using the patient's own sphincters to maintain continence.

The IPAA has a relatively low reoperation rate for complications and high patient satisfaction and is thus currently the procedure of choice for most patients with UC. With the wide adoption of the procedure, the number of patients having a failed IPAA continues to increase over time, with pouch failure rates from 10% to 15% (McLaughlin et al., 2008). A continent ileostomy is currently an option for patients with a failed IPAA when repeat pelvic pouch surgery is not an option (Beart et al., 1979). In addition, the technical improvements to decrease the complication rates of a continent ileostomy in the last three decades have preserved a place for the procedure in the armamentarium of intestinal surgeons that is appropriate for some patients.

Indications

Currently, the continent ileostomy has increasingly become a rare commodity but continues to have a role as a fallback and occasionally as the primary option for individuals who are not candidates due to poor sphincter tone, have low rectal cancer, or do not want an IPAA or in whom IPAA has failed and salvage surgery is not feasible, in a small select number of institutions (Behhrens et al., 1999; Nessar et al., 2006; Wasmuth et al., 2009). In the case of patients who have developed a septic complication leading to pelvic pouch failure due to an anastomotic leak and any abscess or fistula, the IPAA can be modified or converted for use as a continent ileostomy.

Although the majority of patients with a conventional ileostomy live a near-normal life, some patients experience debilitating problems including hernia, prolapse, fistula, stenosis, and leakage (Kock et al., 1977; Nessar et al., 2006). These patients are candidates for the continent ileostomy, especially if stoma revision and relocation have already failed and it is not possible to construct a pelvic reservoir. In addition, psychosocial maladjustment to an end ileostomy may also be a reason to convert to a continent ileostomy. A continent ileostomy provides little to no physiologic improvement but may significantly improve lifestyle and body image. Continence and the lack of an external pouch system may enhance the individual's ability to engage in physical and social activities (Nessar et al., 2006).

Contraindications

Several IBD patients may not be considered for a continent ileostomy. Since the reservoir will not drain itself spontaneously, patients who are unlikely to master pouch intubation for mental, psychological, or physical limitations should not receive a continent ileostomy. Patients will not be eligible for the continent ileostomy if they are at risk for intestinal failure, have a diagnosis of CD of the small bowel and have a high risk for recurrence, or have inadequate small bowel such as in patients who have had an excision of a pelvic pouch, or if their body weight is excessive because excessive mesenteric fat increases the risk of valve dysfunction or slippage (Beart et al., 1979; Handelson et al., 1993; Nessar et al., 2006; Wu & Fazio, 2002).

Surgical Procedure

The continent ileostomy, or Kock pouch, first described by Nils Kock in 1969 as a high-volume, low-pressure intra-abdominal reservoir constructed from the terminal ileum using a double folding technique, was an alternative to an end ileostomy, which allowed patients to maintain continence of stool and flatus without the need for an external stoma appliance (Kock, 1969a,b). The original pouch had a high incidence of incontinence, and therefore, the "nipple valve," an intussuscepted segment of the efferent loop of the pouch, was introduced in 1973 and proved to be the key element in preservation of continence. The pouch consists of a reservoir made out of small bowel and a nipple segment that is created by intussuscepting the efferent 12 cm into itself, followed by the last 8 cm forming the exit conduit and ileostomy segment through the abdominal wall that is flush with the skin (**Fig. 6-12**) (Denoya et al., 2005). It is placed lower on the abdomen than the usual site for an ileostomy since it is not important to locate the stoma away from creases or folds because the use of a pouching system is not anticipated; however, the stoma needs to be located in an area the patient can see to intubate the stoma. The internal pouch is emptied by intermittent self-catheterization when increasing volume of intestinal contents causes the pouch to expand, giving the sensation of fullness to indicate it should be emptied.

Although most patients experience improved quality of life after the operation, the long-term pouch revision and excision rates are high and attributable to slippage of the nipple valve. Subsequent technical modifications included enlargement of the pouch with a third loop, use of mesh that caused fistula development, and stabilization of the nipple valve with staples or a collar segment introduced in 1979 as in the Barnett Continent Ileostomy Reservoir (BCIR) (**Fig. 6-13**) (Barnett, 1984; Denoya et al., 2005; Fazio & Tjandra, 1992; Nessar et al., 2006). Yet, the main problem has persisted, and the valve was predisposed to frequently pull apart, resulting in valve dysfunction with leakage and difficulty to intubate the pouch,

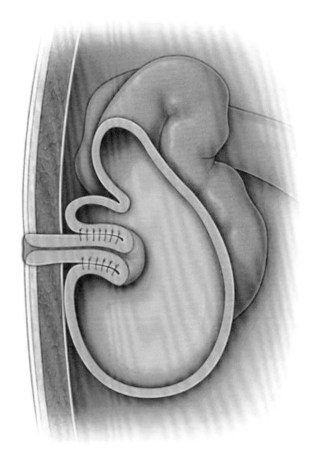

FIGURE 6-12. Continent Ileostomy: Kock Pouch. (Used with permission from Jaffe, R. A., Schmiesing, C. A., Golianu, B. (2019). *Anesthesiologist's manual of surgical procedures.* Philadelphia, PA: Wolters Kluwer.)

stoma prolapse, or combinations thereof requiring reoperations (Fazio & Tjandra, 1992).

Nipple–valve slippage that presents as obstruction or inability to appropriately intubate and evacuate intestinal contents has been recognized as the major reason for operation or pouch failure in the conventional pouch technique. In 2000, the T-pouch continent reservoir design with a nonintussuscepting valve was introduced. The reservoir features a serosal lined antireflux mechanism instead of an intussuscepted valve. A study by Kaiser and associates in 2012 evaluating the first 10 years with 40 patients who had undergone the T-pouch continent ileostomy demonstrated that the valve was less likely to slip, but it is a very complex procedure with inherent surgical risks and requires good patient selection and meticulous surgical technique that still needs long-term results with significant numbers of patients (Kaiser, 2012). However, the study did show improved fecal control and decreased social, sexual, and work restrictions providing patients with a significant level of freedom and normality. While the nipple valve is the

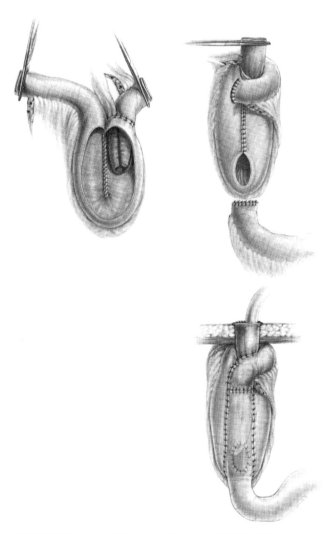

FIGURE 6-13. Barnett Continent Ileostomy. (Used with permission from Corman, M., Nicholls, R. J., Fazio, V. W., et al. (2012). *Corman's colon and rectal surgery.* Philadelphia, PA: Wolters Kluwer.)

key to maintenance of continence, it is also the Achilles heel of the procedure because most complications are related to the valve. Currently, a continent 3-limbed S pouch, BCIR, or the T-pouch procedures are offered to patients in a select few centers as an alternative option to the permanent ileostomy (Beck, 2008; Kaiser, 2012).

Complications with the Continent Ileostomy

Similar postoperative complications that follow any intraabdominal surgery also occur with this procedure. These include obstructions from adhesions, infections, blood clots, suture line leaks, bleeding, etc. Late complications include valve slippage, prolapsed, fistulas, volvulus, perforation hernia, valve stenosis, or pouchitis. There are very few anastomotic leaks and, with the modifications to the valve technique, very few fistulas through the nipple valve. Incontinence caused by nipple valve sliding is the major cause of failure in continent ileostomy and is the result of the unphysiologic construction of the nipple valve.

Therefore, loss of continence is expected in the continent ileostomy after years of intubation. Valve slippage usually occurs in the first 3 months and is less common after 12 months. Symptoms of valve slippage are incontinence to gas or feces or difficulty in intubating the pouch. Weight gain continues to be an ongoing problem with slippage of the valve and needs to be cautioned in these patients with a continent ileostomy (Beck, 2008; Kaiser, 2012).

When a valve cannot be intubated but the pouch remains continent, the patient has a functionally complete bowel obstruction. A pediatric rigid or flexible endoscope can be inserted into the stoma and pouch; gas and pouch contents can be suctioned temporarily decompressing the functional obstruction. A catheter could also be placed to allow for continual drainage until the pouch can be revised surgically (Beck, 2008).

Fistulas and stenosis that threaten pouch function are less frequent. There is a small incidence of ileitis within the pouch (pouchitis), which varies from 10% to 30% and is manifested by an increase in volume of the effluent. The effluent becomes watery, foul smelling, and sometimes bloody. The patient may also develop abdominal pain, distension, fever, and nausea. The complication is thought to be secondary to bacterial overgrowth and is successfully treated with antibiotics (metronidazole and ciprofloxacin) or probiotics to help prevent recurrence. Continuous catheter drainage may be required to avoid stasis of effluent (Beck, 2008).

Revisions or reconstructions are frequent and expected. The revisions are usually successful, and most patients want reconstruction of the pouch to restore their function rather than a definitive conventional ileostomy. With the latest modifications in the creation of the valve, the recurrence rate has dropped from about 20% to 10% (Kaiser, 2012; Wasmuth et al., 2009).

Management of a Continent Ileostomy Catheter Care

An indwelling Medina straight catheter (28 to 32 Fr) is placed in the pouch during surgery and left in to gravity drainage continuously for 2 weeks or more as needed for the pouch to heal. The patient should not experience pressure beneath the pouch, an absence of stool draining from the catheter, or stool leaking around the catheter. If any of these signs occur, the catheter may be kinked and need irrigation or need to be replaced. A split gauze dressing is placed around the indwelling catheter.

KEY POINT

The patient with a continent ileostomy should be taught how to gently irrigate the Medina catheter (generally using no more than 30 cc of warm fluid) to prevent an obstruction that can cause the pouch to retain stool.

It is important to avoid distension of the continent ileostomy pouch in the early postoperative period in order to avoid pressure on the suture line causing a dehiscence and leakage as well as to avoid any stress on the nipple valve resulting in slippage or a leak. The catheter will remain in place for at least 2 to 3 weeks to allow the pouch to heal and mature. After this, the catheter is removed during a postoperative visit and the patient is taught to reinsert the catheter through the stoma into the pouch through the valve. Initially, the catheter is inserted every 2 hours to drain the pouch. The catheter is inserted with decreasing frequency over the next few months as the pouch capacity increases to over 500 mL, and catheterizing will be down to between two and four times per day. The catheter is cleansed and rinsed after each use with soap and water.

How often to drain the pouch varies from person to person, and the patient learns to recognize a feeling of fullness that indicates a need for drainage. The patient is also taught how to irrigate the pouch in case any undigested foods blocking the catheter can be removed and flushed through the catheter. If at any time the patient feels bloated or distended, he/she should drain the pouch. In addition, it is best to empty the continent ileostomy before engaging in physical activity and before bed. The stoma may be covered with a dry gauze dressing or stoma cap.

Diet

After surgery, a dietician should be consulted to give advice on eating and drinking. Immediately after the operation, the patient will start drinking sips of water and once gas and effluent passes through the catheter, the patient can begin to eat low-fiber foods. The patient is usually instructed to add foods one at a time. High-fiber foods and those that cause gas formation are particularly likely to be problematic as the fiber may block the catheter. The patient is advised to chew his/her food very thoroughly as the waste will need to come through the drainage catheter. Foods that are best to avoid are sweet corn, mushrooms, skins and peels, nuts, etc., as these can block the catheter and make it difficult to drain. It is a good idea to drink grape or prune juice to keep the stool thin enough to drain easily. Thick secretions may be thinned by the injection of a little water into the pouch through the catheter. Eventually, patients are able to eat most foods in moderation.

Stoma Care

In the beginning, the stoma may be covered with a dry gauze dressing or stoma cap. It is important to teach the patient to recognize skin irritations as well as methods to prevent irritation of the skin around the stoma. The stoma may secrete a small amount of mucus, which helps with intubation with the catheter. The skin around the stoma should be washed with nonoily soap and water and patted dry as needed. Nonallergenic tape may be used to hold the pad in place.

KEY POINT

Instruct the patient to carry at least two catheters and self-closure plastic bags in case they are unable to cleanse the catheter between pouch emptying, and they can carry the soiled tube in the plastic bag.

Pregnancy and Childbirth

During pregnancy, it may be slightly more difficult to catheterize the continent ileostomy, especially during the third trimester, depending on the size of the baby and its position. If this happens, it may be necessary to leave the catheter in the stoma to gravity drainage during the third trimester.

Other helpful tips for patients with a continent ileostomy are outlined in **Box 6-4**. Patients with a continent ileostomy need yearly follow-up assessment and blood tests to assess for any nutritional deficiencies and pouch problems (**Box 6-5**). Patients should be strongly advised to get a Medic Alert Bracelet or other documentation that they carry with them at all times. This will identify that the patient has a Kock pouch in case of an emergency, and it should contain the following information:

- Internal pouch/continent ileostomy/Kock pouch
- Medina catheter (note size) to be inserted every 4 to 6 hours into the pouch

The continent ileostomy continues to be an alternative for selected patients who have undergone total

BOX 6-4   HELPFUL TIPS FOR PATIENTS WITH A CONTINENT ILEOSTOMY

Carry a catheter at all times.

Inspect stoma site daily for any changes. It should look shiny moist and red.

Inspect the catheter frequently to be sure drainage is flowing freely through the tube and for catheter breakdown and wear. Change the catheter every month.

Irrigate the catheter as instructed by your health care provider with 30 mL of tap water, and let it drain off if the catheter becomes clogged.

If stool becomes too thick and movement through the catheter appears slow or difficult, increase fluid intake to ten to twelve 8-ounce glasses of fluid daily. Include water, juice, and other noncaffeinated beverages.

Do not take laxative preparations that can cause diarrhea and lead to dehydration.

Maintain a stable weight after the procedure to avoid valve slippage problems.

Carry identification that documents the presence of a continent ileostomy.

BOX 6-5   FOLLOW-UP RECOMMENDATIONS FOR A PATIENT WITH A CONTINENT ILEOSTOMY

Yearly outpatient visits with health care provider or APN-led pouch clinic

Annual blood tests

CBC

Urea and electrolytes

Liver function tests

Ferritin

Vitamin B_{12}

Folate

Iron and iron binding

Pouchoscopy with biopsy yearly or every 3 years to evaluate for inflammation or abnormalities per health care provider recommendations

proctocolectomy for whom IPAA and conventional end ileostomy are not possible or desirable. The continent ileostomy is also an alternative for patients when the IPAA fails and repeat pelvic pouch surgery is not an option. Continent ileostomy offers patients freedom from the need for a pouching system with continence provided by a small intestinal valve and unpleasant odors. The procedure needs to be performed by surgeons who are skilled in the procedure and is currently performed in only a few centers in the United States. The main drawback is that reoperation is still commonly required for valve-related problems and these patients are at risk of developing inflammation in the pouch known as pouchitis.

 CONCLUSIONS

There are many surgical options in the management of patients with IBD. The type of surgical intervention is matched to the presenting symptoms as well as the patients' preference and overall health. It takes a coordinated team approach to help patients to understand the surgical procedure as well as the adjustments they will make following surgery to manage their disease.

REFERENCES

Ambe, R., Campbell, L., & Cagir, B. (2012). A comprehensive review of stricturoplasty techniques in Crohn's disease: Types, indications, comparisons, and safety. *Journal of Gastrointestinal Surgery, 16*, 209.

American Society of Colorectal Surgeons. (2019). Retrieved December 29, 2019, from https://www.fascrs.org/patients/disease-condition/minimally-invasive-surgery-expanded-version

Andersson, T., Lunde, O. C., Johnson, E., et al. (2011). Long-term functional outcomes and quality of life after restorative proctocolectomy with ileo-anal anastomosis for colitis. *Colorectal Disease, 13*, 431–437.

Aydinli, H., et al. (2017). 30 day readmission after ileal pouch anal anastomosis surgery: A report from ACS-NSQIP database. AIBD 2017; Poster   001.

Aytac, E., Stocchi, L., Remzi, F. H., et al. (2012). Is laparoscopic surgery for recurrent Crohn's disease beneficial in patients with previous primary resection through midline laparotomy? A case-matched study. *Surgical Endoscopy, 26*, 3552.

Ban, K. A., Minei, J. P., Laronga, C., et al. (2017). American College of Surgeons and Surgical Infection Society: Surgical site infection guidelines, 2016 update. *Journal of the American College of Surgeons, 224*, 59.

Bär, F., Kühbacher, T., Dietrich, N. A., et al.; German IBD Study Group. (2018). Vedolizumab in the treatment of chronic, antibiotic-dependent or refractory pouchitis. *Alimentary Pharmacology and Therapeutics, 47*(5), 581–587.

Barnett, W. O. (1984). Modified techniques for improving the continent ileostomy. *Annals of Surgery, 50*, 66–69.

Barreiro-de Acosta, M., García-Bosch, O., Gordillo, J., et al.; Grupo Joven GETECCU. (2012). Efficacy of adalimumab rescue therapy in patients with chronic refractory pouchitis previously treated with infliximab: A case series. *European Journal of Gastroenterology & Hepatology, 24*(7), 756–758. doi: 10.1097/MEG.0b013e3283525a7b.

Bass, E. M., Del Pino, A., Tan, A., et al. (1997). Does preoperative stoma marking and education by the enterostomal therapist affect outcome? *Diseases of the Colon and Rectum, 40*, 440.

Bauer, J. J., Geiernt, I. M., Salk, B. A., et al. (1986). Proctectomy for inflammatory bowel disease. *American Journal of Surgery, 151*, 157.

Beart, R. W. Jr, Beahrs, O. H., Kelly, K. A., et al. (1979). The continent ileostomy: A viable alternative. *Mayo Clinic Proceedings, 54*, 643–645.

Beck, D. E. (2008). Continent ileostomy: Current status. *Clinics in Colon and Rectal Surgery, 21*(1), 62–70. http://www.ncbi.nlm.nih.gov/pmc/articles/PMC2780187/

Becker, J. M., & Stucchi, A. F. (2009). Treatment of choice for acute severe steroid-refractory ulcerative colitis is colectomy. *Inflammatory Bowel Diseases, 15*, 146.

Behhrens, D. T., Paris, M., & Luttrell, J. N. (1999). Conversion of failed ileal pouch-anal anastomosis to continent ileostomy. *Diseases of the Colon and Rectum, 42*, 490–495.

Bellolio, F., Cohen, Z., MacRae, H. M., et al. (2012). Stricturoplasty in selected Crohn's disease patients results in acceptable long-term outcome. *Diseases of the Colon and Rectum, 55*, 864.

Bergamaschi, R., Pessaux, P., & Arnaud, J. P. (2003). Comparison of conventional and laparoscopic ileocolic resection for Crohn's disease. *Diseases of the Colon and Rectum, 46*, 1129.

Bernstein, C. N., Loftus, E. V. Jr, & Ng, S. C., et al. (2012). Hospitalizations and surgery in Crohn's disease. *Gut, 61*, 622.

Bratzler, D. W., Dellinger, E. P., Olsen, K. M., et al. (2013). Clinical practice guidelines for antimicrobial prophylaxis in surgery. *Surgical Infections, 14*, 73–156.

Browning, S. M., & Nivatvongs, S. (1998). Intraoperative abandonment of ileal pouch to anal anastomosis—The Mayo Clinic experience. *Journal of the American College of Surgeons, 186*, 441–445.

Campbell, L., Ambe, R., Weaver, J., et al. (2012). Comparison of conventional and nonconventional stricturoplasties in Crohn's disease: A systematic review and meta-analysis. *Diseases of the Colon and Rectum, 55*, 714.

Chaudhary, B., Glancy, D., & Dixon, A. R. (2011). Laparoscopic surgery for recurrent ileocolic Crohn's disease is as safe and effective as primary resection. *Colorectal Disease, 13*, 1413.

Cohen, R. D. (2009). How should we treat severe acute steroid-refractory ulcerative colitis? *Inflammatory Bowel Diseases, 15*, 150.

Colombel, J. F., Loftus, E. V. Jr, Tremaine, W. J., et al. (2004). Early postoperative complications are not increased in patients with Crohn's disease treated perioperatively with infliximab or immunosuppressive therapy. *The American Journal of Gastroenterology, 99*, 878.

Cornish, J. A., Tan, E., Teare, J., et al. (2007). The effect of restorative proctocolectomy on sexual function, urinary function, fertility, pregnancy and delivery: A systematic review. *Diseases of the Colon and Rectum, 50*, 1128.

Denoya, P., Schuender, S., & Bub, D. (2005). Delayed Kock pouch nipple valve failure: Is revision indicated? *Diseases of the Colon and Rectum, 51*, 1544–1547.

Dunkar, M. S., Bemelman, W. A., Slors, J. F., et al. (2001). Functional outcome, quality of life, body image, and cosmesis in patients after laparoscopic assisted and conventional restorative proctocolectomy: A comparative study. *Diseases of the Colon and Rectum, 44*, 1800.

Efthymicu, M., Allen, P. B., & Taylor, A. C., et al. (2013). Chromoendoscopy versus narrow band imaging for colonic surveillance in inflammatory bowel disease. *Inflammatory Bowel Diseases, 19*, 2132.

Eshuis, E. J., Polle, S. W., Slors, J. F., et al. (2008). Long-term surgical recurrence, morbidity, quality of life, and body image of laparoscopic-assisted vs. open ileocolic resection for Crohn's disease: A comparative study. *Diseases of the Colon and Rectum, 51*(6), 858–867.

Falcone, R. A. Jr, Lewis, L. G., & Warner, B. W. (2000). Predicting the need for colectomy in pediatric patients with ulcerative colitis. *Journal of Gastrointestinal Surgery, 4*(2), 201–206.

Farouk, R., Pemberton, J. H., Wolff, B. G., et al. (2000). Functional outcomes after ileal pouch-anal anastomosis for chronic ulcerative colitis. *Annals of Surgery, 231*, 919.

Fazio, V. W., & Tjandra, J. J. (1992). Techniques for nipple valve fixation to prevent valve slippage in continent ileostomy. *Diseases of the Colon and Rectum, 35*, 1177–1179.

Fichera, A., McCormack, R., Rubin, M. A., et al. (2005). Long-term outcome of surgically treated Crohn's colitis: A prospective study. *Diseases of the Colon and Rectum, 48*, 963.

Fichera, A., Ragauskaite, L., Silvestri, M. T., et al. (2007). Preservation of the anal transition zone in ulcerative colitis. Long-term effects on defecatory function. *Journal of Gastrointestinal Surgery, 11*, 1647.

Fichera, A., Zoccali, M., & Gullo, R. (2011). Single incision ("scarless") laparoscopic total abdominal colectomy with end ileostomy for ulcerative colitis. *Journal of Gastrointestinal Surgery, 15*, 1247–1251.

Fleming, F., Gartner, W., Ternent, C. A., et al. (2018). The American Society of Colon and Rectal Surgeons clinical practice guideline for the prevention of venous thromboembolic disease in colorectal surgery. *Diseases of the Colon and Rectum, 61*, 14–20

Gaetano, G., Gustavo Kotz, P., & Spinelli, A. (2018). Surgery in ulcerative colitis: When? how? *Best Practice & Research Clinical Gastroenterology, 32–33*, 71–78.

Gaertner, W. B., Decanini, A., Mellgren, A., et al. (2007). Does infliximab infusion impact results of operative treatment for Crohn's perianal fistulas? *Diseases of the Colon and Rectum, 50*, 1754.

Gray, M. (2007). Incontinence-related skin damage: Essential knowledge. *Ostomy/Wound Management, 53*, 28–32.

Halverson, J., & Jarnerot, G. (2009). Treatment of choice for acute severe steroid-refractory ulcerative colitis is remicade. *Inflammatory Bowel Diseases, 15*, 143.

Handelson, J. C., Gottlieb, L. M., & Hamilton, S. R. (1993). Crohn's disease as a contraindication to Kock pouch. *Diseases of the Colon and Rectum, 35*, 840–843.

Hicks, C. W., Hodin, R. A., & Bordeianou, L. (2013). Possible overuse of 3-stage procedures for active ulcerative colitis. *JAMA Surgery, 148*, 658.

Hiroaki, I., Kazushige, K., Keisuke, H., et al. (2015). Comparison of functional outcomes of patients who underwent hand-sewn or stapled ileal pouch-anal anastomosis for ulcerative colitis. *International Surgery, 100*(7–8), 1169–1176. https://doi.org/10.9738/INTSURG-D-15-00012.1.

Holder-Murray, J., & Fichera, A. (2009). Anal transition zone in the surgical management of ulcerative colitis. *World Journal of Gastroenterology, 15*, 769.

Horgan, A. F., & Dozois, R. R. (1999). Management of colonic Crohn's disease. *Problems in General Surgery, 16*, 68.

Hulten, L. (1998). Proctocolectomy and ileostomy to pouch surgery for ulcerative colitis. *World Journal of Surgery, 22*, 335.

Hurst, R., Chung, T. P., Rubin, M., et al. (1998). The implications of acute pouchitis on the long term functional results after restorative proctocolectomy. *Inflammatory Bowel Diseases, 4*, 280.

Hurst, R. D., Molinari, M., Chung, T. P., et al. (1996). Prospective study of the incidence, timing and treatment of pouchitis in 104 consecutive patients after restorative proctocolectomy. *Archives of Surgery, 131*, 497.

Indar, A. A., Efron, J. E., & Young-Fedorak, T. M. (2009). Laparoscopic ileal pouch-anal anastomosis reduces abdominal and pelvic adhesions. *Surgical Endoscopy, 23*, 174.

Jimmo, B., & Hyman, N. H. (1998). Is ileal pouch-anal anastomosis really the procedure of choice for patients with ulcerative colitis? *Diseases of the Colon and Rectum, 41*, 41–45.

Kaiser, A. (2012). T-Pouch: Results of the first year with a nonintussuscepting continent ileostomy. *Diseases of the Colon and Rectum, 55*(2), 155–167.

Kelly, O. B., Rosenberg, M., Tyler, A. D., et al. (2016). Infliximab to treat refractory inflammation after pelvic pouch surgery for ulcerative colitis. *Journal of Crohn's and Colitis, 10*(4), 410–417.

Kock, N. G. (1969a). Intra-abdominal "reservoir" in patients with permanent ileostomy. Preliminary observations on a procedure resulting in fecal "continence" in five ileostomy patients. *Archives of Surgery, 14*, 1–52.

Kock, N. G. (1969b). Intra-abdominal "reservoir" in patients with permanent ileostomy. Preliminary observation on a procedure resulting in fecal continence in 5 ileostomy patients. *Archives of Surgery, 99*, 223–231.

Kock, N. G., Darle, N., Hulten, L., et al. (1977). Ileostomy. *Current Problems in Surgery, 14*, 1–52.

Kono, T., Ashida, T., Ebisawa, Y., et al. (2011). A new antimesenteric functional end-to-end handsewn anastomosis: Surgical prevention of anastomotic recurrence in Crohn's disease. *Diseases of the Colon and Rectum, 54*, 586.

Kornbluth, A., Sachar, D. B., & Salomon, P. (1998). Crohn's disease. In M. Feldman, B. F. Scharschmidt, & M. H. Sleisenger (Eds.), *Sleisenger & Fordtran's gastrointestinal and liver disease: Pathophysiology, diagnosis, and management* (Vol. 2, 6th ed., pp. 1708–1734). Philadelphia, PA: WB Saunders Co.

Kotze, P. G., & Coy, C. S. (2014). The impact of preoperative anti-TNF in surgical and infectious complications of abdominal procedures for Crohn's disease: Controversy still persists. *The American Journal of Gastroenterology, 109*, 139.

Langholz, E. (2010). Review: Current trends in inflammatory bowel disease: The natural history. *Therapeutic Advances in Gastroenterology, 3*(2), 77–86. https://doi.org/10.1177/1756283X10361304

Larson, D. W., Dozois, E. J., Piotrowicz, K., et al. (2005). Laparoscopic-assisted vs open ileal pouch-anal anastomosis: Functional outcomes in a case-matched series. *Diseases of the Colon and Rectum, 48*, 1845.

Leal-Valdivieso, C., Marin, I., Manosa, M., et al. (2012). Should we monitor Crohn's disease patients for postoperative recurrence after permanent ileostomy? *Inflammatory Bowel Diseases, 18*, E196.

Lee, S. S., Kim, A. Y., Yang, S. K., et al. (2009). Crohn's disease of the small bowel: Comparison of CT enterography, MR enterography, and small-bowel follow-through as diagnostic techniques. *Radiology, 251*, 751.

Leinicke, J. A., & Dietz, D. W. (2019). Reoperative surgery in complex Crohn's disease. *Clinics in Colon and Rectal Surgery, 32*(04), 291–299. doi: 10.1055/s-0039-1683918.

Li, G., Ren, J., Wang, G., et al. (2014). Preoperative exclusive enteral nutrition reduces the postoperative septic complications of fistulizing Crohn's disease. *European Journal of Clinical Nutrition, 68,* 441.

Lightner, A. L., Grass, F., McKenna, N., et al. (April 2019). Short-term postoperative outcomes following robotic versus laparoscopic ileal pouch-anal anastomosis are equivalent. *Techniques in Coloproctology, 23*(2). doi: 10.1007/s10151-019-01953-8.

Lightner, A. L., McKenna, N. P., Tse, C. S., et al. (2018). Postoperative outcomes in vedolizumab-treated Crohn's disease patients undergoing major abdominal operations. *Alimentary Pharmacology & Therapeutics, 47,* 573.

Liu, C. D., Rolandelli, R., Ashley, S. W., et al. (1995). Laparoscopic surgery for inflammatory bowel disease. *American Surgeon, 61*(12), 1054–1056.

Maartense, S., Dunkar, M. S., Slors, J. F., et al. (2006). Laparoscopic-assisted versus open ileocolic resection for Crohn's disease: A randomized trial. *Annals of Surgery, 243,* 143.

Malgras, B., Soyer, P., Boudiaf, M., et al. (2012). Accuracy of imaging for predicting operative approach in Crohn's disease. *The British Journal of Surgery, 99,* 1011.

Marchal, L., D'Haens, G., Van Assche, G., et al. (2004). The risk of postoperative complications associated with infliximab therapy for Crohn's disease: A controlled cohort study. *Alimentary Pharmacology & Therapeutics, 19,* 749.

McCLeod, R. S. (1999). Quality of life after surgery for ulcerative colitis. *Problems in General Surgery, 16,* 158.

McLaughlin, S. D., Clark, S. K., Tekkis, P. P., et al. (2008). Review article: Restorative proctocolectomy, indications, management of complications and follow-up: A guide for gastroenterologists. *Alimentary Pharmacology & Therapeutics, 27,* 10.

Menon, A. M., Mirza, A. H., Moolla, S., et al. (2007). Adenocarcinoma of the small bowel arising from a previous stricturoplasty for Crohn's disease report of a case. *Diseases of the Colon and Rectum, 50,* 257.

Michelassi, F. (2014). Crohn's recurrence after intestinal resection and anastomosis. *Digestive Diseases and Sciences, 59,* 1352.

Michelassi, F., Hurst, R. D., Melis, M., et al. (2000). Side-to-side isoperistaltic strictureplasty in extensive Crohn's disease: a prospective longitudinal study. *Annals of Surgery, 232*(3), 401–408.

Michelassi, F., Lee, J., Rubin, M., et al. (2003). Long-term functional results after ileal pouch-anal restorative proctocolectomy for ulcerative colitis: A prospective observational study. *Annals of Surgery, 238,* 433.

Michelassi, F., & Upadhyay, G. A. (2004). Side-to-side isoperistaltic stricturoplasty in the treatment of extensive Crohn's disease. *Journal of Surgical Research, 117,* 71.

Migaly, J., Bafford, A. C., Francone, T. D., et al. (2019). The American Society of Colon and Rectal Surgeons clinical practice guidelines for the use of bowel preparation in elective colon and rectal surgery. *Diseases of the Colon and Rectum, 62,* 3–8.

Miller, A., Berian, J., Rubin, M., et al. (2012). Robotic-assisted proctectomy for inflammatory bowel disease: A case-matched comparison of laparoscopic and robotic technique. *Journal of Gastrointestinal Surgery, 16*(3), 587–594. doi: 10.1007/s11605-011-1692-6.

Myrelid, P., Marti-Gallostra, M., Ashraf, S., et al. (2014). Complications in surgery for Crohn's disease after preoperative antitumour necrosis factor therapy. *The British Journal of Surgery, 101,* 539.

Nasir, B. S., Dozois, E. J., Cima, R. R., et al. (2010). Perioperative anti-tumor necrosis factor therapy does not increase the rate of early postoperative complications in Crohn's disease. *Journal of Gastrointestinal Surgery, 14,* 1859.

Nessar, G., Fazio, W., Tekkis, P., et al. (2006). Long-term outcome and quality of life after continent ileostomy. *Diseases of the Colon and Rectum, 49,* 336–344.

Nguyen, D. L., Parekh, N., Bechtold, M. L., et al. (2014a). National trends and in-hospital outcomes of adult patients with inflammatory bowel disease receiving parenteral nutrition support. *JPEN. Journal of Parenteral Enteral and Nutrition, 40,* 412–416.

Nguyen, G. C., Bernstein, C. N., Bitton, A., et al. (2014b). Consensus statements on the risk, prevention, and treatment of venous thromboembolism in inflammatory bowel disease: Canadian Association of Gastroenterology. *Gastroenterology, 146,* 835.

O'Bichere, A., Wilkinson, K., Rumbles, S., et al. (2000). Functional outcomes after restorative panproctocolectomy for ulcerative colitis decreases an otherwise enhanced quality of life. *The British Journal of Surgery, 87,* 802–807.

Oxford Radcliff Hospitals. (2013). *Colorectal Surgery. Kock pouch operation, information for patients.* Oxford, UK: Oxford Radcliff Hospitals. (Reprint Reviewed 2013). www.uptodate.com

Pandey, S., Luther, G., Umanskiy, K., et al. (2011). Minimally invasive pouch surgery for Ulcerative Colitis: Is there a benefit in staging? *Diseases of the Colon and Rectum, 54,* 306–310.

Pardi, D. S., D'Haens, G., Shen, B., et al. (2009). Clinical guidelines for the management of pouchitis. *Inflammatory Bowel Diseases, 15*(9), 1424–1431.

Parks, A. J., & Nicholls, R. J. (1978). Proctocolectomy without ileostomy for ulcerative colitis. *BMJ, 2,* 85–88.

Pemberton, J. H., Phillip, S. F., Ready, R. R., et al. (1989). Quality of life after Brooke ileostomy and ileal pouch-anal anastomosis. Comparison of performance status. *Annals of Surgery, 209,* 620–628.

Perry-Woodford, Z., & McLaughlin, S. (2008). Recommended follow-up for the ileo-anal pouch patient. *British Journal of Nursing, 17*(4), 220–224.

Peter, J., Zeitz, J., Stallmach, A. (2018). Ustekinumab rescue therapy in a patient with chronic refractory pouchitis. *Journal of Crohn's and Colitis, 12*(8), 1008–1009.

Philpott, J., Ashburn, J., Shen, B. (2017). Efficacy of vedolizumab in patients with antibiotic and anti-tumor necrosis alpha refractory pouchitis. *Inflammatory Bowel Diseases, 23*(1), E5–E6.

Polie, S. W., Dunkar, M. S., Slors, J. F., et al. (2007). Body image, cosmesis, quality of life, and functional outcome of hand-assisted laparoscopic versus open restorative proctocolectomy, long term results of a randomized trial. *Surgical Endoscopy, 21,* 1301.

Qiu, Y., Mao, R., Chen, B. L., et al. (2014). Systematic review with meta-analysis: Magnetic resonance enterography vs. computed tomography enterography for evaluating disease activity in small bowel Crohn's disease. *Alimentary Pharmacology & Therapeutics, 40,* 134.

Randall, J., Singh, B., Warren, B. F., et al. (2010). Delayed surgery for acute severe colitis is associated with increased risk of postoperative complications. *The British Journal of Surgery, 97,* 404.

Recalla, S., English, K., Nazaralli, R., et al. (2013). Ostomy care and management: A systematic review. *Journal of Wound, Ostomy, and Continence Nursing, 40*(5), 489–500; quiz E1–E2, doi: 10.1097/WON.0b013e3182a219a1.

Reese, G. E., Lovegrove, R. E., Tilney, H. S., et al. (2007). The effect of Crohn's disease on outcomes after restorative proctocolectomy. *Diseases of the Colon and Rectum, 50,* 239.

Remzi, F. H., Fazio, V. W., Delaney, C. P., et al. (2003). Dysplasia of the anal transition zone after ileal pouch-anal anastomosis: Results of prospective evaluation after a minimum of ten years. *Diseases of the Colon and Rectum, 46,* 6.

Rutgeerts, P., Geboes, K., Vantrappen, G., et al. (1990). Predictability of the postoperative course of Crohn's disease. *Gastroenterology, 99,* 956–963.

Salvadalena, G., Hendren, S., Muldoon, R., et al. (2015). WOCN Society and ASCRS position statement on preoperative stoma site marking for patients undergoing colostomy or ileostomy surgery. *Journal of Wound, Ostomy, and Continence Nursing, 42*, 249–252.

Sardini, T. C., & Wexner, S. D. (1998). Laparoscopy for inflammatory bowel disease: Pros and cons. *World Journal of Surgery, 22*(4), 370–374.

Selvaseker, C. R., Cima, R. R., Larson, D. W., et al. (2007). Effect of infliximab on short-term complications in patients undergoing operation for chronic ulcerative colitis. *Journal of the American College of Surgery, 204*, 956

Shen, B., Remzi, F. H., Lavery, I. C., et al. (2008). A proposed classification of ileal pouch disorders and associated complications after restorative proctocolectomy. *Clinical Gastroenterology and Hepatology, 6*, 145.

Sher, M. E., Bauer, J. J., Gorphine, S., et al. (1992). Low Hartmann's procedure for severe anorectal Crohn's disease. *Diseases of the Colon and Rectum, 35*, 975.

Similus, C., Purkayastha, S., Yamamoto, T., et al. (2007). A meta-analysis comparing end-to-end anastomosis vs. other configurations after resection in Crohn's disease. *Diseases of the Colon and Rectum, 50*, 1674.

Singh, S., Stroud, A. M., Holubar, S. D., et al. (2015). Treatment and prevention of pouchitis after ileal pouch-anal anastomosis for chronic ulcerative colitis. *The Cochrane Database of Systematic Reviews, 23*, 1–4.

Skowron, K., Lapin, B., Rubin, M., et al. (2016). *Clostridium difficile* infection in ulcerative colitis: Can alteration of the gut-associated microbiome contribute to pouch failure? *Inflammatory Bowel Diseases, 22*, 902–911.

Smith, D. M., Lowenstein, G., Jankovic, A., et al. (2009). Happily hopeless: Adaptation to a permanent, but not to a temporary, disability. *Health Psychology, 28*(6), 787–791.

Strong, S., Steele, S. R., Boutrous, M., et al. (2015). Clinical practice guideline for the surgical management of Crohn's disease. *Diseases of the Colon and Rectum, 58*, 1021.

Subramanian, V., Pollok, R. C., Kang, J. Y., et al. (2006). Systematic review of postoperative complications in patients with inflammatory bowel disease treated with immunomodulators. *The British Journal of Surgery, 93*, 793.

Takayuki, Y., Michele, C., Amy Lee, L., et al. (2020). Up-to-date surgery for ulcerative colitis in the era of biologics. *Expert Opinion on Biological Therapy, 20*(4), 391–398. doi: 10.1080/14712598.2020.1718098.

Tan, J. J., & Tjandra, J. J. (2007). Laparoscopic surgery for Crohn's disease: A meta-analysis. *Diseases of the Colon and Rectum, 50*, 576.

Thorpe, G., McArthur, M., & Richardson, B. (2009). Bodily change following fecal stoma formation: Qualitative interpretive synthesis. *Journal of Advanced Nursing, 65*(9), 1778–1789.

Tran-Minh, M. L., Allez, M., Gornet, J. M. (2017). Successful treatment with ustekinumab for chronic refractory pouchitis. *Journal of Crohn's and Colitis, 11*(9), 1156.

Wasmuth, H., Myrvold, H., & Helge, E. (2009). Durability of ileal pouch-anal anastomosis and continent ileostomy. *Diseases of the Colon and Rectum, 52*(7), 1285–1289.

Wax, J. R., Pinette, M. G., Cartin, A., et al. (2003). Female reproductive health after ileal pouch anal anastomosis for ulcerative colitis. *Obstetrical and Gynecological Survey, 58*, 270.

Williams, L., Armstrong, M. J., Finan, P., et al. (2007). The effect of fecal diversion on the human ileum. *Gut, 56*, 796.

Windsor, A., Michetti, P., Bemelman, W., et al. (2013). The positioning of colectomy in the treatment of ulcerative colitis in the era of biologic therapy. *Inflammatory Bowel Diseases, 19*, 2695.

Wu, J. S., & Fazio, V. W. (2002). Continent ileostomy: Evolution of design. *Clinics in Colon and Rectal Surgery, 15*, 231–243.

Yamamoto, T., & Watanabe, T. (2014). Surgery for luminal Crohn's disease. *World Journal of Gastroenterology, 20*, 78.

Yang, Z., Wu, Q., Wang, F., et al. (2012). Meta-analysis: Effect of preoperative infliximab use on early postoperative complications in patients with ulcerative colitis undergoing abdominal surgery. *Alimentary Pharmacology & Therapeutics, 36*, 922.

Young, R., & Vanderhoof, J. (2012). Pathophysiology of short bowel syndrome. *Uptodate*. Reprint www.uptodate.com

Young-Fadok, T. M., HallLong, K., McConnell, E. J., et al. (2001). Advantages of laparoscopic resection for Crohn's disease. Improved outcomes and reduced costs. *Surgical Endoscopy, 15*, 450.

Zulkowski, K. (2012). Diagnosing and treating moisture-associated skin damage. *Advances in Skin & Wound Care, 25*, 231–236.

QUESTIONS

1. A patient with Crohn's disease is scheduled for bowel resection. What is the guiding principle of surgical management for this condition?
A. Preservation of intestinal length and function
B. Removal of all necrotic intestinal tissue
C. Providing surgical drainage without resection
D. Avoidance of pharmaceutical treatment

2. A WOC nurse is explaining the procedure for laparoscopic ileocolic resection to a patient with Crohn's disease scheduled for surgery. What statement accurately describes an advantage/disadvantage of this procedure over open surgery?
A. A longer hospital stay is required with the laparoscopic approach.
B. The laparoscopic approach shortens the duration of postoperative ileus.
C. The laparoscopic approach increases the incidence of small bowel obstruction.
D. Recurrence rate is slightly higher with the laparoscopic approach.

3. A patient with Crohn's disease develops severe perianal disease and associated sepsis of the rectum and anus. What **initial** procedure would the WOC nurse expect to be scheduled for this patient?
A. Segmental colectomy
B. Diverting stoma
C. Ileocecectomy
D. Primary bowel anastomosis

4. Which patient with Crohn's disease would be the most likely candidate for surgery involving a proctocolectomy with a permanent end ileostomy?
  A. A patient with medically refractory pancolitis
  B. A patient with isolated areas of colonic involvement
  C. A patient who undergoes emergency surgery for a free perforation
  D. A patient with a small bowel to skin fistula

5. What intervention would be appropriate for the WOC nurse to suggest for a patient with Crohn's disease who has a nonhealing perineal wound?
  A. Use of a donut cushion when sitting
  B. Use of a hair dryer to the area
  C. Use of a pressure redistribution seat pad when sitting
  D. Use of cold compresses on the perineum

6. Define the ileal–anal anastomosis procedure.
  A. Removal of colon with an ileal–rectal anastomosis
  B. Reconstruction of an intestinal pouch attached to the anal canal
  C. Michelassi side-to-side isoperistaltic stricturoplasty
  D. Segmental colectomy to remove diseased intestine

7. What treatment approach is viewed as definitive therapy for the patient with ulcerative colitis?

  A. Watch and see approach with topical therapy.
  B. Pharmaceutical and dietary management.
  C. Removal of colon and rectum with end ileostomy.
  D. Stricturoplasty to remove disease.

8. A surgeon is creating an ileal–anal pouch anastomosis using stapled technique. For what postsurgical complication would the WOC nurse monitor this patient?
  A. Cuffitis
  B. Parastomal hernia
  C. Valve complications
  D. Bowel perforation

9. A patient 6 months out from undergoing the final step of the IPAA surgery (stoma closure) tells the nurse: "I've been having cramping in my lower belly with urgency and a lot of watery stools." The patient also complains of being "tired all the time." What potential late complication with an IPAA would the nurse consider?
  A. Anastomotic stenosis
  B. Anastomotic dehiscence
  C. Pouchitis
  D. Pelvic abscess

10. Which postsurgical complication is the major cause of failure in continent ileostomy?
  A. Valve stenosis
  B. Nipple valve sliding
  C. Obstruction from adhesions
  D. Volvulus

ANSWERS AND RATIONALES

1. A. Rationale: It is key to preserve the intestinal length and function because of the high rate of disease recurrence after segmental bowel resection and the possibility of short bowel syndrome with repeated bowel resection and decreased and resultant decreased absorption of nutrients.

2. B. Rationale: The laparoscopic approach shortens the duration of a postoperative ileus because there is less bowel manipulation and less scar tissue formation (adhesions) with this approach.

3. B. Rationale: In order to allow the sepsis in the rectum and anal, a diverting stoma would first be created, followed in the future with a proctectomy (rectum and anus removal).

4. A. Rationale: Because the entire colon, rectum, and anus are involved in a patient with pancolitis and the patient did not respond to medical therapy, a proctocolectomy would most likely be performed.

5. C. Rationale: The use of a pressure redistribution seat pad will redistribute the pressure on the perineal wound to enhance healing.

6. B. Rationale: Reconstruction of an intestinal pouch attached to the anal canal.

7. C. Rationale: Since ulcerative colitis only affects the colon and rectum, a cure is provided when removed.

8. A. Rationale: The stapled technique includes about 2 cm of retained rectal mucosa (called the cuff) that is retained (not removed and could have ulcerative colitis) and could become inflamed.

9. C. Rationale: Symptoms of pouchitis are reported to be similar to active ulcerative colitis: stool urgency, increased watery stools (even when dietary measures are taken to thicken the stools), with or without stool leakage and over all fatigue, all related to pouch inflammation.

10. B. Rationale: A postsurgical complication that is the major cause of failure in a continent ileostomy is value failure due to frequent intubations of the valve.

CHAPTER 7

OTHER CONDITIONS THAT LEAD TO A FECAL DIVERSION

Janice M. Beitz

OBJECTIVE

Describe disease states and conditions that can lead to a fecal stoma.

TOPIC OUTLINE

Introduction 101

Polyposis Syndromes 101
  Familial Adenomatous Polyposis Syndrome 101
    Etiology 101
    Clinical Presentation 101
    Medical Management 102
    Surgical Management 102
  Gardner Syndrome 102
    Etiology 103
    Clinical Presentation 103
    Medical Management 103
    Surgical Management 103
  Peutz-Jeghers Syndrome 103
    Etiology 104
    Clinical Presentation 104
    Medical Management 104
    Surgical Management 104

Diverticular Disease 104
  Etiology 105
  Clinical Presentation 105

  Medical Management 105
  Surgical Management 106

Radiation Enteritis 107
  Etiology 107
  Clinical Presentation 107
  Medical Management 108
  Surgical Management 108

Abdominal/Pelvic Trauma 109
  Etiology 109
  Clinical Presentation 109
  Medical Management 109
  Surgical Management 109

Other Indications 110
  Obstruction 110
  Volvulus 110
  Intussusception 111
    Medical and Surgical Management 111
  Colonic Inertia 111

Conclusion 112

INTRODUCTION

The formation of a fecal diversion is most frequently done for conditions such as colorectal cancer (CRC) or inflammatory bowel disease. However, several other disease states or patient conditions are associated with fecal ostomy formation. These conditions include intestinal polyposis syndromes, diverticular disease, radiation enteritis, abdominal and/or pelvic trauma, and forms of intestinal obstruction (volvulus, intussusception, colonic inertia). Where the fecal diversion is located (colostomy vs. ileostomy) and the nature of its formation (temporary vs. permanent) are often related to the underlying pathology. CRC as an etiologic factor is discussed elsewhere; see Chapter 4.

 POLYPOSIS SYNDROMES

A polyp of the intestine (most often the colon) is a protuberance into the bowel lumen above the surrounding mucosa. Most polyps occur sporadically, but some are part of a genetic polyposis syndrome (Short & Sampson, 2019). Colon polyps are usually asymptomatic but can ulcerate, bleed, cause tenesmus if in the rectum and if large size produce obstruction. Colonic polyps can be neoplastic or nonneoplastic. Colonic polyps can be classified as inflammatory (from localized inflammation such as seen in ulcerative colitis or Crohn's disease), hamartomatous polyps (made of tissue elements normally found at that site but growing in a disorganized mass), serrated polyps (having variable malignant potential), and adenomatous polyps (the most prevalent neoplastic polyps in the colon) (MacRae, 2019).

Inflammatory polyps do not undergo neoplastic transformation, but surrounding dysplasia in inflammatory bowel disease patients can become cancer. Hamartomatous polyps are seen in two polyposis syndromes: juvenile polyposis syndrome (JPS) and Peutz-Jeghers syndrome (PJS) (Chung, 2019a,b). Serrated polyps have variable malignant potential depending on features. Adenomatous polyps are approximately two thirds of all colonic polyps. Some degree of dysplasia exists in all adenomas, so they should be resected completely (MacRae, 2019).

Several polyposis syndromes exist that typify some of these polyp types. The polyposis syndromes can usually be differentiated based on histologic and molecular characteristics of the polyps, involvement of different segments of the gastrointestinal (GI) tract, and alterations in other organs and tissues. Disease severity, cancer risks associated with the disorder, mode of inheritance, and underlying genetic aberration can also help distinguish the disorders (MacRae, 2019). However, some patients present with unexplained polyposis. Despite sequencing of *APC* and/or *MUTYH* genes, many patients still have "unexplained" colorectal polyposis syndromes (Short & Sampson, 2019). The challenge for optimal patient care is evident when geneticists, pathologists, and gastro-enterologists cannot detect specific diagnostic criteria since care approaches differ for the various syndromes. The focus of this discussion will be on more common conditions: familial adenomatous polyposis (FAP), Gardner syndrome, and the less common PJS.

> **KEY POINT**
>
> It is important for the patient and family to be aware of the existing health risks associated with these disorders with polyposis syndromes.

FAMILIAL ADENOMATOUS POLYPOSIS SYNDROME

FAP syndrome was the first polyposis syndrome recognized and is the best investigated. It is one of the CRCs that are known to be associated with familial genetic passage of mutated genes. These disorders include hereditary nonpolyposis colorectal cancer (HNPCC), FAP, PJS, JPS, and MYH-associated polyposis (Samadder et al., 2019a).

Etiology

FAP is an autosomal dominant disorder caused by a mutation in the *APC* (adenomatous polyposis coli) gene located on chromosome 5q21-22 (Samadder et al., 2019a). *APC* is a tumor suppressor gene. On monoallelic mutation analysis (a form of genetic testing), more than 95% of FAP patients display an identifiable mutation. Accurate classification of FAP and other CRC syndromes is imperative given the associated risks, management strategies, and consequent risk to family relatives (Short et al., 2019). The histologic analyses of colorectal polyps in FAP are predominantly adenomatous polyps. FAP is estimated to occur in about 1 in 10,000 individuals usually occurring between 20 and 40 years. FAP accounts for approximately 1% of all CRC cases (Samadder et al., 2019b; Short & Sampson, 2019).

Attenuated FAP (AFAP) is a form of the disease that has lower severity, including delayed onset of polyps, development of fewer polyps (0 to 100 colon adenomas), and lower CRC risk. AFAP is also caused by germline mutation in the *APC* gene. Although FAP (and AFAP) is an inherited disorder, up to 30% of cases of FAP are due to de novo APC mutations (Valle et al., 2019). Genetic testing is necessary to confirm a molecular diagnosis (Samadder et al., 2019a).

Clinical Presentation

The classic clinical presentation of FAP includes the occurrence of hundreds to thousands of adenomatous polyps in the colon and rectum. The sheer number of polyps present in FAP results in nearly a 100% lifetime risk of CRC in untreated persons. Generally, colorectal polyps begin to develop around age 16 years with CRC developing anywhere from 5 to 30 years later (Dinar-vand et al., 2018; Short & Sampson, 2019). Other cancer syndromes have substantial extracolonic manifestations, but when they occur in FAP, the most common scenario is upper GI tract specifically duodenal cancer (Campos et al., 2019; Samadder et al., 2019b).

These intestinal adenomatous polyps are usually dis-covered during endoscopic evaluation for symptoms such as GI bleeding. Conversely, they may be identified during routine screening in people with a known fam-ily history. Clinical diagnosis of FAP requires at least 100 colorectal adenomatous polyps (Samadder et al., 2019b).

Extraintestinal malignancies can be associated with FAP. They include central nervous system tumors (e.g., medulloblastomas), papillary thyroid cancer, and duode-nal cancer. The risk of duodenal or periampullary carci-noma in patients with FAP is estimated to be 100 to 330 times greater than that in the general population, but life-time risk is 12% (Katabathina et al., 2019; Samadder et al., 2019b). The most common extracolonic finding in indi-viduals with FAP is upper GI tract polyps. However, the extracolonic manifestations of FAP can be benign includ-ing duodenal adenomas, gastric fundic gland polyps, and desmoids (Dinarvand et al., 2018; Samadder et al., 2019b).

Although malignancy can occur in childhood and adolescence, malignant degeneration occurs typically by 40 to 50 years of age. The most common age of cancer diagnosis in classic FAP patients is late 30s. The most common cancer location is the rectum followed by the sigmoid and other colon segments (Samadder et al., 2019b). Cancers in other body locations also increase risk. Periampullary cancer (occurring in the duodenum near the ampulla of Vater) and desmoid tumors repre-sent the most common cause of death in FAP patients. Though benign, desmoid tumors cause serious dam-age by local invasion and compression of adjacent body structures (Katabathina et al., 2019).

Medical Management

Genetic testing and counseling are the standard of care for individuals with classic FAP and for at-risk family mem-bers. Genetic evaluation begins with the affected person with the polyposis phenotype and full gene sequenc-ing looking for the *APC* gene mutation (Dinarvand et al., 2018).

For known gene mutation carriers, colorectal screen-ing with flexible sigmoidoscopy or colonoscopy should begin at 12 to 14 years of age. Once polyps are identi-fied, colon screening must be annual (Katabathina et al., 2019). A systematic review supports that registration and screening of FAP patients resulted in a reduction of the CRC incidence and mortality in this hereditary registry of patients (Barrow et al., 2013).

Because of extraintestinal manifestations, screen-ing of the stomach and duodenum is also necessary. Upper endoscopy is recommended every 1 to 3 years

(Katabathina et al., 2019). Since thyroid cancer is a pos-sibility, health care providers should perform thyroid pal-pation and possibly thyroid ultrasonography annually.

Some literature has suggested a role for chemopre-vention against polyps. For example, sulindac, a nonste-roidal anti-inflammatory drug (NSAID), has been shown to cause regression of colorectal adenomas. However, the long-term benefits have been inconsistent; there-fore, chemoprevention is not considered a reasonable alternative to surgery (Samadder et al., 2019b).

Research has also addressed the psychological issues of requisite surveillance for cancer degeneration in persons with FAP and other polyposis syndromes. A systematic review (Gopie et al., 2012) analyzed 32 stud-ies looking at psychological burden of hereditary cancer surveillance (breast, colon, colorectal, melanoma, etc.). For most hereditary cancer syndromes, surveillance was associated with good psychological outcomes. However, distress levels increased in those persons who were at high risk for developing *multiple* tumors.

Surgical Management

Despite frequent colonoscopies and polypectomy, the tumor burden or sheer number of polyps may preclude the continuing use of endoscopy. Total proctocolec-tomy with ileal pouch–anal anastomosis (IPAA) is the pre-ferred surgery. Total colectomy with removal of the rectal mucosa is the goal of therapy (to remove potentially dis-eased tissue) (Ganschow et al., 2019; Katabathina et al., 2019). Total colectomy with ileorectal anastomosis does not offer as clear a benefit as does total colectomy with IPAA since rectal mucosa remains. Annual colonoscopy would be required to follow this retained tissue for polyp development (Dolan, 2019).

A systematic review was conducted examining short- and long-term outcomes after IPAA in pediatric patients. Forty-two papers were reviewed showing acceptable surgical complication and pouch function/incontinence rates. Median stool frequency was between 5 and 5.3 during daytime. IPAA is considered safe with good long-term functional outcomes in pediatric patients (Lightner et al., 2019).

Another study on surgical treatment for FAP done in The Netherlands suggests that surgery can be delayed in selected patients. In a study of 72 FAP patients exam-ined retrospectively, those diagnosed before and after 2000 (when better endoscopy became available) with improved surveillance colonoscopy techniques surgery could be delayed up to 6 years (19 to 24 years) without CRC development. The deciding factor for earlier sur-gery was the identification of large adenomas of >5 to 10 mm (Vasen et al., 2019).

GARDNER SYNDROME

At one time, Gardner syndrome was considered a sep-arate disease from FAP. Today, Gardner syndrome is considered linked to FAP (Dinarvand et al., 2018). Gardner syndrome is an inherited polyposis syndrome that is also associated with germline APC mutation. Gardner syndrome is thought to be a variation in the expressivity of APC mutations rather than being a distinct clinical entity from FAP. In fact, some authors suggest that Gardner syndrome is the full-blown manifestation of the FAP spectrum of clinical features due to the *APC* gene mutation (Samadder et al., 2019a).

KEY POINT

Gardner syndrome usually causes benign tumors to form in many different organs and causes a higher risk of developing CRC and other FAP-related cancers.

Etiology

Gardner syndrome shares characteristics with FAP in that it is due to an autosomal dominant mutation in the *APC* gene. Notably, Gardner syndrome is also associated with formation of adenomatous polyps as opposed to hamartomas that occur in PJS (Baldino et al., 2019). The *APC* gene on chromosome 5q21 is responsible for Gardner syndrome too. The gene encodes a protein that plays a substantive role in cell adhesion and signal transduction. In Gardner syndrome, the APC mutation goes beyond just effects on the colorectum and involves tissue growth in other body areas (hence the tumors and osteomas) (Baldino et al., 2019; Katabathina et al., 2019).

Clinical Presentation

Gardner syndrome has a clinical presentation that is distinct from FAP. In addition to colonic polyposis, Gardner syndrome is associated with osteomas, epidermoid cysts, soft tissue tumors, fibromas, and/or desmoid tumors (Samadder et al., 2019b). In particular, skin manifestations of Gardner syndrome include epidermoid cysts, trichilemmal hybrid, or pilomatricomas developing on the face, scalp, or limbs of patients; something called a nuchal fibroma (diffuse induration and swelling of the back of the neck); and a "Gardner fibroma" area of thick collagen bundles and interspersed fibroblasts located mostly on the trunk (Ponti et al., 2013, pp. 244–245). Osteomas can arise on the mandible and skull. Dental lesions occur in almost one fifth of patients including odontomas, absent, excess, or rudimentary teeth, or multiple caries. It is important to remember that osteoma onset in facial bones and skull precedes GI polyposis (Baldino et al., 2019; Lv et al., 2018). Desmoid tumors do not have a malignant potential since they are locally invasive fibromatoses but can be highly aggressive in growth (Shah et al., 2013). They are associated with a higher mortality and morbidity because they can cause local destruction or tissue blockage. Intra-abdominal desmoid tumors can cause intestinal obstruction, blockage of the ureters,

intestinal hemorrhage, or enterocutaneous fistulae (Katabathina et al., 2019).

Medical Management

Like other polyposis syndromes, endoscopic surveillance is required in Gardner syndrome. Panoramic dental radiographs may detect occult lesions in Gardner syndrome patients.

Prophylaxis regimens for Gardner syndrome have been proposed too. Celecoxib (a COX-2 NSAID) was recommended previously but is of questionable long-term safety due to associated cardiovascular events. Sulindac has also been tested but has a risk of adverse effects on the stomach. With appropriate medical management of GI toxicity (protective coating agents and use of H_2 blockers and proton pump inhibitors), sulindac may be more tolerable in longer usage (Ponti et al., 2013). It should be noted that osteoma formation may *precede* the formation of colon polyps in Gardner syndrome. Persons with a family history should be screened for GI tract involvement if other extraintestinal lesions are identified and genetic counseling is required (Baldino et al., 2019).

Surgical Management

Gardner syndrome is associated with the potential for multiple extraintestinal tissue growth. Consequently, total colectomy is not "curative" therapy. However, surgery may be required if polyps or desmoid tumors obstruct the intestine or if desmoids obstruct the ureters, kidneys, or other vital body systems.

A notable finding in both Gardner syndrome and FAP is the relationship of desmoid tumor formation and trauma. It is hypothesized that abdominal surgery can accelerate or precipitate desmoid formation and growth. The exact pathogenesis of this process is not understood (Katabathina et al., 2019; Xuereb et al., 2017). When small bowel obstruction occurs related to desmoid tumors, several techniques are possible. Intestinal resection, bypass, and strictureplasty have all been used successfully. Desmoids can be locally aggressive and devastating. Desmoids are the cause of death in up to 10% of patients with FAP (Katabathina et al., 2019).

PEUTZ-JEGHERS SYNDROME

PJS is a polyposis syndrome characterized by the formation of hamartomatous polyps in the GI tract as opposed to adenomatous polyps. The hamartomatous syndromes like PJS are much less common than are adenomatous syndromes, approximately 1/10 the frequency (Chung, 2019a,b; Kennedy et al., 2017).

PJS is a rare disease that has an autosomal dominant inheritance pattern. In addition, to the occurrence of hamartomatous polyps in the GI tract, there is usually a family history of PJS and a classical pigmentation finding. The hamartomatous polyps occur most frequently in the small bowel. The characteristic extraintestinal manifestation is mucocutaneous pigmentation (i.e., freckles) of the lips and buccal mucosa (Kennedy et al., 2017; Kumar et al., 2019).

Etiology

Most PJS cases are due to a germline mutation in the nuclear serine–threonine kinase gene *LKBI/STKII* that regulates cell polarization, metabolism, and cell growth and is likely a tumor suppressor gene. The result of the mutation is a truncated protein with no kinase activity (Kennedy et al., 2017; Latchford et al., 2019).

The hamartomas that occur in PJS are macroscopically large and pedunculated. The main histologic characteristic of Peutz-Jeghers polyps is the presence of a central core of bands of smooth muscle covered by mucosa similar to the body region with normal or hyperplastic glandular epithelium. A histologic description of a polyp with these characteristics can assist (along with demonstrable genetic findings) with the diagnosis of PJS (Chung, 2019a,b). They most commonly occur in the small bowel (jejunum most common) but can also occur in the stomach, colon, and, with much less frequency, in the bladder and lungs. They can also occur in the nose, uterus, and gallbladder. While polyps occur most commonly in the small intestine in PJS, the colon is the most frequent site for GI malignancy (Chung, 2019b; Latchford et al., 2019).

Clinical Presentation

PJS usually presents around a median age of 11 years. Classic appearance is altered pigmentation in the form of dark blue to brown macules around the mouth, eyes, nostrils, buccal mucosa, palmar surface of the hands, and genitalia and perianally. It is pigment-laden (melanin) macrophages present in the dermis (Chung, 2019b). Notably, some patients have no pigmentary changes, but 95% of PJS patients have mucocutaneous pigmented lesions (Latchford et al., 2019). When these pigmentary changes do occur, they usually start fading from the third decade onward (Chung, 2019b; Samadder et al., 2019a).

Affected patients usually enter the health care system and begin surveillance after they present with an acute complication. The complications may include abdominal pain due to bowel obstruction, intussusception, volvulus, and rectal bleeding. Once identified, family members should be assessed as well. A definite diagnosis of PJS includes at least two of the following characteristics: (1) hyperpigmentation of the lips or buccal mucosa, (2) two or more hamartomatous polyps in the GI tract, or (3) a PJS family history (Chung, 2019b).

World Health Organization (WHO) criteria differ slightly as definitive diagnosis includes any one of the following: (1) three or more histologically confirmed Peutz-Jeghers polyps, (2) any number of Peutz-Jeghers polyps with a family history of PJS, (3) characteristic prominent mucocutaneous pigmentation with a family history of PJS, or (4)

any number of Peutz-Jeghers polyps and characteristic, prominent mucocutaneous pigmentation (Kennedy et al., 2017; To & Cagir, 2018).

Medical Management

Medical therapy involves ongoing intestinal endoscopic surveillance plus continuous screening for extraintestinal cancer (mammogram, PAP test, testicular ultrasound, etc.) (Chung, 2019b). Endoscopy of both the upper and lower GI tract is recommended. Given PJS's predilection for the small bowel, a small bowel series or capsule endoscopy is usually recommended starting around 8 years of age. Polyps can be removed endoscopically depending on the number of polyps. Surveillance endoscopy should be done every 2 to 3 years (Latchford et al., 2019). Notably, the cancer risks associated with PJS are more significant after 30 years with GI tract cancers having the highest cumulative risk with an average age of 42 years at cancer diagnosis (Chung, 2019b). Ideally, PJS is best managed by specialist centers with expert providers (Latchford et al., 2019).

Surgical Management

Acute surgical intervention is sometimes required for intussusception, volvulus, and small bowel obstruction. CRCs associated with PJS should be managed like other CRCs with segmental resection. Prophylactic colectomy is *not* recommended for PJS given its location in multiple body sites (Kumar et al., 2019). If polyps are above 1.5 cm in size or are suspicious for malignancy, they should be removed endoscopically or, if necessary, surgically (Latchford et al., 2019).

DIVERTICULAR DISEASE

Diverticular disease is a disorder that represents a spectrum of clinical presentation varying from totally asymptomatic and uncomplicated to acute situations requiring emergency surgery with a diversion of fecal stream. Diverticulosis is the term used to describe the presence of colonic diverticula, that is, small sac-like outpouchings of the intestinal wall. Diverticulitis describes when one or more of these diverticula become inflamed. Diverticular disease includes both diverticulosis and diverticulitis. For most people, diverticulosis is discovered only incidentally at colonoscopy or barium enema testing (Pemberton, 2019c). Diverticular disease is a very common GI disorder in the developed world with highest rates in the United States and Europe. Colonic diverticulosis is the most common finding on screening colonoscopies in the United States (Camilleri et al., 2019). By age 80, about 75% of Americans have diverticulosis (Camilleri et al., 2019). Acute diverticulitis is the most common complication of diverticular disease affecting 5% to 15% of patients (Camilleri et al., 2019; DiSiena & Birk, 2018; Pemberton, 2019c; Tursi & Elisei, 2019).

ETIOLOGY

Diverticular disease has been noted to be a disease of aging, that is, acquired over time and is possibly linked to diet. Specifically, diverticulosis is thought to be a "deficiency" disease of Western civilization based on low intake of fiber (Tursi, 2019; Tursi & Elisei, 2019). Painter and Burkitt (1971) originally hypothesized that low-fiber diets resulted in small-volume dry stools that required higher pressures for colonic transit. However, this perspective has been challenged since low fiber intake is not associated with diverticulosis risk (Tursi & Elisei, 2019).

Low fiber theoretically creates the higher luminal pressures that are thought to encourage the mucosa and submucosa to herniate through the bowel wall muscle at the sites where blood vessels perforate the muscle layer (points of greater weakness). Diverticula may develop more in the sigmoid colon because intraluminal pressures are highest in this region (DiSiena & Birk, 2018). The theory provides a logical explanation of why diverticulosis increases with age (Pemberton, 2019c). Note that this etiologic fiber hypothesis has persisted for over 40 years largely without proof. A study by Peery et al. (2012) demonstrated that a high-fiber diet was associated with a *higher* prevalence of diverticula. Conversely, there is some evidence that a high-fiber diet may protect against diverticular disease (i.e., diverticulitis) (Burgell et al., 2013; DiSiena & Birk, 2018; Peery et al., 2013).

In a cross-sectional colonoscopy-based study of 539 people with diverticulosis and 1,569 without it, neither constipation nor a low-fiber diet was associated with an increased risk of diverticulosis (Peery et al., 2013). So findings continue to be mutually contradictory.

Another etiologic perspective relates to the effect of aging on colon tissue. Age-related changes in the connective tissue of the large bowel include an increase in collagen cross-linking and increased elastin; both may contribute to increased colon rigidity (Boynton & Floch, 2013).

Interestingly, when diverticulosis occurs in persons younger than 40 years of age, they tend to be obese and male and the cases are less likely to be complicated; however, emergency operation rates are higher. The diagnosis of diverticulitis should be included in the differential diagnosis of younger male obese patients with lower abdominal pain (Broad et al., 2019a,b; Pilgrim et al., 2013). A cross-sectional study of 23 patients <50 years old demonstrated that risk factors for acute diverticulosis included obesity, male gender, and consumption of alcohol (Pisanu et al., 2013).

Notably, research has demonstrated that nuts and seeds do not increase the risk of diverticulitis or a diverticular bleed (Pemberton, 2019c). Though it was thought that nuts and seeds could obstruct the diverticula and cause a perforation, Strate and colleagues (2008) found

no association in a study that included 47,228 men aged 40 to 75 years.

An evolving concept on the pathogenesis of diverticular disease is the role of genetic susceptibility. It is theorized and is currently being studied whether diverticular disease is heritable. Tursi (2019) suggests that selected genes may affect intestinal neuromuscular function with impaired smooth muscle function and impaired connective tissue support. But the impact of genetic variation on diverticular disease mechanisms still remains unknown.

While inflammation likely does not play a significant role in the pathogenesis of diverticulosis, inflammation is involved in acute diverticulitis. Tursi and Elisei (2019) hypothesize that the inflammation may be due to bowel trauma (fecalith impaction eroding mucosa) or ischemic mechanisms (compression of the vascular structures in the neck of the diverticulum). They suggest both mechanisms may act to the trigger inflammation.

Another possible factor in diverticular disease is theorized to be the gut microbiome. It is hypothesized that dysbiosis of microbes in the gut lumen together with mucosal barrier breakdown and bacterial translocation leading to an inflammatory response (Rezapour & Stollman, 2019). Two other possible risk factors in the literature include smoking and medications. A modest positive association between smoking and diverticulitis has been described. Certain medications increase risk for diverticular disease including NSAIDs, steroids, and opiates (DiSiena & Birk, 2018).

CLINICAL PRESENTATION

Diverticulosis remains asymptomatic in the majority of patients. However, about 20% will experience complications. The two major recognized complications are acute episodes of bleeding and diverticulitis (Pemberton 2019a,e; Tursi & Elisei, 2019).

The symptom presentation in diverticulosis may be subtle and then more pronounced. Patients may report chronic vague GI symptoms including mild abdominal pain, bloating, constipation, and diarrhea or fluctuating bowel habits. Physical examination at this point is usually normal.

When acute diverticulitis strikes, the patient reports abdominal pain in the left lower abdominal quadrant. This presentation occurs because in almost all patients with diverticulosis, the sigmoid and descending colon are involved (Pemberton, 2019d; Tursi & Elisei, 2019).

MEDICAL MANAGEMENT

Symptom management and medical management depend on the state of diverticular disease: diverticulosis versus diverticulitis. Though the fiber hypothesis is not fully supported by research, contemporary diverticulosis medical therapy still targets fiber. In asymptomatic disease that is discovered incidentally, the patient should be counseled to eat a high-fiber diet. Fiber supplements such as psyllium or methylcellulose may also assist with less constipated stool movements.

Most diverticulitis patients can be managed conservatively. For those with mild symptoms and no signs of abdominal complications (e.g., peritoneal signs), they can be treated as outpatients via a clear liquid diet and broad-spectrum antibiotics covering anaerobes, for example, metronidazole 500 mg three times daily or amoxicillin/clavulanate 875/125 mg twice daily plus either ciprofloxacin 500 mg twice daily or trimethoprim–sulfamethoxazole 160/800 mg twice daily for 7 to 10 days or until the patient is afebrile for 72 hours (Broad et al., 2019a; Pemberton, 2019a). A recent retrospective review supported that outpatient treatment for acute uncomplicated diverticulitis was feasible and safe in 50 patients, and they were treated without antibiotics (Azhar et al., 2019).

If symptoms worsen (increasing pain, high fevers, increased white blood cell counts, or peritoneal signs, e.g., rebound tenderness), patients should be hospitalized. Patients should be NPO, be placed on IV fluids, and be given antibiotics covering anaerobic and gram-negative bacteria usually for 5 to 7 days before converting to oral therapy. Commonly used agents include cefoxitin, piperacillin–tazobactam, or ticarcillin–clavulanate (Pemberton, 2019a).

The degree of complexity of diverticulitis can be described using something called the modified Hinchey classification. Based on diagnostic testing and operative findings, the diverticulitis complexity can be placed into one of four stages: stage 1, pericolonic abscess; stage 2, pelvic abscess; stage 3, purulent peritonitis; and stage 4, fecal peritonitis (Hinchey et al., 1978; Pemberton, 2019b). The higher the stage, the more likely a multistage surgery will be used and the higher the associated morbidities. If an abscess is developed related to the diverticulitis, a higher risk of surgical intervention is noted (Pemberton, 2019b; Van De Wall et al., 2013). A colonoscopy should never be done during a diverticulitis attack for risk of bowel perforation. After 6 weeks, it should be done to rule out colon cancer (Lipman, 2018).

SURGICAL MANAGEMENT

Surgical management is usually reserved for those individuals who have had diverticulitis with complications. For persons who have had multiple episodes of diverticulitis, an elective bowel resection of the worst affected parts may be done to ameliorate the likelihood of future attacks. However, prophylactic bowel resection is being questioned for its efficacy in prevention (Lutwak & Dill, 2013; Pemberton, 2019b). Elective surgery for uncomplicated diverticulitis should be done on a case-by-case basis considering patient-specific factors like age, computed tomography (CT)-graded severity, and patients' medical condition (Skoldberg et al., 2019; Turley et al., 2013).

For persons who develop acute diverticulitis with complications (e.g., peritonitis, abscess), emergency surgery will be performed. Commonly, a temporary colostomy and a Hartmann's procedure will be done. Some authors suggest that it is best reserved for Hinchey IV patients (Morini et al., 2019). This approach leaves the anus and rectal stump inside the body closed over with surgical staples. The proximal part of the bowel exits the body in the left lower quadrant as a stoma. When the sepsis resolves (usually 12 to 16 weeks later), the two segments can be reconnected. This approach is usually reserved for patients who are more severely toxic.

Some surgeons do not use the two-step Hartmann's surgery but rather complete it in one step. The diseased segment is removed, the two open bowel ends are cleansed with irrigation, and a primary anastomosis is completed. Sometimes a proximal diversion is used for perforated diverticulitis (Pemberton, 2019b). Both one-stage and Hartmann's procedures can be done laparoscopically (Cassini et al., 2017; Turley et al., 2013). A systematic review by Gaertner et al. (2013) suggests that elective laparoscopic colon resection for diverticular disease is associated with better outcomes and less complications than open colectomy.

Another systematic review examined use of open versus laparoscopic sigmoid resection approaches for treating acute uncomplicated diverticulitis and the use of laparoscopic lavage with resection for treatment of perforated diverticulitis with peritonitis. The authors (Ahmed et al., 2018) found no statistically significant difference in postoperative mortality and morbidity. Both were equally effective. Halim et al. (2019) also conducted a systematic review support for both primary anastomosis and Hartmann's procedure and both acceptable in terms of mortality and wound infection. Increasingly, laparoscopic versus open approaches will be used for both (Kurumboor et al., 2017).

The timing for optimal closure of the colostomy in Hartmann's procedure is much less clear. In a retrospective analysis of a large database of over 1,600 patients who underwent Hartmann's procedure for acute diverticulitis, only 28.3% underwent colostomy closure within a year. Outcomes of the reversal surgery were not influenced by elapsed time from the colostomy creation; optimal timing is unclear and remains at surgeon and patient discretion (Resio et al., 2019). In responding to the Resio et al. publication, Basson (2019) noted that other factors may influence closure timing such as race and socioeconomic status. Bridoux et al. (2017) conducted a multicenter randomized controlled trial (RCT) on diverticulitis patients comparing Hartmann's procedure versus primary anastomosis with diverting stoma. In 102 patients, the primary end point was mortality at 18 months. No difference in mortality was identified. However, the rate of stoma reversal (for the diverting ileostomy) was significantly higher in the primary anastomosis group.

When diffuse peritonitis occurs, "damage control" surgery can be used. This involves laparotomy, resection of the bowel segment affected, copious irrigation of the abdomen, and use of negative pressure wound therapy for the open abdominal wall. The decision to restore continuity or create an end colostomy is postponed for 24 to 48 hours. In the 34 patients studied in the multicenter design, damage control approach was feasible for peritonitis patients and resulted in higher levels of bowel reconstruction (Tartaglia et al., 2019).

 ## RADIATION ENTERITIS

Radiation enteritis, sometimes called radiation enteropathy, is a rare complication of radiation therapy for pelvic malignancy, mainly prostate, rectal, and gynecological cancers. If GI structures are within the radiation therapy field, tissue injury to the GI tract especially the small intestine may occur during treatment or at a variable time following therapy. As more patients survive cancer and radiation is included in multiple cancer care pathways, the incidence of radiation-related GI complications continues to increase (Czito et al., 2019; Kumagai et al., 2018).

KEY POINT

Due to the nature of the treatment, radiotherapy can affect tissue and other organs in the pelvic region. Although they may be called "late effects," some symptoms may occur at any time from during treatment to many years later.

The effects of radiation enteritis can be profound. Over half of patients so affected report that the disorder detrimentally affects their quality of life (Kumagai et al., 2018; Roberts, 2019).

ETIOLOGY

The relationship of radiation enteritis or damage to the intestinal tissue from radiation effects is clear. The radiation damages tissue usually in a dose-dependent fashion. At higher doses, up to 50% of patients may experience radiation enteritis especially in its chronic form (Anwar et al., 2017; Hogan et al., 2013). With radiation exposure, transient mucosal atrophy occurs with stem cell loss and reduced crypt mitoses causing epithelial denudation and dysfunction. Notably, a spectrum of disease exists with some individuals affected more potentially determined by genomic susceptibility to ionizing radiation (Hogan et al., 2013; Roberts, 2019).

Radiation enteritis can develop acutely (usually within 2 weeks of radiation exposure). Tissue damage occurs, and nutrient and fluid loss ensue. Usually, symptoms are self-limiting (Ashburn & Kalady, 2016).

Chronic radiation enteritis most commonly occurs within 18 to 80 months of treatment. However, cases have occurred decades following exposure (Ashburn & Kalady, 2016; Czito et al., 2019). The damage underlying chronic radiation enteritis seems to be mostly related to inflammation, fibrosis, and scar formation (Anwar et al., 2017) **(Table 7-1)**. The intestinal tissue may appear pale, mottled, or telangiectatic. Vascular insufficiency may be present. In its severe form, chronic radiation enteritis may lead to intestinal obstruction or fistula formation (Li et al., 2013).

Patient risk factors may determine susceptibility to intestinal radiation injury. Medical comorbidities such as hypertension, diabetes mellitus, atherosclerosis, inflammatory bowel disease, collagen vascular disorders, and human immunodeficiency virus (HIV) infection may impact individual susceptibility to radiation toxicity. Genetic variations (a patient's genotype) may also play a role in radiotherapy susceptibility (Czito et al., 2019; Roberts, 2019). A person's intestinal microbiome may also play a role in disease pathogenesis (Kumagai et al., 2018; Sokol & Adolph, 2018).

CLINICAL PRESENTATION

Clinical manifestations of GI radiation injury can be acute or delayed. Acute symptoms are related to acute mucosal injury and inflammation. Chronic symptoms derive from fibrosis and vascular sclerosis. Clinical symptoms are also dependent upon the degree and extent of tissue damage plus the location of injury (Czito et al., 2019; Roberts, 2019).

Symptoms of acute and chronic GI radiation injury may include nausea, vomiting, abdominal pain, diarrhea, rectal pain, urgency, fecal incontinence, and bleeding. Chronic radiation enteritis may also be associated with malabsorption, bacterial overgrowth, rapid intestinal transit, and lactose intolerance. Bowel obstruction and fistulization can also occur. Constipation may alternate with diarrhea, and fecal incontinence may occur due to loss of anorectal compliance (Czito et al., 2019; Roberts, 2019).

TABLE 7-1 INTESTINAL TISSUE CHANGES RELATED TO RADIATION ENTERITIS

ACUTE	CHRONIC
Crypt microabscesses	Submucosal fibrosis
Inflammatory cell infiltrate	Lymphatic dilatation
Decreased crypt mitoses	Obliterative endarteritis
Epithelial ulceration and denudation	Tissue ischemia
	Tissue necrosis

Data from Anwar, M., Ahmad, S., Akhtar, R., et al. (2017). Antioxidant supplementation: A linchpin in radiation-induced enteritis. *Technology in Cancer Research & Treatment, 16*(6), 676–691; Ashburn, J. H., & Kalady, M. F. (2016). Radiation-induced problems in colorectal surgery. *Clinics in Colon and Rectal Surgery, 29*(2), 85–91; Czito, B., Meyer, J., & Willett, C. G. (2019). *Overview of gastrointestinal toxicity of radiation therapy.* UptoDate. Retrieved September 15, 2019, from www.uptodate.com; Kumagai, T., Rahman, F., & Smith, A. M. (2018). The microbiome and radiation-induced bowel injury: Evidence for potential mechanistic role in disease pathogenesis. *Nutrients, 10*, 1405, 16 pages. doi: 10.3390/NU10101405.

MEDICAL MANAGEMENT

The evidence base for radiation enteritis medical treatment is limited. Approaches include nutrition therapy, medications (antidiarrheals, anti-inflammatory agents, probiotics, antibiotics, cholestyramine, sucralfate) hyperbaric oxygen therapy (HBOT), and endoscopic management. Management is based on treating the predominant symptoms (Gandle et al., 2019; Roberts, 2019; Wu et al., 2019).

Antidiarrheal drugs like loperamide (preferred) or codeine phosphate can be used to slow diarrhea and transit time, thereby improving bile salt absorption. While these control symptoms, they do not target the etiology (Roberts, 2019).

Anti-inflammatory agents like sulfasalazine and selected steroids (e.g., methylprednisolone), probiotics (VSL#3, a combination of live lactic acid bacteria, and bifidobacteria) (Kumagai et al., 2018), and antibiotics (e.g., metronidazole and doxycycline) have also been tried with limited success. No studies have addressed clinical efficacy with larger samples. Their use therefore may be empirical and based on individual response (Roberts, 2019).

Many symptoms of chronic radiation enteritis are related to bile salt malabsorption. Cholestyramine has been used in selected patients with some success. The drug is not very palatable, and many patients discontinue usage (Roberts, 2019).

Antibiotics can help reduce symptoms in some patients. They are used for patients with evidence of small intestinal bacterial overgrowth (Roberts, 2019).

HBOT has been used in small numbers of patients with some success since it is theorized to facilitate angiogenesis and possibly have an antibacterial effect. However, much research needs to be done to ascertain its true effectiveness (Ashburn & Kalady, 2016; Roberts, 2019; Stacey & Green, 2014).

Endoscopic laser therapy (e.g., argon plasma coagulation) has been used to help symptoms by treating radiation-induced colon telangiectasia and hemorrhages. It has to be used with great care given the risk of perforation in abnormal GI tissue (Ashburn & Kalady, 2016; Stacey & Green, 2014).

Research is investigating the possibility of *preventing* radiation enteritis. Medical approaches like nutrition (diets high in glutamine, arginine, vitamins) and pharmacological therapies like statins (e.g., pravastatin) (Jang et al., 2018) and angiotensin-converting enzyme (ACE) inhibitors (Stacey & Green, 2014) are being tested. An interesting approach is use of circadian rhythm. Less cellular activity occurs in the GI tract during evening hours. Animal models are being used to test if evening radiotherapy is less damaging (Stacey & Green, 2014).

Other areas being researched include use of antioxidant therapy (e.g., vitamins E, C, etc.) on oxidative free radicals in the intestinal tissue to reduce inflammation and damage (Anwar et al., 2017). Substances potentially altering the intestinal microbiome like probiotics (Kumagai et al., 2018), herbal medicine combinations (Murai et al., 2019), and possible herbal radioprotective substances like zingerone (Wu et al., 2019) (an essential oil of ginger) are being studied for their efficacy in both treatment and protection of radiation enteritis (RE); as there is no clinically effective treatment for RE, research is urgently needed.

SURGICAL MANAGEMENT

Radiation enteritis is associated with progressive vasculitis in the bowel wall resulting in ulceration, stenosis, or perforation. Indications for surgical intervention include acute intestinal obstruction, intestinal fistulae, bowel perforation, intestinal bleeding, neoplasm, and malnutrition. Surgery is usually for patients with complicated, prolonged disease (Otterson, 2019). In the past, bowel resection was more frequently used but often resulted in intestinal failure (Kappus et al., 2016; Lenti & DiSabatino, 2019). Contemporary approaches are more conservative. Strictureplasty offers an intestine-preserving method that decreases mortality and morbidity. In the case of chronic radiation enteritis with small bowel obstruction, resection of the blockage is preferred if there is adequate intestinal reserve (Otterson, 2019). The best "surgical" treatment is preventing radiation enteritis from occurring. The choice of incision for the surgery is also an area requiring careful thought. Many surgeons will choose a lower transverse incision to avoid irradiated areas. Laparoscopy would be a logical choice, but dense adhesions may preclude use. Due to the risk of poor wound healing and infection, many surgeons will avoid a large vertical incision (Hogan et al., 2013). If severe malnutrition due to chronic radiation enteritis does not respond to dietary manipulation, antimotility agents, electrolyte correction, probiotics or parenteral nutrition, surgical resection, or small bowel transplantation may be necessary (Otterson, 2019).

When the surgery for radiation enteritis requires a stoma, it should be placed outside of the radiation field. Some patients will have indelible tattoos to guide stoma siting selection. If not marked, the potential stoma site should be designated with a metallic marker before barium or CT imaging studies to reveal whether the stoma site is adjacent to severely damaged intestine (Otterson, 2019).

Prevention of radiation enteritis has been attempted by surgical placement of intestinal slings to keep the bowel away from radiation. Other approaches include physical positioning during exposure so that small bowel segments are not exposed. Another approach is bladder distention during treatment to push small intestine away from the treatment field. Whatever the approach used, a resounding theme pervades the literature on radiation enteritis. *Preventing* damage is optimal treatment though how to best achieve this outcome is unclear. For those people affected, the key is early recognition and referral to a GI specialist. Even with best medical and surgical intervention, prognosis for chronic radiation enteritis is variable. Early mortality is usually due to cancer recurrence. Five-year survival is 70% for noncancer patients as the disease is progressive (Roberts, 2019).

ABDOMINAL/PELVIC TRAUMA

Abdominal and pelvic trauma is usually characterized or divided into two categories: blunt and penetrating. Both forms can cause serious damage to the GI tract and surrounding structures. Notably, pelvic trauma mostly results from high-energy blunt trauma (e.g., motor vehicle accidents), but frail and elderly patients may sustain injury from low-energy mechanisms (e.g., fall). High-energy trauma raises the likelihood of concomitant injuries of the abdominal and pelvic organs and may be associated with serious pelvic fractures (Fiechtl, 2019). In general, penetrating trauma is more likely to result in a fecal diversion especially if the trauma involves the rectum. Fecal diversion remains the mainstay of treatment for rectal trauma to prevent further pelvic contamination and limit sepsis.

ETIOLOGY

The abdomen is divided into three different anatomic sites: the peritoneal space, the retroperitoneal space, and the pelvis (Eckert, 2005). Another schema divides the abdominal cavity into four anatomic zones: anterior abdomen, flanks (right and left), and back (Colwell & Moore, 2019). Any of these areas can be traumatized due to gunshot wounds, stabbing penetrating wounds, or blunt injuries due to seat belts, blast injuries of higher or lower velocity, or rapid deceleration damage. However, penetrating trauma is much more commonly related to intestinal and rectal injuries than blunt (Sarani & Martin, 2019).

CLINICAL PRESENTATION

Patient presentation of abdominal trauma can vary widely depending on etiology and severity of injury. For example, a patient with a gunshot wound (or several) may display loss of consciousness and signs of hypovolemic shock. Conversely, a stab wound victim with a shallow depth injury may display less altered vital signs and be awake and cooperative.

Blunt abdominal trauma that is more common than penetrating may present as bruising and pain or minimal apparent damage. Pieces of equipment like seat belts may leave distinctive marks on the skin. Attention to vital signs is critical in blunt trauma as well. Blunt trauma to the liver, intestine, and other vital structures can become life threatening (Colwell & Moore, 2019; Diercks & Clarke, 2019).

Quality expeditious physical assessment is mandatory as abdominal trauma can affect blood and nerve supply to the extremities. In addition, more hidden injuries to the pelvic area may also be present. Diagnostic imaging will be used to assess the nature and severity of the damage as well (Benjamin, 2019).

Though not a particularly common abdominal/pelvic trauma, the issue of rectal trauma from foreign bodies cannot be ignored. Rectal foreign bodies can represent a variety of objects and can be associated with bowel perforation and delayed injury. Foreign body placement can be voluntary or involuntary (e.g., sexual assault) and sexual versus nonsexual (e.g., "body packing" of illegal drugs). Whatever the cause, patients are usually reluctant to fully disclose their history. Consequently, excellent physical examination including radiologic examination (e.g., abdominal flat plate x-ray) should be used to assess for signs of perforation. Whether the patient requires a diverting stoma depends on the patient's status, degree of injury, and severity of intra-abdominal fecal contamination (Steele & Goldberg, 2019).

MEDICAL MANAGEMENT

Nonoperative management of abdominal trauma is more commonly associated with blunt or nonpenetrating trauma. However, the literature is also describing nonoperative management of penetrating abdominal gunshot wounds (Benjamin, 2019; Varga et al., 2013).

Since World War II, mandatory exploration of the abdomen was the customary approach. As imaging technology has evolved, CT scanning has permitted selective nonoperative management. However, appropriate patient selection is critical to outcomes success (Benjamin, 2019; Colwell & Moore, 2019). Several contraindications are noted for nonoperative management. They include presence of hemodynamic instability, diffuse abdominal pain, peritonitis, or evisceration. In addition, patients who cannot have serial abdominal examinations (e.g., concomitant head or spinal injury) are not good candidates.

Medical management of abdominal trauma includes monitoring of vital signs, appropriate fluid resuscitation as necessary, CT scanning, laboratory testing, ultrasonography, and vigilance for signs of clinical deterioration (e.g., hemodynamic instability, discharge from peritoneum, febrile status) (Diercks & Clarke, 2019).

SURGICAL MANAGEMENT

Modern surgical management of abdominal trauma generally includes the concept of damage control. This process is a staged or stepped approach in which a shortened surgery is used to control immediate life-threatening issues of coagulopathy and hemorrhage, hypothermia, and metabolic acidosis. Physiological restoration then occurs in the intensive care unit with eventual return to the OR for definitive surgery (Benjamin,

2019). For abdominal trauma, damage control laparotomy (DCL) is considered standard of care (Sarani & Martin, 2019).

In the case of intestinal especially colon injury, the trauma surgeon is left with a choice upon return to the OR for definitive repair. The surgeon can do a primary repair of colon discontinuity or create an ostomy for fecal diversion (Benjamin, 2019). While ostomy was considered the gold standard of treatment for decades following World War II, some surgeons decided to try primary repair instead. A recent analysis of the U.S. National Trauma Data Bank shows that there is a definite move away from mandatory fecal diversion to primary colon repair (Hatch et al., 2013). The analysis showed that the overall fecal diversion rate was 9% in the 6,817 patients from 2007 to 2009 who sustained primary colon injuries. Selected factors were associated with diversion: older age, higher injury severity scores, and especially sigmoid colon injury. In addition, U.S. military and worldwide combat operations have demonstrated a change from mandatory fecal diversion or injury exteriorization to the current recommendation of primary repair or resection and reanastomosis (Johnson & Steele, 2013).

Surgical research has added another dimension to when surgeons will or won't divert the fecal stream in colonic injury. Sharpe et al. (2012) reported on the use of a management algorithm in penetrating colon injuries over 15 years in 252 patients with full-thickness colon injuries. More severe destructive injuries associated with pre- or intraoperative transfusion requirements of more than 6 units of packed red blood cells and/or significant morbidities were best managed with fecal diversion.

Another retrospective study examining the years 2000–2010 for surgical patients with colonic injuries and the use of DCL looked at the use of fecal diversion or primary anastomosis (Georgoff et al., 2013). The complication rate in both primary anastomosis patients (*N* = 28) versus diversion patients (*N* = 33) was similar. The authors supported that "a strategy of diversion over anastomosis cannot be strongly recommended" (Georgoff et al., 2013, p. 293).

One factor that can complicate postoperative recovery is the use of open abdomen management of abdominal trauma care whether a diversion is used or not. In a retrospective study of 120 open abdomen patients (35 for hemorrhagic situations), with mean follow-up at 21 months, 30 patients (25%) developed a ventral hernia, 13 patients (11%) experienced an enterocutaneous fistula, and 2 patients experienced bowel obstruction. If trauma care involved use of open abdomen therapy, a high incidence of complications can accompany long-term recovery (Frazee et al., 2013).

An instance in which abdominal trauma will likely involve a fecal diversion is rectal trauma. If the rectal trauma is below the peritoneal reflection, direct repair is usually impossible and the mainstay of treatment is fecal diversion to avoid further contamination (Benjamin, 2019; Steele & Goldberg, 2019).

 ## OTHER INDICATIONS

OBSTRUCTION

Intestinal obstruction or acute bowel obstruction is a generic phrase that covers multiple pathologies both inherent to the GI tract and external to it in the peritoneal cavity. In general, acute mechanical bowel obstruction is observed in the small bowel in 75% of cases and large bowel in 25% of cases. The etiology is often related to age (Karakas et al., 2019). In some instances, bowel obstruction is functional rather than mechanical (called Ogilvie syndrome) (Camilleri, 2019). Given available space, only three disorders will be addressed: volvulus, intussusception, and colonic inertia. The former two are issues related to mechanical or structural forces, while inertia is more functional in nature.

KEY POINT

Tumors, scar tissue (adhesions), or twisting or narrowing of the intestines are mechanical bowel obstructions, and hernias, Crohn's disease (from strictures), and tumors can also block the intestine (Catena et al., 2019; Farkas et al., 2019). For malignant bowel obstruction, colonic stenting can be used as a bridge to surgery (Donlon et al., 2019).

VOLVULUS

Volvulus (from the Latin for "to roll") refers to torsion or twisting of the bowel around its own mesentery. It can affect any area of the GI tract, but colonic volvulus is more common with small bowel volvulus being rare (Amoli et al., 2019; Heo et al., 2019). When volvulus does occur in the colon, it usually affects the sigmoid or cecal segments and less frequently the transverse colon and splenic flexure (Heo et al., 2019). Colonic volvulus accounts for about 3% to 5% of bowel obstruction cases in the United States. However, higher areas of endemicity (prevalent in or peculiar to a particular locality, region, or people) occur across the globe. Africa, the Middle East, and South American rates are much higher; 10% to 50% of bowel obstructions in these regions are due to colonic volvulus (Queneherve et al., 2019). Variations may be due to dietary anatomical, cultural, or infection-related differences (Atamanalp, 2019; Hasnaoui et al., 2019; Heo et al., 2019). When colon volvulus, especially cecal volvulus, occurs in developed countries, adhesions, gynecologic operations, pelvic masses, poor muscle tone, and distal obstruction may be possible causes (Hasnaoui et al., 2019). A characteristic "whirlpool" sign is seen on CT scan with intestinal volvulus (Amoli et al., 2019).

INTUSSUSCEPTION

Intussusception also generates bowel obstruction but in a different way. Intussusception, a disorder that is more common in children (Amuddhu et al., 2018), is the process in which the intestine telescopes back on itself. Ileocolic intussusception represents 90% of all intussusceptions (Mandeville et al., 2012).

The etiology of intussusception is unknown, but the incidence peaks between 3 months and 3 years (Kumar et al., 2019). It is suggested to be due to lymphoid hyperplasia or uncoordinated peristalsis of the intestine. Other possibilities include viral infections especially adenovirus. The blockage can result in bowel necrosis if left untreated. Intussusception is the most common cause of intestinal obstruction in the first 2 years of life (Kumar et al., 2019).

Volvulus and intussusception both present with abdominal pain and vomiting, and a palpable abdominal mass is usually present. In intussusception, bloody stool ("red currant jelly stool") may also be present. However, in intussusception, the four classic signs and symptoms just mentioned present in less than half of patients with the disorder (Kumar et al., 2019). Adults with intussusception present with vaguer symptoms, and diagnosis relies more heavily on diagnostic imaging (Hinton, 2017; Lief et al., 2019).

Medical and Surgical Management

Both medical and surgical interventions may be needed for volvulus and intussusception. Required surgery is dependent upon response to medical intervention and diagnostic studies (Long et al., 2019).

Pillars of management for children with suspected volvulus are initial stabilization with aggressive fluid resuscitation, stomach decompression with a nasogastric tube, and immediate referral to a surgeon (Brandt, 2019; Saliakellis et al., 2013).

Diagnostic studies (e.g., CT scan) are performed on both clinical situations. If obstruction is identified and associated with volvulus, a diagnostic laparoscopy may be considered. If adhesions are noted to be twisting and obstructing the GI tract, then removal of the adhesions and possible bowel resection may be needed, depending on bowel viability (Heo et al., 2019).

In intussusception, patients, mostly children, in this situation can have an abdominal ultrasound scan (the method of choice) (Kumar et al., 2019), or much less commonly, a CT scan can be used. Abdominal radiograph is also possible. In intussusception, a "pseudokidney" sign may be in the abdominal radiograph (Greco et al., 2019).

A retrospective study (Mendez et al., 2012) looked at the effectiveness of abdominal radiographs versus abdominal ultrasound in 6,314 children younger than 3 years from October 1999 to October 2004 who presented to the emergency department with suspected intussusception. Of the sample, 201 underwent radiographic evaluation. Of the 201 study patients, 171 had an abdominal radiograph and 65 had ultrasound, while 145 underwent air enema. The researchers found that RUQ mass, vomiting, and abdominal pain accompanied by a highly suggestive abdominal radiograph were significantly associated with intussusception. The highly suggestive findings included soft tissue mass, bowel obstruction, visible intussusception, and sparse large bowel gas pattern. When surgery is needed for intussusception, indications include peritonitis signs, hemodynamic instability, and unsuccessful nonsurgical reduction (Kumar et al., 2019).

Medical management can include watchful waiting (Kumar et al., 2019) to see if the intussusception will resolve spontaneously (more in small bowel intussusception) or nonsurgical management with air enema reductions to re-expand the bowel (Binkovitz et al., 2019). When the patient fails air enema reduction or has signs of bowel necrosis, surgical intervention is used. Surgery may also be used if the patient displays signs of perforation, shock, or peritonitis (Kumar et al., 2019). Failure to intervene in a timely manner can be fatal (Bogdanovic et al., 2019). If the intussusception is medically or radiologically reduced, a retrospective study of 60 pediatric patients demonstrated outpatient management was safe and preferred by clinicians and families (McLeod et al., 2019). If recurrence of the intussusception occurred, fever was a major risk factor (Ye et al., 2019).

A systematic review and meta-analysis of inpatient admission versus emergency department management of intussusception in children (Amuddhu et al., 2018) analyzed 9 studies comprising over 1,300 patients. There were no statistical differences between recurrence rate and hospital length of stay. They summarized hospital emergency department outpatient management is acceptable as inpatient admission. Another systematic review also supported safety of outpatient intussusception management (Litz et al., 2019).

Factors predictive of postoperative mortality after surgery for colonic (sigmoid), volvulus were increased age, systemic sepsis, and emergent surgery in a retrospective review of a database of over 2,000 surgical patients (Easterday et al., 2019). Another retrospective study on patients with colonic volvulus ($N = 34$) identified that early sigmoid colectomy was associated with lower morbidity, less readmissions, and less complications (Fagan et al., 2019). This need for sigmoid resection in volvulus was noted by Queneherve et al. (2019) in a retrospective study of 83 patients. Those who had endoscopic detorsion of the sigmoid volvulus (rather than surgery) had more volvulus recurrence and higher death rate.

COLONIC INERTIA

Colonic inertia often called slow transit constipation (Naemi et al., 2018; Schiano-DiVisconte et al., 2019) is a functional disorder of the intestine. That is, there is no clear structural abnormality or objective evidence of an underlying pathology but rather a dysfunctional enteric nervous system. Suggested causes include alterations in neurochemistry, neuronal loss, hypoganglionosis, and less numbers of colonic interstitial cells. Colonic inertia can create such poor bowel function that it mimics bowel obstruction. It can be so severe that colectomy is performed though it is considered a controversial treatment (Naemi et al., 2018; Wald 2019a,b).

The mechanism for colonic inertia may be related to an increased level of serotonin or distribution of serotonin in the colonic mucosa. Colonic inertia is associated with altered electrical activity contributing to dysmotility (Naemi et al., 2018; Schiano-DiVisconte et al., 2019).

Clinically, colonic inertia is usually characterized by severe functional constipation with abdominal pain and distention and possibly nausea. Other diagnostic criteria include lack of identified outlet obstruction, delayed colonic transit time identified by the use of radiopaque markers, and manometric demonstrated absent or severely diminished colonic motor activity. Diagnosis for colonic inertia may involve a variety of tests, but the most helpful is the transit time test that determines the speed at which the food moves through the digestive tract (Naemi et al., 2018).

Both medical and surgical approaches are used in the disorder. Dietary changes like high-fiber diet, increasing water intake, avoiding fatty foods, and dairy product avoidance may help some persons that are affected.

Surgical therapy involved colectomy with the small intestine directly attached to the rectum (ileorectal anastomosis). Though the idea of shortening the colon seems to logically make sense, in some patient's symptoms can persist. Though ileorectal anastomosis does not require the use of a diversion that is permanent, some surgeons may consider a temporary diversion to allow healing of anastomoses (Schiano-DiVisconte et al., 2019). A newer approach involves use of sacral nerve stimulation via a minimally invasive procedure. A retrospective cohort study of 21 patients showed promising improvement of the constipation (Schiano-DiVisconte et al., 2019).

CONCLUSION

A variety of conditions can result in a fecal diversion. A review of common disease states that are etiologies for a stoma was presented. Clinical presentation and medical/surgical management were discussed.

REFERENCES

Ahmed, A., Moahammed, A. T., Mattar, O., et al. (2018). Surgical treatment of diverticulitis and its complications: A systematic review and meta-analysis of randomized control trials. *The Surgeon, 16*, 372–383.

Amoli, H., Rahimpour, E., Firoozeh, N., et al. (2019). Midgut volvulus is a rare cause of intestinal obstruction in adults: A case report. *International Journal of Surgery Case Reports, 58*, 41–44.

Amuddhu, S. K., Chen, Y., & Nah, S. (2018). Inpatient admission versus emergency department management of intussusception in children: A systemic review and meta-analysis of outcomes. *European Journal of Pediatric Surgery, 29*(1), 7–13.

Anwar, M., Ahmad, S., Akhtar, R., et al. (2017). Antioxidant supplementation: A linchpin in radiation-induced enteritis. *Technology in Cancer Research & Treatment, 16*(6), 676–691.

Ashburn, J. H., & Kalady, M. F. (2016). Radiation-induced problems in colorectal surgery. *Clinics in Colon and Rectal Surgery, 29*(2), 85–91.

Atamanalp, S. S. (2019). Sigmoid volvulus: The first one thousand-case single center series in the world. *European Journal of Trauma and Emergency Surgery, 45*, 175–176.

Azhar, N., Kulstad, H., Palsson, B., et al. (2019). Acute uncomplicated diverticulitis managed without antibiotics—Difficult to introduce a new treatment protocol but few complications. *Scandinavian Journal of Gastroenterology, 54*(1), 64–68.

Baldino, M. E., Koth, V. S., Nascimento, P., et al. (2019). Gardner Syndrome with maxillofacial manifestation: A case report. *Special Care in Dentistry, 39*, 65–71.

Barrow, P., Khan, M., Lalloo, F., et al. (2013). Systematic review of the impact of registration and screening on colorectal cancer incidence and mortality in familial adenomatous polyposis and Lynch syndrome. *British Journal of Surgery, 100*, 1719–1731.

Basson, M. D. (2019). Decision-making in colostomy closure acceptable vs. optimal safety and selection vs. bias. *JAMA Surgery, 154*(3), 224.

Benjamin, E. (2019). *Traumatic gastrointestinal injury in the adult patient.* UptoDate. Retrieved December 9, 2019, from www.uptodate.com

Binkovitz, L. A., Kolbe, A., Orth, R., et al. (2019). Pediatric ileocolic intussusception: New observations and unexpected implications. *Pediatric Radiology, 49*, 76–81.

Bogdanovic, M., Blagojevic, M., Kuzmanovic, J., et al. (2019). Fatal intussusception in infancy: Forensic implications. *Forensic Science, Medicine and Pathology, 15*, 284–287.

Boynton, W., & Floch, M. (2013). New strategies for the management of diverticular disease: Insights for the clinician. *Therapeutic Advances in Gastroenterology, 6*(3), 205–213.

Brandt, M. (2019). *Intestinal malrotation in children.* UptoDate. Retrieved January 15, 2020, from www.uptodate.com

Bridoux, V., Regimbeau, J. M., Ouaissi, M., et al. (2017). Hartmann's procedure or primary anastomosis for generalized peritonitis due to perforated diverticulitis: A prospective multicenter randomized trial (DIVERTI). *Journal of American College of Surgeons, 225*, 798–805.

Broad, J. B., Wu, Z., Ng, J., et al. (2019a). Diverticular disease management in primary care: How do estimates from community-dispensed antibiotics inform provision of care. *PLoS One, 14*(7), e0219818. doi: 10.1371/journal.pone.0219818.

Broad, J. B., Wu, Z., Xie, S., et al. (2019b). Diverticular disease epidemiology: Acute hospitalizations are growing fastest in young men. *Techniques in Coloproctology, 23*(8), 713–721. doi: 10.1007/s10151-019-02040-8.

Burgell, R. E., Muir, J. G., & Gibson, P. R. (2013). Pathogenesis of colonic diverticulosis: Repainting the picture. *Clinical Gastroenterology and Hepatology, 11*, 1628–1630.

Camilleri, M. (2019). *Acute colonic pseudo-obstruction (Ogilvie's Syndrome).* UptoDate. Retrieved December 10, 2019, from www.uptodate.com

Camilleri, M., Sandler, R. S., & Peery, A. F. (2019). Etiopathogenetic mechanisms in diverticular disease of the colon. *Cellular and Molecular Gastroenterology and Hepatology, 25*, 15–32. doi: 10.1016/J.CMGH.2019.07.007.

Campos, F. Martinez, C., Sulbaran, M., et al. (2019). Upper gastrointestinal neoplasia in familial adenomatous polyposis: Prevalence, endoscopic features, and management. *Journal of Gastrointestinal Oncology, 10*(4), 734–744.

Cassini, D., Miccini, M., Manuochehri, F., et al. (2017). Emergency Hartmann's procedure and its reversal: A totally laparoscopic 2-step surgery for the treatment of Hinchey III and IV diverticulitis. *Surgical Innovation, 24*(6), 557–565.

Catena, F., DeSimone, B., Coccolini, F., et al. (2019). Bowel obstruction: A narrative review for all physicians. *World Journal of Emergency Surgery, 14*, 20, 8 pages. doi: 10.1186/S13017-019-0240-7.

Chung, D. C. (2019a). *Juvenile polyposis syndrome*. UptoDate. Retrieved September 1, 2019, from www.uptodate.com

Chung, D. C. (2019b). *Peutz-Jeghers syndrome: Clinical manifestations, diagnosis and management*. UptoDate. Retrieved August 29, 2019, from www.uptodate.com

Colwell, C., & Moore, E. E. (2019). *Initial evaluation and management of abdominal stab wounds in adults*. UptoDate. Retrieved December 9, 2019 from www.uptodate.com

Czito, B., Meyer, J., & Willett, C. G. (2019). *Overview of gastrointestinal toxicity of radiation therapy*. UptoDate. Retrieved September 15, 2019, from www.uptodate.com

Diercks, D. B., & Clarke, S. (2019). *Initial evaluation and management of blunt abdominal trauma in adults*. UptoDate. Retrieved December 9, 2019, from www.uptodate.com

Dinarvand, P., Davaro, E., Doan, J. V., et al. (2018). Familial adenomatous polyposis an update and review of extra intestinal manifestations. *Archives of Pathology and Laboratory Medicine, 143*, 1–17. doi: 10.5858/ARPA.2018-0570-RA.

DiSiena, M. S., & Birk, J. W. (2018). Diverticular disease: The old, the new, and the ever-changing view. *Southern Medical Journal, 111*(3), 144–150.

Dolan, S. (2019). Familial adenomatous polyposis. *Clinical Journal of Oncology Nursing, 23*(2), 135–138.

Donlon, N. E., Kelly, M. E., Narouz, F., et al. (2019). Colonic stenting as a bridge to surgery in malignant large bowel obstruction: Oncological outcomes. *International Journal of Colorectal Disease, 34*, 613–619.

Easterday, A., Aurit, S., Driessen, R., et al. (2019). Perioperative outcomes and predictors of mortality after surgery for sigmoid volvulus. *Journal of Surgical Research, 245*, 119–126.

Eckert, K. L. (2005). Penetrating and blunt abdominal trauma. *Critical Care Nursing Quarterly, 28*(1), 41–59.

Fagan, P., Stanfield, B., Nur, T., et al. (2019). Management of acute sigmoid volvulus in a provincial center—A 20-year experience. *Management, 132*(1493), 38–43.

Farkas, N. G., Welman, J. P., Ross, T., et al. (2019). Unusual causes of bowel obstruction. *Current Problems in Surgery, 56*, 49–90.

Fiechtl, J. (2019). *Pelvic trauma: Initial evaluation and management*. UptoDate. Retrieved December 9, 2019, from www.uptodate.com

Frazee, R. C., Abernathy, S., Jupiter, D., et al. (2013). Long-term consequences of open abdomen management. *Trauma, 16*(1), 37–40.

Gaertner, W. B., Kwaan, M. R., Madoff, R. D., et al. (2013). The evolving role of laparoscopy in colonic diverticular disease: A systematic review. *World Journal of Surgery, 37*, 629–638.

Gandle, C., Dhingra, S., & Agarwal, S. (2019). Radiation-induced enteritis. *Clinical Gastroenterology and Hepatology, 18*, 1–2. doi: 10.1016/J.CGH.2018.11.060.

Ganschow, P., Treiber, I., Hinz, U., et al. (2019). Functional outcome after pouch-anal reconstruction with primary and secondary mucosectomy for patients with Familial Adenomatous Polyposis (FAP). *Langenbeck's Archives of Surgery, 404*, 223–229.

Georgoff, P., Perales, P., Laguna, B., et al. (2013). Colonic injuries and the damage control abdomen: Does management strategy matter? *Journal of Surgical Research, 181*, 293–299.

Gopie, J. P., Vasen, H. F., & Tibben, A. (2012). Surveillance for hereditary cancer: Does the benefit outweigh the psychological burden? A systematic review. *Critical Reviews in Oncology/Hematology, 83*, 329–340.

Greco, S., Giambelluca, D., Pecoraro, G., et al. (2019). The pseudokidney sign in intussusception. *Abdominal Radiology, 45*(1), 241–242. doi: 10.1007/s00261-019-02113-0.

Halim, H., Askari, A., Nunn, R., et al. (2019). Primary resection anastomosis versus Hartmann's procedure in Hinchey III and IV diverticulitis.

World Journal of Emergency Surgery, 14, 32, 8 pages. doi: 10.1186/S13017-019-0251-4.

Hasnaoui, H., Laytimi, F., Elfellah, Y., et al. (2019). Transverse colon volvulus presenting as bowel obstruction: A case report. *Journal of Medical Case Reports, 13*, 156, 4 pages. doi: 10.1186/S13256-019-2080-1.

Hatch, Q., Causey, M., Martin, M., et al. (2013). Outcomes after colon trauma in the 21st century: An analysis of the U.S. National Trauma Data Bank. *Surgery, 154*, 397–403.

Heo, S., Kim, H., Oh, B., et al. (2019). Sigmoid volvulus: Identifying patients requiring emergency surgery with the dark torsion knot sign. *European Radiology, 29*(10), 5723–5730. doi: 10.1007/s00330-019-06194-9.

Hinchey, E. J., Schaal, P. G., & Richards, G. K. (1978). Treatment of perforated diverticular disease of the colon. *Advances in Surgery, 12*, 85–109.

Hinton, L. (2017). Adult intussusception: A rare but important clinical entity. *ANZ Journal of Surgery, 89*(5), 611–613.

Hogan, N. M., Kerin, M. J., & Joyce, M. R. (2013). Gastrointestinal complications of pelvic radiotherapy: Medical and surgical management strategies. *Current Problems in Surgery, 50*, 395–407.

Jang, H., Lee, J., Park. S., et al. (2018). Pravastatin attenuates acute radiation-induced enteropathy and improves acute radiation-induced enteropathy and improves epithelial cell function. *Frontiers in Pharmacology, 9*, Article 1215, 1–12. doi: 10.3389/FPHAR.2018.01215.

Johnson, E., & Steele, S. R. (2013). Evidence-based management of colorectal trauma. *Journal of Gastrointestinal Surgery, 17*, 1712–1719.

Kappus, M., Diamond, S., Hurt, R.T., et al. (2016). Intestinal failure: New definition and clinical implications. *Current Gastroenterology Reports, 18*, 48, 8 pages. doi: 10.1007/S11894-016-0525-X.

Karakas, D., Yesiltas, M., Gokcek, B., et al. (2019). Etiology management and surgical of acute mechanical bowel obstruction five-year results of a training and research hospital in Turkey. *Ulusal Travma ve Acil Cerrahi Dergisi, 25*(3), 268–280.

Katabathina, V., Menias, C., Khanna, L., et al. (2019). Hereditary gastrointestinal cancer syndromes: Role of imaging in screening, diagnosis and management. *Radiographics, 39*, 1280–1301.

Kennedy, R. A., Thauaraj, S., & Diaz-Cano, S. (2017). An overview of autosomal dominant tumour syndromes with prominent features in the oral and maxillofacial region. *Head and Neck Pathology, 11*, 364–376.

Kumagai, T., Rahman, F., & Smith, A. M. (2018). The microbiome and radiation-induced bowel injury: Evidence for potential mechanistic role in disease pathogenesis. *Nutrients, 10*, 1405, 16 pages. doi: 10.3390/NU10101405.

Kumar, S., Arora, P., & Goswami, P. (2019). Recurrent intestinal obstruction in a patient of Peutz-Jeghers Syndrome. *Journal of Cancer Research and Therapeutics, 15*(1), 252–254.

Kurumboor, P., Kamalesh, N. P., Pramil, K., et al. (2017). Laparoscopic management of colonic diverticular disease and its complications: An analysis. *Indian Journal of Surgery, 79*(5), 380–383.

Latchford, A., Cohen, S., Auth, M., et al. (2019). Management of Peutz-Jeghers syndrome in children and adolescents: A position paper from the ESPGHAN Polyposis Working Group. *Journal of Pediatric Gastroenterology and Nutrition, 68*(3), 42–452.

Lenti, M. V., & DiSabatino, A. (2019). Intestinal fibrosis. *Molecular Aspects of Medicine, 65*, 100–109. doi: 10.1016.J.MAM.2018.10.003.

Li, N., Zhu, W., Gong, J., et al. (2013). Ileal or ileocecal resection for chronic radiation enteritis with small bowel obstruction: Outcome and risk factors. *American Journal of Surgery, 206*, 739–747.

Lief, K., Janakan, G., Clark, C., et al. (2019). Diagnostic challenge of the non-specific presentation of adult intussusception. *BMJ Case Reports CP, 12*(11), e22931, 4 pages. doi: 10.1136/BCR-2019-229931.

Lightner, A. L., Alsughayer, A., Wang, Z., et al. (2019). Short and long-term outcomes after ileal pouch anal anastomosis in pediatrics patients: A systematic review. *Inflammatory Bowel Diseases, 25*(7), 1152–1168.

Lipman, M. (2018). *Avoiding surgery for gut pain*. Consumer Reports (On Health), April 11.

Litz, C. N., Amankwah, E. K., Polo, R. L., et al. (2019). Outpatient management of intussusception: A systematic review and meta-analysis. *Journal of Pediatric Surgery, 54*, 1316–1323.

Long, B., Robertson, J., & Koyfman, A. (2019). Emergency medicine evaluation and management of small bowel obstruction: Evidence-based recommendations. *Journal of Emergency Medicine, 56*(2), 166–176.

Lutwak, N., & Dill, C. (2013). Mild to moderate diverticulitis: What's new on diagnostic approach, treatment, and prevention of recurrence? *Clinical Geriatrics, 21*(7), 6 pages. Retrieved from www.clinicalgeriatrics.com/articles/mild-moderate-diverticulitis-whats-new

Lv, Z., Wang, C., Wu, L., et al. (2018). Identification of a MUTL-Homolog 1 mutation via whole exome sequencing in a Chinese family with Gardner syndrome. *Molecular Medicine Reports, 18*, 987–992.

Macrae, F. A. (2019). *Overview of colon polyps*. UptoDate. Retrieved September 10, 2019, from www.uptodate.com

Mandeville, K., Chien, M., Willyerd, A., et al. (2012). Intussusception-clinical presentations and imaging characteristics. *Pediatric Emergency Care, 28*(9), 842–844.

McLeod, J. S., Gavulic, A. E., Wendt, W., et al. (2019). Intussusception protocol implementation: Single-site outcomes with clinician and family satisfaction. *Journal of Surgical Research, 244*, 122–129.

Mendez, D., Caviness, C., Ma, L., et al. (2012). The diagnostic accuracy of an abdominal radiograph with signs and symptoms of intussusception. *American Journal of Emergency Medicine, 30*, 426–431.

Morini, A., Annicchiarico, A., Romboli, A., et al. (2019). Laparoscopic Hartmann's operation and reversal for acute diverticulitis: Is it really a mini-invasive procedure? *Surgical Innovation, 26*(6), 768–769.

Murai, T., Matsuo, M., Tanaka, H., et al. (2019). Efficacy of herbal medicine TJ-14 for acute radiation-induced enteritis: A multi-institutional prospective Phase II trial. *Journal of Radiation Research, 2019*, 1–6. doi: 10.1093/JRR/RRZ025.

Naemi, K., Stamos, M. J., & Li-Cheng, M. (2018). Massive submucosal ganglia in colonic inertia. *Archives of Pathology and Laboratory Medicine, 142*, 208–212.

Otterson, M. F. (2019). *Surgical approaches to radiation enteritis*. UptoDate. Retrieved September 15, 2019, from www.uptodate.com

Painter, N. J., & Burkitt, L. P. (1971). Diverticular disease of the colon: A deficiency disease of western civilization. *British Medical Journal, 2*, 450–454.

Peery, A. F., Barrett, P. R., Park, D., et al. (2012). A high-fiber diet does not protect against symptomatic diverticulosis. *Gastroenterology, 142*, 266–272.

Peery, A. F., Sandler, R. S., Ahnew, D., et al. (2013). Constipation and a low-fiber diet are not associated with diverticulosis. *Clinical Gastroenterology and Hepatology, 11*, 1622–1627.

Pemberton, J. H. (2019a). *Colonic diverticulosis and diverticular diseases: Epidemiology, risk factors, and pathogenesis*. UptoDate. Retrieved September 1, 2019, from www.uptodate.com

Pemberton, J. H. (2019b). *Clinical manifestations and diagnosis of acute diverticulitis in adults*. UptoDate. Retrieved September 15, 2019, from www.uptodate.com

Pemberton, J. H. (2019c). *Acute colonic diverticulitis: Medical management*. UptoDate. Retrieved September 1, 2019, from www.uptodate.com

Pemberton, J. H. (2019d). *Acute colonic diverticulitis. Surgical management*. UptoDate. Retrieved September 15, 2019, from www.uptodate.com

Pemberton, J. H. (2019e). *Colonic diverticular bleeding*. UptoDate. Retrieved September 20, 2019 from www.uptodate.com

Pilgrim, S. M., Hart, A. R., & Speakman, C. T. (2013). Diverticular disease in younger patients—Is it clinically more complicated and related to obesity? *Colorectal Disease, 15*, 1205–1210.

Pisanu, A., Vacca, V., Reccia, I., et al. (2013). Clinical study—Acute diverticulitis in the young: The same disease in a different patient. *Gastroenterology Research and Practice, 2013*, Article ID 867961, 6 pages. doi: 10.1155/2013/867961.

Ponti, G., Pellacani, G., Seidenari, S., et al. (2013). Cancer-associated genodermatoses: Skin neoplasms as clues to hereditary tumor syndromes. *Critical Reviews in Oncology/Hematology, 85*, 239–256.

Queneherve, L., Dagouat, C., Lerhun, M., et al. (2019). Outcomes of first-line endoscopic management for patients with sigmoid volvulus. *Digestive and Liver Disease, 51*, 386–390.

Resio, B. J., Jean, R., Chiu, A. S., et al. (2019). Association of timing of colostomy reversal with outcomes following Hartmann procedure for diverticulitis. *JAMA Surgery, 154*(3), 218–224.

Rezapour, M., & Stollman, N. (2019). Diverticular disease in the elderly. *Current Gastroenterology Reports, 21*, 46, 10 pages. doi: 10.1007/s11894-019-0715-4.

Roberts, I. (2019). *Diagnosis and management of radiation enteritis*. UptoDate. Retrieved September 15, 2019, from www.uptodate.com.

Saliakellis, E., Borrelli, O., & Thapar, N. (2013). Pediatric GI emergencies. *Best Practice & Research Clinical Gastroenterology, 27*, 799–817.

Samadder, N. J., Giridhar, K., Baffy, N., et al. (2019a). Hereditary cancer syndromes—A primer on diagnosis and management, Part 1: Breast-ovarian cancer syndromes. *Mayo Clinic Proceedings, 94*(6), 1084–1098.

Samadder, N. J., Baffy, N., Giridhar, K., et al. (2019b). Hereditary cancer syndromes—A primer on diagnosis and management, Part 2: Gastrointestinal cancer syndromes. *Mayo Clinic Proceedings, 94*(6), 1099–1116.

Sarani, B., & Martin, N. (2019). *Overview of inpatient management of the adult trauma patient*. UptoDate. Retrieved December 9, 2019, from www.uptodate.com

Schiano-DiVisconte, M., Pasquali, A., Mis, T., et al. (2019). Sacral nerve stimulation in slow-transit constipation: Effectiveness at 5-year follow-up. *International Journal of Colorectal Disease, 34*, 1529–1540.

Shah, K. R., Boland, R., Patel, M., et al. (2013). Cutaneous manifestations of gastrointestinal disease: Part I. *Journal of the American Academy of Dermatology, 68*(2), 189EI–189E21.

Sharpe, J. P., Magnotti, L. J., Weiberg, J. A., et al. (2012). Adherence to a simplified management algorithm reduces morbidity and mortality after penetrating colon injuries: A 15-year experience. *Journal of American College of Surgeons, 214*, 591–598.

Short, E., & Sampson, J. (2019). The role of inherited genetic variants in colorectal polyposis syndromes. *Advances in Genetics, 103*, 183–217.

Short, E., Thomas, L. E., Davies, A., et al. (2019). APC transcription studies and molecular diagnosis of Familial Adenomatous Polyposis. *European Journal of Human Genetics, 28*(1), 118–121. doi: 10.1038/s41431-019-0486-2.

Skoldberg, F., Granlund, J., Discacciati, A., et al. (2019). Incidence and lifetime risk of hospitalization and surgery for diverticular disease. *British Journal of Surgery, 106*, 930–939.

Sokol, H., & Adolph, T. E. (2018). The microbiome: An underestimated actor in radiation-induced lesions? *Gut, 67*(1), 1–2.

Stacey, R., & Green, J. T. (2014). Radiation-induced small bowel disease: Latest developments and clinical guidance. *Therapeutic Advances in Chronic Disease, 5*(1), 15–29.

Steele, S. R., & Goldberg, J. (2019). *Rectal foreign bodies*. UptoDate. Retrieved December 9, 2019, from www.uptodate.com

Strate, L. L., Liu, Y. L., Syngal, S., et al. (2008). Nut, corn, and popcorn consumption and the incidence of diverticular disease. *JAMA, 300*, 907–914.

Tartaglia, D., Costa, G., Camillo, A., et al. (2019). Damage control surgery for perforated diverticulitis with diffuse peritonitis: Saves lives and reduces ostomy. *World Journal of Emergency Surgery, 14*, 19, 6 pages. doi: 10.1186/s13017-019-0238-1.

To, B. A. T., & Cagir, B. (2018). *What are the diagnostic criteria for Peutz-Jeghers Syndrome*. Medscape. Retrieved January 1, 2020, from www.medscape.com

Turley, R. S., Mantyh, C., & Migaly, J. (2013). Minimally invasive surgery for diverticulitis. *Techniques in Coloproctology, 17*(Suppl 1), S11–S22.

Tursi, A. (2019). Current and evolving concepts on the pathogenesis of diverticular disease. *Journal of Gastrointestinal and Liver Diseases, 28*(2), 225–235.

Tursi, A., & Elisei, W. (2019). Role of inflammation in the pathogenesis of diverticular disease. *Mediators of Inflammation, 2019*, Article ID 8328490, 7 pages. doi: 10.1155/2019/8328490.

Valle, L., Vilar, E., Tavtigian, S. V., et al. (2019). Genetic predisposition to colorectal cancer: Syndromes, genes, classification of genetic variants, and implications for precision medicine. *Journal of Pathology, 247*,574–588.

Van de Wall, B., Draaisma, W., Consten, E., et al. (2013). Does the presence of abscesses in diverticular disease prelude surgery? *Journal of Gastrointestinal Surgery, 17*, 540–547.

Varga, S., Zakaluzny, S., & Inaba, K. (2013). Non-operative management of abdominal gunshot wounds. *Trauma, 15*(4), 271–278.

Vasen, H., Ghorbanoghli, Z., De Ruijter, B., et al. (2019). Optimizing the timing of colorectal surgery in patients with Familial Adenomatous Polyposis in clinical practice. *Scandinavian Journal of Gastroenterology, 54*(6), 733–739. doi: 10.1080/00365521.2019.1621930.

Wald, A. (2019a). *Etiology and evaluation of chronic constipation in adults.* UptoDate. Retrieved December 9, 2019, from www.uptodate.com

Wald, A. (2019b). *Management of chronic constipation in adults.* UptoDate. Retrieved December 9, 2019, from www.uptodate.com

Wu, J., Duan, Y., Cui, J., et al. (2019). Protective effects of zingerone derivate on ionizing radiation-induced intestinal injury. *Journal of Radiation Research, 60*(6), 740–746.

Xuereb, S., Xuereb, R., Buhagiar, C., et al. (2017). A case report of desmoid tumour-a forgotten aspect of FAP? *International Journal of Surgery Case Reports, 30*, 122–125.

Ye, X., Tang, R., Chew, S., et al. (2019). Risk factors for recurrent intussusception in children: A systematic review and meta-analysis. *Frontiers in Pediatrics, 7*(145), 1–8. doi: 10.3389/FPED.2019.00145.

QUESTIONS

1. The WOC nurse is counseling the parents of a 5-year-old male patient about their family history of familial adenomatous polyposis (FAP) syndrome. What would the nurse include in the care plan for this family?

A. Begin colorectal screening with colonoscopy at age 12.

B. Once polyps are identified, colon screening should be done every 5 years.

C. Upper endoscopy should be performed every 5 years.

D. Thyroid ultrasonography should be performed every 2 years.

2. A 13-year-old male patient presents with dark blue macules around his mouth, eyes, nostrils, buccal mucosa, hands, and genitalia. What disease state would the WOC nurse suspect?

A. Familial adenomatous polyposis (FAP) syndrome

B. Gardner syndrome

C. Peutz-Jeghers syndrome (PJS)

D. Diverticular disease

3. A WOC nurse is explaining the etiology of diverticular disease to a recently diagnosed patient. What would the nurse list as a possible cause of this disease?

A. Formation of hamartomatous polyps in the gastrointestinal tract

B. Mutation in the APC gene

C. Damage to the intestinal tissue from radiation

D. Low-fiber diet

4. A patient presents with pain in the left lower abdominal quadrant, bloating, and diarrhea. No abdominal masses are found on palpitation. What possible GI disorder is present?

A. Intussusception

B. Volvulus

C. Diverticulitis

D. Colonic inertia

5. The WOC nurse is developing a care plan for a patient diagnosed with radiation enteritis. What is a recommended treatment modality for this disease?

A. Bowel resection

B. Use of anti-inflammatory agents

C. Strictureplasty

D. Fiber supplementation

6. What is considered the standard of care for a patient with abdominal trauma related to an automobile accident?

A. Damage control laparotomy.

B. Ostomy for fecal diversion.

C. Open abdominal surgery.

D. Surgery is not usually warranted.

7. What is a common cause of volvulus occurring in developed countries?

A. Diverticulitis

B. Pancreatitis

C. Radiation enteritis

D. Pelvic masses

8. A 10-year-old girl presents to the emergency department with abdominal pain, vomiting, palpable abdominal mass, and bloody stool. What condition may be present?
A. Volvulus
B. Intussusception
C. Colonic inertia
D. Diverticulosis

9. What medical management technique for intussusception is recommended prior to initiating surgery?
A. High-fiber diet
B. Dairy product avoidance
C. Air enema reduction
D. Antidiarrheal drugs

10. The WOC nurse is counseling a patient diagnosed with colonic inertia. What intervention would the nurse include in a care plan for this patient?
A. Avoiding fatty foods
B. Low-fiber diet
C. Restricting fluids
D. Encouraging consumption of dairy products

ANSWERS AND RATIONALES

1. A. Rationale: Colorectal screening should begin at the age of 12 to 14 years for children with a family history of FAP. Annual screening is done once polyps are identified.

2. C. Rationale: Classic presentation of Peutz-Jeghers syndrome.

3. D. Rationale: Low-fiber diet has been over the years recognized as a theory in contributing to the development of diverticular disease. There are other theories identified in this chapter.

4. C. Rationale: Diverticulitis presents with pain in the lower left abdomen with bloating and diarrhea. The sigmoid and descending colon are common sites for diverticulitis.

5. B. Rationale: Treatment for radiation enteritis is based on symptoms; anti-inflammatory agents, antidiarrheals, probiotics, antibiotics are some management interventions.

6. A. Rationale: Standard of care for a patient with abdominal trauma related to an automobile accident is damage control laparotomy. With colon injury, the surgeon may make the choice of returning the patient to OR for definitive repair.

7. D. Rationale: Pelvic masses are one of the causes of volvulus. Other possible causes can be adhesions, poor muscle tone, gynecologic surgeries, and distal obstruction.

8. B. Rationale: Intussusception symptoms are abdominal pain, vomiting, palpable mass, and bloody stools (described as "red currant jelly" stool). Intussusception occurs when the bowel telescopes back on itself, causing intestinal obstruction.

9. C. Rationale: Air enema reduction is a medical management intervention for intussusception to re-expand the bowel.

10. A. Rationale: Dietary recommendations for colonic inertia can include avoiding fatty and dairy foods and high-fiber foods and increase in water intake.

CHAPTER 8

URINARY DIVERSIONS

Vignesh T. Packiam, Sanjay G. Patel, Ryan P. Werntz, and Gary D. Steinberg

OBJECTIVES

1. Describe disease states and conditions that can lead to a urinary diversion.

2. Discuss incontinent and continent urinary diversions and urinary sphincter saving procedures.

TOPIC OUTLINE

Introduction **118**

Indications for Intestinal Urinary Diversion **118**
  Bladder Cancer 118
    Risk Factors 118
    Presentation 118
    Histopathology 118
    Diagnostic Considerations 118
    Management 120
  Other Malignancies 120
  Benign Indications for Urinary Diversion 120
    Neurogenic Bladder 120
    Radiation Cystitis 120
    Interstitial Cystitis 120
    Trauma 121

Surgical Procedures **121**
  Incontinent Urinary Diversions 121
    Ileal Conduit 121
    Physician Considerations 121
    Patient Considerations 121
    Preoperative Considerations 121
    Surgical Procedure 121
    Postoperative Care 122
    Results 123
    Complications 123
    Colon Conduit 123
    Surgical Procedure 123
    Postoperative Care 123
  Complications 123
    Cutaneous Ureterostomy 124
    Surgical Procedure 124
    Postoperative Care 124
    Complications 124
  Continent Urinary Diversions 124
    Cutaneous Catheterizable
      Urinary Diversion 124
    Indiana Pouch 124
    Physician Considerations 124
    Patient Considerations 124
    Preoperative Considerations 125
    Surgical Procedure 125
    Postoperative Care 125
    Results 126
    Complications 126
  Other Catheterizable Urinary Diversion 126
    Orthotopic Urinary Diversion:
      Neobladder 126
    Physician Considerations 126
    Patient Considerations 126
    Preoperative Consideration 127
    Surgical Procedure 127
    Postoperative Care 127
    Results 128
    Complications 128

Conclusions **128**

INTRODUCTION

Intestinal urinary diversion is a general term used to describe the elimination of urine from the body through a surgically reconstructed intestinal segment. The name of the diversion type typically describes the particular intestinal segment utilized or the name of the institution at which it was developed (e.g., ileal conduit, Indiana pouch, ileal neobladder). Continent urinary diversions allow for control of urinary elimination, whether this is via the urethra or a continent catheterizable channel on the skin. Meanwhile, an incontinent urinary diversion is a surgically reconstructed reservoir or channel with an incontinent stoma on the skin. A wide variety of diversions have been developed to utilize bowel segments since the late 1800s, and the techniques have evolved with time.

Early urinary diversions involved bringing the ureters or bladder directly to the skin, which could result in stenosis at the skin level. Ureterosigmoidostomy involved anastomosis of the ureters to the sigmoid colon, with the anal sphincter providing continence, but resulted in increased risk of pyelonephritis and colon cancer, and thus has largely been abandoned as a diversion choice. In the 1950s, Bricker popularized and developed the ileal conduit in which urine drained from a budded stoma that was constructed on the patient's abdomen. The ileal conduit resulted in improved patient quality of life and reduced rates of stomal stenosis. More recently, continent diversions have improved the cosmesis of urinary diversion as patients eliminate their urine via small catheterizable channel on their abdomen or void via their native urethra (Pannek & Senge, 1998). **Table 8-1** summarizes the most common incontinent and continent urinary diversions, which will be discussed further in this chapter.

 INDICATIONS FOR INTESTINAL URINARY DIVERSION

There are both benign and malignant indications for intestinal urinary diversion. Urinary diversion is most commonly utilized when the bladder has to be removed due to malignancy. Less commonly, urinary diversion is utilized to divert urine from the bladder for benign indications due to severe bladder dysfunction, incontinence, bladder pain, or bleeding. In instances of benign urinary diversion, consideration must be taken to remove the bladder as some patients may develop pyocystis or infection in the native bladder. Pyocystis develops when the secretions of the native bladder accumulate and develop into an infection because there is no flow of urine through the bladder to eliminate these secretions. Pediatric conditions leading to a urinary diversion will be covered in Chapter 15.

BLADDER CANCER

Bladder cancer is the fourth most common cause of cancer death in men in the United States with a 3:1 male-to-female ratio (Bladder Cancer Support Society, 2014).

The average age at diagnosis is approximately 70 years. The most common histologic subtype of bladder cancer is urothelial carcinoma of the bladder. Bladder cancer requiring removal of the bladder is the most common indication for performing an intestinal urinary diversion.

Risk Factors

Several risk factors for bladder cancer have been implicated. The most common cause is cigarette smoking, which is a potent source for carcinogens that concentrate in the urine. Environmental exposure to chemicals (blue aniline dyes, chemicals in dye, paint, petroleum, rubber, and textile industries) has been implicated in the development of bladder cancer. Patients with chronic indwelling catheters or exposure to *Bilharzia* (parasite) have an increased risk of developing squamous cell carcinoma of the bladder.

Presentation

More than 80% to 90% of cases of bladder cancer present with gross hematuria, which is typically painless and intermittent. Twenty to thirty percent of patients present with irritative voiding symptoms such as urgency/frequency and dysuria (pain with urination). Diagnosis of bladder cancer is often delayed, as patients are commonly misdiagnosed as having routine urinary tract infections, which is associated with advanced disease.

Histopathology

Bladder cancer arises from the inner lining of the bladder known as the mucosa. The aggressiveness of bladder cancers is characterized by both their Grade (microscopic appearance of their cancer) and their Stage, or invasiveness (depth of penetration into the bladder). The bladder has several layers. From innermost to outmost, the layers are mucosa → submucosa → muscle → perivesical fat (fat surrounding the bladder). Low-grade superficial tumors are generally limited to the mucosal layer and have low risk of invasion to the deeper layer of the bladder and disease progression. On the other hand, higher-grade tumors have the potential to infiltrate the layers of the bladder in a stepwise manner resulting in patient morbidity and mortality (mucosa → submucosa → muscle → perivesical fat → lymph nodes → distant metastases → death). (See **Fig. 8-1**.)

Diagnostic Considerations

Patients who present with gross or microscopic hematuria typically undergo a standard urologic evaluation with imaging (contrast-enhanced CT scan of the kidneys, ureter, and bladder), urine cytology, and endoscopic evaluation of the urethra and bladder using a cystoscope. Once a bladder tumor is identified, patients are taken to the operating room where the bladder tumor is resected using a cystoscope that is placed through the patient's urethra into the bladder. The resection allows for the microscopic determination of the histology (cell type), grade, and stage (depth of penetration of the tumor into the bladder wall). Resection of the tumor is diagnostic,

TABLE 8-1 COMMON INCONTINENT AND CONTINENT URINARY DIVERSION

TYPE	PROCEDURE	INDICATIONS	ADVANTAGES	CONTRAINDICATIONS/DISADVANTAGES
Incontinent				
Ileal conduit	Segment of small intestine isolated. Proximal end closed, ureters implanted into segment, and distal end to skin	Need for urinary diversion: Bladder cancer, urinary fistula, neurogenic bladder, refractory cystitis, inability to manage continent reservoir	Simplest segment of bowel to use Familiar to urologists Lowest complication rate	Large body habitus may limit ability of stoma to reach skin level Prior radiation to the bowel Renal deterioration Hyperchloremic hypokalemic metabolic acidosis Need to wear pouching system for urine collection
Colon conduit	Same as ileal conduit but colon used in place of small bowel	Same as ileal conduit, but favored if small bowel disease is present or in history of pelvic radiation	Less risk of stomal stenosis	Renal deterioration Hyperchloremic hypokalemic metabolic acidosis Need to wear pouching system for urine collection Larger stoma (than ileal conduit)
Continent				
Orthotopic neobladder	Isolated, detubularized segment of ileum is used. Ureters implanted, and distal portion is connected to urethra to allow voiding	Same as ileal conduit, but patient selection is critical Cancer-free urethra Functional sphincter	Improved cosmesis: No stoma Voiding per urethra	Renal deterioration Must have urethra uninvolved with cancer Risk of: Incomplete emptying requiring catheterization Incontinence
Indiana pouch	Isolated, detubularized segment of ileocecal region used. Ureters implanted. Ileocecal valve used as continence mechanism. The patient will catheterize through abdominal wall stoma	Same as ileal conduit, but patient selection is critical	No pouching system needed Smaller stoma, which can be covered with dressing	Renal deterioration Must carry catheter at all times Patient must be capable of intermittent, self-catheterization Inability to catheterize is urologic emergency

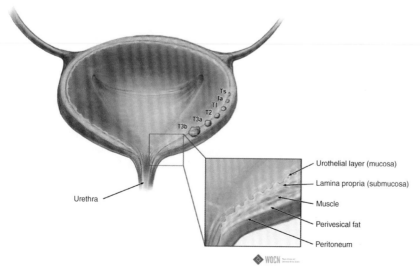

Urethra

Ts
Ta
T1
T2
T3a
T3b

Urothelial layer (mucosa)
Lamina propria (submucosa)
Muscle
Perivesical fat
Peritoneum

FIGURE 8-1. Bladder Cancer Low-Grade Upper Right to High-Grade Tumor Invasion, Lower Right.

prognostic, and therapeutic. Complete resection has been associated with improved survival.

Management

Patients with lower-grade and noninvasive bladder tumors are candidates for minimally invasive management, which includes endoscopic resection and administration of intravesical therapies including immunotherapy such as Bacille Calmette-Guérin (BCG) and chemotherapy such as mitomycin C and gemcitabine. After complete resection, these patients undergo close surveillance with frequent (every 3 to 6 months) cystoscopic evaluation of their bladder to identify recurrent tumors.

Once patients develop muscle invasive bladder cancer, endoscopic management is associated with inferior outcomes. Thus, in patients who are suitable operative candidates, the gold standard treatment for select high-grade nonmuscle invasive, or muscle-invasive bladder cancer is radical cystectomy. In male patients, the bladder, prostate, and pelvic lymph nodes are removed; in female patients, the bladder, uterus, fallopian tubes, ovaries, and anterior vagina are removed. This surgery has traditionally been performed using a low midline incision from the umbilicus to the pubic symphysis. Neoadjuvant chemotherapy, or chemotherapy, can be administered prior to the performance of radical cystectomy in select patients.

In select patients, or those who are not suitable operative candidates, alternative management strategies include "trimodal therapy," which entails maximal endoscopic resection of tumor with the administration of radiation and chemotherapy. There are also approaches that utilize only some or one of these components, but these are considered as inferior oncologic strategies compared to radical cystectomy.

With the increased experience with robot-assisted laparoscopic techniques, urologists are adopting the use of robot-assisted laparoscopic cystectomy and urinary diversion. From a technical standpoint, robotic cystectomy and urinary diversion has a steep learning curve that requires an experienced perioperative care team. Despite these challenges, the benefits of robot cystectomy with intracorporeal diversion are mixed, and the exact role of this technique is still being investigated. The pros of robotic cystectomy with intracorporeal diversion (as is the case with any laparoscopic surgery) include decreased blood loss, lower risk of transfusion, and quicker functional recovery times (due to the use of smaller incisions). The cons of the robotic techniques include increased cost and increased operative times. From a complication standpoint, there does not seem to be any clear advantage of a minimally invasive versus open approach to urinary diversion; however, there may be a trend toward fewer wound-related complications with a minimally invasive approach. Further randomized trials comparing intracorporeal and extracorporeal

diversion are needed to define the advantages and disadvantages of robotic techniques for cystectomy and urinary diversions.

OTHER MALIGNANCIES

Less common oncologic indications for removal of the bladder include gynecologic malignancy (vagina and uterus) and rectal malignancy, which can locally invade the bladder and require cystectomy and urinary diversion in some patients.

BENIGN INDICATIONS FOR URINARY DIVERSION

Neurogenic Bladder

Neurogenic bladder is a generalized term describing bladder dysfunction caused by neurologic impairment of the central and peripheral nervous system, which innervates the bladder. Several conditions can result in neurogenic bladder and include stroke, multiple sclerosis, spinal cord trauma, diabetes, and postsurgical injury (radical hysterectomy, rectal surgery, spine surgery). These patients can have several bladder manifestations, namely, urinary incontinence, urinary retention, detrusor overactivity (irritable bladder), or high-pressure storage of urine. In a majority of cases, conservative medical and surgical management is adequate to treat neurogenic bladder; however, in severe cases, urinary diversion can be utilized as a last resort.

Radiation Cystitis

Patients who undergo radiation to their pelvis for treatment of malignancy (prostate, rectum, cervix/uterus) may develop incapacitating symptoms as a result of radiation-induced damage to the bladder and sphincter. This bladder damage can result in urinary incontinence, refractory bleeding, poorly compliant bladder, or painful bladder sensations with filling (Ratner, 2001). In cases refractory to medical management, urinary diversion is employed to divert the urine away from the bladder. These patients typically undergo ileal conduit diversions, since complication rates are higher in more complex continent diversions, especially in patients who have undergone radiation.

Interstitial Cystitis

Interstitial cystitis is a painful disorder of the bladder with unknown etiology. Patients typically present with pelvic/bladder pain with associated bladder symptoms (urgency, frequency, nocturia). These patients have negative findings in laboratory and urine studies and oftentimes have small ulcerations or petechial hemorrhage on cystoscopy. Only in refractory cases do these patients undergo urinary diversion and are good candidates for both incontinent and continent urinary diversions. After surgery, some patients continue to experience pelvic pain, and it is of paramount importance that these patients have appropriate preoperative counseling.

Trauma

Severe pelvic trauma resulting in partial or complete disruption of the urethra from the bladder may cause scarring and subsequent stricturing of the urethra. Patients with a severely strictured urethra, who fail attempts to reconstruct the urethra, typically drain their bladder with indwelling suprapubic catheters, which must be changed every 4 weeks to minimize infection and clogging. Some patients opt to have urinary diversion to avoid the use of an indwelling catheter.

Trauma involving the urinary sphincter can result in severe incontinence, which can be quite distressing to patients and negatively affect their quality of life. Furthermore, continuous leakage of urine results in perineal and sacral tissue breakdown and can negatively impair healing of sacral pressure injury in patients with limited mobility and confined to their beds. Continent and incontinent urinary diversions are often performed depending on the patient's preferences and physical limitations.

SURGICAL PROCEDURES

INCONTINENT URINARY DIVERSIONS

Ileal Conduit

Incontinent urinary conduit in the form of an enterocutaneous (bowel to skin) stoma is a mainstay of urinary diversion. The ileum remains the most common segment of intestine used to create a conduit as it has the lowest complication rate and is most familiar to urologists. The ileal conduit may be the least cumbersome urinary diversion to manage from a patient perspective, as it only requires minor care of the stoma site and changing of the ostomy pouching system every 3 to 4 days. From a surgical perspective, the ileal conduit is the easiest to construct and requires shorter operative times.

Physician Considerations

Several factors are considered preoperatively when deciding what type of urinary diversion to construct for a patient. For patients with diseased intestine or multiple previous bowel resections, it is often preferred to maintain as much intestinal length as possible. Incontinent diversion requires shorter lengths of bowel (approximately 10 to 12 cm) compared to continent diversion (50 to 60 cm). Continent diversions are more technically challenging and may increase operative time, complication rate, and reoperation rate, compared to ileal conduit.

A history of prior pelvic radiation is a consideration when choosing the segment of bowel to use, as the ileum and sigmoid colon may have been included in the radiation field. A transverse colon conduit may be considered in these circumstances.

Patient Considerations

Patient-specific factors are also important to consider. Undergoing urinary diversion can drastically alter body image. Patients who have ileal conduits must be willing to accept having a stoma on their abdomen and wearing a pouching system to collect their urine. For continent cutaneous diversions, a minimal dressing is often placed over the small catheterizable stoma allowing patients to conceal their stoma. Patients with orthotopic urinary diversion or neobladders void via their urethra and do not have a visible stoma on their abdomen, which improves cosmesis.

Patients who undergo continent diversion need to have sufficient general health, manual dexterity (i.e., ability to perform self-catheterization), motivation, and understanding to reliably manage their diversions. Patients who lack these qualities are better candidates for ileal conduit diversion, which is significantly easier to manage.

Regardless of continent or incontinent diversion choice, multiple studies have been performed without clear consensus of superior quality of life in patients with continent or incontinent urinary diversions (Yang et al., 2016).

Preoperative Considerations

Preoperative medical and cardiac clearance is performed to ensure that patient comorbidities are optimized before undergoing any intestinal urinary diversion. Specifically to urinary diversion, a preoperative consultation by the WOC nurse is critical for an optimal outcome. The visit is important for patient education, choice of preferred diversion type, and determination and marking of stoma site (Salvadalena et al., 2015). The preoperative placement of stoma site markings is critical, as the patient is in a supine position intraoperatively and the determination of an optimal stoma site can be unclear.

Some urologists have historically used a mechanical and/or antibiotic preoperative bowel regimen. The goal has been to decrease intestinal bacterial load in an effort to limit infectious complications. Mechanical preparations may include GoLytely, Fleet, Miralax, or magnesium citrate. These bowel preparations have largely been abandoned as they can hinder post-operative return of bowel function and cause dehydration. However, patients undergoing Indiana Pouch urinary diversion still often undergo a bowel preparation in efforts to empty the colon prior to reconstruction and limit fecal contamination. The colon has bacteria that can lead to increased infection rates if gross fecal contamination occurs during the operation. All patients receive preoperative intravenous antibiotics immediately before surgery, which are usually stopped within 24 hours.

Surgical Procedure

The most distal 12- to 15-cm segment of ileum just proximal to the ileocecal valve is typically spared given its importance for bile salt and vitamin B_{12} absorption. A 10- to 12-cm segment of ileum proximal to this is identified. Transillumination of the mesentery is performed to ensure adequate blood supply to the segment. Surgical staplers are used to transect the bowel at each end of the conduit to isolate segment, and an anastomosis is performed to reestablish continuity of the bowel. It is important to maintain orientation of the conduit so that peristalsis is in the direction of urine flow.

Ureterointestinal anastomosis is most commonly performed in a refluxing manner near the proximal portion of the conduit over a stent, which aids in healing. There is some controversy over refluxing versus nonrefluxing anastomosis with some favoring nonrefluxing in an attempt to limit transmission of pressure and bacteria to the upper urinary tracts. While the nonrefluxing type is more technically challenging, it also has a higher stricture rate. There is no clear consensus as to an overall benefit of one method over the other (Kristjánsson et al., 1995).

There are a variety of methods to manage the proximal end of the conduit. Some surgeons suture and/or excise the staple line in order to prevent urine from contacting the staples in an effort to prevent future stone formation. The distal portion of the conduit is delivered through the skin, and the staple line is excised. The stoma is matured with multiple sutures to form a rosebud appearance (**Fig. 8-2**). This elevated rosebud-shaped stoma prevents urine from directly contacting the skin when a pouching system is applied.

Particularly in obese patients with a thick, short mesentery, an end loop ileal conduit can be performed. This allows creation of an ileal conduit with less tension, which may be required in these patients. If performed, a small rod is left in place temporarily through the mesentery at the skin level to prevent stomal retraction.

> **KEY POINT**
>
> A loop end (sometimes called an end loop Turnbull stoma) stoma will have a rod or support bridge under the bowel for support until healing takes place. The removal of the rod will depend upon the patient's potential to heal and the amount of tension over the rod. The time the rod remains in place can vary from 5 days to 3 weeks after surgery.

Postoperative Care

The ureterointestinal anastomoses are performed over ureteral stents in order to maintain patency and allow proper healing. The distal aspect of a stent exits the stoma and can be a variety of colors or sizes. They are often sutured into place within the conduit and empty directly into the pouching system. The stents are typically left in place anywhere from 5 days to 2 weeks after surgery depending upon the surgeon's preference. They are sometimes formally removed, or they may fall out on their own after disintegration of the absorbable sutures keeping them in place. Care must be taken with initial appliance changes to not dislodge the stents. Some surgeons additionally may leave a catheter in the stoma to ensure adequate healing and drainage during the initial postoperative period.

> **KEY POINT**
>
> Many surgeons will cut one stent on an angle to designate the right or left ureter (typically the left stent is cut on an angle). If the stents require shortening for easier application of the appliance, a close examination of the stents should be performed prior to shortening (be sure to keep the cut on an angle).

Additionally, a closed suction, Jackson-Pratt or Blake drain, is normally placed during surgery near the ureteroileal anastomosis and attached to bulb suction. This acts to diagnose and drain any urine leakage. This drain is typically removed before discharge as long as no significant leak is identified.

Some surgeons leave a nasogastric tube in place after surgery, which is removed at some point before initiating diet. Most practitioners await return of bowel function before starting any substantial oral intake. However, many high volume institutions are placing patients on an enhanced recovery after surgery pathway (ERAS), with principles of reduced use of opioids, no bowel prep, no nasogastric tube, early feeding, and early ambulation. This is thought to hasten the return of bowel function and

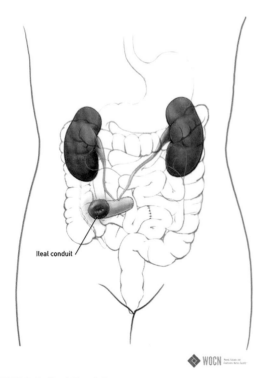

Ileal conduit

FIGURE 8-2. Ileal Conduit.

decrease both the length of stay and complication rates. Early ambulation is critical in the prevention of deep vein thrombosis. A typical uncomplicated postoperative stay can be between 5 and 10 days.

Early postoperative education is important for patients and their caregivers, who must learn to care for a new ostomy. Inpatient visits by the WOC nurse can avoid common pitfalls, which can minimize morbidity associated with incontinent urinary diversion.

Results

Ileal conduit urinary diversion is a complicated surgical procedure. Perioperative mortality ranges from 1% to 3% in large series in high-volume centers (Zhang et al., 2019). Morbidity is significant, and complications include ileus, bowel leak, urine leak, infection, ureteral stricture, and stomal complications such as stenosis or hernia. Perioperative complication rate is reported in the range of 25% to 45% (Zhang et al., 2019).

Complications

Stomal complications are common after incontinent urinary diversion. These include stomal stenosis, prolapse, retraction, and parastomal hernia. Stomal stenosis can sometimes be managed with catheterization but may necessitate revisional surgery. Retraction of the stoma may lead to difficulty in fitting of the pouching system, which may result in skin irritation or urine leakage. Parastomal hernia may be prevented by creating an appropriately sized fascial opening during surgery as well as placing the ostomy through the belly of the rectus abdominis muscle. An end loop stoma has a lower risk of stomal stenosis but a higher risk of parastomal hernia.

The ureterointestinal anastomoses may also be a source of complications, including stricture or leak. Due to the more extensive mobilization of the left ureter, the left side is more commonly affected. Management of ureterointestinal stricture can be performed endoscopically with dilation/incision of the stricture with placement of ureteral stent; however, the most definitive and successful management strategy is open surgical revision. A fraction of these strictures may represent urothelial cancer as the ureteral margin may be a site of disease recurrence (Fichtner, 1999).

Infectious complications are common, especially in the initial period after urinary diversion. These may be in the form of abdominal abscess, urine leak, bowel leak, pyelonephritis, or wound infection. Treatment includes antibiotics and adequate drainage of any infectious collection. Patients with incontinent bowel diversion will commonly have chronic bacteriuria, and a majority of asymptomatic patients will have positive urine cultures. These patients are oftentimes treated inappropriately with repeated rounds of antibiotics resulting in multidrug-resistant organisms. Antibiotics should be reserved for patients with other clinical signs of infection. See appendix D for obtaining a sample of urine from an ileal conduit.

The distal ileum is active in the absorption of vitamin B_{12} and bile salts. Vitamin B_{12} deficiency can potentially develop years after urinary diversion. Some practitioners routinely monitor and replace it as needed, often in the form of injection. If malabsorption of bile salts occurs, patients can experience a fatty diarrhea.

As bowel segments used for diversion are still metabolically active, resultant electrolyte and acid–base disturbances have been described for different bowel segments. For ileum, patients experience a hyperchloremic hypokalemic metabolic acidosis (Vasdev et al., 2013).

Over time, chronic renal insufficiency is not uncommon for patients with urinary diversions. This may be secondary to chronic obstruction, recurrent infections, or chronic exposure of the upper urinary tracts to bacteria.

Urolithiasis is another common complication. These may be in the form of calcium oxalate stones, the type most common in the general population, but chronic bacterial colonization can also cause magnesium ammonium phosphate stones to form. Stones may be located in the renal pelvis, in the ureter, or along the proximal ileal staple line if this was not excluded or excised during surgery. Retained foreign material from surgery such as stent fragments or permanent suture in contact with urine can act as a nidus for stone formation and should be avoided. These patients may be more complicated to treat with conventional methods given the altered anatomy of the urinary tract.

Colon Conduit

The use of colon for urinary diversion may be preferable in patients with prior pelvic radiation as portions may have been spared from the radiation field. The transverse colon is outside most radiation templates and is appropriate for use. A colon conduit urinary diversion may also be preferable in a patient with an existing colostomy for stool as it can obviate the need for bowel anastomosis and its associated morbidity.

Surgical Procedure

Sigmoid or transverse colon is most commonly used for creation of a colon urinary conduit. The steps are similar to creation of an ileal conduit. Directionality is maintained, and identification of adequate blood supply is critical. The segment of colon is taken out of continuity, and a bowel anastomosis is performed as previously described.

Postoperative Care

Immediate postoperative care is similar to an ileal conduit.

Complications

The stoma is slightly larger secondary to the caliber of colon, and therefore, stomal stenosis is less common.

Otherwise, complications are similar. Patients with colonic urinary diversion also may experience a hyperchloremic hypokalemic metabolic acidosis.

Cutaneous Ureterostomy

While cutaneous ureterostomies have largely been performed historically, there has recently been renewed and increased interest in this technique for select patients. There are several potential advantages of this approach. First, the operation is simplified in patients with multiple prior abdominal surgeries. Particularly in the setting of a solitary kidney, only a single new anastomosis is required. The perioperative course recovery can be hastened due to the lack of a bowel anastomosis. Furthermore, all the long complications of utilizing intestine that have previously been discussed are avoided. This can be a good option for elderly patients with advanced bladder cancer as well as a more palliative option in other situations where a physician wants to take every effort to limit complications.

Surgical Procedure

Cutaneous ureterostomy involves anastomosis of one or more of the ureters directly to the skin (**Fig. 8-3**). There can be a single ureterostomy, bilateral ureterostomies, or the ureters can be sewn together with a single ureterostomy to the skin.

Postoperative Care

Immediate postoperative care is similar to an ileal conduit.

Complications

The major downside of a cutaneous ureterostomy is the risk of stomal stenosis. Therefore, these patients often remain stent dependent. This can be associated with dislodged stents, and more frequent urinary tract infection and pyelonephritis. This type of diversion can be particularly challenging for placement of the ostomy appliance, as they are typically completely flush to the skin and can be difficult to get a good seal with the ostomy appliance.

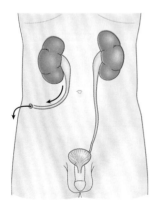

FIGURE 8-3. Ureterostomy.

CONTINENT URINARY DIVERSIONS

Cutaneous Catheterizable Urinary Diversion

Cutaneous catheterizable urinary diversions involve the creation of an intestinal reservoir with an intestinal channel (catheterizable channel) that is brought from the reservoir to the skin. A variety of bowel segments can be used to create the reservoir (colon, ileum) as well as the catheterizable channel (colon, ileum, appendix). Generally, the continence between the reservoir and catheterizable channel is provided by preexisting anatomic (i.e., ileocecal valve) or surgically constructed valves. The catheterizable channel must be catheterized several times during the day to empty the reservoir. It is imperative that any patient undergoing catheterizable continent urinary diversions has adequate mental capacity and hand–eye coordination to perform catheterizations multiple times per day.

While most urinary diversions entail mucous production by the intestinal segment, this is particularly relevant for patients with continent urinary diversions. Mucous production can be more substantial within the initial 30 days after surgery, as the intestinal villi begin to slough when exposed to urine. In patients with continent urinary diversion, frequent irrigation is important in order to remove mucous through the catheter. Irrigation serves to both prevent infections and ensure efficient drainage of the diversion.

Indiana Pouch

The Indiana pouch has become the predominant urinary diversion for patients who desire a continent catheterizable urinary diversion. Compared to orthotopic neobladders, patients do not need to have a patent urethra or a functional urinary sphincter. Indiana pouches can be performed in instances where the small intestinal segments are unable to reach the urethra in patients planned to undergo orthotopic neobladders; Indiana pouches are used as second-line continent urinary diversion in these instances (Rowland, 1996).

Contraindications for continent catheterizable channels include hepatic dysfunction, compromised intestinal function (i.e., previous surgery, radiation, inflammatory bowel disease), and renal failure (serum creatinine >1.7).

Physician Considerations

Indiana pouches are constructed from the terminal ileum, ileocecal valve, and right colon, and thus, these segments must be present (no prior resection, no significant disease burden, i.e., Crohn's disease) in order to perform this diversion. Furthermore, the ileocecal valve must be functional as incompetence of this valve may result in leakage of urine from the valve (incontinence).

Patient Considerations

With any continent catheterizable diversion, patients must have both the mental capacity and motivation to maintain their urinary diversion, which requires frequent self-catheterizations and occasional irrigation of mucus from the reservoir of the Indiana pouch. Sufficient manual dexterity to perform self-catheterization is also critical. From a cosmetic standpoint, patients must accept the appearance of the catheterizable channel; however, the small stoma of the catheterizable channel can be easily concealed with a dressing (Lee et al., 2014).

Preoperative Considerations

Patients should undergo evaluation and stoma marking by the WOC nurse. This is an opportunity to determine the patient's motivation, manual dexterity, and mental capacity. Selection of stoma site is determined on the right lower quadrant with consideration of belt line, skin folds, and ease of visualization by the patient.

Surgical Procedure

The Indiana pouch is created from 10 to 12 cm of ileum (catheterizable channel), the ileocecal valve (continence mechanisms), and the right colon (reservoir). This segment of bowel is mobilized and discontinued from the remaining small and large bowel. Bowel continuity is reestablished by anastomosis of the ileum to the transverse colon using surgical staplers (**Fig. 8-4**).

Next, the right colon is detubularized by incising it along its length to disrupt the muscular connections of the bowel. Care is taken to avoid incising the ileocecal valve and terminal ileum. The ureters are passed through the posterior wall of the detubularized right colon and are secured to the inside of the pouch. These ureteral anastomoses are refluxing. Lastly, ureteral catheters or stents are placed into the ureters to protect the anastomoses and aid in their healing.

The detubularized right colon is folded over in a clamshell fashion and sutured closed, thus forming the reservoir for urine. Once closed, a 24-Fr Malecot catheter is placed into the reservoir through a stab wound, and the ureteral stents are passed out of the reservoir.

The distal ileum forms the catheterizable channel and is tapered over a 14- to 16-Fr catheter by stapling on the antimesenteric side of the bowel to remove excess bowel. The reservoir is filled with normal saline via the Malecot catheter to make sure that ileocecal valve maintains continence preventing urine leaking from the reservoir.

The tapered ileum is then brought to the skin and secured while maintaining a straight path for catheterization.

Postoperative Care

The ureterointestinal anastomoses are performed over ureteral stents in order to maintain patency and allow proper healing. These stents are externalized and drain to gravity and are typically left for 1 to 2 weeks after which time they are pulled out if there is no evidence of urinary leak. A Jackson-Pratt or Blake drain is placed near the reservoir to drain excess fluid and monitor for urinary leak. The Jackson-Pratt or Blake drain is typically removed prior to discharge from the hospital if there is no evidence of urinary leak.

The 24-Fr Malecot catheter is used to drain the reservoir of the Indiana pouch during the immediate postoperative period. Irrigation of the reservoir is performed intermittently during the first several days after surgery to clear mucous and is titrated to a frequency that makes the mucus manageable. Initially, irrigation is with 30 to 60 mL of normal saline three times or more until irrigant is clear. This process should be performed four times per day and can be spaced out accordingly. The irrigant is introduced into the pouch and allowed to flow out without suction from the syringe.

KEY POINT

The patient and a family member should be taught how to irrigate the pouch prior to discharge. The patient should be discharged with a dependent drainage collector to use at night and a leg bag to use during the day.

A 16-Fr Foley is placed through the catheterizable channel into the reservoir and capped. This catheter maintains the patency of the catheterizable channel and is kept in place for at least 2 to 3 weeks after surgery.

Once the patient is ready to perform self-catheterization (2 to 3 weeks after the operation), the patient is taught to use clean technique and catheterize the pouch every 2 to 4 hours. The patient starts with self-catheterization every 2 hours for 1 week, then every 3 hours for week 2 to 3, and then every 4 hours for week 4 and onward. The patient can increase catheterization if he/she has an increase in fluid intake. During this initial learning period, the Malecot catheter is capped, but it can be uncapped and drained should the patient encounter difficulty in catheterizing.

Once the patient has proven the ability to perform intermittent catheterization, the Malecot catheter is

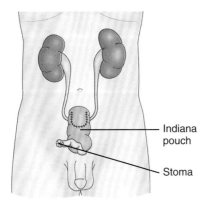

Indiana pouch

Stoma

FIGURE 8-4. Indiana Pouch.

removed. Some urologists choose to perform a poucho-gram whereby the reservoir is filled with contrast and x-ray imaging is performed to ensure that there is no uri-nary leak prior to removal of the Malecot catheter.

A small dressing or Band-Aid can be placed over the catheterizable stoma site for protection. With time, the reservoir will expand between 300 and 500 mL. The patient will achieve increased independence as the fre-quency between catheterization increases.

Early postoperative education is important for patients and their caregivers, who must learn to care for the new continent catheterizable urinary diversion. Inpa-tient visits by the WOC nurse can avoid common pitfalls, which can minimize morbidity associated with continent catheterizable urinary diversion.

KEY POINT

The patient should be instructed to carry at least two cath-eters with him or her at all times along with self-closing plastic bags in which the used catheters can be placed if unable to cleanse the tube after each use.

Patients should obtain medical alert bracelets or other identifying information carried with them at all times to inform other caregivers of the catheterizable channel in the event of an emergency.

Results
The primary objective of a continent urinary diversion is to maintain continence, with a low-pressure, high-volume reservoir, which allows urine to exit via catheterization at reasonable intervals. With time, the capacity of the Indiana pouch increases to 300 to 500 mL, and the incidence of urinary incontinence at 1 year is <2% (Rowland, 1996).

Complications
Similar to patients undergoing ileal conduit diversion, morbidity is significant, and complications include ileus, bowel leak, parastomal hernia, urine leak, infection/pouchitis, urinary stone formation, metabolic alterations (metabolic acidosis, B_{12} deficiency), and ureteral stricture (Kouba et al., 2007; Vasdev et al., 2013). Strictures of the stoma or catheterizable channel can make catheteriza-tion difficult and often requires endoscopic incision or dilation. Rupture of the pouch can occur in patients due to poor compliance with catheterization and can be life threatening.

OTHER CATHETERIZABLE URINARY DIVERSION
While the Indiana pouch is the most predominantly uti-lized catheterizable urinary diversion, several other cath-eterizable urinary diversions have been developed over the years. In a Miami pouch, the bowel segments used

are the same as the Indiana pouch, however, cutting the ascending colon and folding it into a U shape and construct the reservoir. The Koch pouch is constructed by folding 60 cm of ileum into a U shape and creating proximal and distal nipple valves. The ureters are anas-tomosed to the proximal valve, and the distal valve is brought to the skin as a catheterizable stoma. In a Mitro-fanoff procedure, the appendix is used as the cath-eterizable channel. The proximal end is tunneled into the mucosa of the reservoir, which serves as the conti-nence mechanism, and the distal end of the appendix is brought to the skin.

Orthotopic Urinary Diversion: Neobladder
Orthotopic urinary diversion, also called a neobladder, involves the creation of a low-pressure, high-volume res-ervoir that is anastomosed to the urethra. Patients rely on their urinary sphincter for continence and void by relaxing their sphincter and pelvic floor in combination with increasing intra-abdominal pressure by perform-ing Valsalva or Credé maneuver. A minority of patients will develop hypercontinence (inability to empty) and will need to perform intermittent self-catheterization to ade-quately empty their neobladder.

Orthotopic urinary diversion is created in patients who want improved cosmesis (no stoma) and wish to void per urethra. Neobladder diversions are occasionally performed on patients with a large body habitus where bringing a conduit or continent catheterizable channel to the skin is technically difficult.

Similar to continent catheterizable diversion, abso-lute contraindications for orthotopic urinary diversions include hepatic dysfunction, compromised intestinal function (e.g., previous surgery, radiation, inflammatory bowel disease), and renal failure (serum creatinine >1.7). Specific to orthotopic urinary diversion, patients should have a competent urinary sphincter and no evidence of urethral obstruction (Lee et al., 2014).

Physician Considerations
Orthotopic urinary diversions typically are constructed from 50 to 60 cm of ileum, and thus, these segments must be present (no prior resection) and healthy (no inflam-matory bowel disease, no radiation damage) in order to perform this diversion. In oncologic cases, patients must have no disease at the bladder neck or urethra and have a low risk of cancer recurrence. Having a history of prior pelvic radiation significantly increases the complexity of the surgery and the complication rate postoperatively and must be considered prior to performing a neoblad-der diversion.

Patient Considerations
Patients must be motivated and mentally capable of per-forming the more rigorous maintenance of their neoblad-der compared to ileal conduit diversion. Maintenance includes scheduled voiding every 2 to 3 hours and

performing self-catheterizations if needed to empty their reservoir or irrigate mucus that may accumulate within the reservoir. Patients with poor mental capacity, social support, and general health should undergo ileal conduit diversion.

Preoperative Consideration

In the event that during the surgical procedure it is determined an orthotopic urinary diversion cannot be created, patients should undergo evaluation and stoma siting by the WOC nurse to mark for either a continent catheterizable channel or ileal conduit. This is another opportunity to determine the patient's motivation, manual dexterity, and mental capacity.

Similar to patients undergoing ileal conduits and continent catheterizable channels, some urologists choose to employ a mechanical and/or antibiotic preoperative bowel regimen. All patients receive preoperative intravenous antibiotics immediately before surgery, which are typically stopped within 24 hours.

Surgical Procedure

In male patients, the bladder and prostate are removed, while in female patients, the bladder, anterior vagina, uterus, fallopian tubes, and ovaries are removed. In both instances, care is taken to perform meticulous dissection near the urethra and urinary sphincter to preserve continence. In female patients who elect for an orthotopic neobladder, sparing the anterior vagina wall, uterus, and ovaries can be performed. This helps maintain support for the neobladder as well as the more optimal urethral voiding angle. An additional concern in female patients with neobladders is formation of vesicovaginal fistula that may form between the suture line of the neobladder and the suture line of the vagina.

Reservoirs are typically created from 50 to 60 cm of ileum, which is mobilized and discontinued from the remaining bowel. Continuity of the bowel is reestablished using bowel staplers. Next, the bowel is detubularized by incising it on the antimesenteric side.

There are two main types of orthotopic neobladders that are commonly performed: the Studer and Hautmann neobladders. The main differences between these diversions are the shape the bowel is folded when constructing the reservoir. In a Studer diversion, the bowel is folded over in a U configuration (**Fig. 8-5**), while in a Hautmann diversion, the bowel is folded to create an M or W configuration.

After the posterior plate of the reservoir is sutured, the ureters are anastomosed to the neobladder in an end-to-side fashion over a stent, which is placed up the ureter to protect the anastomosis and aids in healing. The anterior plate of the reservoir is next closed with suture. The ureteral stents are brought out of the neobladder, and a 24-Fr Malecot catheter is placed through the skin into the neobladder and secured.

Lastly, a small buttonhole opening is created in the most dependent portion of the neobladder, which is used as the anastomosis to the urethra.

Postoperative Care

The ureteral stents are externalized and allowed to drain to gravity. They are typically left for 1 to 2 weeks after which time if there is no evidence of urinary leak, they are removed. A Jackson-Pratt or Blake drain is placed near the reservoir to drain excess fluid and is typically removed prior to discharge from the hospital if there is no evidence of urinary leak.

The 24-Fr Malecot catheter is externalized and is used to drain and irrigate the reservoir of the neobladder during the immediate postoperative period. Irrigation of the reservoir is performed intermittently during the first several days after surgery and is titrated to a frequency that makes the mucus manageable.

A 22-Fr Foley is placed through the urethra into the reservoir and is also used to drain and irrigate the neobladder. The catheter aids in the healing of the anastomosis between the neobladder and urethra. It is kept in place for at least 2 to 3 weeks after surgery.

At or about 3 weeks post op the Malecot tube is capped, the urethral foley is removed, and the patient is instructed to void every 2 to 3 hours for about 3 weeks and return to the outpatient area to have creatinine and BUN done as well as check for post residual void. The Malecot can be removed at this time or can be left in place for uncapping if the patient encounters difficulty in

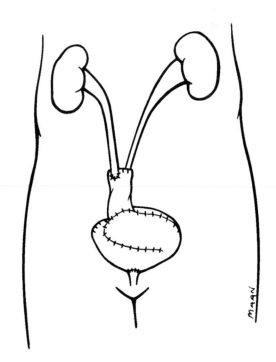

FIGURE 8-5. Studer Neobladder. (Used with permission from Fischer, J. E. (2018). *Fischer's mastery of surgery* (7th ed.). Philadelphia, PA: Wolters Kluwer.)

emptying the neobladder. The 24-Fr Malecot catheter is removed once the patient is comfortable and proficient at emptying their neobladder per the urethra.

If the post residual void is reasonable (<100 cc) and creatinine is normal, they can extend their voids to every 4 hours as long as they don't leak. Some clinicians have the patients see the pelvic floor physical therapy before surgery to do Kegels, and the physical therapist may follow them for several months.

Emptying of the neobladder relies on relaxation of the urethral sphincter and pelvic floor in combination with increasing intra-abdominal pressure by performing Valsalva or Credé maneuver. Patients should be taught how to perform self-intermittent catheterization if they are unable to completely empty their neobladder or need to irrigate accumulated mucus. Patients should also perform pelvic floor exercises to aid in strengthening their urinary sphincter and pelvic floor. Patients often develop nighttime incontinence and need to set an alarm clock to one to two times per night to empty their neobladder and prevent overflow incontinence.

As with continent catheterizable urinary diversion, patients with neobladders should wear medical alert bracelets stating that they have a "continent internal urinary diversion."

Results

There is a general improvement with continence from 6 to 12 months when the neobladder increases in capacity to around 300 to 500 mL. Daytime continence rates are generally >90% based on the results from pooled series with nighttime continence rates of 80% to 90% (Steers, 2000). Failure to empty the neobladder has been reported to be 4% to 25% necessitating intermittent self-catheterization (Nagele et al., 2006; Steers, 2000).

Complications

As with any bowel diversion, morbidity is significant, and complications include ileus, bowel leak, urine leak, infection, urinary stone formation, metabolic alterations (metabolic acidosis, B_{12} deficiency), and ureteral stricture. These have been described in the ileal conduit section.

Specific to orthotopic neobladder procedures, there is a low risk of reservoir perforation and typically occurs in patients with noncompliance in emptying their neobladder or obstruction of their neobladder. Contracture of the bladder neck can occur in patients and requires endoscopic dilation or incision. Infections of the pouch, known as pouchitis, can often occur causing pain, fever, malaise, and hematuria and requires antibiotic treatment. Recurrence of cancer at the urethra requires urethrectomy and conversion of the orthotopic neobladder to a cutaneous catheterizable channel or ileal conduit.

 ## CONCLUSIONS

Urinary intestinal diversion has evolved over the years with several different diversion options available to patients. Careful preoperative and postoperative counseling by physicians and WOC nurses are imperative to ensure that each patient selects the appropriate diversion and is predicated upon on assessment of the patient's health status, disease burden, and physical, psychological, social, and financial status.

REFERENCES

Bladder Cancer Support Society. (2014). Retrieved December 20, 2019, from http://bladdercancersupport.org/bladder-cancer-help/bladder-cancer-facts/statistics?gclid=CN_qhJyEnsACFYk7Mgod-TywAMA.

Fichtner, J. (1999). Follow-up after urinary diversion. *Urologia Internationalis, 63*(1), 40–45.

Kouba, E., Sands, M., Lentz, A., et al. (2007). Incidence and risk factors of stomal complications in patients undergoing cystectomy with ileal conduit urinary diversion for bladder cancer. *The Journal of Urology, 178*(3 Pt 1), 950–954.

Kristjánsson, A., Wallin, L., & Månsson, W. (1995). Renal function up to 16 years after conduit (refluxing or anti-reflux anastomosis) or continent urinary diversion. 1. Glomerular filtration rate and patency of uretero-intestinal anastomosis. *British Journal of Urology, 76,* 539–545.

Lee, R. K., Abol-Enein, H., Arani, W., et al. (2014). Urinary diversion after radical cystectomy for bladder cancer: Options, patient selection, and outcomes. *BJU International, 113*(1), 11–23.

Nagele, U., Kuczyk, A., Aristotelis, G., et al. (2006). Radical cystectomy and orthotopic bladder replacement in females. *European Urology, 50,* 249–257.

Pannek, J., & Senge, T. (1998). History of urinary diversion. *Urologia Internationalis, 60*(1), 1–10.

Ratner, V. (2001). Interstitial cystitis: A chronic inflammatory bladder condition. *World Journal of Urology, 19*(3), 157–159.

Rowland, R. G. (1996). Present experience with the Indiana pouch. *World Journal of Urology, 14,* 92–98.

Salvadalena, G., Hendren, S., McKenna, L., et al. (2015). WOCN Society and AUA position statement on preoperative stoma site marking for patients undergoing urostomy surgery. *Journal of Wound, Ostomy, and Continence Nursing, 42,* (3), 253–256.

Steers, W. D. (2000). Voiding dysfunction in the orthotopic neobladder. *World Journal of Urology, 18*(5), 330–337.

Vasdev, N., Moon, A., & Thorpe, A. C. (2013). Metabolic complications of urinary intestinal diversion. *Indian Journal of Urology, 29*(4), 310–315.

Yang, L. S., Shan, B. L., Shan, L. L., et al. (2016). A systematic review and meta-analysis of quality of life outcomes after radical cystectomy for bladder cancer. *Surgical Oncology, 25*(3), 281–297.

Zhang, J. H., Ericson, K. J., Thomas, L. J., et al. (2019). Large single institution comparison of perioperative outcomes and complications of open radical cystectomy, intracorporeal robot-assisted radical cystectomy and robotic extracorporeal approach. *Journal of Urology, 203*(3), 512–521. https://doi.org/10.1097/JU.0000000000000570

QUESTIONS

1. A patient with refractory cystitis is scheduled for surgery for a urinary diversion. Which diversion is a good choice for this patient as it involves the simplest segment of bowel and has the lowest complication rate?
   A. Ileal conduit
   B. Colon conduit
   C. Orthotopic neobladder
   D. Indiana pouch

2. Which disease state is the most predominant indication for performing an intestinal urinary diversion?
   A. Neurogenic bladder
   B. Refractory cystitis
   C. Bladder cancer
   D. Urinary fistula

3. Which patient would the WOC nurse place at greatest risk for bladder cancer?
   A. A patient who has diabetes mellitus
   B. A patient who smokes two packs of cigarettes a day
   C. A patient who drinks a six pack of beer a day
   D. A patient who has experienced trauma involving the urinary sphincter

4. A patient with an identified bladder tumor would most likely undergo which diagnostic procedure to formulate a prognosis and manage the tumor therapeutically?
   A. Contrast-enhanced CT scan of the kidneys
   B. Bladder tumor resection
   C. Endoscopic evaluation of the urethra and bladder
   D. Urine cytology

5. A WOC nurse evaluating the urine studies of a patient notes that the patient has petechial hemorrhage as a finding of cystoscopy. Which bladder disorder would the nurse suspect?
   A. Bladder cancer
   B. Neurogenic bladder
   C. Interstitial cystitis
   D. Trauma to the bladder

6. A surgeon is performing a neobladder diversion for a patient who has bladder cancer. What amount of bowel length would be required to create this type of diversion?
   A. 10 to 15 cm
   B. 15 to 30 cm
   C. 40 to 50 cm
   D. 50 to 60 cm

7. The most distal 12- to 15-cm segment of ileum just proximal to the ileocecal valve is typically spared during the surgical procedure for an ileal conduit given its importance for bile salt and
   A. Vitamin B_{12} absorption
   B. Calcium absorption
   C. Vitamin C absorption
   D. Protein absorption

8. Which complication of an incontinent urinary diversion can sometimes be managed with catheterization but may necessitate revisional surgery?
   A. Prolapse
   B. Retraction
   C. Parastomal hernia
   D. Stomal stenosis

9. Which urinary diversion is the predominant urinary diversion for patients who desire a continent catheterizable urinary diversion?
   A. Indiana pouch
   B. Colon conduit
   C. Orthotopic urinary diversion
   D. Mitrofanoff procedure

10. The WOC nurse is evaluating a patient for an orthotopic urinary diversion. What is a major patient consideration for creating this type of diversion?
   A. Ease of maintenance
   B. Improved cosmesis
   C. No need for self-intermittent catheterization
   D. Low risk of infection of the pouch

ANSWERS AND RATIONALES

1. A. Rationale: Ileal conduit has the lowest complication rates and has the shortest OR time compared to continent diversions and the colon conduit.

2. C. Rationale: Bladder cancer is the most common condition that requires a urinary diversion.

3. B. Rationale: People who smoke are at a high risk to develop bladder cancer.

4. B. Rationale: Bladder tumor resection should be performed to determine the pathology of the tumor and to develop the treatment plan.

5. C. Rationale: Small ulcerations or petechial hemorrhage are a finding via cystoscopy in the patient with interstitial cystitis.

6. D. Rationale: Continent urinary diversion requires 50 to 60 cm of bowel length compared to 10 to 12 cm for an ileal conduit.

7. A. Rationale: The 12 to 15 cm of the ileum closet to the ileocecal valve are usually spared because of the importance of vitamin B_{12} absorption along with bile salt.

8. D. Rationale: Stomal stenosis is an ileal conduit complication that may be managed with a catheterization; however, surgery maybe indicated to revise the stoma.

9. A. Rationale: The Indiana pouch is a continent catheterizable urinary diversion. The colon conduit is an incontinent urinary diversion managed with a pouch system. Mitrofanoff procedures is a catheterizable diversion but not as common as the Indiana pouch. With the orthotopic diversion, the person is able to void through the urethra.

10. B. Rationale: The orthotopic neobladder advantage is improved cosmesis with no stoma.

CHAPTER 9

FECAL AND URINARY STOMA CONSTRUCTION

Linda Jean Stricker, Barbara Hocevar, and Sherief Shawki

OBJECTIVE

Discuss construction of fecal and urinary stomas.

TOPIC OUTLINE

Introduction   **131**

Stoma Construction Surgical Technique   **132**
    Stoma Maturation   132
    Stoma Construction Types   132
        End Stoma   132
        Loop Stoma   133
        Loop–End Stoma   135

Fecal Stoma Construction   **136**
    Small Bowel   136
        Duodenostomy   136
        Jejunostomy   136
        Ileostomy   136

    Hydration Concerns   136
    Large Bowel   137
        Cecostomy   137
        Colostomy   137
        Mucous Fistula   137

Urinary Stoma Construction   **138**
    Types   138
        Ureterostomy   138
        Ileal Conduit   139
        Jejunal Conduit   139

Conclusions   **139**

INTRODUCTION

The word stoma comes from the Greek word for mouth. Generally speaking a stoma is a surgically created opening that connects a hollow viscus, most commonly the gastrointestinal tract (GIT) to the abdominal wall skin. A stoma can be created from any part of the GIT, in which case the effluent will represent the GIT-type content respective of that portion. The more distal in the GIT, the more formed stool is excreted. However, the higher the location in the GIT the more fluid, electrolytes, and chemical contents (e.g., bile, pancreatic fluids, enzymes) are excreted as well as increase higher volume. Alternatively, a piece of the distal alimentary tract may be resected and used as a conduit, to which both ureters are connected (hand-sewn anastomosis), for urinary excretion. This conduit acts as a passage way for urine to exit the body in lieu of urinary bladder.

Writings about spontaneous stomas occur throughout history, and many of these stomas were originally the result of battle-related wounds or disease. Over the years, surgical techniques improved as did techniques for stoma construction. These advancements enhanced a surgeon's ability to treat disease or repair and minimize the effects of trauma, thereby saving lives (Wu, 2012). Optimizing quality of life and maintaining good health are now primary goals for a person with an ostomy.

Preoperative stoma site marking, ideal stoma construction, and the promotion of self-care through the fitting and management of the ostomy system contributes to enhanced quality of life for the individual with a stoma.

Classifications of stomas include temporary or permanent, construction type of the stoma and the anatomical location (**Table 9-1**). Temporary stomas usually remain in place for 3 to 6 months but may become permanent for 20% to 50% of individuals (Forgione & Cataldo, 2003; Pine & Stevenson, 2014; Wexner et al., 1993; Whitehead et al., 2014). An example would be a patient with an ostomy after bowel resection that chooses to keep the stoma rather than undergoing another operation to restore bowel continuity or a person who is a poor surgical candidate. Stomas are also identified by the type of surgical construction: end, loop, and loop–end. Abdominal stomas are also identified as fecal and urinary.

 ## STOMA CONSTRUCTION SURGICAL TECHNIQUE

STOMA MATURATION

Initially, stomas were created flush to skin level which made them very hard to manage. This technique resulted in severe peristomal skin destruction as stomas were very difficult to manage due to leaking of the ostomy pouching system. The concept of a spouted (nonskin level) stoma was introduced in 1913. At that time, the bowel was raised above the skin level, leaving its outer layer (serosa) exposed to the atmosphere. Since this is not the physiological environment for the bowel, significant inflammatory reaction called "serositis" would occur after surgery. As a result of serositis, there is massive edema of the stoma with a risk for partial or complete obstruction, diarrhea, fluid and electrolyte imbalances, and dehydration (Kaidar-Person et al., 2005; Martin & Vogel, 2012; Wu, 2012). Eventually, these stomas would self-mature. Maturation refers to the eversion of the bowel segment to expose the mucosa at the time of stoma construction (**Fig. 9-2**). Stomas not matured at surgery undergo self-maturation, a process that occurs when the inflamed and gummy serosal surfaces adhere to each other, causing a gradual eventual eversion of the stoma (Doughty, 2004).

Self-maturation or eversion of the bowel is a gradual process taking approximately 4 to 6 weeks. The stoma will look the same at the end of this process as a matured stoma. An unmatured stoma is difficult for patients to deal with due to the dramatic appearance. The concept of eversion or primary maturation introduced by Dr. Bryan Brooke in 1952 paved the way for increased survival for the majority of individuals requiring ostomy surgery; this technique is referred to as a Brooke stoma (Kaidar-Person et al., 2005; Martin & Vogel, 2012; Wu, 2012). In primary maturation, the intestinal segment is brought through the predesignated site and everted or folded back on itself, similar to cuffing a sleeve. The matured stoma will expose the inner mucosal lining of the bowel with a beefy red, shiny, and moist surface. There are no sensory nerve endings in the stoma. Stretch receptors are located within the intestinal wall so a stretch feeling may be felt as bowel content exits the stoma. This can be experienced with a sigmoid colostomy that may pass a large formed stool.

STOMA CONSTRUCTION TYPES

> **KEY POINT**
>
> There are three stoma construction types: end, loop, and loop–end (**Table 9-2**).

End Stoma

An end stoma means that the part of bowel used to create the stoma is disconnected from bowel downstream. The surgeon prepares and mobilizes the intestinal segment with mesentery to be used and brings the segment through the predetermined abdominal aperture to create the stoma (**Fig. 9-1**). The aperture is two finger-breadths in size, or about 2 to 3 cm in length, in order to minimize the risk of herniation or prolapse (Forgione & Cataldo, 2003; Garofalo, 2012; Martin & Vogel, 2012; Pine & Stevenson, 2014; Saunders & Hemingway, 2008; Stocchi, 2012; Whitehead & Cataldo, 2017). The application of sterile dressings or drapes to the surgical site protects the incision from possible fecal contamination;

TABLE 9-1 STOMA CLASSIFICATIONS			
LENGTH OF TIME	CONSTRUCTION STOMA TYPE	ANATOMIC LOCATION	
Temporary	End	Fecal	Urinary
Permanent	Loop	Colon	Conduit + bowel segment used
	Loop–end	Ileum	Ileum
	Continent	Jejunum	Sigmoid colon
		Duodenum	Jejunum
			Continent diversion

TABLE 9-2 STOMA CONSTRUCTION TYPES

TYPE OF STOMA*	FEATURES
End	One stoma with one opening
Loop	One stoma with two openings
	Proximal or functioning opening
	Distal or nonfunctioning opening
Loop–end	One stoma with two openings
	Used in patients with thick abdominal
	walls and possible vascular
	compromise if created as an end
	stoma

*Anatomic location dictates type, amount, and quality of effluent.

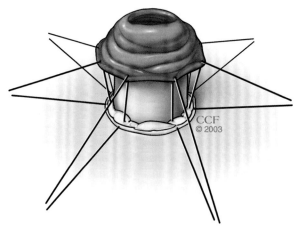

FIGURE 9-2. Stoma Maturation. Absorbable sutures are placed through the full thickness of the bowel wall and secured to the subcuticular (dermal) layer of skin only. Full-thickness suturing of the skin (through the epidermis) can result in tracking of mucosal cells through the epidermis, resulting in mucosal implants. (Reprinted with permission, Cleveland Clinic Center for Medical Art & Photography © 2014. All Rights Reserved.)

maturation of the stoma follows. The edge of this intestinal segment is everted using four equidistant sutures placed through the entire bowel wall followed by suturing through the subcuticular (dermal) layer of the respective quadrant in the stoma aperture (**Fig. 9-2**). This is done to prevent seeding of the epidermis with mucosal cells, which can result in peristomal mucosal implants (Whitehead & Cataldo, 2017).

It is important that the matured piece of bowel is well vascularized, properly oriented (not twisted), and under no tension to avoid retraction (Martin & Vogel, 2012; Saunders & Hemingway, 2008; Whitehead & Cataldo, 2017; Wu, 2003). Once full eversion is accomplished, additional sutures are added to complete the process, and the newly created stoma is ready for the appropriate pouching system (Garofalo, 2012). End ileostomies should protrude from the skin approximately 2 to 3 cm (Martin & Vogel, 2012; Stocchi, 2012; Whitehead & Cataldo, 2017). The formation of a spout should

prohibit the effluent from going beneath the pouching system (**Fig. 9-3**). End colostomies should protrude 0.5 to 1.0 cm above the skin, but flush construction may also occur (Garofalo, 2012; Martin & Vogel, 2012; Saunders & Hemingway, 2008; Whitehead & Cataldo, 2017). In this case, there is less concern about skin irritation (as mentioned above) as the well-formed stool should not leak between the skin and the pouching system.

Loop Stoma

The loop stoma is one stoma with two openings, proximal (stool will pass from this opening) and distal (leading to the divert section). In general, loop stoma construction usually protects a distal anastomosis, put distal diseased/inflamed bowel out of function, or diverts from a downstream obstruction. After completion of the surgery on the

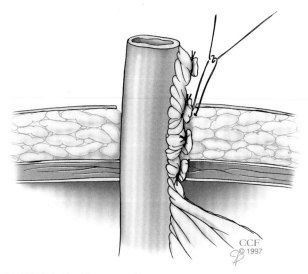

FIGURE 9-1. End Ileostomy. The end of the ileum is brought through the preselected stoma site. (Reprinted with permission, Cleveland Clinic Center for Medical Art & Photography © 2014. All Rights Reserved.)

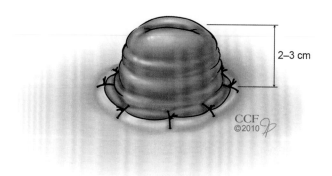

FIGURE 9-3. Matured End Ileostomy. The stoma ideally protrudes 2 to 3 cm above skin level. This helps to protect the skin from stomal output and makes for easier pouching. (Reprinted with permission, Cleveland Clinic Center for Medical Art & Photography © 2014. All Rights Reserved.)

distal intestinal anastomosis, the surgeon brings a loop of intestine, usually located 12 to 15 cm from the ileocecal valve for an ileostomy (Martin & Vogel, 2012; Whitehead & Cataldo, 2017), through a predetermined site on the abdomen. It is important that the proximal and distal ends of the intestine are properly identified in order to maintain appropriate anatomic orientation. In some instances, the distal limb is marked with a catgut (brown) suture, and the proximal limb is marked with a blue (Vicryl) suture "(brown for the earth [i.e., {sic}, down or distal] and blue for the sky [i.e., {sic}, upward or proximal])" (Martin & Vogel, 2012, p. 25). A plastic rod, tubing, or similar device may be placed under the loop of intestine to provide support in order to prevent early retraction of the stoma (**Fig. 9-4**).

After closing the abdominal wounds, sterile dressings or towels are used to cover the surgical incision(s) to avoid contamination when opening the bowel to create the stoma. The intestine is then cut open about 5/8ths of its circumference. The intestine remains joined along its mesenteric or inside edge, and maturation of the two cut edges creates one stoma with two openings (**Figs. 9-5 and 9-6**). The proximal opening is the functional lumen through which effluent will pass. The distal lumen leads to the lower intestine; a small quantity of mucus will occasionally pass from the distal lumen or anus. The proximal lumen usually protrudes more from the abdomen than the distal lumen (Whitehead & Cataldo, 2017) (**Fig. 9-7**). This is important to allow the effluent to flow into the pouching system, minimizing the chance of leakage.

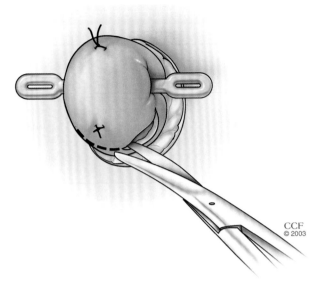

FIGURE 9-5. Loop Ileostomy Construction. The appropriate area of the intestine is opened from one side to the other, leaving intact intestine on the underside. (Reprinted with permission, Cleveland Clinic Center for Medical Art & Photography © 2014. All Rights Reserved.)

The rod under the stoma stays in place for 2 to 7 days depending on whether the case is laparoscopic or open, the amount of tension present on the rod, and surgeon preference (Garofalo, 2012; Martin & Vogel, 2012; Pine & Stevenson, 2014; Stocchi, 2012). The rod commonly remains in place for 2 days following a laparoscopic

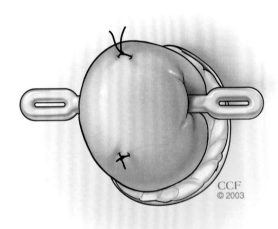

FIGURE 9-4. Loop Ileostomy Construction. Note the placement of sutures (each would be in a different color) that help maintain appropriate orientation of the proximal and distal portions of the intestine. The loop of the small bowel is brought out through the predetermined stoma site, and a rod is placed underneath the intestine and on top of the skin in order to provide support to the intestinal loop. (Reprinted with permission, Cleveland Clinic Center for Medical Art & Photography © 2014. All Rights Reserved.)

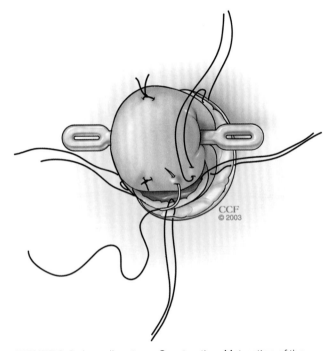

FIGURE 9-6. Loop Ileostomy Construction. Maturation of the stoma: Note the placement of the sutures through full thickness of the intestinal wall and the subcuticular (dermal) layer of the skin. (Reprinted with permission, Cleveland Clinic Center for Medical Art & Photography © 2014. All Rights Reserved.)

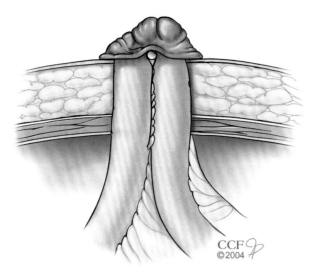

FIGURE 9-7. Matured Loop Ileostomy. The proximal (afferent) limb of the stoma is the protruding end, and the distal (efferent) limb is flush to skin level. (Reprinted with permission, Cleveland Clinic Center for Medical Art & Photography © 2014. All Rights Reserved.)

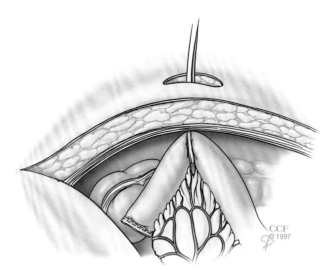

FIGURE 9-8. Loop–end Ileostomy Construction. Distal intestine is removed or left dormant. The proximal end of the intestine is stapled closed. The vascular arcade is protected with this technique. (Reprinted with permission, Cleveland Clinic Center for Medical Art & Photography © 2014. All Rights Reserved.)

creation of the stoma and 3 days following conventional surgery. As with an end stoma, it is important to bring the intestine used to create the stoma through the abdominal opening with as little tension as possible, with a good blood supply, and with normal anatomical orientation of the mesentery.

KEY POINT

End stoma construction results in one stoma with one opening.

Loop–End Stoma

In certain situations, an end type of stomas is required, although it is hard to bring a true "end" of the bowel as a stoma to reach the skin level. However, a loop of bowel, just proximal to the end, can reach without tension. In these cases, the terminal end of the bowel is closed, and the stoma is created as loop stoma hence the name loop–end (Martin & Vogel, 2012; Stocchi, 2012; Wu, 2003). Externally, there is no difference in how a loop or loop–end stoma looks. With loop–end construction, the distal lumen leads to a blind pouch. The blind segment is usually short and will produce mucus. A loop–end ileal conduit uses this type of construction and is discussed in more detail under ileal conduits. Loop–end construction is used when the person has a thick abdominal wall, shortened mesentery, or a combination, and there is concern about adequate blood supply to the distal end of the stoma (**Figs. 9-8 and 9-9**). Additionally, when there is a need for a permanent stoma and a loop stoma is already present, the distal limb can be transected and the stoma converted to loop–end construction (Martin & Vogel, 2012; Stocchi, 2012; Wu, 2003).

KEY POINT

Loop–end stoma is sometimes called Turnbull loop–end stoma.

Double-barrel ostomy construction is seen rarely; when it is, it usually occurs with colostomies. Two stomas are created in proximity to each other, resembling the end of a double-barrel shotgun, hence the name. The proximal stoma is functional, and the distal stoma

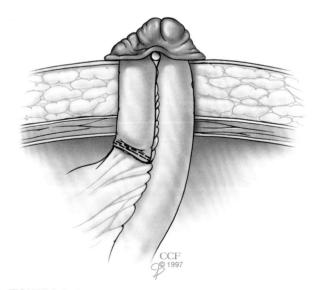

FIGURE 9-9. Loop–end Ileostomy Construction. A loop of intestine above this staple line is brought through the premarked site, and a loop of ileum is matured. This creates one stoma with a proximal, functioning lumen and a short distal segment. (Reprinted with permission, Cleveland Clinic Center for Medical Art & Photography © 2014. All Rights Reserved.)

serves as a mucous fistula (Saunders & Hemingway, 2008). Double-barrel construction prevents any effluent from flowing into the distal stoma (mucous fistula). Indications for this type of stoma construction include massive infection and situations of distal obstruction where the bowel above the obstruction needs venting. Leaving a blind loop in the abdomen increases the risk for perforated viscus; there needs to be a way for the mucus to exit the bowel. Depending on how far apart the stomas are, pouching can be difficult.

FECAL STOMA CONSTRUCTION

SMALL BOWEL

Duodenostomy

Duodenostomies, that is, stomas in the duodenum, are rarely done. This type of stoma sometimes indicates an abdominal catastrophe. Essential care of a duodenostomy consists of peristomal skincare and management of high-volume output as the later can result in dehydration and electrolyte disturbances. The location of these stomas is in the midline and near body creases, which is a direct result of limited bowel length secondary to the initial catastrophic event; this location creates significant pouching challenges. These patients tend to require much emotional support as minimal preoperative education is performed due to the emergent nature of surgery. Pouching considerations are the same as with jejunostomies which are discussed below.

Jejunostomy

The location of jejunostomies is usually in the left upper quadrant of the abdomen. Creation of this stoma type is generally done to protect a distal anastomosis, or as a result of an abdominal catastrophe, such as an embolism to the superior mesenteric artery (SMA). Fifteen percent of emboli tend to settle at the origin of the SMA. The remainder will settle distally to the SMA's origin at its first major branch, which is the middle colic artery, thus sparing ischemia to the upper jejunum (Oldenburg et al., 2004; Pearl & Gilani, 2018). Jejunostomies produce high volumes of liquid output (Bafford & Irani, 2013; Martin & Vogel, 2012; Rombeau, 2012); chunks of food can be seen in the output if the person is taking food orally. These stomas typically begin function on days 1 to 3 postoperatively. The initial output is a dark green viscous liquid. The output from a jejunostomy is neutral to slightly alkaline with a pH ranging from 7 to 9 and contains activated digestive enzymes.

When jejunal effluent contacts the skin, the activated enzymes digest the epidermis, rapidly exposing the dermis. Peristomal moisture-associated skin damage is moist, red, and painful with a burning, stinging sensation, particularly when effluent comes in contact with the denuded area. Issues of concern are protection of the peristomal skin from stoma output, containment of high-volume output, and management of fluid and electrolyte disturbances (Colwell et al., 2011; Gray et al., 2013; Krapfl & Zurcher, 2010). Individuals with jejunostomies run the risk of dehydration and may require total parenteral nutrition to maintain proper nutrition and fluid intake; use of medication to slow intestinal motility is common (Parekh & Seidner, 2012). Suggested for use with liquid output are pouching systems with extended wear skin barriers, which have components that withstand liquid output better than do regular wear skin barriers (Goldberg et al., 2010). High-volume output pouches are standard. Placing pouches to constant drainage during sleeping hours helps to decrease excessive pull on the pouching system and allows patients to sleep undisturbed. The output has minimal odor.

> **KEY POINT**
>
> Duodenostomy and jejunostomy are rare and usually created following a catastrophic event.

Ileostomy

Ileostomies, usually located in the right lower quadrant, have output that ranges from a liquid to a mushy (applesauce or pudding) consistency depending upon the location in the ileum. The more proximal the ileostomy, that is, the closer the stoma is to the stomach, the more liquid the output and the greater the enzyme content. Ileostomies begin to function from 1 to 3 postoperatively. The initial effluent is usually a dark green liquid with a viscous appearance, later turning brown in color with liquid to mushy character. There is potential for significant peristomal moisture-associated skin damage if the effluent contacts the peristomal skin. The preference is for extended wear skin barriers (Goldberg et al., 2010; Registered Nurses' Association of Ontario [RNAO], 2009). Drainable pouches are the norm; if an individual has high-volume output, the recommendation is to use high-volume output pouches.

Hydration Concerns

Special consideration needs to be given to stomas that have high volume output; this occurs when there is <200 cm of small bowel to the stoma such as occurs with jejunostomies, impaired bowel function, gastrointestinal infections particularly *Clostridium difficile*, abrupt withdrawal of steroids, intra-abdominal abscess, or in those with multiple small bowel resections (Arenas et al., 2015; Raju et al., 2018; Smith & Boland, 2013). High volume output can also be found in newly formed ileostomies in the early postoperative period (Raju et al., 2018; Smith & Boland, 2013). Stomas with high volume output present unique challenges. High volume output in stomas varies in the literature from 1,000 mL to 2,000 mL/24 hours (Goodey & Colman, 2016; Smith & Boland, 2013; Stankiewicz et al., 2019; Vries et al., 2017). Output over 1,200 mL/24 hours over time is known to result in dehydration, electrolyte depletion, and renal failure, which can lead to acute kidney disease (Arenas et al., 2015; Goodey & Colman, 2016; Smith & Boland, 2013). Fluid loss, as well as sodium and magnesium losses are of particular concern. It is not unusual for a person with an ileostomy to have high volume output for approximately 2 weeks after surgery (Goodey & Colman, 2016; Medlin, 2012; Murken & Bleier, 2019; Smith & Boland, 2013) and with many individuals discharged from the hospital early (from 3 to 5 days postoperatively), education to prevent dehydration and readmission is vital. Education may include measurement of output (both urinary and stomal) for 2 weeks post-discharge with documentation of the volume; at least 1,200 mL of urine/24 hours to assure good kidney health (Bridges et al., 2019). Individuals must notify their health care provider if the ostomy output is over 1,200 mL/24 hours or if they have signs or symptoms of dehydration (Steinhagen et al., 2017). They also need to be educated on the need to limit hypotonic fluids such as water, regular sports drinks, and tea as these pull more sodium into the lumen of the bowel, increasing sodium loss through the stoma (Goodey & Colman, 2016; Medlin, 2012; Smith & Boland, 2013; Yang & Boushey, 2014). In order to replace this loss, oral rehydration solutions are recommended and can be purchased or made at home (Goodey & Colman, 2016; Medlin, 2012; Stankiewicz et al., 2019). A multidisciplinary team is necessary to manage these patients (Yang & Boushey, 2014); referral to a registered dietitian nutritionist who is familiar with high volume output stomas is desirable (Goodey & Colman, 2016; Medlin, 2012). In general, people with high volume output stomas should avoid simple sugars and take in low fiber starchy foods such as potatoes and white bread, rice, and pastas with normal intake of fats; an increased salt intake is also helpful (Medlin, 2012; Smith & Boland, 2013; Yang & Boushey, 2014). Medications are also prescribed to decrease the volume of fluid in the intestine as well as to slow transit time. Medications include proton pump inhibitors, histamine-2 receptor antagonist, and antimotility agents in particular loperamide and if needed, codeine (Vries et al., 2017) (see Chapter 14 for more information).

LARGE BOWEL

Cecostomy

Cecostomies are rarely done, and when they are done, it is as a tube cecostomy. The tube cecostomy acts to decompress the colon, treat cecal volvulus, or manage perforation of the cecum when resection is not an option (Garofalo, 2012; Saunders & Hemingway, 2008). A large-bore tube or catheter is inserted into the cecum, secured

to the skin, and connected to gravity drainage. The output is liquid with particles, is malodorous, and frequently clogs the drainage tubing even with irrigation (Garofalo, 2012). Leakage around the catheter or tube is very common, and peritubular moisture-associated skin damage can occur.

Colostomy

Ascending colostomies are another rare type of stoma. They have output similar to cecostomies in that it is semiliquid with a strong odor secondary to the effects of colonic bacteria (Martin & Vogel, 2012). The effluent can cause considerable tissue destruction to the peristomal skin. Fluid and electrolyte imbalances are also a concern.

Transverse colostomies may be in the right upper quadrant, midabdomen, or left upper quadrant depending upon where in the transverse colon, the stoma creation occurs. The stool is a liquid to a pasty consistency and usually malodorous. They are generally created for protection of an anastomosis or to relieve a distal obstruction and are often constructed as part of an emergent surgery (Garofalo, 2012). Stomal prolapse, particularly of the distal lumen in loop transverse colostomies, and hernia formation are common problems seen in transverse colostomies. Pouching can be problematic, should these problems occur.

The location of a descending or sigmoid colostomy is usually in the left lower quadrant, unless patients body habitus is not suitable hence will be in left upper quadrant. The stool is a pasty to a formed consistency; the stool is not as irritating to the skin as ileostomy effluent but can still cause peristomal moisture-associated skin damage (**Fig. 9-10**). Depending upon how often the stoma functions, an individual will use either a drainable pouch or closed-end pouch. A closed-end pouch is recommended if the stoma functions once to twice a day. Individuals with a descending or sigmoid colostomy may choose to irrigate the stoma to control its activity. Irrigation entails instilling water into the bowel at the same time every day in order to stimulate the bowel to function. This procedure is discussed in more detail in Chapter 14.

Odor and gas are a concern for the individual with a colostomy (Goldberg et al., 2010; Registered Nurses' Association of Ontario [RNAO], 2009). Use of filtered pouches; pouch deodorant; or oral, intestinal deodorizing medications can assist in odor and gas control. Dietary measures also are used to deal with gas and odor (see Chapters 10, 13, and 14 for more information).

Mucous Fistula

The mucous fistula is formed when the distal end (downstream) of a section of defunctionalized bowel is brought through the abdominal wall and a stoma is

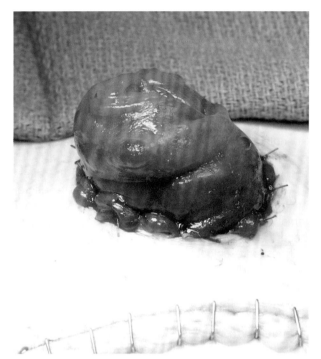

FIGURE 9-10. Matured End Colostomy. Note the degree of stomal eversion and presence of sutures to secure mucocutaneous junction. (Reprinted with permission, Cleveland Clinic Center for Medical Art & Photography © 2014. All Rights Reserved.)

created (Pine & Stevenson, 2014). See **Figure 9-11**. The output from a mucous fistula is mucus, sometimes mixed with small amounts of blood depending on the reason for its formation. A classic example of a mucous fistula occurs when a patient has toxic megacolon. The surgery

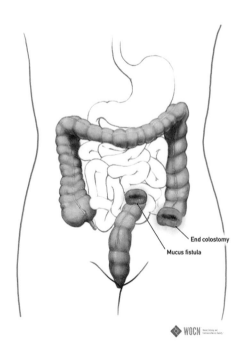

End colostomy

Mucus fistula

FIGURE 9-11. Mucous Fistula.

initially performed is a subtotal colectomy, also known as total abdominal colectomy. In this surgery, the colon is removed, and the rectum with the adjacent part of sigmoid colon remains in place; it is known as the rectal stump.

The method used to manage the top of the rectum depends on the integrity of the rectal tissues. Sometimes, stapling or suturing the top of the rectum closed and placing it immediately under the skin with incisional closure occurs when rectal tissues are relatively healthy. In this way, finding the top of the rectal stump is easy when a person undergoes further surgery. Additionally, if the top of the rectum opens, the drainage becomes a nuisance rather than a crisis, as the pus and blood drain onto the abdomen and not into the peritoneal cavity. Alternately, if tissue integrity is poor, formation of a stoma from the top of the rectal stump serves as an exit point for the pus and blood of the retained rectum. This stoma is the mucous fistula, which tends to produce small amounts of drainage. Initially, a pouch can be applied over a mucous fistula, and consideration of use of absorbent dressings occurs as drainage decreases. It is normal for the individual to feel the need to have a bowel action or pass mucus and a small amount of blood through the anus. Education on this point needs to occur, so individuals are not frightened or confused when it happens.

URINARY STOMA CONSTRUCTION

> **KEY POINT**
>
> The purpose of any urinary stoma is to divert the urinary stream. They function immediately upon creation. These diversions are usually permanent, but some can be temporary.

TYPES

Vesicostomies are generally a temporary diversion constructed for young children, and usually closed before toilet training age. In this procedure, an opening is created above the symphysis pubis, the bladder opened, and the bladder mucosa approximated to the skin (Patel & Fergany, 2012). Containment of the urine is commonly done with diapering if the child is at an age where this is acceptable. Protecting the peristomal skin is needed to prevent peristomal moisture-associated skin damage (Gray et al., 2011). Products used to protect the skin include liquid skin barriers, cyanoacrylate-based monomer, or petrolatum-based products. It is difficult to obtain a predictable seal with pouching, so not a common management option.

Ureterostomy

The role of the ureterostomy is limited. In this procedure, the ends of the ureters are brought onto the abdomen or flank and sutured to the skin. These stomas are very tiny, <7/8 inch, and tend to become stenotic. Ureterostomies are also freely refluxing, so there is a danger of increased urinary tract infections and hydronephrosis (Kaefer et al., 2014). (See Fig 8-3.) Ureterostomy is considered when a patient is not a candidate for another type of urinary diversion.

Ileal Conduit

The most common urinary diversion is the ileal conduit (Colombo & Naspro, 2010; Morrison & Kielb, 2017). The right lower quadrant is the usual location for ileal conduits. In ileal conduit surgery, if removal of the bladder is necessary, the cystectomy is completed first. Resection of a 12- to 18-cm segment of ileum, about 10 to 15 cm from the ileal-cecal valve is resected. This segment remains attached to the mesentery preserving its blood and nerve supply. Gastrointestinal continuity is then restored through an ileal to ileal anastomosis.

The proximal end of the resected ileal segment is sutured closed. The ureters are anastomosed to the bottom of ileal segment, and the distal end is used to create a stoma. Ileal conduits can have either end or loop—end construction depending on reach as described above (Colombo & Naspro, 2010; Morrison & Kielb, 2017; Patel & Fergany, 2012) **(Fig. 9-12)**.

It is important to have a healthy and patent ureteroileal anastomosis with optimum integrity. Therefore, the surgeon ensures adequate blood supply to the distal ureters, avoids ureteral kinking or twisting, has clear ureteral margins if cancer was the underlying reason for surgery, and maintain a tension-free anastomosis (Patel & Fergany, 2012). At the time of construction, ure-

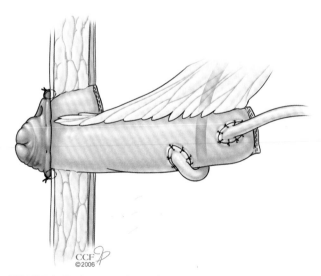

FIGURE 9-12. Loop—end Ileal Conduit. A short segment of ileum is resected from the gastrointestinal tract along with its mesentery. A loop of ileum is brought through the premarked stoma site and matured in the usual manner. The ureters are implanted at the proximal end of this segment. (Reprinted with permission, Cleveland Clinic Center for Medical Art & Photography © 2014. All Rights Reserved.)

teric stents will pass through the ureteroileal anastomosis (both left and right) and exit through the stoma. Depending on surgeon preference, the stents remain in situ for about 6 to 10 days. There may be a catheter left in the conduit to facilitate urinary drainage in the early postoperative period while healing takes place. (Colombo & Naspro, 2010). Urine flows almost continuously from these stomas (Registered Nurses' Association of Ontario [RNAO], 2009). Urostomy pouches with urinary drainage spouts are used, allowing ease of drainage and the ability to connect to leg or bedside urinary drainage bags.

KEY POINT

An extended wear skin barrier is recommended for an ileal conduit pouching system.

Jejunal Conduit

When it is not feasible to use ileum as a conduit, jejunum or a segment of colon may be used. Jejunal conduits lead to electrolyte disturbances that are characterized by hyponatremia, hypochloremia, hyperkalemia, acidosis, and azotemia. Clinically, individuals present with nausea, vomiting, dehydration, anorexia, lethargy, and muscle weakness. Treatment of electrolyte disturbances includes hydration and salt and bicarbonate replacement. In colon conduits, the ureters are able to be implanted in a nonrefluxing manner secondary to the thicker musculature of the colon (Patel & Fergany, 2012).

 CONCLUSIONS

Surgical creation of a stoma is often as important to patient survival and quality of life as managing the disease process or traumatic event. The ability for a person (or caregiver) to self-manage his or her ostomy care is directly dependent on many factors, including preoperative stoma site selection and the quality of stoma construction. These factors will provide a mechanism for a reliable and predictable pouch seal that contains effluent and odor and minimizes the chances for stomal and peristomal skin complications (Erwin-Toth et al., 2012; Salvadalena, 2016). Stoma construction types include end, loop, and loop—end. Determining the type of stoma construction depends on the intestinal anatomic location used, abdominal wall thickness, whether the stoma is temporary or permanent, and the disease process involved.

REFERENCES

Arenas, V. J., Lopez-Rodriguez, C., Abiles, J., et al. (2015). Protocol for the detection and nutritional management of high-output stomas. *Nutrition Journal, 14*(45). doi: 10.1186/s12937-015-0034-z.

Bafford, A., & Irani, J. (2013). Management and complications of stomas. *Surgical Clinics of North America, 93*(1), 145–166. doi: 10.1016/j.suc.2012.09.015.

Bridges, M., Nasser, R., & Parrish, C. (2019). High output ileostomies: The stakes are higher than the output. *Practical Gastroenterology,* 20–33. Retrieved from https://practicalgastro.com/wp-content/uploads/2019/10/Parrish-September-2019.pdf

Colombo, R., & Naspro, R. (2010). Ileal conduit as the standard for urinary diversion after radical cystectomy for bladder cancer. *European Urology Supplements, 9*(10), 736–744. doi: 10.1016/j.eursup.2010.09.001.

Colwell, J., Ratliff, C., Goldberg, M., et al. (2011). MASD part 3: Peristomal moisture-associated dermatitis and periwound moisture-associated dermatitis. A consensus. *Journal of Wound, Ostomy, and Continence Nursing, 38*(5), 541–553. doi: 10.1097/WON.0b013e31822acd95.

Doughty, D. (2004). History of stoma creation and surgical advances. In J. Colwell, M. Goldberg, & J. Carmel (Eds.), *Fecal & urinary diversions. Management principles* (pp. 3–17). St. Louis, MO: Mosby.

Erwin-Toth, P., Hocevar, B., & Stricker, L. (2012). Wound, ostomy, and continence/enterostomal therapy (WOC/ET) nursing. In V. Fazio, J. Church, & J. Wu (Eds.), *Atlas of intestinal stomas* (pp. 75–84). New York, NY: Springer.

Forgione, P., & Cataldo, P. (2003). Colostomy. *Operative Techniques in General Surgery, 5*(4), 264–272. doi: 10.1053/j.optechgensurg.2003.10.004.

Garofalo, T. (2012). Colostomy: Types, indications, formation, and reversal. In V. Fazio, J. Church, & J. Wu (Eds.), *Atlas of intestinal stomas* (pp. 127–145). New York, NY: Springer.

Goldberg, M., Aukett, L., Carmel, J., et al. (2010). *Management of the patient with a fecal ostomy: Best practice guideline for clinicians.* Mount Laurel, NJ: Wound, Ostomy and Continence Nurses Society.

Goodey, A., & Colman, S. (2016). Safe management of ileostomates with high-output stomas. *British Journal of Nursing (Stoma Supplement), 25*(22), S4–S9.

Gray, M., Black, J., Baharestani, M., et al. (2011). Moisture-associated skin damage: Overview and pathophysiology. *Journal of Wound, Ostomy, and Continence Nursing, 38*(3), 233–241. doi: 10.1097/WON.0b013e318215f798.

Gray, M., Colwell, J., Doughty, D., et al. (2013). Peristomal moisture-associated skin damage in adults with fecal ostomies. A comprehensive review and consensus. *Journal of Wound, Ostomy, and Continence Nursing, 40*(4), 389–399. doi: 10.1097/WOCN, 0b013e3182944340.

Kaefer, M., Misseri, R., Frank, E., et al. (2014). Refluxing ureteral reimplantation: A logical method for managing neonatal UVJ obstruction. *Journal of Pediatric Urology, 10*(5), 824–830. https://doi.org/10.1016/j.jpurol.2014.01.027.

Kaidar-Person, O., Person, B., & Wexner, S. (2005). Complications of construction and closure of temporary loop ileostomy. *Journal of the American College of Surgeons, 201*(5), 759–773. doi: 10.1016/j.jamcollsurg.2005.06.002.

Krapfl, L., & Zurcher, S. (2010). High volume output from a jejunostomy. *Journal of Wound, Ostomy, and Continence Nursing, 37*(6), 662–664. doi: 10.1097/WON.0b013e3181fac09e.

Martin, S., & Vogel, J. (2012). Intestinal stomas. Indications, management, and complications. *Advances in Surgery, 46*(1), 19–49. doi: 10.1016/jyasu.2012.04.005.

Medlin, S. (2012). Nutritional and fluid requirements: High-output stomas. *British Journal of Nursing (Stoma Care Supplement), 21*(6), S22–S25.

Morrison, C., & Kielb, S. (2017). Use of bowel in reconstructive urology: What a colorectal surgeon should know. *Clinics in Colon and Rectal Surgery, 30,* 207–214. doi: https://doi.org/10.1055/s-0037-1598162.

Murken, D., & Bleier, J. (2019). Ostomy-related complications. *Clinics in Colon and Rectal Surgery, 32,* 176–182. doi: https://doi.org/10.1055/s-0038-1676995.

Oldenburg, W. A., Lau, L. L., Rodenberg, T., et al. (2004). Acute mesenteric ischemia. A clinical review. *Archives of Internal Medicine, 164,* 1054–1062.

Patel, A., & Fergany, A. (2012). Urinary stomas. In V. Fazio, J. Church, & J. Wu (Eds.), *Atlas of intestinal stomas* (pp. 213–229). New York, NY: Springer.

Parekh, N., & Seidner, D. (2012). Medical management of the high-output enterostomy and enterocutaneous fistula. In V. Fazio, J. Church, & J. Wu (Eds.), *Atlas of intestinal stomas* (pp. 97–109). New York, NY: Springer.

Pearl, G., & Gilani, R. (2018). Acute mesenteric arterial occlusion. *UpToDate®.* Retrieved on November 5, 2019, from www-uptodate-com.ccmain.ohionet.org/contents/acute-mesenteric-arterial-occlusion?search=Acute%20mesenteric%20occlusion&source

Pine, J., & Stevenson, L. (2014). Ileostomy and colostomy. *Surgery (Oxford), 32*(4), 212–217. doi: 10.10161/j.mpsur.2014.01.007.

Raju, D., Sheshagiri, N., Kadarapura, S., et al. (2018). A systematic approach in the management of a high output ileostomy resulting in a favorable clinical outcome. *Anesthesiology Case Reports, 1*(1), 1–3. Retrieved from https://www.pulsus.com/scholarly-articles/a-systematic-approach-in-the-management-of-a-high-output-ileostomy-resulting-in-a-favorable-clinical-outcome.pdf

Registered Nurses' Association of Ontario (RNAO). (2009). Ostomy care and management. US National Guideline Clearing House. Retrieved from https://search.ebscohost.com/login.aspx?direct=true&db=nrc&AN=5000013298&site=ede-live

Rombeau, J. (2012). Physiologic and metabolic effects of intestinal stomas. In V. Fazio, J. Church, & J. Wu (Eds.), *Atlas of intestinal stomas* (pp. 59–67). New York, NY: Springer.

Salvadalena, G. (2016). Peristomal skin conditions. In J. Carmel, J. Colwell, & M. Goldberg. (Eds.), *Wound Ostomy and Continence Nurses Society Core curriculum Ostomy management.* Philadelphia, PA: Wolters Kluwer.

Saunders, R., & Hemingway, D. (2008). Intestinal stomas. *Surgery (Oxford), 26*(8), 347–351. doi: 10.1016/j.mpsur.2008.05.001.

Smith, L., & Boland, L. (2013). High output stomas: Ensuring safe discharge from hospital to home. *British Journal of Nursing (Oncology Supplement), 22*(5), S14–S18.

Stankiewicz, M., Gordon, J., Rivera, J., et al. (2019). Clinical management of ileostomy high-output stomas to prevent electrolyte disturbance, dehydration and acute kidney injury: A quality improvement activity. *Journal of Stomal Therapy Australia, 39*(1), 8–10.

Steinhagen, E., Colwell, J., & Cannon, L. (2017). Intestinal stomas—Postoperative stoma care and peristomal skin complications. *Clinics in Colon and Rectal Surgery, 30,* 184–192. doi: https://doi.org/10.1055/2-0037-1598159.

Stocchi, L. (2012). Ileostomy. In V. Fazio, J. Church, & J. Wu (Eds.), *Atlas of intestinal stomas* (pp. 85–95). New York, NY: Springer.

Vries, F., Reeskamp, L., Ruler, O., et al. (2017). Systematic review: Pharmacotherapy for high-output enterostomies or enteral fistulas. *Alimentary Pharmacology & Therapeutics, 46*(3), 266–273.

Wexner, S., Taranow, D., Johansen, O., et al. (1993). Loop ileostomy is a safe option for fecal diversion. *Diseases of the Colon & Rectum, 36*(4), 349–354. doi: 10.1007/BF02043937.

Whitehead, A., & Cataldo, P. (2017). Technical considerations in stoma creation. *Clinics in Colon and Rectal Surgery, 30,* 162–171. doi: https://doi.org/10.1055/s-003701598156.

Whitehead, A., Seah, A., & Cataldo, P. (2014). Technical tips for difficult stomas. In S. Steele, J. Maykel, B. Champagne, et al. (Eds.), *Complexities in colorectal surgery* (pp. 147–156). New York, NY: Springer. doi: 10.1007/978-1-4614-9022-7_9.

Wu, J. (2003). Ileostomy. *Operative Techniques in General Surgery, 5*(4), 257–263. doi: 10.1053/j.optechgensurg.2003.10.003.

Wu, J. (2012). Intestinal stomas: Historical overview. In V. Fazio, J. Church, & J. Wu (Eds.), *Atlas of intestinal stomas* (pp. 1–37). New York, NY: Springer.

Yang, I., & Boushey, R. (2014). Short bowel syndrome. In S. Steele, J. Maykel, B. Champagne, et al. (Eds.), *Complexities in colorectal surgery* (pp. 447–462). doi: 10.1007/978-1-4614-9022-7_29.

QUESTIONS

1. A patient is scheduled for surgery for the creation of an end ileostomy. What technique would the surgeon perform to prevent seeding of the epidermis with mucosal cells resulting in mucosal implants?
   A. A plastic rod, tubing, or similar device is placed under the loop of intestine to provide support.
   B. Two stomas are created in proximity to each other, resembling the end of a double-barrel shotgun.
   C. The well-vascularized bowel segment is brought through a predetermined three-fingerbreadth abdominal aperture to create the stoma.
   D. Eversion is performed using four equidistant sutures through the entire bowel wall and suturing through the subcuticular (dermal) layer of the adjacent skin.

2. What type of stoma construction would the surgeon most likely choose for a patient scheduled for ileal conduit who has a thick abdominal wall with a shortened mesentery?
   A. Loop–end stoma
   B. Double-barrel stoma
   C. End stoma–loop stoma

3. In the emergency department, a patient is diagnosed with an embolism to the superior mesenteric artery (SMA). Which of the following ostomy type is the most likely outcome?
   A. Gastrostomy
   B. Ileostomy
   C. Jejunostomy
   D. Cecostomy

4. The WOC nurse is describing the ileostomy to a new nurse. What statement accurately describes an aspect of this diversion?
   A. The stoma is usually located in the left lower quadrant.
   B. The more proximal the ileostomy, the more liquid the output.
   C. Ileostomies begin to function within 1 week postoperatively.
   D. The effluent is usually a light yellow liquid with viscous appearance.

5. What is a common complication when a loop transverse colostomy is created?
   A. Stomal prolapse
   B. Leakage around the catheter or tube
   C. Tissue destruction to the peristomal skin
   D. Fluid and electrolyte imbalances

6. The creation of a fecal stoma with a mucous fistula may be indicated in which of the following conditions?
   A. Rectal polyps
   B. Stomal prolapse
   C. Stomal hernia
   D. Toxic megacolon

7. What complication would the WOC nurse assess for in a patient with an ureterostomy?
   A. Hydronephrosis
   B. Electrolyte disturbance
   C. Dehydration
   D. Septicemia

8. Which procedure is the most common urinary diversion?
   A. Vesicostomy
   B. Ureterostomy
   C. Ileal conduit
   D. Cystectomy

9. The WOC nurse is explaining the procedure for constructing an ileal conduit to a patient scheduled for the surgery. Which statement by the nurse adequately describes a step in this procedure?
   A. Resection of an 8- to 10-cm segment of ileum occurs.
   B. Gastrointestinal continuity is restored through an ileal to ileal anastomosis.
   C. The distal end of the resected ileal segment is sutured closed.
   D. Ileal conduits must end in a loop–end construction to allow free flow of urine.

10. A support rod is placed under a loop stoma to prevent which of the following stoma complications?
   A. Prolapse
   B. Retraction
   C. Stenosis
   D. Necrosis

ANSWERS AND RATIONALES

1. D. Rationale: When maturing the stoma, the sutures are placed through the subcuticular layer of skin to prevent implanting stoma tissue into the dermis.

2. A. Rationale: loop–end construction is used when a person has a thick abdominal wall (easier to get above the skin), shortened mesentery, or a combination, and there if there is concern about adequate blood supply to the distal end of the stoma.

3. C. Rationale: The majority of emboli to the superior mesenteric artery (SMA) settle distally to the SMA's origin at its first branch, causing ischemic injury to the ileum, sparing ischemia to the upper jejunum: a jejunostomy is created.

4. B. Rationale: The more proximal the stoma, the more liquid the output.

5. A. Rationale: Stoma prolapse, particularly in the distal lumen, is a common problem seen in loop transverse colostomies.

6. D. Rationale: A classic example of the creation of a mucous fistula can occur when a patient has toxic megacolon. The involved colon is resected and the end brought out as a stoma and the remaining section end brought to the skin for drainage.

7. A. Rationale: Ureterostomies are freely refluxing which means the urine can flow upward toward the kidney, so there is an increased risk for urinary tract infections and hydronephrosis.

8. C. Rationale: The most common urinary diversion is the ileal conduit.

9. B. Rationale: After a 12 to 18 cm segment of ileum is resected, gastrointestinal continuity is restored through an ileal–ileal anastomosis and the proximal end of the ileal segment is sutured.

10. B. Rationale: A rod is used to provide support in order to prevent early retraction of the stoma; the rod supports the bowel while healing takes place.

CHAPTER 10

PREOPERATIVE PREPARATION OF PATIENTS UNDERGOING A FECAL OR URINARY DIVERSION

Margaret T. Goldberg and Mary F. Mahoney

OBJECTIVE

Describe preoperative preparation of a patient undergoing a fecal and/or urinary diversion including stoma site marking.

TOPIC OUTLINE

Introduction **144**
  Significance of Preoperative Education 144
    Preoperative Ostomy Education 144
Post Discharge Education **145**
Patient Assessment **146**
  Planned Procedure, Diagnosis, Prognosis, and
    Treatment Plan 146
  Major Concerns of Patient and Family/
    Significant Others 146
  Barriers to Self-Care 147
    Psychological 147
    Physical 147
    Cognitive 147
    Understanding Fears 147
  Learning Style/Learning Level 147
  Patient Support Systems 148
Guidelines for Preoperative Education **148**
  Explanation of Planned Procedure 148
    Anatomy and Physiology 148
    Surgical Procedure 148
    Overview of Lifestyle Modifications 149
    Diet 149
    Activity 149
    Clothing 149
    Medications 149
    Travel 149

Pouching Systems 149
Emptying 150
Importance of Peristomal Skin
  Management 150
Obtaining and Paying for Supplies 150
Psychological Issues 150
Sexuality 150
Acknowledgment of Normal Stages of
  Adjustment 150
Ostomy Visitor 151
Professional Counseling 151
Bowel Prep 151
Stoma Siting **152**
  Rationale 152
  Procedure Guidelines 153
    Stoma Site Marking Procedure 154
    Considerations in Stoma Site Marking 154
    Unique Stoma Marking Considerations:
      Marking for Two Stomas 155
    Moving the Stoma 155
    Thin Patient 155
    Creases and Folds 156
    Scars 156
    Distension 156
    Pregnancy 156
    Pendulous Breasts 156
    Tattoos 156

Contractures, Kyphosis, or Scoliosis 156
Spiritual Beliefs 156
Difficult Stoma Siting Using Computed
    Tomography 156
Continent Stoma Marking 157
Wheelchair 157
Brace or Leg Prosthesis 157
Pain/Limited Mobility 157

Special Equipment/Work Belts 157
Radiation 157
Marking During Surgery 157
Infants and Children 157
Teenagers 157
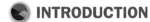 **Documentation 158**
Conclusions 158

INTRODUCTION

SIGNIFICANCE OF PREOPERATIVE EDUCATION

Preoperative Ostomy Education

Patients who receive preoperative ostomy education experience better recovery, possibly a shorter hospital stay, and fewer postoperative complications (WOCN, 2010). Preoperative education can assist in alleviating the patients' fears and anxieties associated with surgery and help them understand the adjustments that they will need to make for living with a stoma. Barreira (2018) concluded that in a group of similar patients, preoperative education was a decisive factor for a much faster recovery of the physical and instrumental autonomy of the ostomy care compared to an unprepared group.

The United Ostomy Associations of America's (UOAA): Ostomy and Continent Diversion Patient Bill of Rights adopted in 2017 identifies the needs and expectations of the person undergoing ostomy surgery (see Appendix L). The counseling must include the following:

- Preoperative stoma site marked by a medical professional following Standards of Care (established by the Wound, Ostomy, and Continence Nurses Society™, American Society of Colon & Rectal Surgeons and American Urological Association position statement)
- Explanation of surgical procedure and the rationale for surgery
- Discussion of ostomy/continent diversion management
- Impact of surgery on activities of daily living such as physical adaptation, clothing choices, exercise, possible changes in sexual activity and treatment, and dietary needs
- The opportunity to talk with someone who has been through ostomy or continent diversion surgery
- The opportunity to discuss the emotional impact of surgery
- Counseling in a language and at a level of understanding that is comfortable for the patient

Joint statements by the Wound, Ostomy, Continence Nurses Society™ (WOCN), American Society of Colorectal Surgeons (ASCRS), and the American Urologic Association (AUA) state that ostomy education and stoma site selection should be performed preoperatively for all patients when

an ostomy is a possibility (Salvadalena et al., 2015a,b). The ASCRS state in their clinical practice guideline for ostomy surgery that ostomy education should have a preoperative and postoperative component and should involve a specialized provider, such as a wound ostomy continence (WOC) nurse when possible (Hendren et al., 2015). Several large retrospective studies have shown that preoperative education by an ostomy nurse was associated with fewer stoma-related complications (23% vs. 32% without the education) and significantly decreased postoperative skin and leakage problems (Klink et al., 2011). A number of studies have reported on questionnaires of patients with ostomies, showing that ostomy nurse teaching was highly valued by patients and was associated with better psychosocial adjustment (Coggrave et al., 2012; Haugen et al., 2006). Preoperative education for the patient undergoing the creation of a fecal or urinary diversion is an important and necessary part of the plan of care. Preoperative education for both the patient and the family (when possible) should include stoma explanation, and site marking, the surgical procedure and postoperative stoma management is highly recommended by the World Council of Enterostomal Therapists (WCET, 2014).

The reduction in the length of the hospital stay for patients after stoma surgery, due to enhanced recovery after surgery (ERAS) protocols/pathways, as well as minimally invasive procedures, results in decreased time for education while hospitalized. Laparoscopic surgery combined with ERAS allowed more than 60% of patients of colorectal surgery patients to be discharged within 72 hours in a review by Chand et al. (2016). Since patients are recovering from surgery during their shortened stay, learner readiness may not be present. Alternatives to bedside teaching now include some web-based resources. In 2017, Pittman et al. evaluated no-cost web-based resources and found that while the content can be variable, they may be a cost-effective way to provide education and support, and a positive aspect was the 24-hour availability of the ostomy information. Planning for the educational experiences might include a prehospital visit with the patient and caregiver(s). See **Box 10-1** for Teaching Strategies and methods. The WOCN® recommends coordination of care across care settings among all disciplines who provide care to the person with an ostomy (WOCN, 2017). The institution of a preoperative stoma education group class for patients anticipating

BOX 10-1	TEACHING STRATEGIES AND METHODS

Verbal instruction

Printed instructional sheets or booklets (many ostomy manufacturers provide comprehensive instruction booklets, the United Ostomy Associations of the America [UOAA] has printed information, or the place of nurse's employment may provide instruction sheets)

Photos

Illustrations or diagrams

Plain paper with pen to draw diagrams. Models made by the nurse or manufactured models such as VATA anatomical health care models (http://www.vatainc.com) or The Anatomical Apron by Joy (http://www.apronsbyjoy.com)

Actual pouch system demonstrations

Videos of people changing the ostomy pouch or sharing testimonials

Valid Web sites (such as manufacturer or UOAA Web sites)

---

the creation of a fecal stoma was found by Stokes et al. (2017) to significantly reduce peristomal complications. The pre op stoma educational class was 2 hours, and the American College of Surgeons Ostomy Home Skills Kit was used to teach the patients and their significant others. Patients and their partners or caregivers were given a hands-on tutorial regarding care of a fecal stoma. Topics included the pre- and postoperative interventions patient, diet changes, instructions regarding symptoms of dehydration due to ileostomy dysfunction, and examples of various pouching systems and accessory supplies. Current reimbursement issues which may restrict a pre and post discharge visit and decreased face time with patients while hospitalized, call for varied and creative methods to accomplish necessary patient education.

POST DISCHARGE EDUCATION

O'Flynn (2018) states that the continuity of care for the rehabilitation of patients with stomas is the weakest link in community services. It has been recognized that after discharge, there are insufficient numbers of outpatient ostomy clinics to provide continued education to the person with a new ostomy and prevent or treat complications after the person is discharged from the hospital (WOCN, 2017). An article describes the use of an evidence-based and content validated ostomy algorithm for use in home care (Bare et al., 2017). Designed to assist the nurses in home care with limited experience in ostomy care, the algorithm was found to improve clinical outcomes and increase patient satisfaction. Colwell et al. (2016) published outcome criteria for discharging the new ostomy patient from home health care developed by expert ostomy nurse clinicians based on known evidence and basic principles. Eighteen statements of minimum criteria for discharge from home health care were developed and are in **Box 10-2**.

BOX 10-2	THE MINIMUM DISCHARGE CRITERIA FROM HOME CARE FOR THE NEW PATIENT WITH AN OSTOMY

1. Patient/caregiver is able to identify when to empty gas or effluent from the pouch.
2. Patient/caregiver is able to demonstrate the correct way to empty the pouch.
3. Patient/caregiver is able to identify when to remove and replace the closed end pouch
4. Patient/caregiver demonstrates how to remove and replace closed-end pouch.
5. Patient/caregiver is able to verbalize when to change pouching system based on an established wear time. Wear time should be established for patient-specific situations prior to discharge.
6. Patient/caregiver is able to provide a return demonstration of how to change the pouching system including removal, cleansing, and application.
7. Patient/caregiver is able to identify the appearance of normal peristomal skin.
8. Patient/caregiver is able to identify the normal appearance of the stoma.
9. Patient/caregiver is able to describe changes in stoma appearance that require the patient to seek medical attention.
10. Patient/caregiver is able to describe the changes in the skin surrounding the stoma that require the patient seek medical attention.
11. Patient/caregiver is able to describe or demonstrate the management of skin irritation surrounding the stoma.
12. Patient/caregiver is able to describe the expected volume, consistency, and character of the stoma output.
13. Patient/caregiver is able to describe changes in stoma output that require the patient to seek medical attention.
14. Patient/caregiver is able to verbalize the importance of and demonstrates measuring the stoma and altering the skin barrier opening to accommodate changes in the stoma size.
15. Patient/caregiver is able to describe a plan for obtaining ostomy supplies.
16. Patient/caregiver is able to discuss issues related to living with an ostomy and identify resources.
17. Patient/caregiver is able to describe diet and fluid guidelines according to the type of stoma.
18. Patient/caregiver is able to identify resources to access a certified WOC nurse.

Colwell, J. C., et al. (2016), Outcome criteria for discharging the patient with a new ostomy from home health care: A WOCN Consensus Conference. *Journal of Wound, Ostomy and Continence Nursing, 43*(3), 239–273.

This chapter covers the development of a plan of care for preoperative education for the person anticipating ostomy surgery and the principles of stoma site marking.

KEY POINT

Support and education in the preoperative period by a WOC nurse has been found to be effective in improving recovery after ostomy surgery.

PATIENT ASSESSMENT

The development of a plan of care for the preoperative education of the patient undergoing ostomy surgery will include the diagnosis that necessitated the surgical procedure, the type and date of surgical procedure, the patient's understanding of the upcoming procedure, any limitations to learning such as inability to read, physical limitations, and the presence or absence of a support system. Other important assessments include religious affiliation, culture, family, employment status, and medical/surgical history.

PLANNED PROCEDURE, DIAGNOSIS, PROGNOSIS, AND TREATMENT PLAN

Prior to the preoperative educational session, the WOC nurse should determine the reason for the surgical procedure, the type of surgical procedure that will be performed (**Table 10-1**), and the expected patient prognosis. See also Appendix A for surgical procedures.

General postoperative care should be reviewed with the patient and include the probable location of the incision or incisions and the type of tubes they may have such as IVs, abdominal drains, and a urinary catheter. Describe how pain will be managed and the importance of early ambulation. Be sure that the patient understands that he or she may be NPO until bowel function has returned as indicated by the presence of gas in the pouch.

Use the teach-back method to evaluate the patient's understanding. Suggested examples to ask the patient are as follows: "I want to be sure that I explained your ostomy surgery correctly. Can you tell me what your stoma will look like and how it will function?" or "We have covered a lot of information about ostomy surgery today. Can you tell me three things that you learned about your ostomy surgery?"

Some manufacturers of ostomy equipment provide kits for ostomy education to WOC nurses or are available online. The American College of Surgeons (ACS, 2016) Ostomy Home Skills kit was developed to encourage self-care skills and is available to patients and nurses at https://www.facs.org/education/patient-education/skills-programs. See Appendix B resources for a list of manufacturers that provide ostomy education materials.

KEY POINT

Patients who feel well prepared for ostomy surgery experience better postoperative adjustment to ostomy. When providing preoperative ostomy education, it is key that instruction is by a specialty nurse such as a WOC nurse, with a focus on self-care of the ostomy and/or assistance of a caregiver as needed.

MAJOR CONCERNS OF PATIENT AND FAMILY/SIGNIFICANT OTHERS

Since the adjustment capabilities of the patient are affected by the support of their spouse or partner (WOCN®, 2017), with the patient's approval, they should be included in the educational process and may contribute to their understanding and ability to provide support.

Start the preop educational session by asking the patient and support person to describe their understanding of the surgical procedure. This will provide

---

TABLE 10-1 SURGICAL PROCEDURE, TYPE OF OSTOMY, TYPICAL LOCATION		
SURGICAL PROCEDURE	TYPE OF OSTOMY	TYPICAL STOMA SITE LOCATION
Abdominal perineal resection	Permanent end colostomy Rectum removed Perineal surgical incision	Left side
Hartmann's procedure	Temporary (in certain situations may be permanent) end colostomy or ileostomy Rectum is retained.	Left or right side
Ileal pouch anal anastomosis	Stage one: temporary end ileostomy Stage two: temporary loop ileostomy	Right side
Proctocolectomy	Permanent end ileostomy	Right side
Low anterior resection (LAR)	Temporary loop ileostomy	Right side
Subtotal colectomy	Temporary end or loop ileostomy	Right side
Sigmoid colectomy	Temporary loop ileostomy	Right side
Continent ileostomy (Kock pouch)	Continent stoma	Right side
Cystectomy (ileal conduit or colon conduit)	Urostomy	Right side if ileal conduit, left side if colonic conduit
Continent urine reservoir (Indiana reservoir)	Continent intestinal stoma	Right side

an awareness of what they may have heard or retained when speaking to the health care team; Weiss (2003) has demonstrated that 40% to 80% of the medical information patients receive is forgotten immediately and nearly half of the information retained is incorrect. Establishing what information the patient knows helps to gain an understanding of his or her grasp of the upcoming procedure and identifies any educational gaps to be addressed during the preoperative session.

The patient and family should be asked what, if anything, they know about living with an ostomy. Encourage them to share concerns they have regarding the upcoming surgery and describe anyone they may have known with an ostomy. This question facilitates the conversation regarding the patient's worries and possible misconceptions of ostomy care. The patient may have a relative or friend who had a bad experience with an ostomy, and this is a good time to allay any unnecessary fears.

For example, it is not uncommon that an elderly relative may have had an ostomy, and the pouching system was not effective, causing odor or leakage. This can provide the nurse with the opportunity to explain that ostomy equipment available today is much improved from the past. Describe that the patient may have been unknowingly in the presence of someone with an ostomy, but since there are no visible signs (odor, bulging under the clothes), the ostomy is not readily apparent. Many times, people will discover a friend or acquaintance who has an ostomy that they haven't disclosed. Patients who are anxious about a certain aspect of the ostomy will have difficulty learning at the preoperative session. In addition to coping with ostomy surgery, many patients are simultaneously faced with a potentially terminal diagnosis or life-changing disease. Patients facing emergency surgery are often in pain, and there may be limited time for the WOC nurse to provide preoperative education.

BARRIERS TO SELF-CARE

Psychological
There is a good deal of psychological stress when a patient has been diagnosed and told about the need for surgery. Patients should be encouraged to express fears, concerns, worries, disgust, and potential embarrassment regarding the upcoming surgery that will result in the creation of an ostomy (Dorman, 2009). Patients' fears can be unfounded and may be easily dealt with calmly and with correct information. For instance, some patients think their diets will be changed markedly in the presence of an ostomy, and this is not necessarily true. Other people think their clothing must be loose to accommodate the pouching system and that everyone will know they have an ostomy. Alleviating these fears can help the patients cope with all of the changes they will be facing. A visit with a person with an ostomy could be beneficial and a visit with a trained ostomy visitor can

be arranged (with the patient's permission) by contacting the UOAA (see Appendix B for resources).

Physical
The WOC nurse should assess the patient's physical abilities. Note if the patient has physical conditions such as arthritis or stroke that could affect his or her ability for self-care. Does the patient have visual limitations that will need to be considered when teaching the patient how to manage his or her stoma? Inadequate coordination and function as seen in Parkinson disease and post-stroke weakness are also barriers to self-care (Dorman, 2009). Reinforce to the patient that self-care can be awkward and frustrating in the beginning, but confidence is gained with experience as patients develop new skills to perform the tasks of emptying and changing the pouching system.

Dorman (2009) indicates that the physical and emotional disabilities of the surgery may have an impact on the ability to perform ostomy care. If there are disabilities that render self-care difficult or impossible, a caregiver must be identified and included in the pre- and postoperative teaching sessions.

Cognitive
Many people have difficulty reading and understanding medical information. Reinforce that the patient and family can call the ostomy nurse with questions after surgery and discharge. Suggest that the patient start a notebook to write down questions in order to remember to ask the WOC nurse or the doctor. The patient can keep all notes regarding the surgery, phone numbers, Web sites, and other information gathered in this special notebook. For the person who may have problems grasping all of the preoperative information, the family member or support person should be included. People with low literacy skills tend to use family or friends to assist the interpretation of the medical information shared (Weiss, 2003).

Understanding Fears
According to the UOAA (2008), odor control and leakage are two major concerns of the ostomy patients, and these need to be addressed during the preoperative education. An explanation of how odor is managed (the pouching system is odor proof and will only have odor when emptying the pouch) should be provided in a manner that the patient's fears are alleviated. Describe to the patient how his or her fear of leakage will be addressed, by instructing the patient in how a pouch seal is maintained. Dietary, clothing, and sexual issues can all be discussed and the patient helped to understand that these challenges are normal and fairly easily managed.

LEARNING STYLE/LEARNING LEVEL
Patients should be asked if they are comfortable with learning by reading or if they prefer another way of learning such as photos, video, or audio instruction. Asking

> **BOX 10-3   POUCHING OVERVIEW**
>
> Pouches are available in different sizes, shapes, and materials.
> Features include one- and two-piece systems.
> Pouching systems are odor proof.
> Usual wear time is four days (Richbourg et al., 2007).
> Follow-up with the ostomy nurse should be done on a routine
> visit and as needed.

in a shame-free manner will more likely elicit an honest response (Weiss, 2003). If reading is not their preferred manner of learning, offer other methods, for example, watching a demonstration video, practicing on a model, or working with the nurse on emptying and changing their pouch as many times as possible. See **Box 10-1** for teaching methods and **Box 10-3** for pouching overview.

PATIENT SUPPORT SYSTEMS

The WOC nurse should determine the patient's emotional support system. This would be a person who can be available during the preoperative visit and at several postoperative sessions as well as follow-up visits and someone the person can call when he or she needs to talk. It is important to include the patient's support system in the preoperative as well as the postoperative education sessions. When patients are in crisis, specifically facing ostomy surgery, absence of social support may result in poor coping and adapting behaviors (Nichols, 2011).

While it is ideal to meet with the patient several weeks prior to surgery, time may be limited and the appointment may be the same day as the surgery. Factor this timing into the amount of education shared with the patient as you might need to limit the provision of information to addressing the patient's greatest fears and providing basic information on the skills the patient will need to acquire after surgery. Educational materials regarding the specific type of ostomy planned should be provided. This may include printed instructional sheets or booklets, photos, illustrations, models, pouches, and/or videos (see Appendix B for patient education resources).

 GUIDELINES FOR PREOPERATIVE EDUCATION

> **KEY POINT**
>
> Preoperative education should include: (1) brief discussion of anatomy and physiology, (2) description of surgical procedure, (3) overview of modifications, (4) introduction to the pouching system and (5) a focus on psychological preparation.

The 2017 WOCN Clinical Guideline: Management of the Adult Patient with a Fecal or Urinary Ostomy recommends that preoperative education includes the following:

- A brief discussion of the anatomy and physiology of the gastrointestinal and/or urinary tract
- A description of the planned surgical procedure
- A brief overview of lifestyle modifications
- An introduction to the pouching system
- A focus on psychological preparation

EXPLANATION OF PLANNED PROCEDURE

Anatomy and Physiology

Begin with a simple review of the anatomy and bodily functions. Take time for this review because patients often do not have a clear understanding of how their bodies work or how (where) organs are positioned in the abdomen. Explain the physiology of the abdominal organs, particularly the roles of the gastrointestinal and genitourinary systems. Use a diagram or a model to illustrate the changes associated with the planned surgery (resources are in Appendix B). A 3D model helps to reinforce the concepts of the anatomy inside the abdomen. Explain that the actual stoma does not come off or have the ability to move around like the model.

The effect of the surgery on other organs inside the abdomen needs to be explained; many individuals need to be assured that the body can continue to function despite the loss of a portion of the intestinal tract or the bladder. For example, the nurse must be very clear that the patient undergoing urostomy surgery will have a section of the intestine used for urine drainage, but the intestine will be reconnected to function as the normal passageway for stool.

Surgical Procedure

A brief review of the procedure to reinforce what the surgical team has discussed with the patient is recommended referring to the anatomy and physiology that was reviewed. This will allow the patient in simple terms to understand what body part maybe resected, reconnected or diverted.

The WOC nurse should describe how the stoma is created, if the diversion is permanent or temporary, the appearance of the stoma, and expectations of the stoma output. It is important that the patient understand that the stoma will be red and moist and will have no sensation. Many patients have expressed that since the stoma is red, they associated red with pain or infection. Diagrams or models help to demonstrate the surgical creation of the stoma. An easily accessible method to describe the maturation of a stoma is to suggest that the stoma is matured just as a turtleneck that is everted. The lining of the mouth is much like the appearance of the stoma: red and moist. The use of analogies is helpful to describe the expected output from the stoma (e.g., ileostomy output is similar to pudding or oatmeal consistency). Patients should be instructed to assess their own peristomal skin area at every pouch change and encouraged to recognize changes and report them to their ostomy nurse (Colwell et al., 2019).

Overview of Lifestyle Modifications

Many people anticipating ostomy surgery are not sure what adjustments they will need to make. The following should be considered: diet may be restricted to low residue after surgery until healing has taken place, they will learn how to empty and change their pouching system while hospitalized, they will not be proficient in pouch management at the time of discharge but should have follow-up at home with a home care nurse and if possible a WOC nurse, they may have several incisions that will prevent them from heavy lifting for 6 to 8 weeks, they will be discharged with some ostomy products, and they will receive supportive information such as written instructions, booklets, and Web sites.

Diet

Many patients assume that they will need to alter their diet following ostomy surgery. The patient needs to know that he or she may have a restricted diet after surgery up to approximately 6 weeks. Most people with ostomies will not have to follow a diet once surgical healing has taken place; however, foods may have the same effects as they had prior to surgery. EATING WITH AN OSTOMY: A Comprehensive Nutrition Guide for Those Living with an Ostomy (Burgess 2020) is a free booklet that describes some dietary effects of ostomy and is available to patients and nurses from the United Ostomy Associations of America Web site.

Activity

Determine whether the patient is concerned about resuming normal activity after surgery. Explain that the pouching system should not interfere with activity, and give specific examples of how the patient can integrate the ostomy into his or her lifestyle. Patients often wonder if the pouch can get wet. Assure the patient that typically a daily shower is acceptable, and in some cases, submersion under water for a length of time such as swimming or hot tub may require waterproof tape, applied around the barrier edges "picture framing". Prior to bathing, the seal should be checked. Patient may be advised to "test" pouch seal by submerging in a bathtub to be sure their pouching system will hold up in a pool.

Clothing

Discuss the patient's current clothing and determine if there are any challenges the patient will encounter. Most people are able to return to their former clothing styles after surgery. Be sure that the patient understands that it will not be necessary to wear baggy loose clothing to conceal the pouch (see Chapter 13).

Medications

Some medications or nutritional supplements may change the color, odor, or consistency of the stool or urine. Certain medications may not be completely absorbed (see Chapters 13 and 14 for more information). For example, in a patient with an ileostomy, time release capsules are not recommended as they may pass through the stoma without breaking down. Medications may need to be converted to liquid or gel form to get the full benefit of the medicine.

Travel

Be sure the patient knows that there are no limitations to travel with the ostomy. Patients should carry ample amount of supplies with them when they travel and to be aware that certain screening processes, when flying, may note the presence of a pouch and require a personal screening. These screenings are usually very professional, in private with two of the same sex officers, and the TSA staff will be discreet to limit embarrassment. This is done for everyone's safety and is conducted as efficiently and quickly as possible. The UOAA has a travel card that can be carried while traveling that explains some of the conditions associated with an ostomy; copies can be obtained from http://www.ostomy.org/uploaded/files/travel_card/Travel_Card_2011b.pdf. However, most TSA agents are trained to conduct searches appropriately and privately if needed.

KEY POINT

Technical difficulties of managing the ostomy is negatively correlated with psychosocial adjustment.

Pouching Systems

Use the same or similar pouching system that will be used after surgery to demonstrate to the patient how the pouch is applied, removed, and emptied. This might be a good time to hand the pouch to the patient and see if he or she can open and close the bottom of the pouch and suggest that they practice this skill at home. The American College of Surgeons kit (see Appendix B) has two practice stomas, one that can be used at the preop session, with the WOC nurse demonstrating how to measure the stoma, cut the pouch, and place the pouch over the stoma model. The second model can be used at home for practice by the patient. This is a great opportunity for the patient to begin to see how they will manage their stoma after surgery.

The WOC nurse will provide the patient with an overview on changing the pouching system (**Box 10-3**). Patients should understand that they will plan a pouching system change on a routinely scheduled basis possibly two times per week. They will practice changing the pouch while in the hospital but may not acquire the skills prior to discharge and in most cases will have home care nursing to continue to work toward independence in stoma care. Be sure the patients understand that they will go home with ostomy supplies and written instructions to use as they work toward acquiring the necessary skills.

KEY POINT

Important considerations in pouching system selection include stoma type and location, abdominal contours, lifestyle, personal preference, visual acuity, and manual dexterity.

Emptying

Instruct the patient/caregiver that the first skill to be learned before discharge is how to empty the pouch. As the stoma does not have nerves, there is no sensation of output, and the pouch needs to be checked for filling. Describe approximately how many times in 24 hours they will need to check for filling and recommend emptying when 1/2 to 1/3 full (see Watch & Learn videos: *"Instructions on how to open a pouch and empty it"* and *"How to empty a different type of pouch"*). Instruct that most people sit on the toilet and direct the pouch contents into the toilet. If unable to sit on the toilet, the pouch can be emptied into a container that is then emptied into the toilet. The patient with a fecal stoma may wipe the outside and/or inside of the pouch tail with toilet tissue, apply deodorant (if used), and close (**Figure 13-1**). If the patient has a urostomy, the pouch may be connected to large capacity drainage system at night. Help the patient to visualize how to accommodate these changes in the home setting.

Importance of Peristomal Skin Management

Be sure the patient understands that the skin around the stoma should not be reddened or sore and must be maintained intact to avoid problems with the pouch seal. Patients need to understand the principles of ostomy care to prevent skin irritation or redness and to apply a pouching system securely. The skin around the stoma should be healthy, and the pouching system should not leak between planned changes. Some patients do not seek assistance for signs of peristomal skin breakdown. Erwin-Toth et al. (2012) revealed that 61% of participants had signs of peristomal skin disorder upon inspection by the WOC nurse. If possible, reinforce the availability of the WOC nurse for follow-up care; one method is to provide a discharge packet with a follow-up appointment after discharge with the ostomy outpatient clinic. Current care should be communicated to home health nurses for appropriate follow-up.

Obtaining and Paying for Supplies

Instruct the patient that most insurances cover the majority of the cost of ostomy supplies. Since insurance coverage varies, the patient should check with the insurance provider to verify coverage of the ostomy supplies and to determine if there is a preferred vendor. The patient also

needs to know that they may need a prescription to obtain ostomy supplies. Medicare usually provides coverage of 80% for necessary supplies with a prescription; however, Medicare Part B will not cover supplies while home health care services are in place, Colwell et al. (2016). The home care agency is contracted by Medicare to provide both nursing services and all ostomy supplies. Once home care is discontinued, the patient can purchase ostomy supplies that will be reimbursed by Medicare. See Appendix J for listing of supplies and CMS codes.

Psychological Issues

As noted above, this is a good time to ask the patient about their fears and concerns, and to start to address with them how the health care team will work with them to help to reduce their fears.

Sexuality

Chapter 14 describes the potential impact of an ostomy on body image and sexual function.

The topic of sexuality may be difficult for the patient to broach but is usually a concern, and it is important that the nurse assesses the patient's need to learn about sexuality with an ostomy and to help identify the need for further counseling. The PLISSIT counseling model (described in Chapter 14) highlights some levels of sexual counseling. The WOC nurse is encouraged to intervene at the permission and limited information level where the patient is given permission to acknowledge the need for the discussion, and in the explanation phase, some simple suggestions for initial sexual encounters after surgery such as emptying the pouch and checking the seal, clothing options, for example, and the patient should be encouraged to ask specific questions.

Patients and their significant others need reassurance that sexual enjoyment can still be a part of their lives, despite the alteration in physical changes (Junkin & Beitz, 2005). Challenges identified in a small (*n* = 14) Turkish study include changes in sexual life, body image, and fear and anxiety during sexual intercourse. The author suggested that sexual counseling be offered within the first 3 months after surgery and continued as long as the necessary (Vural et al., 2016).

KEY POINT

The stoma itself should not be used for sexual intimacy, as it is easily damaged and is not an erogenous area.

Acknowledgment of Normal Stages of Adjustment

Adjustment to a new stoma requires a period of time to incorporate the stoma into the patients' life and to acquire the necessary skills to manage the stoma. Chapter 14 describes the stages of adjustment. Patients should understand that adjustment to an altered body image and function takes time and energy. They should also be aware that the WOC nurse will be available for consultation after discharge for any challenges that arise.

Ostomy Visitor

Patients facing ostomy surgery are at various levels of acceptance. Patients may feel ready to accept the upcoming changes, but most patients need further assistance. One suggestion is to refer the patient to a trained visitor who has an ostomy or to refer the patient to an ostomy support group before the ostomy surgery. There are local and national ostomy support groups affiliated with the UOAA, and local groups can be found by consulting https://www.ostomy.org/support-group-finder/. The people in these groups have experienced the physical and emotional stressors associated with disease, surgery, body image changes, and lifestyle changes associated with an ostomy. Some local chapters or groups offer Ostomy Education Days to provide all patients with ostomies the opportunity to learn more about having an ostomy, receive encouragement, and see new supplies at a vendor fair. Despite advances in ostomy pouch system technology, many patients still experience problems with psychosocial adjustment.

Many patients relate that the personal turning point in learning to accept the ostomy was the moment he or she met another person with a similar ostomy. Seeing the trained visitor or another person with an ostomy in regular clothing, sharing experiences, and hearing the recovery stories can help patients and families to move toward acceptance. Another method to connect with people with an ostomy is to seek information on qualified Web sites. The UOAA has videos sharing patients' stories. The ostomy manufacturers also have education and tools for patients and families (see resource list in Appendix C). Most patients eventually learn to live a healthy lifestyle with an ostomy.

Professional Counseling

There are times when a patient is unable to cope with an ostomy in a healthy manner. The patient's primary care provider may be able to offer assistance in the form of counseling, but it may be necessary to refer the patient and/or family to a clinical psychologist or psychiatrist for expert consultation regarding issues with coping. Patients may be reluctant to make an appointment with a specialist due to the stigma of mental illness. The nurse should help the patient and/or family understand that people need help to overcome the barriers for healthy recovery. It is not a failure for the patient to see the specialist; it is a negative outcome if the patient fails to follow up with a professional and does not learn to live with the ostomy in a healthy manner. Assessment and identification of psychosocial issues the patient faces is a challenge for the nurse and primary care provider. The WOC nurse should identify any other education the patient will need. For example, the patient undergoing a temporary ileostomy for ileal pouch anal anastomosis (IPAA) may be ready to have information regarding diet, sphincter exercises, and skin care.

Bowel Prep

Most facilities have developed a preoperative bundle to decrease the risk of surgical site infections. Components of the preoperative bundle will include preoperative bathing with chlorhexidine, smoking cessation, and optimal blood glucose control and in some cases, MRSA screening, bowel preparation, and antibiotic (oral) administration (Ban et al., 2017; Zywot et al., 2017).

Cleansing is done with a chlorhexidine preparation usually the day before surgery and the morning of surgery, done by the patient prior to arrival at the hospital. If the patient has a history of smoking, cessation is strongly advised 4 to 6 weeks before surgery, and optimal glucose control is advised as well. Oral antibiotics are taken the day before surgery and will be given intravenously in the immediate preoperative period.

Review the method of bowel preparation prior to surgery. Be sure to check with the surgeon regarding the current methods to prepare for surgery. Some surgeons require mechanical bowel preparation (MBP) and others consider MBP potentially harmful (Yang et al., 2013). The solutions do not clean out the colon completely and leave a watery residue. Studies have indicated that infection rate for operations without MBP is equal to or in some cases, less than operations done with the bowel preparation (Ellis, 2010).

A recent review concluded that the majority of colorectal surgeons employ a combination of oral antibiotic bowel preparation (ABP), MBP, and parenteral antibiotics prior to colorectal surgery (McChesney et al., 2019). The American Society of Colon and Rectal Surgeons Clinical Practice Guidelines for the Use of Bowel Preparation in Elective Colon and Rectal Surgery (Migaly et al., 2019) strongly recommend MBP along with preoperative oral antibiotics for elective colorectal resections based on moderate quality evidence, and Fry (2016) concluded that these are the standard of care for elective colon surgery. However, he calls for refinement in methods of bowel preparation and additional clinical investigations to further enhance outcomes. Combined MBP/ABP were found by Klinger et al. (2019) to result in significantly lower rates of SSI, organ space infection, wound dehiscence, and anastomotic leak than no preparation and a lower rate of SSI than ABP alone.

Since the type of bowel preps used will depend upon the surgical team, it is important to determine their preferred type of prep. There are many different types of MBP, and some are used alone or in combination.

The bowel preparation usually involves dietary restriction and mechanical cleansing of the gastrointestinal tract with the use of a bowel preparation. Typically, the patient is on clear liquids for one to two days before surgery and begins the mechanical bowel prep the day before surgery. Examples of MBPs are polyethylene glycol (PEG) electrolyte solution; laxatives (mineral oil, agar, and phenolphthalein); mannitol; glycerin enemas (900-mL water containing 100-mL glycerin); sodium phosphate (NaP) solution; bisacodyl (10 mg) and enemas; diets, low residue, nonresidue, and with clear liquids; and saline enema per rectum (Guenaga et al., 2011).

The most common solutions used prior to colorectal surgery are the PEG solution and the NaP solution. The PEG solution is an osmotic laxative. The large-volume solution causes watery diarrhea to cleanse the stool out of the colon. The PEG laxative solution also contains electrolytes to prevent dehydration and other serious side effects that may be caused by fluid loss as the colon is emptied. Patients complain of the salty taste, nausea, abdominal fullness, discomfort, and vomiting that may be associated with this preparation. The NaP solution is a low-volume, hyperosmotic liquid. The effectiveness of oral NaP solution is generally similar to or significantly better than PEG solution in patients preparing for colorectal surgery. Typically, oral NaP solution is significantly more acceptable to patients than is the PEG solution due to the low volume but may cause electrolyte imbalances and dehydration (Ellis, 2010; WOCN, 2011).

KEY POINT

Stoma site marking may reduce the incidence of complications and improve self-care.

STOMA SITING

The term *stoma siting* refers to identification and marking the optimal location for the stoma on the patient's abdomen. A pouching system has an adhesive seal that in order to be effective should be placed on skin around a stoma that is flat with minimal creases and in an area that the patient can visualize to support self-care. Stoma siting is vital to the patient's quality of life with an ostomy since poor stoma positioning will greatly affect the patient's quality of life (McKenna et al., 2016). Marking the proposed stoma site prior to surgical intervention was introduced by Turnbull and Gill in the 1950's (Doughty, 2008) and quickly emerged as best practice in the medical and nursing fields. Stoma siting is also an expectation of the person about to undergo planned or potential ostomy surgery as outlined in the Ostomy and Continent Diversion Patient Bill of Rights (UOAA, 2018; see Appendix L). The position statements authored by the WOCN®, The American Society of Colon and Rectal Surgeons, and the American Urological Association on Preoperative Stoma

site marking recommends stoma site marking all patients who are scheduled for surgery that may result in a stoma (Salvadalena et al., 2015a,b).

RATIONALE

Person et al. (2012) found that preoperative stoma site marking results in significantly better QOL, improved patients' confidence and independence, and lower rates of postoperative complications, irrespective of the type of stoma. McKenna et al. (2016) compared the quality of life of patients in receiving preoperative stoma marking to those that did not receive preoperative marking and found that the group that were marked had a higher quality of life following surgery compared to the group that did not have stoma site marking before surgery. Preoperative stoma site marking not only decreases stoma-related complications, including pouch leakage and peristomal dermatitis, but also accelerates patient's pouch management independence and eases the psychological adjustment of living with and caring for an ostomy (Wasserman & McGee, 2017). The World Council of Enterostomal Therapists (2014) notes that preoperative education should include explanation of the surgical procedure, stoma site marking, and postoperative management. The WOCN® Clinical Guideline: Management of the Adult Patient with a Fecal or Urinary Ostomy (Wound Ostomy Continence Nurses Society, 2017) notes selection of a suitable stoma site helps ensure the patient has an optimal quality of life and that poor placement of the stoma can result in stomal and peristomal complications. It is clear that preoperative stoma site marking is the guideline of clinical experts.

Despite the strong evidence that stoma site marking should be done for every patient who may have ostomy surgery, not all ostomy patients receive stoma site marking. Richbourg et al. (2007), in an ostomy patient survey, noted that <50% of respondents had been seen by an ostomy nurse prior to surgery for stoma siting. Pittman et al. (2008) found that 71% of stoma complications were related to a poor stoma location and in a separate study noted that <67% of patients were marked preoperatively (Pittman, 2011).

"The ideal stoma site is located below the umbilicus, within the rectus muscle, away from scars, creases, bony prominences, umbilicus, and belt line, on the summit of the infra-umbilical fat mound, and visible to the patient" (WCET, 2014). See **Figures 10-1 and 10-2**.

The choice of the proposed stoma site is a guide for the surgeon, as the location of the stoma may need adjustment if issues are encountered during surgery. The patient should understand that this is a proposed stoma site, and the actual site may be in a different location depending upon the findings at the time of surgery.

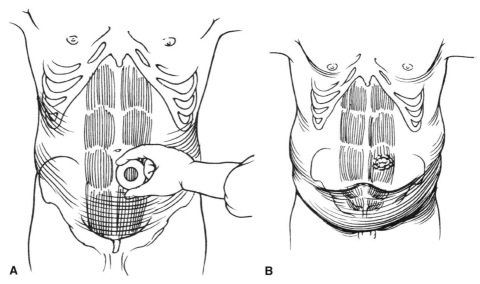

FIGURE 10-1 Stoma Site Through Rectus Muscle. **A.** The usual site for a stoma is on the apex of the infra-umbilical bulge. **B.** In obese patients, the stoma is located on the upper abdomen, where it is visible and on flat skin. (Fischer, J. E., Jones, D. B., Pomposelli, F. B., et al. (2011). *Fischer's mastery of surgery*. Philadelphia, PA: Wolters Kluwer.)

PROCEDURE GUIDELINES

Preoperative stoma site selection and marking needs to be performed by a person who is trained in the procedure such as a colorectal surgeon, urologist, a WOC nurse, or an educated and experienced clinician (WOCN®, 2017).

The patient's medical record should be reviewed before stoma marking. Knowing the patient's background

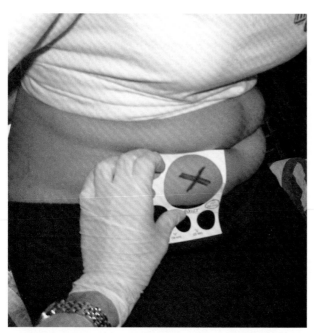

FIGURE 10-2. The Stoma Site is Located Below the Umbilicus, Within the Rectus Muscle, Away from Scars, Creases, Bony Prominences, Umbilicus, and Belt Line, on the Summit of the Infra-umbilical Fat Mound, and Visible to the Patient. (Courtesy of Jane Carmel, MSN, RN, CWOCN.)

helps to anticipate abdominal plane issues such as habitus of the abdomen, scars from previous surgeries, or radiation treatments that may alter the area that can be used as a stoma site. Understanding the patient's disease process will help to determine if the patient may gain weight (possible in the case of Crohn's disease or ulcerative colitis) or lose weight (possible in the case of cancer) after surgery. After the information is gathered, schedule an appointment with the patient. Explain that the surgeon has asked the patient to meet with a WOC nurse before the procedure to learn about the surgery, the expectations of the surgery, the care after surgery, and the stoma site marking. Encourage the presence of patient's spouse or partner if possible. Allow an hour or longer based on the patient's needs for the education, questions, and marking.

The information the ostomy nurse teaches during the preoperative session regarding the anatomy, physiology, and bowel preparation should coincide with the information the surgeon shared. The nurse needs to notice nonverbal cues that the information is too much or at too high level for the patient to understand. The nurse also needs to be attentive to the patient's emotional needs as the patient may need to stop to cry or gather composure to be ready to learn more. The focus is not to provide copious information; the goal is to help the patient understand the implications of the surgery at the level he or she is ready to understand. Cronin (2012) suggests that during stoma site marking, the time spent with the patient explaining and allowing plenty of opportunity for questions is hugely beneficial to the patient. If possible, scheduling multiple, short sessions before surgery, will help the patient to absorb the information being given.

Stoma Site Marking Procedure

The WOC nurse should begin by explaining the procedure (how and why) and obtain verbal consent or written consent, based on institutional policy.

Gather items needed for the procedure: surgical marker, transparent film dressing, and flat skin barrier. If a preoperative kit is used, open kit and lay out all supplies to be used.

Explain the stoma marking procedure to the patient and encourage patient or partner participation and input.

1. In a warm, private room, carefully examine the patient's abdominal surface. Begin with the patient fully clothed in sitting position with feet on the floor. Observe for the presence of belts, braces, and any other ostomy pouch systems. Ask patients if they are employed in an industry in which they wear clothing in or around the waist area such as a carpenter with a tool belt. This information will be helpful when choosing a stoma site as the patient may need to change their clothing or use protective devices to shield the stoma.

2. Examine the patient's exposed abdomen in various positions (standing, lying, sitting, and bending forward) to observe for creases, valleys, scars, folds, skin turgor, and contour. The abdominal physical planes are affected by age, previous surgeries, and treatments.

3. With the patient lying on their back, identify the rectus muscle. This can be done by asking the patient to do a modified sit-up (raise the head up off the bed). If the rectus muscle cannot be seen because of obesity, use the nipple line to determine the outer edge of the rectus muscle. Placement within the rectus muscle can help to prevent peristomal hernia formation.

4. In a sitting position, choose an area that is visible to the patient, through the rectus muscle and in a flat area that is 2 to 3 inches in size, away from bony prominences and the umbilicus. Identify the apex of the infra-umbilical bulge (if present) while sitting and consider the apex as a possible site (**Fig. 10-3**).

5. If the abdomen is obese, consider the placement in the upper abdominal quadrants to allow the patient to visualize and care for the stoma.

6. For the patient with a soft protuberant abdomen, the belt line is typically well below the lower abdominal fold (see Appendices F and G for marking the obese abdomen). Marking the site below the fold will result in the inability of the patient to visualize the stoma and lack the flat surface area needed for a secure seal of the pouching system. Mark the stoma site in an upper quadrant on a flat surface, where it is visible to the patient and on a smooth plane for better pouch adhesion (**Fig. 10-4**).

Once the mark is chosen, ask the patient to place a finger on the mark to indicate that he or she can visualize the stoma to provide self-care. Explain to the patient why that particular area has been selected and determine their understanding and agreement with the stoma mark. Discuss rationale for placement, that is, where they can see it as patient must be in agreement. The patient may want to fasten shirt and trousers to check the site in relation to clothing.

Clean the desired site with alcohol and allow to dry. Mark the selected site with a surgical marker/pen. Cover with transparent film dressing (Salvadalena et al., 2015a,b).

Considerations in Stoma Site Marking

If there are two viable locations for the stoma placement, consider marking both and numbering by preference. Chart in the patient's medical record the reason for choosing the two sites, and if possible, have a conversation with the surgeon before surgery. Watt (1982)

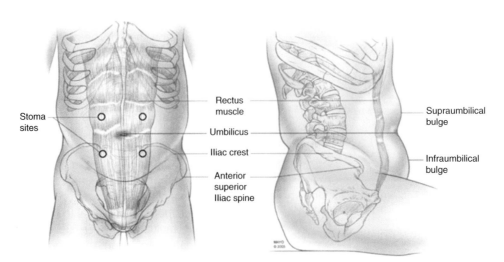

FIGURE 10-3. Supra- and Infra-umbilical Bulges. (Fischer, J. E., Jones, D. B., Pomposelli, F. B., et al. (2011). *Fischer's mastery of surgery.* Philadelphia, PA: Wolters Kluwer.)

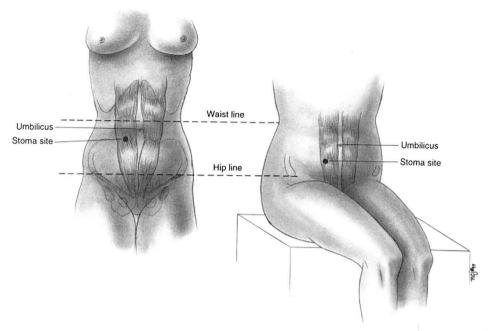

FIGURE 10-4. Stoma Site Marking. (From Hurst, R. (1999). Proctocolectomy with ileostomy, abdominal colectomy with ileostomy, and abdominal colectomy with ileoproctostomy. In F. Michelassi & J. W. Milsom (Eds.), *Operative strategies in inflammatory bowel disease* (p. 157). New York, NY: Springer-Verlag.)

suggested that marking several sites with a preferential ranking on the abdomen gave the surgeon more than one option to use during the surgery with the best option ranked first. Colwell and Folkedahl (2001) concurred with this guidance to mark several stoma sites.

For some patients who have abdomens with many creases and folds that will not be visible to the surgeon in a flat position (as when the patient is on the operating table), consider noting areas that would be inadvisable to place the stoma. This can be done by marking the word "no" in creases or skin folds that would make pouching a stoma difficult or impossible.

Unique Stoma Marking Considerations: Marking for Two Stomas

Occasionally, a patient may need to be marked for two stomas, a urinary stoma and a fecal stoma. The goal of marking two stomas on the same abdomen is to mark the stomas at different abdominal heights if possible. If one of the pouching systems needs an ostomy belt, the variation in height will allow the use of the belt without interfering with the other ostomy pouch. When marking the two stomas at the same time, it is preferable to mark the urostomy at least 1 inch higher.

For individuals who already have a stoma and now need to be marked for another stoma, use the general principles of stoma siting and allow ample surface area for the pouching system barrier in relation to the other stoma and offset the height of the stoma sites in the event that one of the stoma sites would require a belt.

Moving the Stoma

Patients may need to have the original stoma moved to another site. Typically, this is due to a hernia at the original site, but there may be other reasons. The patient commonly is more participative for this site marking because he or she is familiar with the pouching systems and where he or she likes to have the stoma. Discuss the site with the patient and accommodate his or her wishes if possible. Explain that the new site will have a new stoma and that the pouching system may need to be changed. The new stoma will be edematous and require resizing for the pouch system, as the stoma changes in shape and size after surgery.

Thin Patient

There are several considerations for a thin patient. One consideration is the patient with a small amount of adipose tissue. A thin patient may have lost weight due to lengthy illness. The mark should be positioned according to anticipated weight gain. The goal is to avoid marking the site in an area where a crease may develop. It may help to gently squeeze the skin of the infra-umbilical fold and mark away from the crease of the fold.

Another consideration is the patient who is thin with loose, wrinkly skin over a firm abdomen musculature. This is a challenge because the mark may be placed but the loose skin moves easily and the mark will move with the skin. In this case, the nurse must contact the surgeon and be very clear on the placement of the stoma site in relation to the patient's abdomen. It may help to assess the patient together with the surgeon.

Creases and Folds

People of all body types have creases and folds to take into consideration. It is imperative to watch the patient's abdomen as the patient moves from standing to sitting to lying and as the patient bends over. Mark the site on the outer curve of a crease to avoid placement in a location that would be difficult to get a pouch to seal.

Scars

Note any scars and the texture of the scar. Some scars are soft, and the stoma location may be safely placed near the scar. However, scars may also be firm or sinewy and may cause uneven pouching surface or tension on the pouching surface. The firm, sinewy scars should be avoided in the peristomal plane.

Distension

Patients with distension are often seen prior to emergent surgical situations, for example, bowel blockage. Ask the patient to describe what his or her abdomen generally looks like. Inspect carefully for signs of creases that are not currently present due to the distension, such as discolored skin tones or light wrinkles. Take these areas into account when selecting a site. If the outer edge of the rectus muscle cannot easily be determined, use the nipple lines as a marker for the edge of the rectus muscle. Keep in mind the abdomen distension will decrease and the mark will become more midline as the swelling recedes. Mark the site ample distance from the midline to accommodate the ostomy pouch system.

Pregnancy

The pregnant patient faces similar challenges as the patient with distension. Marking the site requires careful consideration. Ask the patient about her normal habitus and inspect for signs such as discoloration of the skin or small wrinkles that indicate the location of a crease to avoid. The rectus muscle is generally not palpable. Mark the stoma site fairly lateral, as the site will migrate toward midline after the baby is born.

Pendulous Breasts

Women with pendulous breasts may experience problems if the breast covers the stoma site. Ask the patient to apply and remove her bra during the stoma marking session to assess the changes. The patient may need to wear her bra during ostomy care in order to see the site. If the breast completely covers the pouching system, this may interfere with the procedure to change and empty the pouching system, and a new site may need to be considered.

Tattoos

Patients may have tattoos on their abdomen. When choosing the site, be sure to explain to the patient that you are choosing the best site based on obtaining a secure pouch seal. When the patient has a tattoo, do not hesitate to mark on the tattoo if it is in the best interest of the patient. Be sure the mark is visible and contact the surgeon to explain the situation and the patient's response to the mark. Piercings should be avoided, and the jewelry should be worn during the marking. The patient will be instructed to remove the pierced jewelry before surgery.

Contractures, Kyphosis, or Scoliosis

Patients with bony structural changes such as contractures, kyphosis, or scoliosis pose unique problems for stoma siting because the body alignment distorts the abdominal plane and may limit the space for an ostomy pouch. The goals are to select a site where a pouch will adhere and where the patient can perform the self-care. While visualization is optimal, the patient may need to learn techniques to adjust to lack of seeing the stoma. It may benefit the patient to wear an ostomy pouch after the stoma marking to confirm the stoma site.

Spiritual Beliefs

Patients may have strong spiritual beliefs that require the stoma site to be in a specific location. For example, patients of the Muslim faith may request stoma to be located on the left side. In a letter to the Journal of Wound, Ostomy Continence Nursing Editor, Iqbal et al. (2013) explain that Muslim patients report that the left-sided stoma is more compliant with their spiritual beliefs and is easier to manage during the ritual of sacred washing (refer to Chapter 14). The nurse should discuss the implications with the patient and consult with the surgeon regarding the patient's wishes and the safety to have the stoma placed on the left side. Consider marking several sites with the preferences numbered.

Difficult Stoma Siting Using Computed Tomography

Craig et al. (2007) share an excellent case study that involved team work to determine the site marking in a difficult case. The team reported the patient had undergone multiple abdominal procedures. The standard surgical procedure is to perform a laparotomy to identify the bowel segment that is mobile enough to reach the skin surface. The laparotomy often requires extensive adhesiolysis (the process of cutting adhesions between two abdominal structures), and the stoma site is often at the mercy of the length of the bowel. In this case study, the patient was assessed by the WOC nurse and marked with several potential sites away from scars. The patient then had a computed tomography (CT) examination with the medical team present. Areas in the abdomen were identified with radiopaque markers and rescanned to confirm the positions over the bowel. The final stoma site was then chosen by the WOC nurse based on the available sites. The patient had successful construction of a loop colostomy.

Continent Stoma Marking

Verify the type of continent stoma the surgeon will perform. Mark the continent stoma site in a location that follows the guidelines of general stoma site marking. Be sure the site is visible to the patient and in a location that the patient is able to manage the stoma drainage procedure. Ideally, mark the location on a smooth abdominal plane. In the event the patient would need to pouch the stoma, it is ideal to have a location that allows pouch adherence.

Wheelchair

Assess the patient in his or her own wheelchair with clothing removed from the abdomen to visualize the area. Sitting on the examination table is not the same posture the patient will assume in their wheelchair. Discuss activities and watch the patient use the chair to note any changes in abdomen contour. The site chosen for a person in a wheelchair is slightly higher than normal. This allows better visualization and usually a better abdominal plane. The person may have a large abdomen because of the lack of strength of the abdominal muscle, and the abdomen may rest directly on the thigh (Colwell & Folkedahl, 2001).

Brace or Leg Prosthesis

Assess the patient while they are wearing the brace. Determine if the brace will cause undue pressure or shearing of the pouching system. Consult with the surgeon if the site may interfere with the brace in order to choose a location that will allow the patient to be independent with care.

Pain/Limited Mobility

The patient may be in too much pain or be unable to assume the positions required for stoma siting. Sitting position may be simulated with raising the head of the bed.

Special Equipment/Work Belts

Patients may have careers or hobbies that require the use of belts or other apparatus that may need to be considered as the stoma is marked. Ask the patient to bring the belt or apparatus to the stoma siting appointment to show the nurse where the item comes in contact with the abdomen. The patient should also perform movements that mimic the activity necessary while wearing the item. For example, police and carpenters need to wear thick, heavy leather belts and the stoma mark may be better sited above this belt to avoid compression and possible dislodgement of the pouch.

Radiation

Areas treated with radiation should be avoided for stoma marking if possible. Radiation treatments cause narrowing of the capillaries and can increase the risk of mucocutaneous separation as the stoma heals after surgery. Radiation causes skin changes in the epidermis to be dry and fragile and easily traumatized by the adhesives of the pouch barrier (Erwin-Toth et al., 2012).

Marking During Surgery

In emergent situations prior to surgery, the patient is usually able to sit up or be assisted to sit to visualize the abdominal planes and detect skin creases or folds. However, there are occasions the surgeon needs to create a stoma during the operative case. See **Box 10-4** for stoma marking tips during the surgical case. The best suggestion is to squeeze the abdomen to identify the infra and supra umbilical folds and to place the stoma at the apex of either area and away from the umbilicus and laparotomy incision if present.

Infants and Children

Babies have special needs due to the small abdomen. Newborns often have a large umbilical cord area, and the baby may have tubes or access sites also on the abdomen. Avoid marking close to the umbilical cord, because once the cord falls off, the surface will be uneven (Boarini, 1988). It is important to choose a site that has enough surface for a pouch barrier and avoid these obstacles. Discuss the site with the surgeon if necessary. Explain the requirement of space needed to accommodate the barrier of the pouching system. See Chapter 15 for discussion of pediatric ostomy management.

Teenagers

Teenagers have many different styles of body type. The guidelines followed for adults can be followed for teenagers. Consider that the teen will grow and develop over the years and that the stoma will need to be placed

---

BOX 10-4   TIPS FOR STOMA SITE MARKING DURING SURGERY

Most abdomens appear flat when body is supine.

The main goals are to avoid placing the stoma in a crease and to place the stoma high enough for the patient to see the stoma.

Try to find a flat area that is 2 to 3 inches in size, away from bony prominences and the umbilicus.

The abdomen can be gently squeezed to identify the natural infraumbilical and supraumbilical folds in order to find the infraumbilical bulge.

Look for signs of belt lines or creases by skin discoloration and small wrinkles in the skin. Avoid placing the stoma along these lines.

The ideal placement is on the infra-umbilical bulge, but in more obese patients, the supra-umbilical bulge may be more appropriate (**Fig. 10-1**).

Allow ample room between the midline incision (if this is the type of incision used for the procedure) and the stoma site for the pouching system adhesive.

accordingly. The teen may want the mark as low as possible, but the nurse must place the mark in the best interest of the teen for the future years. Teens may have a narrow abdomen, and it will be difficult for the mark to avoid the midline, iliac crest, and costal margin. Belt line and style of clothing can be a challenge to meet their needs for ideal stoma siting

 ## DOCUMENTATION

Document the preoperative educational and marking session thoroughly. Include ostomy teaching information covered, tools used for education, the consent of the patient to mark for the stoma, and the stoma site marking procedure. Document the location of the site using anatomic markings such as the umbilicus or document in an image placed in the patient's record in the event the stoma mark fades and surgeon is unable to locate during surgery. Document patient teach-back, the materials that were sent home with patient, and note the patient's response to teaching. It is important to document the patient's agreement on the stoma site marking. Note referrals for further education or counseling if the patient has time for these interactions before surgery.

 ## CONCLUSIONS

The preoperative counseling session(s) should include physical and emotional assessment and help to determine resources of ongoing support for the patient. This preoperative education helps to alleviate the patient's fears and anxieties associated with the potential surgery. In addition, stoma site marking prior to surgery has been found to prevent problems associated with a poor pouch system seal. The WOCN® Clinical Guideline: Management of the Adult Patient with a Fecal or Urinary Ostomy (Wound Ostomy Continence Nurses Society, 2017) conclude that "The person who is well prepared for the challenges that the new ostomy brings will have a less protracted period of adjustment."

REFERENCES

American College of Surgeons. (2016). Skills Programs. Retrieved from https://www.facs.org/education/patient-education/skills-programs

Ban, K. A., Minei, J. P., Laronga, C., et al. (2017). American college of surgeons and surgical infection society: surgical site infection guidelines, 2016 update. *Journal of the American College of Surgeons, 224*(1), 59–74.

Bare, K., Drain, J., Timko-progar, M., et al. (2017). Implementation of an evidence-based and content validated standardized ostomy algorithm tool in home care. *Journal of Wound, Ostomy, and Continence Nursing, 44*(3), 262–266.

Barreira, S. I. R. (2018). The role of stoma nurse in preoperative education. An analysis on the recovery time of the autonomy of the person with ostomy. *Clinical Nutrition ESPEN, 25*, 198–199.

Boarini, J. H. (1988). Principles of stoma care for infants. *Journal of Enterostomal Therapy, 16*(1), 21–25.

Burgess, J. (2020). *Eating with an Ostomy: A comprehensive nutrition guide for those living with an ostomy*. United Ostomy Associations of America. Retrieved from https://www.ostomy.org/wp-content/uploads/2020/07/Eating_with_an_Ostomy_2020-07.pdf

Chand, M., De'Ath, H. D., Shahnawaz, R., et al. (2016). The influence of peri-operative factors for accelerated discharge following laparoscopic colorectal surgery when combined with an enhance recovery after surgery (ERAS) pathway. *International Journal of Surgery, 25*, 59–63.

Coggrave, M. J., Ingram, R. M., Gardner, B. P., et al. (2012). The impact of stoma for bowel management after spinal cord injury. *Spinal Cord, 50*, 848–852.

Colwell, J. C., & Folkedahl, B. (2001). Stoma site selection in a patient with multiple enterocutaneous fistulae. *Journal of Wound, Ostomy, and Continence Nursing, 28*(2), 113–115.

Colwell J., Bain K. A., Hansen A. S., et al. (2019). Guidelines for assessment of peristomal body profile, ostomy patient engagement and patient follow up: results of an international ostomy consensus. *Journal of Wound, Ostomy, and Continence Nursing, 46*(6), 497–504.

Colwell, J. C., Kupsick, P. T., & McNichol, L. L. (2016). Outcome criteria for discharging the patient with a new ostomy from home health care. *Journal of Wound, Ostomy, and Continence Nursing, 43*(3), 1–5.

Craig, E., Garner, J., & Amin, S., (2007). Stoma siting using CT guidance in a multiply scarred abdomen. *Techniques in Coloproctology, 11*(3), 281–282.

Cronin, E. (2012). What the patient needs to know before stoma siting; an overview. *British Journal of Nursing, 21*(22), 1234–1237.

Dorman, C. (2009). Ostomy basics: The nurse's personal feelings toward ostomies play a role in patient outcomes. [RN], 22–27. Retrieved from www.rnweb.com.

Doughty, D. (2008). History of ostomy surgery. *Journal of Wound, Ostomy, and Continence Nursing, 35*(1), 34–38.

Ellis, C. N. (2010). Bowel preparation before elective colorectal surgery: What is the evidence? *Seminars in Colon and Rectal Surgery, 21*(3), 144–147.

Erwin-Toth, P., Thompson, S., & Davis, J. (2012). Factors impacting the quality of life of people with an ostomy in North America: Results from the Dialogue Study. *Journal of Wound, Ostomy, and Continence Nursing, 39*(4), 417–422.

Fry, D. E. (2016). Antimicrobial bowel preparation for election colon surgery. *Surgical Infections, 17*(3), 269–274.

Guenaga, K. F., Matos, D., & Wille-Jorgensen, P. (2011). Mechanical bowel preparation for elective colorectal surgery. *The Cochrane Database of Systematic Reviews,* (9), CD001544.

Haugen, V., Bliss, D. Z., & Savik, K. (2006). Perioperative factors that affect long-term adjustment to an incontinent ostomy. *Journal of Wound, Ostomy, and Continence Nursing, 33*(5), 525–535.

Hendren, S., Hammond, K., Glasgow, S. C., et al. (2015). Clinical practice guidelines for ostomy surgery. *Diseases of the Colon and Rectum, 58*(4), 375–387.

Iqbal, F., Zaman, S., & Bowley, D. M. (2013). Stoma location requires special considerations in selected patients. *Journal Wound Ostomy Continence Nursing, 401*(6), 565–566.

Junkin, J., & Beitz, J. (2005). Sexuality and the person with a stoma implications for comprehensive WOC nursing practice. *Journal of Wound, Ostomy, and Continence Nursing, 32*(2), 121–128.

Klinger, A. L., Green, H., Monlezun, D. J., et al. (2019). The role of bowel preparation in colorectal surgery results of the 2012–2015 ACS-NSQIP Data. *Annals of Surgery, 269*(4), 671–677.

Klink, C. D., Lioupis, K., Binnebösel, M., et al. (2011). Diversion stoma after colorectal surgery: loop colostomy or ileostomy? *International Journal of Colorectal Disease, 26*, 431–436.

McChesney, S. L., Zelhart, M. D., Green, R. L., et al. (2019). Current U.S. pre-operative bowel preparation trends: a 2018 survey of the American Society of Colon and Rectal Surgeons members. *Surgical Infections, 21*(1), 1–8. Retrieved from https://www.liebertpub.com/doi/abs/10.1089/sur.2019.125

McKenna, L. S., Taggart, E., Stoelting, J., et al. (2016). The impact of preoperative stoma marking on health-Related Quality of life. *Journal of Wound, Ostomy, and Continence Nursing, 43*(1), 57–61.

Migaly, J., Bafford A. C., Todd D. F., et al. (2019). The American Society of Colon and Rectal Surgeons Clinical Practice Guidelines for the use of bowel preparation in elective colon and rectal surgery. *Diseases of the Colon and Rectum, 62*, 3–8.

Nichols, T. R. (2011). Social connectivity in those 24 months or less post-surgery. *Journal of Wound, Ostomy, and Continence Nursing, 38*(1), 63–68.

O'Flynn, S. K. (2018). Care of the stoma: complications and treatments. *British Journal of Community Nursing, 23*(8), 382–387.

Person, B., Ifargan, R., Lachter, J., et al. (2012). The impact of preoperative stoma site marking on the incidence of complications, quality of life, and patient's independence. *Diseases of the Colon and Rectum, 55*(7), 783–787.

Pittman, J. (2011). Characteristics of the patient with an ostomy. *Journal of Wound, Ostomy, and Continence Nursing, 38*(3), 271.

Pittman, J., Rawl, S., Schmidt, C., et al. (2008). Demographic and clinical factors related to ostomy complications and quality of life in veterans with an ostomy. *Journal of Wound, Ostomy, and Continence Nursing, 35*(5), 493–503.

Richbourg, L., Thorpe, J. M., & Rapp, C. G. (2007). Difficulties experienced by the ostomate after hospital discharge. *Journal of Wound, Ostomy, and Continence Nursing, 34*(1), 70–79.

Salvadalena, G., Hendren, S., McKenna, L., et al. (2015a). WOCN Society and AUA position statement on preoperative stoma site marking for patients undergoing urostomy surgery. *Journal of Wound, Ostomy, and Continence Nursing, 42*(3), 253–256.

Salvadalena, G., Hendren, S. K., Mckenna, L., et al. (2015b). WOCN Society and ASCRS position statement on preoperative stoma site marking for patients undergoing colostomy or ileostomy surgery. *Journal of Wound, Ostomy, and Continence Nursing, 42*(3), 249–252 .

Stokes, A. L., Tice, S., Follett, S., et al. (2017). Institution of a preoperative stoma education group class decreases rate of peristomal complications in new stoma patients. *Journal of Wound, Ostomy, and Continence Nursing, 44*(4), 363–367.

United Ostomy Associations of America (UOAA). (2008). Controlling odor. Columbus Discovery. Retrieved from http://www.ostomy.org

United Ostomy Associations of America (UOAA). (2018). Inspire excellence! Practices for Ostomy Nurses to utilize and support ostomy and continent diversion patient Bill of Rights. Advocates for a Positive Change. Retrieved from http://www.ostomy.org

Vural, F., Harputlu, D., Karayurt, O., et al. (2016). The impact a ostomy on the sexual lives of persons with stomas. *Journal of Wound, Ostomy, and Continence Nursing, 43*(4), 381–384.

Wasserman, M. A., & McGee, M. F. (2017). Preoperative considerations for the ostomate. *Clinics in Colon and Rectal Surgery, 30*, 157–161.

Watt, C. (1982). Stoma placement. In D. Broadwell, & B. Jackson (Eds.), *Principles of ostomy care.* St. Louis, MO: Mosby.

Weiss, B. (2003). *Health literacy. A manual for clinicians* (2nd ed.). Chicago, IL: American Medical Association Foundation and American Medical Association.

World Council of Enterostomal Therapists. (2014). In K. Zulkowski (Ed.), *WCET International Ostomy Guideline.* Osborne Park, Australia: WCET.

WOCN. (2011). *Bowel prep for patients with a colostomy.* Mt. Laurel, NJ: WOCN. Retrieved from www.wocn.org

Wound Ostomy Continence Nurses Society. (2010). *Best practice guideline for clinicians. Management of the adult patient with a fecal ostomy.* Mt. Laurel, NJ: WOCN. Retrieved from www.wocn.org

Wound Ostomy Continence Nurses Society. (2017). *Clinical guideline: Management of the adult patient with a fecal or urinary ostomy.* Mt. Laurel, NJ: WOCN. Retrieved from www.wocn.org

Yang, L., Chen, H., Welk, B., et al. (2013). Does using comprehensive preoperative bowel preparation offer any advantage for urinary diversion using ileum? A meta-analysis. *International Urology and Nephrology, 45*(1), 25–31.

Zywot, A., Lau, C. S., Fletcher, S., et al. (2017). Bundles prevent surgical site infections after colorectal surgery: Meta-analysis and systematic review. *Journal of Gastrointestinal Surgery, 21*, 1915–1930.

QUESTIONS

1. A patient is scheduled for surgery for an abdominal perineal resection (APR). What type of stoma will be created during this procedure?
   A. Temporary end colostomy or ileostomy
   B. Permanent end colostomy
   C. Permanent end ileostomy
   D. Temporary loop ileostomy

2. The WOC nurse can help patients with their fears and concerns as they face surgery for an ostomy by
   A. Telling them the ostomy isn't so bad and could be a lot worse
   B. Advise them to keep quiet about their fears and they will feel better soon
   C. Providing the opportunity for a visit with a trained ostomy visitor
   D. Explain that nurses can deliver stoma care so the patient doesn't have to

3. The WOC nurse is teaching a patient with a new stoma about pouching systems. Which teaching point accurately describes an important aspect of using a pouching system?
   A. There are two- and three-piece pouching systems available.
   B. Pouching systems are not odor proof and may have an odor.
   C. Follow-up with an ostomy nurse is usually scheduled on an emergency basis.
   D. The usual wear time for a pouch is 4 days.

4. If the surgeon is siting the stoma during the case in the OR, what advice would you give for general information for stoma site marking?
   A. Ideally, the stoma should be placed on the apex of the abdominal infra-umbilical bulge.
   B. If possible, the stoma should be placed in a crease.
   C. The stoma should be placed over wrinkles if possible for more available skin.
   D. Placement in the incision line allows for ease of pouching.

5. The patient with ulcerative colitis who is being prepared for a surgical procedure to create a permanent end ileostomy should receive preoperative education that includes the following:
   A. Instructing patients that they will need to change their clothing style after this surgery.
   B. They may be a candidate for ostomy irrigation and not need to wear a pouching system.
   C. Help the patient to understand that they can live a full life without a colon and rectum.
   D. Reinforcing to the patient that self-care is simple with few steps to follow.

6. The WOC nurse helps prepare the patient for ostomy surgery by
   A. Determining the patient's emotional support system
   B. Meeting with the patient undergoing elective surgery 5 weeks prior to surgery
   C. Administering mechanical bowel prep prior to surgery
   D. Explaining that the stoma will be red and dry and will have minimal sensation

7. The WOC nurse counsels patients regarding lifestyle issues following stoma surgery. What statement accurately describes an important teaching tip?
   A. Patients with an ostomy should take a tub bath instead of a shower.
   B. Most patients will not have to follow a special diet once healing takes place.
   C. Travel on airplanes is prohibited with an ostomy appliance.
   D. Most patients need to modify their clothing to accommodate the pouch.

8. The first skill the patient with a colostomy should learn before discharge is
   A. How to clean the stoma
   B. How to measure the stoma
   C. How to empty the pouch
   D. How to connect the pouch to a leg bag

9. The WOC nurse should include the preoperative education sessions for an 80-year-old gentleman scheduled for an ileal conduit
   A. Stoma complications
   B. Pouch system demonstration
   C. List of foods that cause flatus
   D. List of medications to avoid

10. The WOC nurse has a consult for stoma site marking for a patient scheduled for an ileal conduit. Where should the stoma most likely be marked?
   A. Right abdomen
   B. Left abdomen
   C. Suprapubic
   D. Near the umbilicus

ANSWERS AND RATIONALES

1. B. Rationale: APR surgery includes the resection sigmoid colon, rectum, and anus, and creation of end colostomy. This is a permanent fecal diversion.

2. C. Rationale: The opportunity to meet with a trained visitor or another person with an ostomy in regular clothing, sharing experiences, and hearing the recovery stories can help patients and families to move toward acceptance.

3. D. Rationale: Patients should be taught that the pouching system wear time should be predictable and is expected to maintain a seal for up to 4 days. If leakage occurs in <2 days, follow-up with an ostomy nurse is advised.

4. A. Rationale: Ideally, the stoma should be placed on the apex of the abdominal contour infra-umbilical fat mound and be visible to the patient.

5. C. Rationale: It is important that the patient understands that once healed, they can return to their pre-illness baseline with few restrictions.

6. A. Rationale: Encouraging the patient's emotional support system to assist the patient in learning and performing self-care is key to patient's adjustment to ostomy.

7. B. Rationale: Usually patients are able to return to prior diet after stoma edema has subsided.

8. C. Rationale: Patients must first learn to empty pouch because they need to empty the pouch frequently when at home and should not rely on another person to be available to do so.

9. B. Rationale: The pouching system and its ease of use may help allay fears and concerns the patient has about self-care.

10. A. Rationale: It is likely that the stoma will be placed on the right side of the abdomen since the ileum is used which, the end of which is located on the right side of the abdomen.

CHAPTER 11

POSTOPERATIVE NURSING ASSESSMENT AND MANAGEMENT

Janice Colwell and Kathleen Hudson

OBJECTIVE

Plan for postoperative nursing assessment and management following surgical procedures that result in a fecal and/or urinary diversion.

TOPIC OUTLINE

Postoperative Assessment **162**

Stoma Assessment **163**
    Anatomic Location and Function 163
    Stoma Construction/Type 165
    Stoma Assessment 167

    Stoma Mucosa 167
    Stoma Structure 168
    Peristomal Skin 168

Postoperative Planning **168**

Conclusions **169**

POSTOPERATIVE ASSESSMENT

Following the surgical procedure to create an intestinal stoma, a thorough patient assessment and understanding of the surgical procedure must be completed in order to plan care. The surgical report should be read to determine the type of surgical procedure performed as well as any intraoperative findings such as the type of stoma created, presence of advanced disease, existence of adhesions, and/or unusual findings not anticipated before the surgical event (Sonia, 2013). It is important to determine if a minimally invasive surgical approach (such as laparoscopic or robotic approach) has been used as this may contribute to a reduced length of stay (Carmichael et al., 2017).

This information will be necessary to support the patient after surgery. The immediate postoperative notes should be read to understand the patient's first 24 hours

after surgery, noting pain management and participation in ambulation, coughing, deep breathing, and potential discharge date. Self-care ostomy management will need to be started as soon as the patient can concentrate on the acquisition of new skills; understanding his or her response to pain management as well as his or her ability to participate in routine postoperative activities may help in knowing when teaching can begin. It is more than likely that the first postoperative teaching session will start within 24 hours after surgery.

Postoperative patient assessment includes the following:

- *Incisional integrity* noting the type of closure (primary, left open to heal by secondary intention, staples, stitches, liquid bonding agent). If the wound has been approximated and closed, examine the incision and if present the dressing for drainage. Wearing gloves, gently palpate either side of the incision noting the firmness or lack of firmness of the tissue, the temperature of the skin, as well as any oozing that might be present while examining the area. Note the color of the skin at the incision and compare to the area outside of the surgical area. If the wound is healing by secondary intention, note the approximate size of the wound, the depth, the quality of the tissue as well as the type of dressing, and the presence of wound drainage (color, amount, presence of odor).

- *Presence of abdominal drains* noting the insertion site for drainage at the skin/drain interface, the amount of drainage (number of gauze pads used and how often changed), and quality of drainage. Assess how the drain is secured (with or without sutures). Assure that the drainage tube has the suction source intact and that the container is emptied when at least three fourths full and that the amount emptied is captured in the intake and output record.

- *Presence of a urinary catheter.* Urinary catheters should be removed within 24 hours of elective colonic or upper rectal resection. Urinary catheters should be removed 48 hours after mid-rectal/lower rectal resections (Carmichael et al., 2017). It is advisable to consult with the surgical team on the removal of the urinary catheter.

- Note the amount and frequency of *pain medication* and the patient's response to pain medications.

- Assess for the presence or absence of *bowel sounds*. Using a stethoscope, listen in the four abdominal quadrants for the presence of bowel activity. Examine the ostomy pouch for the presence of gas; trapped air in the pouch is one sign that bowel activity has returned.

- Gently *palpate the abdomen* noting firmness and excessive tenderness as indicated by the patient's response.

- Assess the *respiratory status* by listening to breath sounds and encourage the use of the incentive spirometer, deep breathing, and coughing.

- Patient's *overall response* to the surgery and recovery. It is important to determine the patient's understanding of his/her role in the postoperative recovery and to educate the patient on meeting goals to help move toward recovery. The patient should be ambulating several times in 24 hours and spending time out of bed to decrease the incidence of postoperative complications and increase strength and endurance. Remind the patient that he or she will need to learn how to empty his or her pouch prior to discharge as well as have a good understanding of how the pouching system will be changed.

- Review of the daily *intake* (IV fluids and when started oral intake) and *output* (urinary, stool, and, if present, drainage collected in drainage collectors).

KEY POINT

Examine the periwound skin and/or incisions and determine the amount of space between the wound/incisions and the outer footprint of the ostomy pouching system. This information will help in determining the appropriate pouching system to avoid injury to the new surgical wound/incision.

Diet: Once bowel activity has returned, the diet is resumed. For most patients, a clear liquid diet is ordered and the patient instructed to sip a small amount of fluid to determine if he or she can tolerate fluid. If the patient is part of the enhanced recovery after surgery (ERAS) protocol, he or she should be offered a regular diet immediately after elective colorectal surgery, monitoring for diet tolerance if consistent with the facility's protocol (Carmichael et al., 2017). Since gas is an issue after abdominal surgery, avoiding a straw is suggested as well as encouraging ambulation to help peristalsis. If the liquid diet is first introduced to the patient and tolerated, a low-residue diet is ordered; suggest to the patient that they should eat small frequent meals and to chew all foods well. A fecal stoma will be edematous after surgery, and a low-residue diet will allow the stool to pass through the stoma (Prinz et al., 2015). The patient with a colon or ileal conduit has a bowel anastomosis (where the conduit was excised) and because of potential edema at the anastomosis, a low-residue diet is preferred.

KEY POINT

As the patient resumes oral intake, discourage the use of a straw as using a straw can increase the intake of air causing bloating and excessive gas.

STOMA ASSESSMENT

Although the surgical report should describe the type of stoma constructed, a thorough assessment of the stoma should be performed. Assessments will include the anatomic location of the stoma (where in the GI or urinary system), the function of the stoma (volume and consistency), and the type of stoma (the configuration-end, loop or end loop) (**Tables 11-1 and 11-2**).

ANATOMIC LOCATION AND FUNCTION

Review the operative report, the history and physical, and other pertinent notes to understand from what section of the intestine the stoma was created. The function of the fecal stoma will depend upon the location in the GI tract; closer to the end of the colon the output will be less in volume and thicker in consistency. A fecal stoma will generally start to function 1 to 3 days after surgery, commonly earlier when the patient undergoes a laparoscopic surgical procedure. Gas followed by liquid is the

TABLE 11-1 PATIENT WITH A NEW FECAL STOMA: ASSESSMENT PARAMETERS	
Anatomic location (most likely obtained from OR report/chart)	Small intestine: jejunum, ileum Large intestine: ascending, transverse, descending, sigmoid Amount (cm) of intestine above stoma
Function	Presence of gas: note pouch inflation Volume, color, and consistency of effluent
Construction	End: single lumen (opening) Loop or end loop: double lumens (openings), determine which opening is the proximal and distal lumen. Note presence of support bridge.
Stoma assessment	Stoma mucosa: Color: deep red Edema: lack of normal folds, creases, taut tissue firm to touch Protrusion: above skin, at skin, below skin Lumen/os location: center, off center, even with skin, below skin Mucocutaneous junction: Junction of stoma/skin: intact Junction of stoma/skin: not intact—separation between stoma and skin, a mucocutaneous separation Percentage of junction that is separated Approximate depth of separation Type of tissue in separation (see Chapter 16)

TABLE 11-2 PATIENT WITH A NEW URINARY STOMA: ASSESSMENT PARAMETERS	
Anatomic location (most likely obtained from OR report/chart)	Small intestine: ileal conduit Large intestine: colonic conduit
Function	Volume and color of urine, presence of mucus in urine
Construction	End: single lumen (opening) End loop: observe presence of support bridge Stents: check end of each, note cut (even or slanted) and presence/location of sutures around stents into stoma
Stoma assessment	Stoma mucosa: Color: deep red Edema: lack of normal folds, creases, taut tissue firm to touch Protrusion: above skin, at skin, below skin Lumen/os location: center, off center, even with skin Mucocutaneous junction: Junction of stoma/skin: intact Junction of stoma/skin: not intact—separation between stoma and skin Percentage of junction that is separated Approximate depth of separation Type of tissue in separation (see Chapter 16)

initial output of both a small and large bowel fecal stoma. A urostomy will begin to function immediately with the presence of mucus and blood-tinged urine.

A jejunostomy, an opening into the jejunum, will have liquid stoma output, and the volume can be as high as 2,400 mL in 24 hours. An ileostomy is an opening into the last portion of the small intestine, the ileum. The output will vary but is generally about 1,200 mL in 24 hours (Orkin & Cataldo, 2007), and while dietary choices can influence the output, it should vary between a thick liquid to a semipasty consistency (like oatmeal). A colostomy is an opening into any section of the colon, and the activity of the colostomy will depend upon the location of the stoma in the colon; closer to the rectum, the output will be pasty to almost formed because the stool has had time to sit in the colon and more fluid is absorbed. Thus, a right-sided colostomy (ascending) will have stoma output similar to that of an ileostomy, a transverse colostomy

will have pasty to semisolid stool, and a left-sided colostomy (descending and sigmoid) will have a semisolid to formed stool depending on how close the stoma is to the end of the colon. Colostomy volume will vary from 600 to 1,000 mL in 24 hours depending on the anatomic location. However, after surgery each of the above-noted stomas will have variable function, starting liquid and moving toward "normal" depending on oral intake, medications, and past medical/surgical history. A person who has lost some of the small bowel from other surgeries will have an alteration in the type and volume of stoma output. Examples of diagnoses that can alter stoma function can include Crohn's disease, previous radiation to the abdomen, ischemic disease, medications, and concurrent treatment such as chemotherapy.

A high-output fecal stoma, usually a jejunostomy or ileostomy, can cause dehydration, slow the rehabilitative process, and in severe cases cause metabolic issues. It is important that ostomy output be carefully measured during the postoperative period, and if the volume of output exceeds what is considered to be the normal amount, a plan of care will need to be worked out that will include ruling out a partial or intermittent bowel obstruction, abdominal sepsis, enteritis (such as *Clostridium difficile*), or sudden drug withdrawal (opiates or corticosteroids). The plan of care may include the following: the use of isotonic fluids, restriction of hypo- and hypertonic fluids, dietary restrictions of high-sugar foods and fluids, dietary inclusions of starch-based foods, and/or the use of antisecretory and antimotility drugs (Baker et al., 2011; WOCN®, 2017). Others may need to be on parenteral infusions (WOCN®, 2017). A person with a high-output ostomy may have reduced wear time of the skin barrier due to the high liquid output increasing the erosion of the skin barrier. This can be addressed by using an extended-wear skin barrier with a high-output pouch system and/or using accessory products to prevent erosion of the skin barrier and preventing skin injuries/leakage (WOCN®, 2017).

A urostomy can be created from a segment of the colon or ileum. The most common approach is to use the terminal ileum (ileal conduit), but in some cases, the colon is used (colon conduit). The function of a urostomy depends upon kidney function and hydration, but minimal output should be 800 mL/24 hours. It is important to remember that since the intestine is used to make a conduit, there will be at least initially a large amount of mucus expelled from the stoma. The intestinal mucosa secretes mucus to lubricate the intestinal contents and continues to secrete mucus when diverted. For most people with a urostomy, the volume of mucus is high for the first few months and is reported to decrease over time. In the postoperative period it is suggested that the urostomy pouch be connected to a drainage collector when in the bed, but can be removed from the bedside drainage collector when ambulating and the patient learns how to empty the pouch and use the adapter to connect to the bedside drainage collector (WOCN®, 2017).

An ileal or colon conduit will have stents that are placed at the time of the ureter/conduit anastomosis, the purpose of which is to protect the anastomosis (**Fig. 11-1**). The length of time that the stents remain in place will depend upon the integrity of the anastomosis, the patient's ability to heal, and the surgeon's preference. Note the number of stents (one for each ureter) and the securement device (sutures from the stents to the stoma). Should a stent push out of the stoma before the planned removal, the urology team needs to be notified.

It is important not to rely on the location of the stoma on the abdominal wall to indicate the type of stoma. While it is likely in many cases if the ileum is used the stoma should be on the right side of the abdomen, the physical location of the stoma should be correlated with the medical record/operative report and consultation done with the surgical team to verify the anatomic location of the stoma.

STOMA CONSTRUCTION/TYPE

The type of stoma constructed by the surgeon will depend on the etiology of the medical or surgical problem and

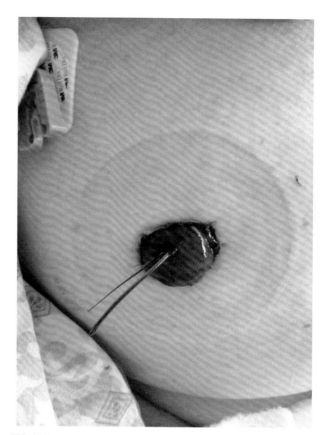

FIGURE 11-1. Urostomy with Stents. (Courtesy of Janice Colwell, APRN, CWOCN, FAAN.)

the patient's anatomy. The type of stoma needs to be assessed, as the structure of the stoma will impact the choice of pouching system.

An *end stoma* is created by dividing the intestine, bringing the proximal end of the intestine through the abdominal wall, maturing the stoma once outside of the abdominal wall to attach to the skin (see Chapter 9) **Figure 11-2**. Any portion of the GI tract can be used to create an end stoma. The distal end of the intestine can be removed or closed off. Surgical interventions that create an end stoma include the abdominal perineal resection (see Chapter 6), proctocolectomy (see Chapter 6), or a bowel resection and the creation of a Hartmann's pouch. A Hartmann's pouch is the resection of the colon or intestine, the creation of a stoma and the oversewing of the remaining colon, and creating a Hartmann's pouch aslo referred to as the Hartmann's procedure (**Fig. 11-3**).

KEY POINT

The patient with a Hartmann's pouch may pass old stool from the rectum if the bowel was not cleansed prior to the operation. Advise patients that they may feel pressure at the rectum and they should sit on the commode to pass any old stool; the feeling that the rectum needs to be emptied may occur every few days and mucous maybe passed.

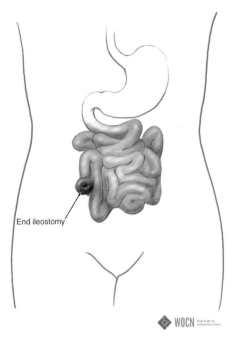

FIGURE 11-2. End Stoma.

A *loop stoma* is created in the small or large intestine by mobilizing the side of the intestine up through the abdominal wall, making a transverse incision on the intestine, and maturing the mucosa (see Chapter 9). A support bridge or rod may be placed under and in many cases around the stoma, and the intestine is attached to the abdominal wall. There are two support bridges that are typically used by surgeons, a soft silicone support bridge or a firm rigid plastic support bridge (McTigue

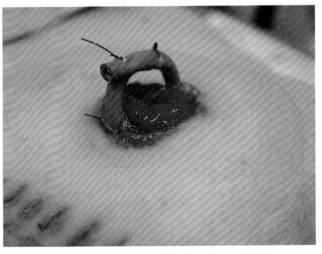

FIGURE 11-4. Loop Ileostomy with Rubber Support Bridge. (Courtesy of Janice Colwell, APRN, CWOCN, FAAN.)

et al., 2019). If a support bridge is used it should be the soft silicone-based support bridge (**Fig. 11-4**) as the conventional rigid plastic rods (**Fig. 11-5**) can cause intestinal necrosis, increased pain, peristomal skin complications, and difficulty obtaining a consistent seal of the ostomy appliance (Langenbach et al., 2011; McTigue et al., 2019). There is little evidence to support using a support bridge when creating a loop stoma, but many surgeons choose to place one to attempt to decrease the retraction of the stoma (Hendren et al., 2015; Speirs et al., 2006). Surgical indications for creation of a loop stoma include protection of a distal anastomosis, diversion of an obstruction below the stoma, and diversion of an anastomotic leak. Most loop stomas are created as a temporary stoma but can become permanent depending upon the patient's condition.

Support bridges are left in place until the stoma heals to the abdominal skin, and the time frame can

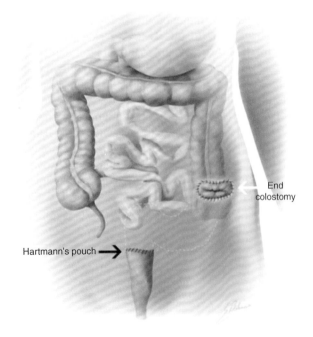

FIGURE 11-3. Hartmann's Procedure.

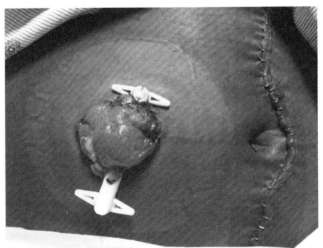

FIGURE 11-5. Loop Colostomy with Plastic Stoma Bridge. (Courtesy of Paulina Petrishka, MSN, APN, CNP.)

vary depending upon the surgical technique, the reason for creation, and the amount of tension of the support bridge on the skin and the ability of the patient to heal. The support bridge should be removed when there is little tension of the stoma on the abdominal wall and when the stoma has healed to the abdominal wall. The time frame for use of the support bridge can be as little as 1 day and as long as a month (McTigue et al., 2019). The decision for removal should be a joint decision between the surgeon and the WOC nurse. After explaining the procedure to the patient, the support bridge is removed by clipping the sutures that were placed during surgery and the suture location will vary by surgeon. After the sutures are removed, the bridge is slipped out from under/around the stoma. If there are openings in the skin where the bridge or sutures were located, skin barrier powder can fill the defect until healing takes place.

In infrequent cases, when the intestine is resected, both ends of the intestine are brought to the skin, the proximal or functioning stoma as well as the distal or nonfunctioning stoma. The distal end is considered a *mucous fistula* (**Fig. 11-6**) as there will be no active stool from this opening, yet mucus on occasion may be present. One indication for this type of diversion may be a distal obstruction, and the mucous fistula can allow any drainage to be expelled since nothing can get beyond the obstruction. Care of the mucous fistula depends on the type and amount of drainage. If the colon was not cleaned out prior to the surgical intervention, old stool may drain for a short time period and the use of a pouch would be indicated. Once the segment is no longer passing stool, a dry dressing can be placed over the stoma to protect the patient's clothes from mucus.

An *end loop ileostomy*, sometimes referred to as a Turnbull end loop (see Chapter 9, Figs. 9-8 and 9-9), is an option when the thickness of the abdominal wall does not allow for an easy passage of an end ileostomy such as in the obese patient. The end section of the small bowel is closed, and a loop of the segment is then used to make the stoma. A support bridge can be placed under the stoma until healing takes place.

A urostomy can be constructed from the small or large intestine (see Chapter 8). The term urostomy defines that there is an opening that drains urine; the type of stoma will be an ileal or colon conduit, or an ureterostomy. An ileal or colon conduit uses the ileum or colon to make a passage for the urine to exit the body (Fig. 8.2). An ureterostomy uses the ureters, either each brought to the skin in two separate stomas or one ureter anastomosed to the other and a single ureter brought out as a stoma (Fig. 8.3). The ureterostomy is rarely created but if used is generally performed as a temporary diversion (Rhee et al., 2012). A vesicostomy is an uncommon form of urinary diversion characterized by a small opening in the anterior bladder wall that is brought to the skin for bladder drainage.

The *end loop urinary stoma (also called a Turnbull loop urostomy)* can be used to create a urostomy in an obese patient with short mesentery as described above for a fecal diversion.

STOMA ASSESSMENT

The following variables are included when assessing a stoma:

- *Stoma mucosa*: color, presence of edema, and texture
- *Stoma structure*: size, shape, protrusion, location of the lumen, and mucocutaneous junction
- *Peristomal skin*: integrity and abdominal contours: creases and folds

Stoma Mucosa

A newly created stoma will be red, moist, and edematous, and the mucosa will be shiny and taut with fluid (**Fig. 11-7A**). As the stoma heals, there will be a texture to the stoma and creases and folds will be visible (**Fig. 11-7b**). Most stomas are a deep red with the exception of an ureterostomy that generally is a pale pink. If the stoma is a dark red to purple or there is dark nonvascular tissue present, this can indicate a blood flow problem and the surgical team should be consulted, see Chapter 17 for stoma necrosis.

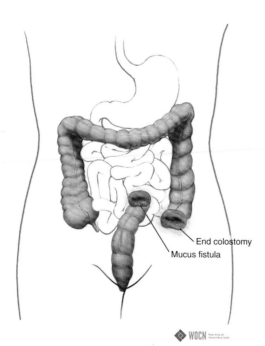

End colostomy
Mucus fistula

WOCN

FIGURE 11-6. Mucous Fistula.

> **KEY POINT**
>
> Advise the patient with a new fecal diversion that because of the postoperative edema the patient may hear noise as stool and gas pass from the stoma.

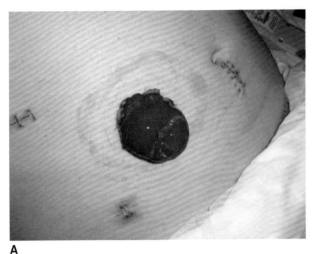

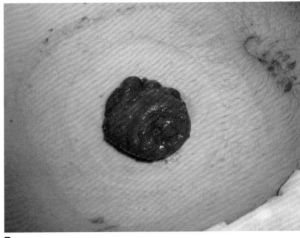

A

B

FIGURE 11-7. Edematous Stoma. **A.** Postoperative edema. **B.** Two-week postoperative resolving edema. (Courtesy of Janice Colwell, APRN, CWOCN, FAAN.)

Stoma Structure

The stoma should be assessed and reevaluated periodically during the postoperative period for the size and shape as well as protrusion, because stoma edema will reduce slowly for the first 6 to 8 weeks after creation. The size and shape will help to determine the size of the opening in the skin barrier of the pouching system (see Chapter 12). Preferably, all stomas should protrude at least 2 cm above the skin to allow the stool or urine to drain into the pouching system (WOCN®, 2017). When there is inadequate stoma protrusion or if the stoma is flush to the skin or retracted, there may be effluent leakage under the seal and a specific pouching system should be considered (see Chapter 12). Ideally, the *stoma lumen* (**Fig. 11-8**) would be at the top apex of the stoma to allow the urine or stool to exit the stoma and drain directly into the pouching system; determine the location of lumen or os by looking at the stoma in a sitting and lying position as the lumen may change as the

body contours change. A lumen that is even with the skin will need special consideration in choosing the pouching system (see Chapter 12). Evaluate the *mucocutaneous junction* (skin–stoma junction) for presence and type of sutures as well as note any gaps between the stoma and skin (called a mucocutaneous separation see Chapter 17) that can indicate delayed or poor healing.

Peristomal Skin

The peristomal skin should be evaluated for any alterations in the skin integrity. Ideally, the skin should be intact, free from any injury. When a pouching system is first removed, the peristomal skin may be pink, but this should resolve quickly. Examine the skin in good lighting to determine if there is a partial or full skin loss, papules or pustules, or other alterations in the skin integrity. Skin loss can indicate a poor pouching system seal, prolonged wear time, inappropriate use of product, or sensitivity to a product (see Chapter 16). The abdominal contours are examined with the patient standing, bending, lying flat, and sitting. The area around the stoma can change in each position, and knowing the presence of creases or folds in each of these positions can help determine the correct skin barrier shape or the use of accessories (see Chapter 12). The stoma should be assessed as the patient changes positions, as the stoma shape or size that can also change as the abdominal contours change.

🔘 POSTOPERATIVE PLANNING

The patient (or a family member or significant other) will need to acquire the skill of emptying the ostomy pouch prior to discharge, and the teaching of this skill should start within 24 hours after surgery. This skill should be return demonstrated by the patient or family member or significant other (Prinz et al., 2015). The teaching session should be planned immediately after surgery, working with the patient to determine if he or she would like or

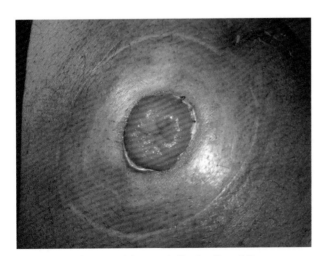

FIGURE 11-8. Stoma with Lumen in Center, Top of Stoma. (Courtesy of Janice Colwell, APRN, CWOCN, FAAN.)

needs a second person involved in the stoma care education (see Chapter 13).

 CONCLUSIONS

Postoperative management of the patient undergoing a fecal and/or urinary diversion will include a thorough assessment of the patient's overall status as well as a special focus on the stoma, the peristomal skin, and the stoma functioning. Once all of the assessments are complete, the data can be reviewed and a plan of care developed. The goal is to plan care that will include the choice of the best pouching system and the instruction of the patient and his or her designee in self-care and a successful rehabilitation of the person with a stoma.

REFERENCES

Baker, M. L., Williams, R. N., & Nightingale, J. M. (2011). Causes and management of a high output stoma. *Colorectal Disease, 13*(2), 191–197.

Carmichael, J. C., Keller, D. S., Baldini, G., et al. (2017). Clinical practice guidelines for enhanced recovery after colon and rectal surgery from the American Society of Colon and Rectal Surgeons and Society of American Gastrointestinal and Endoscopic Surgeons. *Diseases of the Colon & Rectum, 60*, 761–784.

Hendren, S., Hammond, K., Glasgow, S. C., et al. (2015). Clinical practice guidelines for ostomy surgery. *Diseases of the Colon & Rectum, 58*(4), 375–387. https://doi.org/10.1097/DCR.0000000000000347

Langenbach, M. R., Sauerland, S., Issa, E., et al. (2011). Loop ileostomy and colostomy: A comparison between supporting plastic rods and epicutaneous or subcutaneous silicon drains. *Surgical Science, 2*(5), 252–256. https://doi.org/10.4236/ss.2011.25056

McTigue, T., Lei, J., Kowalski, M. O., et al. (2019). Stoma bridge types and their impact on patient outcomes: A retrospective analysis and prospective global survey of surgical practice. *Journal of Wound, Ostomy, and Continence Nursing, 46*(4), 309–313. https://doi.org/10.1097/WON.0000000000000543

Orkin, B. A., & Cataldo, P. A. (2007). Intestinal stomas. In B. G. Wolf, J. W. Fleshman, D. E. Beck, et al. (Eds.), *The ASCRS textbook of colon and rectal surgery* (pp. 622–630). New York, NY: Springer.

Prinz, A., Colwell, J. C., Cross, H. H., et al. (2015). Discharge planning for a patient with a new ostomy: Best practice for clinicians. *Journal of Wound, Ostomy, and Continence Nursing, 42*(1), 79–82. https://doi.org/10.1097/WON.0000000000000094

Rhee, C. H., Yerkes, E. B., & Rink, R. C. (2012). Incontinent and continent urinary diversions. In A. G. Coran, A. Caldamone, N. Scott Adzick, et al. (Eds.), *Pediatric surgery* (7th ed., pp. 1487–1496). St. Louis, MO: Elsevier, Mosby.

Sonia, C. (2013). Care of surgical patients. In P. A. Potter, A. G. Perry, P. A. Stockert, et al. (Eds.), *Fundamentals of nursing* (8th ed., pp. 1254–1295). St. Louis, MO: Elsevier, Mosby.

Speirs, M., Leung, E., Hughes, D., et al. (2006). Ileostomy rod—Is it a bridge too far? *Colorectal Disease, 8*(6), 484–487. https://doi.org/10.1111/j.1463-1318.2005.00923.x

Wound, Ostomy and Continence Nurses Society™. (2017). *Clinical guideline: Management of the adult patient with a fecal or urinary ostomy*. Mt. Laurel, NJ: Author.

QUESTIONS

1. A nurse is performing an assessment of a postoperative patient following the creation of a urinary diversion. Which assessment technique has the nurse performed correctly?
   A. Wearing gloves, the nurse gently palpates either side of an approximated and closed incision.
   B. The nurse empties the drainage tube container when it is completely full and records the drainage on the I&O record.
   C. The nurse uses deep palpation to assess the firmness and tenderness of the patient's abdomen
   D. The nurse checks that the patient has been ambulating at least once in 24 hours and spends time out of bed to increase endurance.

2. The WOC nurse is assessing the stoma of a patient with a new fecal diversion. Which assessment data indicate a finding of edema?
   A. The stoma is a deep purple color.
   B. The stoma is taut and firm to the touch.
   C. The lumen location is off center.
   D. The skin at the junction of the stoma is not intact.

3. The WOC nurse is assessing the stoma of a patient with a new urinary diversion. Which data represent a normal postoperative finding?
   A. The stoma is retracted.
   B. Mucus is present in the urine.
   C. There is partial skin loss.
   D. The stoma is a dark purple color.

4. The WOC nurse is reviewing the operative report of a patient with a new fecal diversion. Which type of stoma function would the nurse expect to find based on this report?
   A. The fecal stoma will generally start to function within 1 to 3 days after surgery.
   B. When a patient undergoes a laparoscopic surgical procedure the fecal stoma will generally function later than when the patient undergoes a laparotomy.
   C. Initial fecal stoma output resembles pudding or oatmeal consistency.
   D. A low-output fecal stoma, usually a jejunostomy or ileostomy, can cause dehydration.

5. Based on the location of the fecal stoma in the GI tract, the nurse would expect which finding regarding the stoma output in a patient with an established fecal diversion?
   A. The output from an ileostomy will vary but is generally about 500 mL in 24 hours.
   B. A jejunostomy will have liquid stoma output, and the volume can be as high as 3,400 mL in 24 hours.
   C. Colostomy volume will vary from 300 to 500 mL in 24 hours depending on the anatomic location.
   D. With a colostomy that is close to the rectum, the output will be pasty to almost formed because the stool has had time to sit in the colon.

6. The nurse is planning care for a patient who has ileostomy output that far exceeds what is considered to be the normal amount. What intervention is expected in this situation?
   A. The use of hypo- and hypertonic fluids
   B. Dietary inclusions of high sugar foods and fluids
   C. The use of isotonic fluids
   D. The restriction of starch-based food

7. The WOC nurse is assessing a patient with a new urostomy. Which normal finding would the nurse expect?
   A. Minimal output should be 800 mL/24 hours.
   B. The urine will be clear with mucus.

C. Two stents at the outer side of the stoma attached to the skin.
D. The location of the stoma determines the type of stoma created.

8. Which type of stoma construction would be most commonly found in an obese patient with a short mesentery who requires the creation of an ileostomy?
   A. End stoma
   B. Loop stoma
   C. End loop ileostomy
   D. Mucous fistula

9. Which surgical intervention most commonly results in a loop stoma?
   A. Abdominal perineal resection
   B. Diversion of an obstruction below the stoma
   C. Proctocolectomy
   D. Creation of a Hartmann's pouch

10. Which teaching point would the WOC nurse consider a priority for a postoperative patient who has undergone a fecal and/or urinary diversion?
    A. Teaching the patient and/or significant other how to empty the ostomy pouch
    B. Making referrals for follow-up care and psychiatric counseling
    C. Determining if the patient needs a second person involved in stoma care
    D. Teaching the patient to reduce the number of meals consumed per day

ANSWERS AND RATIONALES

1. **A. Rationale:** Wearing gloves, gently palpate either side of the incision noting the firmness or lack of firmness of the tissue, the temperature of the skin, as well as any oozing that might be present while examining the area. Deep palpation is neither necessary nor warranted in this situation.

2. **B. Rationale:** An edematous stoma has a lack of normal folds, creases, and will have taut tissue that is firm to touch.

3. **B. Rationale:** It is important to remember that since the intestine is used to make a conduit, there will be at least initially a large amount of mucus expelled from the stoma. The intestinal

mucosa secretes mucus to lubricate the intestinal contents and continues to secrete mucus when diverted. For most people with a urostomy, the volume of mucus is high for the first few months and is reported to decrease over time.

4. **A. Rationale:** A fecal stoma will generally start to function 1 to 3 days after surgery, earlier when the patient undergoes a laparoscopic surgical procedure. Gas followed by liquid is the initial output of both a small and large bowel fecal stoma.

5. **D. Rationale:** The activity of the colostomy will depend upon the location of the stoma in the colon; closer to the rectum, the output will be

pasty to almost formed because the stool has had time to sit in the colon, more fluid is absorbed, and the stool is more formed.

6. **C. Rationale:** The plan of care may include the following: the use of isotonic fluids, restriction of hypo- and hypertonic fluids, dietary restrictions of high-sugar foods and fluids, dietary inclusions of starch-based foods, and/or the use of antisecretory and antimotility drugs.

7. **C. Rationale:** An ileal or colon conduit will have stents that are placed at the time of the ureter/conduit anastomosis, the purpose of which is to protect the anastomosis site and prevent urine from leaking into the abdominal cavity.

8. **C. Rationale:** An end-loop ileostomy is an option when the thickness of the abdominal wall and lack of mesentery (blood flow to the intestine) does not allow for an easy passage of an end ileostomy such as in the obese patient. The end section of the small bowel is closed, and a loop of the segment is then used to make the stoma.

9. **B. Rationale:** Surgical indications for creation of a loop stoma include protection of a distal anastomosis, diversion of an obstruction below the stoma, and diversion of an anastomotic leak.

10. **A. Rationale:** The patient (or a family member or significant other) will need to acquire the skill of emptying the ostomy pouch prior to discharge, and the teaching of this skill should start within 24 hours after surgery. This skill should be return demonstrated by the patient or family member or significant other. The teaching session should be planned immediately after surgery working with the patient to determine if he or she would like or needs a second person involved in the stoma care education.

CHAPTER 12

SELECTION OF POUCHING SYSTEM

Janice Colwell and Kathleen Hudson

OBJECTIVES

1. Describe factors to consider when selecting pouching systems.

2. Differentiate among product options when selecting pouching systems based on the patient assessment.

TOPIC OUTLINE

Introduction **172**

Skin Barriers **173**
Solid Skin Barrier   173
Wear Time   175
Solid Skin Barrier Shapes   175
Convex Product Characteristics   176

Assessment/Clinical Considerations
for Use of Convexity **176**
Use of Convexity: Other Considerations   177
Outer Diameter Skin Barrier Shape   178
Fit of the Solid Skin Barrier   178
Accessory Skin Barrier Products   180
Skin Barrier Paste   180
Skin Barrier Powder   180
Skin Barrier Ring   181
Skin Barrier Strip Paste   181
Elastic Skin Barrier Strip   181
Liquid Barriers   181

Ostomy Pouches **182**
One-Piece Pouching System   182

Two-Piece Pouching System   183
Pouch Features   183
Drainable Pouch for Fecal Stoma
Management   183
Drainable Pouch for Urinary Stoma
Management   184
Nondrainable Pouches   184
Pouch Length   184
Pouch Films   184
Gas Management   185

Pouching Accessory Products **185**
Belt   185
Adhesive Products   185
Pouch Covers   185
Pouch Liners   185
In-Pouch Deodorant Liquids   185
Oral Odor Eliminators   186
Absorbent Products   186

Conclusions **186**

INTRODUCTION

The principles that guide the selection of a pouching system are (1) consistent wear time: the ability to maintain the pouch seal for a predictable amount of time (no leakage between the application and removal of the pouching system); and (2) intact peristomal skin: when the pouching system is removed, the peristomal skin is undamaged (WOCN, 2017).

The pouching system is defined as the products used to collect the stoma effluent, which will provide a secure predictable seal and protect the peristomal skin (Wound Ostomy and Continence Nurses Society [WOCN]), (WOCN, 2017). Pouching systems vary among people with an ostomy, and the product choices will depend upon a thorough assessment of the patient, his or her stoma, peristomal skin, and his or her self-care abilities coupled with a good understanding of ostomy products. When the patient has a new stoma, he or she has many reservations and a leading fear is leakage and a negative impact on quality of life (Pittman et al., 2008). In a study by Richbourg et al. (2007) of patients with an ostomy that encountered leakage, 62% reported a reduction in enjoyable activities and depression or anxiety. Additional findings from this study included fear of leakage that kept 47% of the sampled ostomates from leaving their home one or more times per week. It is imperative that the most appropriate pouching is chosen for the person with an ostomy and education on how to utilize the pouching system is provided. Periodic review of the fit of the pouching system (Colwell et al., 2019), wear time, and utilization should be done, keeping in mind that as a person's abdomen changes (loss or gain of weight, abdominal surgery, changing contours due to aging), the stoma and the surrounding area can change and an alteration in the pouching system may need to be considered. The pouching system products include skin barriers, pouches, and accessory products.

SKIN BARRIERS

Skin barriers are available in several configurations—flat or convex, precut opening or cut to fit, moldable or stretch to fit, solid sheet integrated with the pouch (a one-piece pouching system), a solid sheet with a flange/coupling mechanism attached (a two-piece pouching system), paste, powder, ring, strip, and liquid. Skin barriers provide skin protection and the solid skin barriers also provide adhesion; each is unique in its use and purpose (**Table 12-1**).

SOLID SKIN BARRIER

The solid skin barrier is the interface between the skin and the pouch; it provides the seal (adhesion) and protects the peristomal skin (**Fig. 12-1**). Solid skin barriers contain many ingredients including hydrocolloids, carboxymethyl cellulose (CMC), adhesives, pectin, gelatin, and polymers. The purpose of the hydrocolloid is to absorb moisture and maintain the skin barrier seal. The CMC combines with moisture to form a strong gel, providing erosion resistance, and has a high absorption capacity to keep the skin dry. The adhesive provides the seal between the skin barrier and the peristomal skin. The pectin helps ensure that the skin's pH is maintained close to the skin's pH of around 5.5 to help decrease the risk of invading microorganisms. Hydrocolloids are water-loving compounds, meaning they draw moisture from the skin. If moisture (e.g., from perspiration-transepidermal water loss) is allowed to collect on the skin, the adhesive seal may be weaker or lost; thus, absorbing some moisture helps to maintain the seal.

Moisture from the stoma (stool or urine) is absorbed by the hydrocolloid, and if an excessive amount of moisture is absorbed, the hydrocolloid may erode (the hydrocolloid over saturates and loses structural integrity) and is less adhesive. The erosion depends upon several factors, the volume and moisture content of the stoma output, the skin moisture, the use of accessory products (see below), and the type of skin barrier. Thus, the person with a high-output ileostomy with loose watery stool will note that skin barrier erosion occurs faster than does a person with a pasty infrequent stool. The area of absorption/erosion will turn a whitish color making it easy to monitor how much moisture is absorbed (**Fig. 12-2**). By examining the back of the skin barrier upon removal, the nurse and patient can assess if the amount of absorption is excessive, indicating the need for decreased wear time or use of an accessory such as a barrier ring or strip.

There are two categories of skin barrier materials, regular wear and extended wear. The difference between these two types of skin barriers depends upon the product ingredients: the extended wear barrier has lower absorption and a higher level of adhesion, generally providing longer wear time (Colwell, 2004). Some skin barriers are infused with ceramide, aloe vera, and Manuka honey and are thought to benefit peristomal skin. Ceramide is a component of the stratum corneum of the epidermal layer and helps to prevent excessive water loss and provide support as a barrier against entry of microorganisms (Colwell et al., 2018). Aloe is a succulent plant best known for treating skin injuries. Manuka honey has been shown in laboratory studies to have antibacterial properties and may suppress inflammation and stimulate cell growth (Burlando & Cornara, 2013). There is limited information on the effect of the infused ingredients on the peristomal skin; one study noted a suggestion that ceramide-infused skin barriers reduce the effects of skin stripping (Nichols et al., 2019), and another noted a reduction in peristomal skin complications and a cost saving (Colwell et al., 2018). It is suggested that because aloe acts as a humectant, this may help to moderate skin hydration (Salts Web site accessed November 30, 2019). Findings in one study suggest the use of Manuka honey in a pouching system skin barrier had a positive effect on peristomal skin (Roveron, 2017).

Skin barriers are pressure sensitive, and the bond depends upon the barrier making full contact with the skin surface and is achieved by applying gentle pressure upon application. Applying pressure will ensure that the skin barrier adhesive flows onto the skin contours: skin barriers are pressure sensitive adhesives.

TABLE 12-1 SKIN BARRIERS

SKIN BARRIER TYPE	INDICATIONS FOR USE	CONSIDERATIONS	TIPS
Solid skin barrier	Protection of the peristomal skin from stoma effluent, integrated into most pouching systems.		Determine the size (stoma opening) and shape (flat or convex) to match the stoma and peristomal assessment. Apply gentle pressure to enhance the seal of the skin barrier/skin seal.
Paste	Prevent undermining of stoma effluent under pouch seal. Fill in uneven areas.	If the product contains alcohol, will cause stinging if applied to denuded skin. Can be difficult to squeeze tube for application. Do not use for a person with urostomy.	Can use as "caulk" around the edge of the skin barrier next to stoma to enhance the seal. Use a moist finger to adjust paste; touching paste with a dry finger will cause the paste to stick to the finger.
Powder	Absorbs moisture of denuded peristomal skin providing a surface to apply pouching system.	Too much powder left on the peristomal skin can cause pouch seal failure.	Sprinkle the denuded area liberally with powder; brush off excess before pouching system application. Consider sealing with a nonalcohol liquid skin barrier film.
Ring	To enhance the seal with a second layer of solid skin barrier. To provide "soft" convexity to a flat pouching system or enhance the convexity of a convex pouching system. Convex rings can be used to provide soft convexity and improve seal.	When placed around a slightly protruding stoma, can be too high a "rise" and may not allow stoma effluent to drain over the ring into the pouch; consider the use of a slim barrier ring in this instance. Can be used in place of paste on denuded skin, as there is no alcohol to cause stinging.	Stretch the inner diameter of the ring to the size of the stoma opening; place either around the stoma or on the back of the pouch seal. Use on an oval stoma when the pouching system that is used has a round opening; will cover the exposed skin.
Strip	Use around a stoma to enhance the seal as a second skin barrier. Small pieces can be used to fill in uneven areas of the peristomal skin.	Requires manual dexterity to work the strip into the sizes and shapes needed. Can be used in place of paste if there is irritated skin; will not cause further irritation.	Small pieces can be pulled off and rolled into the exact size of the area that needs to be filled or evened out.
Elastic barrier strips	Used to enhance the seal on the outer edge of the pouching system.	May not be needed if the pouching system seal remains intact for the wear time.	Can assist in people who have shifts in the peristomal skin such as the person with a peristomal hernia that causes the peristomal skin to move.
Liquid skin barrier film	Used to protect fragile peristomal skin from stripping. Used to seal skin barrier powder to enhance seal.	Select skin barriers will not adequately adhere when a liquid skin barrier is on the skin; check manufacturer's recommendation. Skin barriers with an alcohol base will cause stinging upon application to denuded skin.	Allow liquid skin barrier to dry before pouching system application. The use of a liquid barrier spray can facilitate application onto denuded skin by providing a dry surface.

KEY POINT

When teaching a patient to apply a solid skin barrier, suggest that he or she hold the hand over the skin barrier as this will apply even pressure of the skin barrier to the peristomal skin.

A unique solid skin barrier available in a ring, sheet, or paste is created from karaya, a vegetable gum produced from tree sap. Karaya has adhesive properties, is acidic in nature, and absorbs moisture rapidly. As karaya absorbs moisture, the adhesive bond is loosened. The use of a karaya skin barrier may be considered when the peristomal skin is damaged from an alkaline environment (such as in crystal buildup on the peristomal skin of a person with a urostomy) or when a patient reports a contact dermatitis from other synthetic skin barriers (karaya is a natural product). A karaya skin barrier seal does not generally last as long as a hydrocolloid seal.

Silicone skin barriers, another type of skin barrier, are manufactured in a ring or paste. They contain a cross-linking of polymers providing a moisture-resistant matrix and do not erode. Moisture from perspiration and transepidermal water loss can travel through the silicone matrix managing

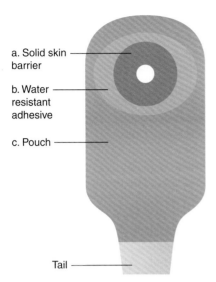

a. Solid skin barrier

b. Water resistant adhesive

c. Pouch

Tail

FIGURE 12-1. Pouching System.

perspiration. Silicone seals have elastic and adhesive properties to form a seal–skin bond and because they do not erode will not leave adhesive residue on the peristomal skin.

WEAR TIME

When considering how a solid skin barrier erodes over time, the challenge becomes how to decide when is the appropriate time to replace the skin barrier (**Box 12-1**). Changing too soon may lead to medical adhesive–related skin injury (McNichol et al., 2013) stripping the skin because the adhesive seal was still intact. Changing too late could mean that the stoma effluent can make contact with the skin because the hydrocolloid eroded or the adhesive seal completely failed and there was leakage under and beyond the pouch adhesive. Average wear time has been reported to be 4 days; however, wear time due to skin barrier erosion is variable and should be determined on a case-by-case basis (Richbourg et al., 2008).

The underside of the skin barrier (the adhesive surface toward the skin) should be examined after removal following several days of wear. The evaluation of the skin barrier integrity starts at the opening that was fitted to the stoma skin junction. The skin barrier material will appear saturated and swollen (**Fig. 12-2**). If the skin barrier opening is larger than it was on application, this indicates the ability of the stoma output to make contact with the skin and cause skin injury. If the skin barrier material shows discoloration or undermining of the stoma output, this indicates a break in the seal, with possible skin injury and loss of the entire seal. These observations require a decision to be made to decrease wear time, consider a different type of skin barrier, or use an accessory product.

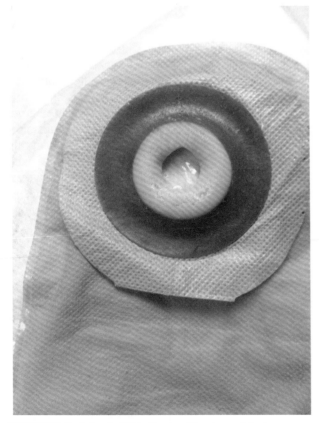

FIGURE 12-2. Saturated Skin Barrier. (Courtesy of Janice Colwell, APRN, CWOCN, FAAN.)

KEY POINT

Assessment of the underside of the seal should be done at each pouch change by both the clinician and the patient.

SOLID SKIN BARRIER SHAPES

Solid skin barriers are available in several shapes. One distinction is a flat or convex skin barrier; this refers to the shape of the underside of the skin barrier (the adhesive surface toward the skin). A flat skin barrier (**Fig. 12-3B**) has a level or even adhesive surface.

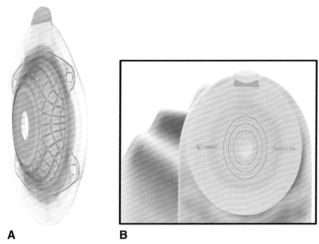

A   **B**

FIGURE 12-3. Convex (**A**) and Flat (**B**) Skin Barrier.

A convex skin barrier's adhesive surface is curved or rounded, and the amount of curvature varies between products. (Hoeflok et al., 2012). A convex skin barrier (**Fig. 12-3A**) can have a minimal amount of curvature (light, flexible or soft convexity) to a maximum amount of curve (deep convexity). Convex skin barrier options can also include convexity located next to the skin barrier opening as well as some that extend outward onto more of the skin barrier. Another distinction is flexible or soft versus firm convexity. A flexible or soft convex skin barrier can bend and move with the body; a firm convex skin barrier does not bend; rather it remains rigid helping to keep creases or folds flat. The challenge is deciding which type of convexity will meet the patient's needs. There are several considerations when deciding when to use a flat or convex skin barrier. The peristomal skin should be examined when the person is lying, standing, and sitting; the sitting position is recommended because it allows optimal assessment of abdominal contours and the position of the stoma within the abdomen (Hoeflok et al., 2017). The area is examined for the presence of creases and/or folds. If the area around the stoma is flat in all positions, a flat barrier should be successful in maintaining the skin barrier seal (WOCN, 2017). Assess the stoma and examine the amount of protrusion and the location of the stoma opening or os. If there is inadequate protrusion or the os is at or below the peristomal skin, a convex skin barrier may help the stoma to protrude above the skin barrier enhancing the skin barrier seal. Because convex skin barriers have several considerations for use the following section describes the characteristics, assessment and clinical considerations for use of convexity in managing the patient with an ostomy.

CONVEX PRODUCT CHARACTERISTICS

There is no industry standard for defining convex skin barrier features. Multiple convex pouching systems are available with various characteristics, many described as firm and soft convexity (Hoeflok et al., 2017), while others describe convexity depth as shallow, medium and deep (Young, 1992). Firm convex products are thought to support and stabilize the abdominal contours via rigidity and soft convex products are known for their flexibility and patient comfort (Hoeflok et al., 2017). Rolstad and Boarini (1996) define convexity by measuring product depth, suggesting that shallow is <1/16th of an inch, medium is >1/16th inch but <1/4 inch and deep is >1/4th. Another characteristic of the convexity is the location on the skin barrier, measuring the width of the plateau or where the curvature occurs (Colwell, 2019). This feature is significant because the effect of convexity can be enhanced if placed close to the base of the stoma (Hoeflok et al., 2017) that retracts or the os is at or below skin level. There has been some discussion in the literature about the amount of tension that a convex system can apply to the peristomal skin (flattening creases), altering the stoma protrusion (for a stoma with less than ideal protrusion) but this nomenclature has not been used by product manufactures (Hoeflok et al., 2012). It is important to understand the convex features of the product line you are using for your ostomy patient population.

ASSESSMENT/CLINICAL CONSIDERATIONS FOR USE OF CONVEXITY

The determination of matching stoma and peristomal characteristics to the type of convexity is a clinical decision. If when examining the patient sitting without a pouching system in place, creases and folds are noted, these can compromise the seal and a convex barrier can help to flatten the creases. Note if the peristomal skin is flaccid. The convex shape can help to keep the peristomal skin flat/even or stabilize flaccid peristomal skin to enhance the seal. The degree of convexity depth (depending upon the product characteristics) is matched to the depth of the creases and the amount of pressure/tension that may be needed to keep the peristomal skin flat and provide an adequate skin barrier seal.

In some cases, a flexible convex skin barrier is considered when there are deep creases on a soft abdomen and the rigid convexity appears to pop off the creased area. A second consideration for the use of convexity would be a stoma that does not protrude above the skin barrier causing a seal problem, that is, the stoma effluent discharges under the skin barrier (WOCN, 2017). A convex adhesive barrier can apply pressure directly around the stoma to help with stoma protrusion (WOCN, 2017). It is advisable that the location of the convexity be close to the base of the stoma to help with the stoma protrusion. The amount of convexity depth will depend upon the protrusion or lack of protrusion of the stoma. A third consideration for the use of convexity may be when the lumen of the stoma is near or flush to the skin or in some cases under the skin. In some cases, the stoma has adequate protrusion but the lumen is off to the side close to the skin, and the stoma output drains under the skin barrier (**Fig. 12-4**). The convex skin barrier can help the stoma lumen protrude up over the skin barrier edge. Other assessment considerations for the use of convexity include type of output from the stoma (Hoeflok et al., 2017) (a liquid output can undermine a seal), loop stomas (frequently the proximal stoma does not have adequate protrusion above the skin), unacceptable wear times, and telescoping stoma (the pulling inward of the stoma when functioning) (WOCN, 2017).

In 2017 (Hoeflok et al., 2017) an international consensus was convened of ostomy nurse specialists to provide guidance for consideration of convex pouching system usage. **Table 12-2** provides a listing of the 26 statements that provide guidance for use of convex pouching systems.

USE OF CONVEXITY: OTHER CONSIDERATIONS

Convexity can be considered for use in the postoperative period if a consistent pouching system seal is not obtainable. Historically there has been some concern about causing a mucocutaneous separation from the pressure of the convexity; however, if a seal cannot be obtained, the outcome of a mucocutaneous separation can be managed with topical care (see Chapter 16) but a poor seal will adversely affect the peristomal skin integrity and the adaptation of living with a stoma (Colwell et al., 2017). The above noted consensus agreed that in the immediate

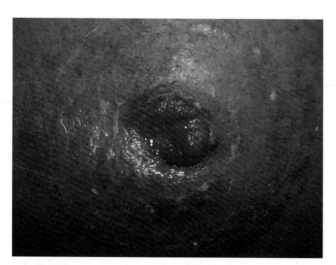

FIGURE 12-4. Stoma with Lumen off to Side, Discharging Stoma Effluent onto Skin. (Courtesy of Janice Colwell, APRN, CWOCN, FAAN.)

TABLE 12-2 CONSENSUS STATEMENTS
Product characteristics
Some convex products are firm.
Some convex products are soft.
A belt can be used to enhance the effect of convexity.
The effect of convexity can be enhanced if placed close to the base of the stoma.
Patient assessment
To best assess the need for convexity, the pouching system must be removed.
The best position for assessment for convexity is the sitting position.
Assessment for convexity includes type of output (such as formed, semiformed, and loose or liquid).
Assessment for convexity includes the location of the stoma opening, stoma height, whether the stoma telescopes, and location of distal lumen in the loop or double-barrel stoma.
Assessment for convexity includes abdominal tone, contour of peristomal region, and the presence of peristomal skin disorders.
An ostomy patient using convexity must be reassessed based on individual needs.
An ostomy patient using convexity must be reassessed based on clinician judgment.
Assessment of harmful effects of convexity (such as ulceration, pain) is needed with each pouching system change.
Indications
Convexity can be used with colostomy, ileostomy, and urostomy.
Liquid output can be an indicator for convexity to prevent or manage leakage.
Stoma opening at the level of the skin can be an indicator for convexity.
A protruding stoma can require convexity.
With a firm peristomal region, soft convexity can be a better option than firm convexity.
With a soft peristomal region, firm convexity can be a better option than soft convexity.
People with peristomal skin disorders can require convexity.
In the immediate postoperative period, convexity can be considered.
The stoma care nurse is best prepared to advise patients and health care providers on the appropriate use of convexity.
Loop stomas with the distal opening at skin level can be an indicator for convexity.
Stoma opening that is off center can be an indicator for convexity.
A stoma opening below the level of the skin can be an indicator for convexity.
Convexity can be used to manage enterocutaneous fistulae.

postoperative period, convexity can be considered (Hoeflok et al., 2017).

There are convex barrier rings that can be used to provide the primary source of convexity or to enhance the convexity of existing convex skin barriers. A belt may be used to enhance the effect of convexity (Hoeflok et al., 2017) to stabilize or enhance the pressure of the convexity to the adhesive seal.

Contraindications to the use of convexity may include the use for a person with a peristomal hernia, peristomal varices, and peristomal pyoderma (see Chapter 16).

OUTER DIAMETER SKIN BARRIER SHAPE

A second characteristic of a solid skin barrier's shape refers to the outer diameter, and the considerations are round, square, or oval. Round skin barriers are circular, a square skin barrier is rectangular, and oval is elliptical (**Fig. 12-5**). Considerations for use of a round, square, or oval skin barrier are the location of the stoma, if there are skin folds near the stoma that are horizontal (examine the patient sitting, standing, and lying). In some cases, an oval skin barrier can cover more area in the crease than a flat or round skin barrier. In other cases, a round skin barrier may be preferable when there are creases or folds at the edge of the skin barrier, as the use of round skin barrier can avoid creases where a square skin barrier may lie at the edge of the crease causing the outer seal to loosen.

FIT OF THE SOLID SKIN BARRIER

The opening in the solid skin barrier should be the size of the stoma (WOCN, 2017) (**Fig. 12-6**). If the stoma is oval, then the opening should be oval; if the stoma has an irregular shape the opening should be the same irregular shape, and if the stoma is round the opening should be round. The skin barrier should prevent stoma effluent from contacting the peristomal skin;

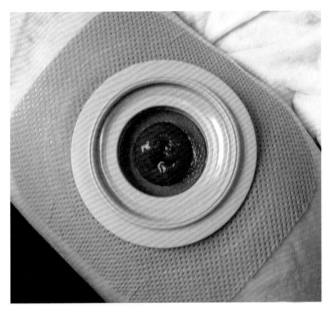

FIGURE 12-6. The Skin Barrier Fits to the Skin–Stoma Junction. (Courtesy of Janice Colwell, APRN, CWOCN, FAAN.)

thus, the opening should fit at the stoma–skin junction. The options to provide this seal include a cut to fit barrier, a precut round barrier, and a moldable/stretch-to-fit barrier. A cut-to-fit skin barrier has either no opening or a small opening that can be used to start to cut the skin barrier to fit. The opening can be cut to any shape or dimension. A precut skin barrier will have predetermined sizes. The moldable/stretch-to-fit skin barrier can be fitted to the stoma by rolling or stretching the barrier so it hugs the base of the stoma (Szewczyk et al., 2014).

Benefits of the cut-to-fit skin barrier include the ability to change the skin barrier opening as the stoma changes, such as in the immediate postoperative period; the ability to cut the stoma size to match the shape of the stoma, for instance an irregular stoma; and the ability to offset the stoma opening to avoid other structures (incisions, drains). A measuring guide with round shapes or a custom template (for an oval stoma) can be made of the stoma shape and used to cut out additional skin barriers (**Fig. 12-7**). An adjustment of the template should be made as the stoma shape changes. A precut opening in the skin barrier can be used for a round stoma, for a stoma in which the size/shape is not thought to change, or for a person who prefers not to cut or may not be able to cut the opening. However if the precut opening does not fit the stoma (in the case of an oval or irregular stoma shape), the peristomal skin may need protection, which can be provided with an accessory; see below. A measuring guide can be used to determine the size of the stoma, and the opening in the skin barrier can be obtained to that size. A newly created stoma should be measured at least every 2 weeks until the size stabilizes.

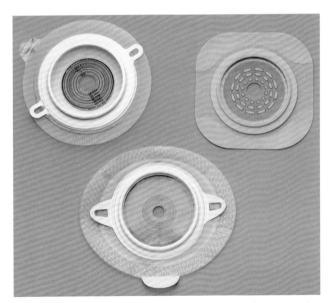

FIGURE 12-5. Skin Barrier Outer Shapes, Circular, Square, and Oval.

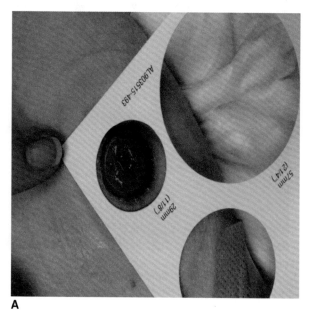

A   **B**

FIGURE 12-7. Use of Measuring Guide. **A.** Too large. **B.** Good fit.

A moldable/shape-to-fit barrier (**Fig. 12-8**) can be used to stretch the opening to the approximate size of the stoma. The moldable/shape-to-fit skin barrier may be of benefit to someone who does not want to or is unable to cut the skin barrier opening, or if it is anticipated that the stoma size will change over time.

If the stoma is oval or an irregular shape, consider the use of a small piece of clear plastic that can be held over the stoma to trace the shape; the shape can be cut out and traced onto the back of the skin barrier (**Fig. 12-9**) Save the backing (release paper) from the skin barrier to use for the next pouching system change (see Watch & Learn videos: 📷 "*How to cut out a one-piece pouching system*", 📷 "*How to measure a stoma to make the same*

size opening for the pouch" and 📷 "*How to make an oval stoma template for cut to fit pouch*").

Pouching a stoma with a support bridge can present a challenge because in some instances a support bridge can be sutured to the peristomal skin. Because the peristomal skin should be covered by the skin barrier on the pouching system, the opening in the skin barrier may be difficult to cut. A custom template can be used to go around the support bridge (plastic sheet held up over the stoma and the sutured support bridge; use a felt tip marker and trace the shape onto the plastic; cut out and use as a template). Keep in mind that you

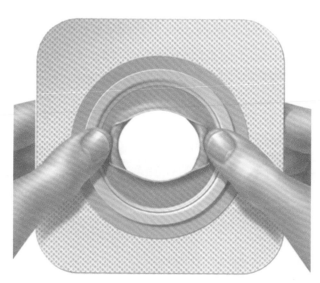

FIGURE 12-8. Moldable Skin Barrier. (Courtesy of and copyright ConvaTec Incorporated.)

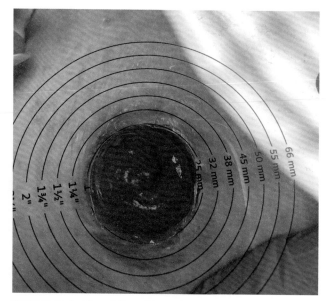

FIGURE 12-9. Use of Clear Plastic Sheet to Make Custom Template.

might have to use a large skin barrier, larger than you might normally use if just pouching the stoma in order to accommodate the support bridge, which can extend out from the stoma some distance. In some instances, a two-piece pouching system can be easier to use (the stoma and support bridge can be seen easier than when the pouch is in place). If making a template to go around the support bridge is difficult, using a thin or slim barrier ring around the stoma and bridge might be another option. If the bridge has several sutures at the end (such as an X rod), consult with the surgeon to see if one or two of the sutures could be removed for easier application of the pouch. Keep in mind that pouching over the support bridge may not be a good option as the skin barrier would not be flat and leakage might occur.

ACCESSORY SKIN BARRIER PRODUCTS

Skin Barrier Paste

Skin barrier paste is an adhesive hydrocolloid mixture available in a tube. It can be used to enhance the seal of the pouching system by caulking the edge of the skin barrier closest to the stoma to help to prevent undermining of the seal (**Fig. 12-10**) and/or to fill uneven areas around and near the stoma to facilitate the seal of the solid skin barrier (WOCN, 2017). Paste is available with and without alcohol, and alcohol-containing paste should be used with caution in the person with denuded peristomal skin because the alcohol can cause stinging upon application to injured peristomal skin. Paste is not recommended for use in management of the person with a urostomy as urine quickly erodes the paste, negating any benefit.

If after application the paste needs to be adjusted or smoothed, wet a gloved finger or a gauze pad and use to adjust. If paste is touched with a dry pad or gloved finger, it will stick to the dry surface, and you will not be able to easily make the necessary adjustment.

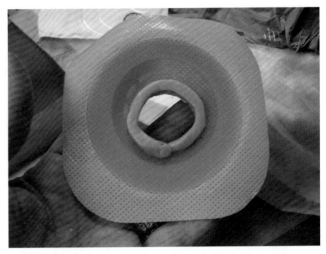

FIGURE 12-10. Skin Barrier Paste Placed at the Edge of Skin Barrier Opening to Caulk Seal. (Courtesy of Janice Colwell, APRN, CWOCN, FAAN.)

SKIN BARRIER POWDER

Skin barrier powder is a hydrocolloid that can be used to absorb moisture and can be utilized to treat denuded peristomal skin. The affected area is sprinkled with skin barrier powder, the powder gently rubbed or patted over the denuded skin, and the excess brushed off (**Fig. 12-11**). The powder will absorb some of the skin moisture helping to secure a seal. Karaya powder, another type of skin barrier powder, is an acidic gum/sap that can be sprinkled on denuded peristomal skin, which may assist in helping to secure the pouching system seal.

One way to treat denuded skin is to apply skin barrier powder to the denuded skin as described above and seal the powder using a liquid skin barrier film. There are two types of liquid skin barriers films, those with alcohol and those without (see below). The liquid skin barriers films with alcohol will cause a stinging sensation to denuded skin and the nonalcohol version is preferred. This method of treating the denuded skin is known as

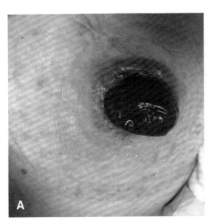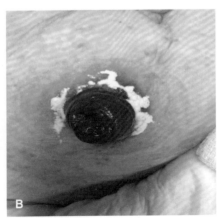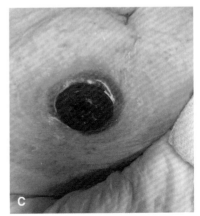

FIGURE 12-11. Denuded peristomal skin (**A**), skin barrier powder applied to denuded skin (**B**), excess brushed off (**C**).

crusting and creates a dry pouching surface to allow for good adhesion of the solid skin barrier (Colwell et al., 2017). In some instances several layers of powder and liquid skin barrier are applied.

SKIN BARRIER RING

A skin barrier ring is an adhesive hydrocolloid washer that can be used around the stoma to enhance the seal by providing additional solid skin barrier and/or to level out the area around the stoma (WOCN, 2017). There are several types of hydrocolloid rings: flat/thin (approximately 2.3 to 1.5 mm), flat/thick (approximately 4.2 to 4.5 mm), and convex (**Fig. 12-12**). A thin barrier ring might be considered when the stoma has minimal height as a thicker barrier ring might provide too high of a seal and prevent the stoma effluent from getting into the pouch. Barrier rings are available with various inner openings, and the inner diameter can be stretched to the stoma size and shape. A convex barrier ring that is presized round or oval can be used to provide convexity on a flat pouching system or to increase convexity on a convex pouching system. A barrier ring will be fitted around the stoma and can be applied directly to the skin before the skin barrier application or on the back of the skin barrier at the edge next to the stoma before application.

SKIN BARRIER STRIP PASTE

A skin barrier strip paste is a band of adhesive hydrocolloid that can be used to fit around a stoma to enhance the seal, or pieces can be used to fill in uneven areas such as wrinkles or dips in the peristomal area.

ELASTIC SKIN BARRIER STRIP

An elastic skin barrier strip is a piece of hydrocolloid with elastic that is used to secure the outer seal of the pouching system. Unlike other hydrocolloid products, it is not used directly around the stoma to secure a seal at the interface of the stoma and the pouching system; rather it is used around the outer edge of the barrier for extra security.

LIQUID BARRIERS

Liquid barriers have two categories: barrier films, a polymer delivered via a solvent, and skin protectants, cyanoacrylates. The purpose of the liquid barrier is to provide skin protection from stoma effluent or adhesive stripping,

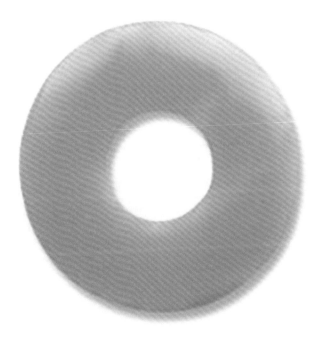

FIGURE 12-12. Skin Barrier Ring. (Courtesy of and copyright ConvaTec Incorporated.)

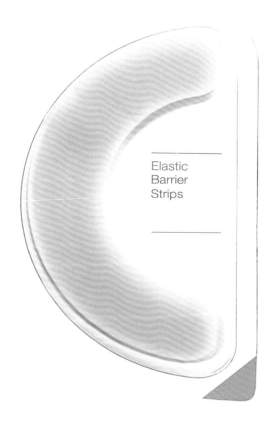

Elastic Barrier Strips

FIGURE 12-13. Elastic Skin Barrier Strip. (© Coloplast Corp. Reprinted With Permission-All Rights Reserved).

to provide a relatively dry skin surface or in some cases to seal skin barrier powder (WOCN, 2017). The barrier is wiped over the area that requires protection and allowed to dry. Some clinicians use the powder in a technique called crusting (see above). Some liquid barrier films may contain alcohol that could cause a stinging sensation when applied; a no-sting skin barrier film without alcohol is available and can be used on denuded peristomal skin. When applied, the liquid barrier should be dry before application of the pouching system. Liquid barriers are available as a pledget, a spray, a foam applicator on a stick, or an ampule. Check with the manufacturers of solid hydrocolloid skin barriers, as in some instances, the seal of the solid skin barriers can be decreased with the use of a liquid barrier.

OSTOMY POUCHES

The ostomy pouch collects and contains the stoma effluent. The pouch material is odor proof and will not allow odor to penetrate the pouch film. The type of pouch utilized will depend upon the stoma function as well as personal preference. The options for pouches include the following:

- One piece: skin barrier and pouch as one unit (**Fig. 12-1**)
- Two piece: skin barrier with flange/coupling and pouch as two separate parts (**Fig. 12-14**), either floating flange or attached flange (**Fig. 12-15A**) or snap/locking or adhesive coupling (**Fig. 12-15B**)
- Drainable, either fecal (**Fig. 12-16**) with integrated or add-on closures or urinary (**Fig. 12-17**) with taps, valves, and/or plugs for closures
- Nondrainable closed (**Fig. 12-18**)
- Various lengths and variable capacity (**Fig. 12-19**)
- Films: clear, ultra-clear, opaque (**Fig. 12-19**)
- Material on the back side (toward the patient's body) only, material on both sides of the pouch:
- Gas management, filters to allow gas to escape while deodorized

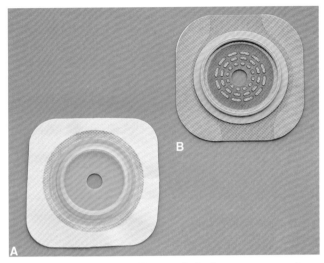

FIGURE 12-15. Two-Piece Flanges. **A.** Stationary snap coupling. **B.** Floating flange coupling.

ONE-PIECE POUCHING SYSTEM

A one-piece pouching system is constructed with the solid skin barrier and the pouch as one unit; the pouch is heat sealed onto the skin barrier (**Fig. 12-1**). One-piece pouching systems are available with the following skin barrier options: convex/flat, precut/cut to fit/moldable, extended/regular wear, outer diameter round, oval, or square. The pouches are available with the following options: drainable/nondrainable, various lengths, clear/opaque film, and material on the back and or front of the pouch, with or without a gas filter, and with the following closures: integrated, separate and a tap, valve or plug. Most one-piece pouching systems have a water-resistant material framing the solid skin barrier, providing protection of the solid skin barrier when showering or immersing the pouching system in water such as bathing or water sports. Considerations of using a one-piece pouching system are as follows: a flat peristomal pouch profile as compared to many of the two-piece pouching systems (WOCN, 2017), only a single seal (no risk of

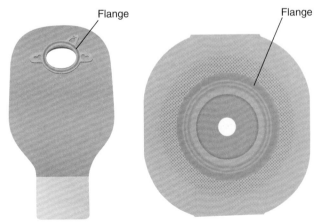

FIGURE 12-14. Two-Piece Pouching System, Flange, and Pouch.

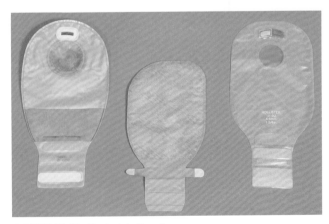

FIGURE 12-16. Drainable Pouches.

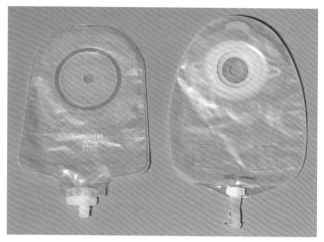

FIGURE 12-17. Urinary Pouches with Tap.

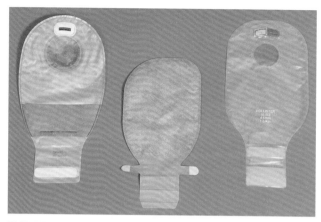

FIGURE 12-19. Various Pouch Lengths and Pouch Films.

detachment of skin barrier from the pouch), and if the stoma is located in a deep crease or skin fold (a one-piece system may be more flexible than a two-piece pouching system and provide a more consistent seal) (WOCN, 2017).

TWO-PIECE POUCHING SYSTEM

A two-piece pouching system consists of a solid skin barrier with a mechanism that accepts the pouch (**Fig. 12-14**). The solid skin barrier has the characteristics noted above: convex/flat, precut/cut to fit/moldable, extended/regular wear, and outer diameter round, oval, or square. The pouch connects to the skin barrier in one of three ways, with a plastic flange that either is fixed to the solid skin barrier (**Fig. 12-15A**) or a plastic flange that floats above the skin barrier (**Fig. 12-15B**) or with a resealable adhesive coupling. The plastic flange has a rim attached to the skin barrier and a channel or plastic ring on the pouch; the two snap together with pressure to make the connection (**Fig. 12-15A**). Other two-piece systems use a

connection in which the skin barrier flange can be pulled up from the skin barrier (a floating flange) (**Fig. 12-15B**) and the connection made by pinching the two pieces together. The adhesive coupling system has a flat thin piece of soft material on the skin barrier and the pouch has an adhesive seal; the seal is placed over the landing zone on the skin barrier to make the connection.

The solid skin barrier in a two-piece system is available both with and without a water-resistant frame on the outer edge of the skin barrier. All two-piece pouching systems have belt tabs on either the pouch or the skin barrier. Considerations in using a two-piece pouching system are ability to center the skin barrier around the stoma with no pouch in place providing easy visualization (WOCN, 2017), being able to change the pouch without removing the skin barrier, capability to use a pouch liner, profile of the plastic flange under clothing (some wearers do not like the potential visibility of flange), and security of the pouch and flange connection (see below).

> **KEY POINT**
>
> A two-piece pouching system allows the patients to change pouches without changing the skin barrier, for instance wearing a shorter pouch during the day when they can empty as needed and switching to a longer pouch at night while sleeping.

POUCH FEATURES

Drainable Pouch for Fecal Stoma Management

The end of the drainable pouch can be opened to allow stool to be drained: the end of the pouch has a tail that is sealed with a closure device. The pouch is drained when one-third to half full (WOCN, 2017). When the pouch tail is opened, the stool is drained and the end wiped clean and reclosed. The types of closures include the following:

- A rubber or plastic clamp: placed at the end of the pouch, the pouch is folded over the closure and the

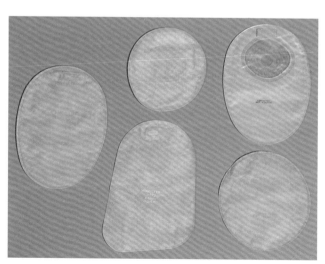

FIGURE 12-18. Nondrainable (Closed-End) Pouch.

clamp is snapped closed; a similar clamp uses a rubber band to make the closure. This was a common closure on pouches manufactured before 1980.

- Integrated closure/interlocking: the pouch tail is rolled up several times and the plastic interlocking fasteners are pinched closed.
- Velcro closure: the pouch tail is rolled up several times and the tabs of Velcro are smoothed together.
- Some or all of the above closures can be tucked away under the pouch to avoid any discomfort of the pouch closure against the skin.

The type of closure will depend upon the patient's preference as well as ability to easily open and close the system.

A drainable pouch can be considered for use by a person who has liquid stool that requires the pouch to be emptied more than twice per day (volume of more than 400 mL). The person with a drainable pouch can sit on the toilet far enough back that the water can be seen, the closure opened, and the pouch contents drained. The tail is wiped and the pouch closed (**Fig. 12-20**) (see Watch & Learn videos: ▦ *"Instructions on how to open a pouch and empty it"* and ▦ *"How to empty a different type of pouch"*).

Drainable Pouch for Urinary Stoma Management
Urostomy pouches have a tap that allows urine to be emptied (**Fig. 12-17**). The types of taps on the bottom of the pouches for a urinary pouch include a cap that is removed and the pouch drained and the cap replaced, and/or a valve that is twisted or a plug that is pulled out to allow emptying. All urinary systems are drainable, and a feature on a urostomy pouch not found in fecal pouches is an antireflux valve that prevents the urine from refluxing to the top of the pouch and eroding the skin barrier seal, and some urostomy pouches have chambers that distribute the urine throughout the pouch to prevent bulging. A urinary pouching system can be connected to dependent drainage at night with the use of an adapter that attaches the end of the pouch to the dependent drainage collector. Most dependent drainage collectors (or nighttime drainage systems) are closed systems and should be used for 14 days and discarded. If the type of drainage system used can be opened, it can be cleansed if necessary with a commercially made solution called a cleanser/decrystallizer or a solution made of one part white vinegar and three parts water for cleansing (United Ostomy Associations of America, Inc., 2017).

Nondrainable Pouches
Nondrainable pouches are closed and will require removal when the pouch is more than one-third to half full (WOCN, 2017) (**Fig. 12-18**). They are used in the management of fecal stomas with low output that is under 400 mL/24 hours, and for people who irrigate and need a pouch in between irrigation. The pouch is either removed from the skin when using a one-piece closed end system or removed from the skin barrier when using a two-piece system and the pouch is discarded; a new pouch is replaced. Many manufacturers of the two-piece systems provide opaque disposable bags to use in discarding the used pouch. The one-piece closed-end pouches have a gentle skin barrier that should not cause peristomal skin trauma when removed once or more in 24 hours.

Pouch Length
Drainable and urostomy pouches are available in several lengths from 9 to 16 inches (**Fig. 12-19**). Some manufacturers have a high-output pouch that can hold more volume than the standard drainable pouches. The end of most high output pouches has a tap on the end allowing the user to attach to dependent drainage as needed. Nondrainable pouch lengths can vary from 3 inches (used primarily by people who irrigate or for intimacy) to 12 inches.

Pouch Films
Pouch film is available as clear on both sides (body side and front), clear on the front, material on the body side, opaque on both sides, material and/or textile on both sides (**Fig. 12-19**), or material on both sides with a viewing "window," a slit in the material that will allow inspection of the stoma or output. The type of film used will depend on the location of use; for instance right after surgery, the ability to see the stoma and the stoma output is important and a clear pouch may be chosen (WOCN, 2017).

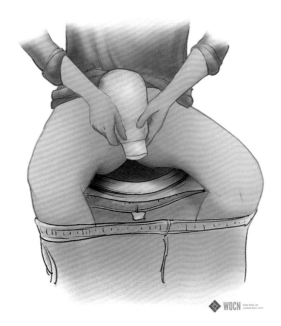

FIGURE 12-20. Pouch Emptying.

Some people who use a pouch with material or textile find that the material is slow to dry after water submersion (bathing or swimming). You can advise your patient to use a towel or a blow dryer on low to dry or if using a two-piece pouching system, to use a pouch just for showering and remove the pouch after showering allowing it to dry until the next shower.

Gas Management

Some pouches have an integrated gas filter that can allow gas to pass from the pouch through a gas deodorizing filter and exit the pouch. The filters are generally at the top of the pouch, containing a membrane both inside and outside of the pouch with the charcoal between. The challenge for a pouch filter is that the charcoal can become plugged when moist, which happens frequently with stool and humidity in the pouch. Thus, the life of most gas filters is 24 to 36 hours.

A gas vent is an external device that can be placed on the pouch and a hole is made through the pouch film under the vent. The vent has a plug that remains closed until the gas needs to be vented, the plug is opened, the nondeodorized gas is vented, and the vent is closed.

Be sure that your patients know when they use a gas vent the gas is not deodorized and they need to consider where and when they vent the gas.

Instruct your patient to empty gas that does not vent through the filter or plug to prevent ballooning of the pouch and possible adhesive failure. Ballooning is a term to describe when the pouch fills up with gas; the pouch is airtight, and when gas fills the pouch it can inflate the pouch usually called ballooning. Never poke a hole in the pouch to allow the gas to vent; this will cause odor to escape as well.

 ## POUCHING ACCESSORY PRODUCTS

BELT

Some pouching systems have belt tabs (one or two on each side) that allow the wearer to use a belt, fitting the belt into the belt tab(s) located on the either side of the pouch adhesive or flange, bringing the belt around the body, and attaching to the belt tab(s) on the each side (**Fig. 12-21**). The belt is worn snug to the body to apply pressure to the pouching system to enhance the seal. When using a convex pouch, the use of a pouching system belt can help to apply pressure to the convexity and add to the seal.

Belts come in several lengths, and most are adjustable. The belt should fit snug against the abdomen to apply pressure but not so firm as to damage the skin.

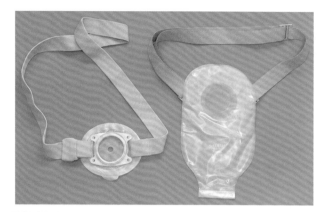

FIGURE 12-21. Pouching with Belt Tabs.

ADHESIVE PRODUCTS

There are several ostomy adhesive products that can be used to supplement the seal of the pouching system. They include adhesive sprays applied to the back of the pouching system seal, cement adhesives that are placed both on the pouch seal as well as on the skin, and adhesives that are painted on the pouching system seal. Some of the ostomy adhesive products contain latex and are flammable.

POUCH COVERS

Pouch covers can be used to cover or conceal the pouch. The covers can absorb moisture or perspiration between the pouch and skin, decrease rustle (noise of the plastic against the skin), and for some are used during intimacy to conceal the pouch.

POUCH LINERS

Pouch liners can be used to line the inside of a two-piece pouching system to collect the stoma output. When the pouch requires emptying (approximately one-third full), the pouch is detached from the skin barrier flange, and the liner is removed and deposited into a toilet (the liner is biodegradable). A new liner is inserted into the same pouch and reapplied to the flange.

IN-POUCH DEODORANT LIQUIDS

In-pouch deodorant liquids and tablets are available to use to decrease or eliminate odor. When a pouch is properly sealed there should be no odor; however, there will be odor when emptying stool, and an in-pouch odor eliminator can be placed in the pouch upon pouch application and after each emptying. The in-pouch deodorants are available as liquid, allowing drops to be placed into the pouch, or as a lubricating solution that can also be placed in the pouch. The lubricating deodorant is squirted into the pouch to lubricate the inside of the pouch to not only eliminate odor but also facilitate stool drainage. The liquid deodorant or odor eliminator will not harm the stoma, but may contain a dye that can change the color of the stool. The majority of the in-pouch deodorizers/eliminators are indicated for use with fecal stoma pouch management.

ORAL ODOR ELIMINATORS

Oral odor eliminators are over-the-counter pills that are taken to reduce or eliminate odor from stool. The dose is titrated until results are achieved; as many as four pills a day may be needed to be effective. The two main products contain the following ingredients, bismuth subgallate or chlorophyllin copper complex (known to cause a green discoloration of stool).

ABSORBENT PRODUCTS

Absorbent products contained in a packet, sachet, pill, or crystals can be placed into the fecal stoma pouch to turn the effluent into a gel-like substance. The liquid stool is converted into a gel and diverts a high-liquid fecal output away from the pouching system seal and can decrease the noise of the liquid stool in the pouch.

The choice of a pouching system is a decision that is made after a thorough assessment of the following characteristics: the location of the stoma on the abdomen, the amount of stoma protrusion, the location of the lumen of the stoma, the function of the stoma (volume and consistency of the effluent), the peristomal skin integrity, and the peristomal skin geography (flat, creased, soft, or firm tissue). Once pouching options are decided, the patient is educated about the rationale for the suggested pouching system, and an assessment of the patient's abilities to work with the recommended pouching system is done. In some cases, the system chosen may not work, because the patient does not have the ability to handle the products due to physical or cognition issues. A family member, a significant other, or an assistive worker may need to be educated on the use of the pouching system. Another deciding factor on the choice of a pouching system may be reimbursement. If the desired product is not reimbursed or has poor reimbursement, and the purchase of the items needed cause a hardship for the patient, an alternative product may be needed. It is advisable for the person with a stoma to become familiar with what coverage is available for reimbursement of his or her pouching systems. See Appendix J.

CONCLUSIONS

Consistent wear time, intact peristomal skin, and patient personal preference drive the decision of the type of pouching system a person with a stoma should use. Each of the attributes of a pouching system must be considered as an assessment of the patient's stoma, peristomal skin, abilities, and financial support is done (WOCN, 2017). Reevaluation should be done periodically as the person's body habitus changes such as following an illness and weight gain or loss.

REFERENCES

Burlando, B., & Cornara, L. (2013). Honey in dermatology and skin care: A review. *Journal of Cosmetic Dermatology, 12*(4), 306–313.

Colwell, J. C. (2004). Principles of ostomy management. In J. C. Colwell, M. T. Goldberg, & J. E. Carmel (Eds.), *Fecal and urinary diversions: Management principles* (pp. 240–262). St. Louis, MO: Mosby.

Colwell, J. C. (2019, September 26). Convexity: Where did it come from and where are we now. WOCN Continuing Education Center webinar.

Colwell, J. C., Bain, K. A., Steen Hansen, A., et al. (2019). International consensus results: Development of practice guidelines for assessment of peristomal body and stoma profiles, patient engagement and patient follow-up. *Journal of Wound, Ostomy, and Continence Nursing, 46*(6), 497–504.

Colwell, J. C., McNichol, L., & Boarini, J. (2017). North America wound, ostomy, and continence and enterostomal therapy nurses current ostomy care practice related to peristomal skin issues. *Journal of Wound, Ostomy, and Continence Nursing, 44*(3), 257–261.

Colwell, J. C., Pittman, J., Raizman, R., et al. (2018). A randomized controlled trial determining variance in ostomy skin condition and the economic impact (ADVOCATE trial). *Journal of Wound, Ostomy, and Continence Nursing, 45*(1), 37–42.

Hoeflok, J., Kittscha, J., & Purnell, P. (2012). Use of convexity in pouching a comprehensive review. *Journal of Wound, Ostomy, and Continence Nursing, 40*(5), 506–512.

Hoeflok, J., Salvadalena, G., Pridham, S., et al. (2017). Use of convexity in ostomy care results of an International Consensus Meeting. *Journal of Wound, Ostomy, and Continence Nursing, 44*(1), 55–62. Retrieved November 30, 2019 from https://www.salts.co.uk/en-gb/products/closed/harmony-duo-with-flexifit-and-Aloe-1

McNichol, L., Lund, C., Rosen, T., et al. (2013). Medical adhesives and patient safety: State of the science: Consensus statements for the assessment, prevention, and treatment of adhesive-related skin injuries. *Journal of Wound, Ostomy, and Continence Nursing, 40*(4), 365–380.

Nichols, T., Houser, T., & Grove, G. (2019). Comparing the skin stripping effects of three ostomy skin barriers infused with ceramide, honey or aloe. *The Journal of Stomal Therapy Australia, 39*(2), 14–18.

Pittman, J., Rawl, S. M., Schmidt, C. M., et al. (2008). Demographic and clinical factors related to ostomy complications and quality of life in veterans with an ostomy. *Journal of Wound, Ostomy, and Continence Nursing, 35*(5), 493–503.

Richbourg, L., Fellows, J., & Arroyave, W. (2008). Ostomy pouch wear time in the United States. *Journal of Wound, Ostomy, and Continence Nursing, 35*(5), 504–508.

Richbourg, L., Thorpe, J. M., & Rapp, C. G. (2007). Difficulties experienced by the ostomate after hospital discharge. *Journal of Wound, Ostomy, and Continence Nursing, 34*(1), 70–79.

Rolstad, B. S., & Boarini, J. (1996). Principles and techniques in the use of convexity. *Ostomy/Wound Management, 42*(1), 24–26, 28–32.

Roveron, G. (2017). An analysis of the condition of the peristomal skin and quality of life in ostomates before and after using ostomy pouches with Manuka honey. *World Council of Enterostomal Therapists Journal, 37*(4), 22–25.

Szewczyk, M. T., Majewska, G., Cabral, M. V., et al. (2014). The effects of using a moldable skin barrier on peristomal skin condition in persons with an ostomy: Results of a prospective, observational, multinational study. *Ostomy/Wound Management, 60*(12), 16–26.

United Ostomy Associations of America, Inc. (2017). *Urostomy fact sheet.* Retrieved November, 2019, from http://www.ostomy.org/ostomy_info/factsheets/facts_urostomy_en.shtml

Wound Ostomy and Continence Nurses Society. (2017). *Clinical guideline: Management of the adult patient with a fecal or urinary ostomy.* Mount Laurel, NJ: Author.

Young, M. J. (1992). Convexity in the management of problem stomas. *Ostomy/Wound Management, 38*(4), 53–60.

QUESTIONS

1. The WOC nurse is assessing the seal of a skin barrier for a patient with an ileostomy. The peristomal skin is intact but slightly reddened. The nurse notes that the skin barrier material is undermined with stool. What could this finding indicate?
   A. Excessive wear time that allowed skin exposure to the effluent
   B. Peristomal skin infection that caused erosion to the skin barrier
   C. The need to utilize a one-piece pouching system
   D. The use of an opaque pouching system to prevent undermining

2. The WOC nurse assessing the peristomal skin of a patient in a sitting position notes that there are creases and folds in the peristomal skin. What shape of skin barrier would the nurse recommend for this patient?
   A. Flat
   B. Convex
   C. Firm
   D. Cut to fit

3. What factor(s) determine the size and shape of the opening of a solid skin barrier?
   A. Size and shape of the stoma
   B. Amount of effluent from the stoma
   C. Patient desired wear time
   D. Condition of peristomal skin

4. For which patient would the use of skin barrier paste be contraindicated?
   A. A patient with an irregular-shape stoma
   B. A patient with a urostomy
   C. A patient with an ileostomy
   D. A patient with folds in the peristomal skin

5. A WOC nurse assesses the area around a patient's stoma and notes that it is not level on the lateral side next to the stoma. The following products are available; which product would be the best option for this patient?
   A. Skin barrier powder
   B. Skin barrier paste
   C. Liquid skin barrier
   D. Karaya powder

6. The WOC nurse is helping a patient with a new urinary diversion choose a pouching system. The stoma is located in an area that is hard for the patient to visualize, and a two-piece pouching system is recommended. What is an advantage of this type of system?
   A. It accommodates a flat peristomal profile.

B. There is no risk of detachment of skin barrier from the pouch.
   C. It allows for application of the skin barrier without the pouch obstructing the view.
   D. It is the best fit when a stoma is located in a deep crease or skin fold.

7. For which patient would a nondrainable pouch be the best option?
   A. A patient with a colostomy with formed to semiformed stool once a day
   B. Any patient with a urostomy and an excessive amount of mucus most of the day
   C. A patient who has liquid stool requiring pouch emptying at least two times per day
   D. A patient with an ileostomy who has at least 1,000 cc of output in a day

8. A WOC nurse is counseling a patient with a colostomy about gas management for his pouching device. What teaching point accurately describes gas control features?
   A. A gas vent allows deodorized gas to be vented through a plugged opening.
   B. Some pouches have a gas filter at the bottom of the pouch to control gas.
   C. Most pouches with gas filters are effective for 24 to 36 hours.
   D. All pouches allow gas to dissipate naturally within the pouch itself.

9. When assessing the fit of the skin barrier to the stoma, what guides the size of the skin barrier opening?
   A. The opening in the skin barrier should be 1/8" larger than the stoma.
   B. The opening should fit to the stoma–skin junction with no skin showing.
   C. The opening should have slits cut into to adjust to stoma size changes.
   D. The opening should be cut slightly smaller than the stoma.

10. The WOC nurse is teaching a patient with a fecal diversion about accessory products available for use. Which statement accurately describes one of these products?
   A. A once-a-day oral pill is available to reduce or eliminate odor from stool.
   B. Absorbent crystals can be placed in the pouch to turn effluent into a gel.
   C. Liquid pouch deodorant should be applied to the stoma.
   D. Pouch liners can be used to cover or conceal the pouch.

ANSWERS AND RATIONALES

1. A. Rationale: Excessive wear time allows the stool to erode the skin barrier, which can then allow the stool to injure the peristomal skin and cause pouch seal failure.

2. B. Rationale: A convex pouching system can help to flatten the peristomal skin in the area of the creases and folds and provide a consistent seal.

3. A. Rationale: The size/shape of the solid skin barrier of a pouching system provides protection to the peristomal skin and should fit to the skin–stoma junction.

4. B. Rationale: A patient with a urostomy should not use paste, as it does not maintain its shape or seal because urine can melt the paste soon after applied.

5. B. Rationale: Skin barrier paste could be used to fill in or level the uneven area before the pouching system application. The other products will not fill in an uneven area.

6. C. Rationale: Since it is hard for the patient to see the stoma, using a two-piece skin barrier will allow the patient to center the pouch over the stoma and then apply the pouch.

7. A. Rationale: The patient with a colostomy with semiformed stool once a day would benefit from the closed-end pouch. The patient can detach the pouch from the skin barrier and discard instead of trying to empty the semiformed to formed stool.

8. C. Rationale: Gas can be passed from the pouch filter but has a life that rarely extends longer than 36 hours, so to keep a vented pouch the patient should be instructed to change the pouch every 24 to 36 hours.

9. B. Rationale: The opening in the skin barrier should fit to the stoma–skin junction to allow all of the peristomal skin to be covered to prevent the stoma output from making contact with the skin.

10. B. Rationale: The liquid stool is converted into a gel and diverts a high-liquid fecal output away from the pouching system seal and can decrease the noise of the liquid stool in the pouch.

CHAPTER 13

POSTOPERATIVE EDUCATION FOR THE PATIENT WITH A FECAL OR URINARY DIVERSION

Jane Carmel and Margaret T. Goldberg

OBJECTIVE

Distinguish specific ostomy care needs when educating patients and caregivers.

TOPIC OUTLINE

- **Introduction** **189**
- **Patient Education** **190**
- **Assessing Readiness** **190**
- **Pouching Principles** **191**
  - How to Empty 191
  - When to Empty 192
  - Indications for Pouch Change 192
  - Preparing Equipment 192
  - Assessing Peristomal Skin 193
  - Measuring Stoma 193
  - Peristomal Skin Cleansing 193
  - Removal of Pouching System 193
  - Placement of Pouching System 193
  - Problem Identification, When to Seek Assistance 193
- **Living with a Stoma** **194**

Where and When to Obtain Supplies 194
Bathing 194
Clothing 194
Sexual Concerns 195
Dietary Concerns 195

- **Dietary Concerns** **196**
  - Ileal Conduit 196
  - Ileostomy 196
    - Colostomy 196
    - Odor 197
    - Pelvic Exenteration 197
  - Medications 197
  - Physical Activities 197
  - Follow-Up Care 197
  - Support Groups 198
- **Conclusions** **198**

INTRODUCTION

Body image changes and the physical alterations that come with ostomy surgery require major adjustments by the patient. Learning to adapt to these changes as well as acquiring necessary skills for stoma care can present a number of challenges. The ability to care for the stoma and its output are crucial steps toward the rehabilitation of the person with the new ostomy.

Patient education has become even more challenging in recent years due to changes in health care and the decreasing lengths of hospital stay, limiting the time available to present the necessary information. The enhanced recovery after surgery (ERAS) program was developed to improve patient's recovery, lower complication rates, and promote early discharge (Jones, 2017). Postoperative ERAS colorectal protocols include early ambulation, removal of urinary catheter, early oral nutrition, and discharge criteria (Pedziwiatr et al., 2018). ERAS program consists of preoperative education to provide information on what to expect during the hospital stay, review of the surgery, and discharge expectations.

Shortened hospital stays, however, impact the time provided for ostomy education. However, it is also thought that preoperative education has an effect on length of hospital stay (WCET, 2014). Comprehensive education delivered by a wound ostomy continence (WOC) nurse can result in a positive adjustment to the ostomy, not only immediately but also long term (Collado-Boira et al., 2018; Fingren et al., 2018; Merandy, 2016).

It remains the most important function of the WOC nurse to provide instructions for self-care and encouragement and support to the person having ostomy surgery.

PATIENT EDUCATION

Patients should leave the hospital with optimal ostomy survival skills. There is no specific research on required postoperative education for the person with an ostomy before being discharged home. The WOCN® Society (2017) and the American Society of Colon and Rectal Surgeons (ASCRS) (Hendren et al., 2015) developed clinical guidelines for ostomy care. Recommendations for the discharge teaching plan included basic ostomy skills, complications, and activities of daily living (WOCN®, 2017). Culture and sexual issues were also addressed along with follow-up care after discharge from the hospital.

The Joint Commission (2012) requires that the patient's learning needs, abilities, preferences, and readiness to learn are assessed. The assessment should consider cultural and religious practices, emotional barriers, desire and motivation to learn, physical and cognitive limitations, language barriers, and financial implications of care choice.

It is important to include any family member that the patient wishes to receive instruction, for in many cases having a "backup" to assist with the ostomy care after discharge will be needed. Zhou et al. (2017) describe the importance of the support of the patient's partner on the adjustment capabilities of the patient and including the partner in the instruction process may contribute to his or her understanding and acceptance of the ostomy.

There are many methods for teaching ostomy self-care, and the ostomy nurse needs to assess the patient to identify his or her learning style. The "teach back" method is one approach that can assess the person's understanding and ability to perform skills required to be independent in their ostomy care. Some teaching methods include demonstration and return demonstration, video, illustrations, pamphlets, anatomical apron, and PowerPoint presentations. The education sessions should not last longer than 1 hour. Pouresmail et al. (2019) described using a wearable stoma simulator. This device

was developed for the patient with culture and religious practice that does not accept touching urine or stool. (See Chapter 14.)

ASSESSING READINESS

Components of a learning assessment should include the patient's cultural and spiritual beliefs, emotional barriers, desire and motivation to learn, physical or cognitive limitations, and barriers to communication. A patient's readiness to learn can be affected by physical or psychological comfort such as pain, fatigue, anxiety, anger, or fear. In view of existing time constraints, teaching might begin with encouraging the patient to recognize the need to participate in his or her care. Asking the patient their views of living with the stoma and function, and how the ostomy nurse can assist them to assume the necessary tasks that came with the stoma, can be a beginning of their recognition of their need for learning.

While it may seem in these days of shortened lengths of hospital stay that consideration of learner readiness may seem unproductive. The patient who does not recognize the need to learn, or is depressed or angry may not be amenable to learning. Recognition of these issues allows the WOC nurse to implement interventions that lead the patient to understand the need for learning and acquiring new skills. Merandy et al. (2017), discussed delaying education until the person is ready, as late as postoperative day 4. The ostomy nurse needs to be able to provide other education methods, in order to engage the reluctant patient in learning survival ostomy skills before discharge.

Preoperative education may be very limited or not be available in many situations as patients may not arrive at the hospital until just prior to surgery. Emergency surgery may result in a fecal diversion that the patient was not prepared for or seen preoperatively by a WOC nurse. Some patients find that they cannot remember any ostomy teaching preoperatively and little postoperatively, due to anxiety and surgical pain.

The skill set recommended by the WOCN® Society Ostomy Consensus Statement (2007) is described as the abilities of the postoperative patient to perform the actions listed in **Box 13-1**. Teaching the elder patient may require a longer time to learn, and relating ostomy teaching to previous learning or experiences helps the aged patient gain the necessary knowledge and skills without any extraneous facts. Many factors can delay the older person from becoming independent in ostomy care:

BOX 13-1   SKILL SET FOR THE POSTOPERATIVE OSTOMY PATIENT

Manipulate pouch clip or spout
Empty the pouch
Remove and apply a pouching system
Additional skills if possible
　Bathing
　Clothing
　Activity restrictions
　Influence of medications on ostomy function
　Dietary considerations
　Peristomal skin care
　Monitoring for complications
　Sexual function (Colwell & Beitz, 2007)
　Option for colostomy irrigation

KEY POINT

A convex skin barrier may be useful if the stoma is flush with the skin or has soft abdominal turgor or the stoma is retracted below skin level. Convexity is available in several degrees of depth and flexibility: light, soft, firm, medium, or deep. The WOC nurse should assess for depth and flexibility of convexity.

chronic illnesses, limited physical conditions and mental status changes. The goal for the older person is to become independent in ostomy care. They may view the ostomy as the last threat to their independence. Teaching illiterate patients should involve verbal explanations, pictures, videos, audio tapes models, and demonstrations. Arrows showing the flow of the procedure in pictures can be helpful. It is also important to recall that illiteracy does not imply a lack of intelligence and these patients self-esteem should be protected.

(This is discussed more in Chapter 14.)

POUCHING PRINCIPLES

Regardless of type of ostomy, there are principles that apply when managing a stoma with a pouching system. The pouching system should provide the person with an ostomy-consistent wear time and containment of stoma output and protection of the peristomal skin.

There are one- and two-piece types of pouching systems with both flat and convex skin barriers. The skin barrier is the part of the system that attaches to the skin; it should fit snugly around the stoma so that no peristomal skin will be exposed. Skin barriers are available as precut or cut to size to accommodate the stoma, which is irregularly shaped or is still shrinking. There are also barriers that may be molded to fit around the stoma without cutting. The pouch contains the output from the stoma and can be drainable and emptied several times per day as needed or may have a closed end where the pouch is removed and replaced rather than emptied. Pouch closures may be a separate clip or integrated into the pouch, closing with a spout or a hook and loop closure. There are many accessory products that are usually used to solve problems such as liquid skin barriers used to protect peristomal skin or paste, strips, or rings used to "caulk" around a stoma where the skin surface is uneven. See Chapter 12 for an in-depth discussion on pouching systems and the principles of pouching.

While general instructions for stoma care are described, over time and when back at home in his or her own environment, the person with the new ostomy is encouraged to find a comfort level with this care and make the techniques and practices his or her own. The WOC nurse might instruct in current practices, but in order to incorporate the ostomy into his or her life, the patient may fine-tune some of these new procedures until they work well for him or her.

HOW TO EMPTY

There are many ways of emptying a pouch, and while the WOC nurse will instruct patients on methods of emptying, the person will adjust the practices to suit his or her lifestyle, along with ease of performing the tasks. Once the patient is comfortable enough to rework the instructions into his or her routine, it is a sign of the beginning of adjustment to the stoma.

Emptying the pouch into the toilet after placing toilet tissue in the bowl to prevent splash back is the most common way to empty pouches. Sitting on the toilet emptying the pouch between the legs and in the case of a fecal ostomy, cleaning the bottom edge with toilet tissue is a practice used by many people while others turns the end of the pouch back on to itself to form a cuff with a pouch that uses a clamp. Fecal drainable pouch with a Velcro closure requires the patient to unroll and then pinch open the end to empty. Some people find it easier to face the toilet and empty the pouch down into the bowl, while others use a two-piece system, detach the pouch from the skin barrier and empty into the toilet, and then replace the pouch on the flange. Emptying a urostomy pouch requires opening the tap and direct the urine to flow into the toilet. This is an area that the patient can adjust to his or her own comfort level; front facing, back facing, or standing, patient preference can be accepted and can help the patient to feel some control over his or her care. See **Figure 13-1**.

Some people with a fecal ostomy wish to rinse out the pouch, either with each emptying or daily, although this is not necessary, as long as the tail edge of the pouch is kept clean. The practice of frequently rinsing a pouch every time it is emptied can actually weaken the adhesive seal. Pouches are manufactured to be odor proof, which means they will contain the odor in the pouch; however, when the pouch is emptied, there may

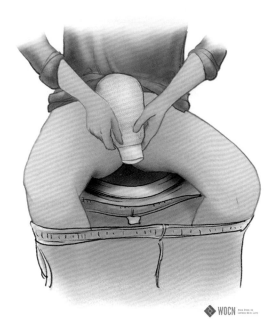

FIGURE 13-1. Emptying a Pouch.

be unpleasant odors. Pouches are available with gas filters that are charcoal and allow gas to escape from the pouch while absorbing odor. These do not perform as well when the output from the stoma is very liquid, as in an ileostomy, as the liquid stool may clog the filter. There are in-pouch deodorants, odor eliminators, and systemic pill deodorants that can assist in the elimination of odor when emptying pouch. Prior to emptying, an odor eliminator spray can also be used. (See **Box 13-2** for simple pouch emptying instructions.)

BOX 13-2   INSTRUCTIONS FOR POUCH EMPTYING

1. Sit on the toilet, as far back as possible.
2. Hold up the pouch and remove/open the bottom of the pouch (clamp, closure or plug tip).
3. Pinch open the end of the fecal pouch, turn the end of the pouch over the water, and release the contents. Allow the stool to drain; push stool out if necessary. If a urostomy pouch, open the tap, aim into the toilet, and allow urine to drain.
4. Place a piece of toilet paper into the toilet and drain pouch into the toilet (reduces splash back).
5. Clean end of the outlet with toilet paper or wipe—rinsing pouch is not necessary.
6. Close the end of the pouch or fasten plug tip. If needed, in-pouch deodorant may be used at this time.

Based on Doughty, D. (2005). Principles of ostomy management in the oncology patient. *Supportive Oncology, 3*(1), 59–69; Bak, G. P. (2008). Teaching ostomy patients to regain their independence. *American Nurse Today, 3*(3), 30–34.

WHEN TO EMPTY

This is typically the first skill the person with a new ostomy must learn. It is the most frequent task they will have to perform with the ostomy, sometimes four, five, or six times daily with an ileostomy or urostomy, less often with a colostomy. It is very important that this skill be acquired before the patient leaves the hospital, and he or she should be able to demonstrate his or her ability to check the pouch for filling, empty, and close the end spout or use the clip successfully.

Since there is no sensation of urine or stool coming through the stoma, the patient must get into the habit of feeling the pouch to see how full it is. The pouch should be emptied when it is half to one-third full to avoid strain on the adhesive seal, or sooner if the person finds this uncomfortable (see Watch & Learn videos: *"Instructions on how to open a pouch and empty it"* and *"How to empty a different type of pouch"*). As noted, as soon as he or she is able, the patient should be responsible for checking the filling of the pouch and alerting to the need for emptying. As recovery continues, patients should be responsible for pouch emptying before discharge from the hospital, since they will be as soon as they get home.

INDICATIONS FOR POUCH CHANGE

Most pouching systems are routinely changed twice per week (every 3 or 4 days) or any time there is evidence of leakage or skin irritation. Usually itching, burning, and feeling of moistness under the skin barrier are indicators that there is moisture in contact with the skin under the barrier. Leakage outside the edges of the barrier should never be "fixed," repaired, or taped over. Doing this merely traps the effluent onto the skin and will result in skin irritation or peristomal irritant dermatitis. Pouching systems should be changed as soon as possible whenever leakage is noted.

Many people with an ostomy will change the pouching system prior to sexual activity to ensure a leak-free experience, and others may find that religious observations require a clean pouch; otherwise, most people establish a routine so that the pouching system is changed prior to any signs of leakage.

PREPARING EQUIPMENT

Before removing the pouch, the patient should assemble all the necessary equipment at hand so that they do not have to look for items once the pouch is removed and while the stoma is functioning. Most people keep their supplies together on a shelf or in a box or bag for all of their ostomy equipment, including the pouching system and any accessory products they are using: paste, belt, tape, or scissors. If the stoma has been recently created, a measuring guide may be used to recheck the stoma circumference since it will shrink postoperatively. After a month or so, if stoma size is stable, a presized barrier may be ordered. If not using a presized skin barrier, it is best to trace the size from the measuring guide onto the paper on the back of the skin barrier, and cut out the skin barrier and apply paste or barrier ring (if used) prior to removing the pouch. Most pastes contain alcohol, so allowing the alcohol to dry before application of the skin barrier helps to protect the skin from the effects of the alcohol.

ASSESSING PERISTOMAL SKIN

The skin around the stoma should not look very different from the rest of the skin. While the pouch is off, examine the area for any redness, rashes, or open skin areas. Inspect outer edges of where adhesive tape attaches to barrier for any signs of skin irritation.

When removing the pouching system, examine the adhesive side of the skin barrier to see if there is any erosion especially around the stoma opening and teach the patient to do the same. This might indicate that the pouching system has been in place for too long. If there are any changes to the peristomal skin such as breakdown, erosion, or rashes, instruct the patient to contact the WOC nurse for an appointment. It has been noted that many patients accept skin breakdown under the barrier as normal; they should be instructed that this is cause for a follow-up visit with the WOC nurse.

MEASURING STOMA

The stoma will shrink for some time after surgery due to decreasing edema. This means the patient will have to resize the stoma opening of the skin barrier until the size stabilizes. Usually the stoma should be measured for 4 to 6 weeks postoperatively, until the stoma edema has resolved and the patient finds the size does not change for a few pouch changes. Most ostomy equipment comes with measuring guides that allow placing the openings over the stoma to facilitate selection of the correct stoma size. If the stoma size is not round, usually the WOC nurse will send home a pattern for the patient to trace onto to the skin barrier, but the patient must assess that the pattern remains the correct size while the stoma continues to shrink (see Watch & Learn videos: *"How to measure a stoma to make the same size opening for the pouch"* and *"How to make an oval stoma template for cut to fit pouch"*).

PERISTOMAL SKIN CLEANSING

There are many products available for cleaning and protecting peristomal skin; however, soap is not recommended for routine care for the peristomal skin area (Washula, 2017). If soap is used, it should be rinsed off thoroughly. Soap with oils should be avoided, as they may interfere with the pouch adhesion. Most people use warm water and a paper towel that can be disposed rather than washcloths that require laundering. The area should be wiped with warm water and patted dry. The stoma does not need to be cleaned; if stool is present, it

can be removed with toilet tissue. If the peristomal area has a large amount of hair growth, clipping with an electric razor should be considered, in case the hair interferes with adhesion of skin barrier or causes discomfort upon pouching system removal.

REMOVAL OF POUCHING SYSTEM

Some people remove the pouch in the shower and wash the peristomal skin with mild, nonoily soap and water. Others prefer to remove the pouching system in the bathroom and apply the system they have laid out ready for application. A gentle removal of the barrier by using a "push pull" technique from the top down helps to protect the peristomal skin from mechanical injury. Adhesive remover wipes or sprays releasers can be used to break the seal and will provide less discomfort with removing the barrier.

PLACEMENT OF POUCHING SYSTEM

If the person received preoperative stoma site marking, the stoma location should be visible and application of the pouching system easily accomplished. Many people apply the skin barrier while standing, in order to insure a flat abdominal area. Sitting can be considered if the abdomen is flat and the stoma area easy to see. For most people, it is important that the area around the stoma be as flat as possible to enhance the pouching system seal.

The spout part of the pouch is usually in the 6 o'clock position, which allows the effluent to fall to the bottom of the pouch and ease of emptying into the toilet. If the patient wears a belt, this is the position that keeps the belt tabs in the 3 and 9 o'clock locations. This again can vary with patient preference.

PROBLEM IDENTIFICATION, WHEN TO SEEK ASSISTANCE

Many issues with stoma management do not occur until the patient is at home, attempting to integrate the new ostomy into his or her actual existence. Some of the challenges the person with an ostomy commonly faces after discharge from the hospital include pouch leakage, skin irritation, odor, depression, or anxiety. Fear of an accident can result in social isolation and delay in returning to work. Merandy (2016) identified adaptation factors that affected the person with a urinary diversion. In this study, patients identified the need for more education, support, and resources once discharged. Because of this, the author recommends WOC nurses remaining in contact with their patients by follow-up postoperative discharge calls, and/or a postoperative appointment at an outpatient ostomy clinic. The ostomy outpatient clinics are an excellent resource for people, regardless of how long they have their diversion. These clinics provide the patient with assistance in incorporating the ostomy into their lives and dealing with problems associated with a new or well-established ostomy.

BOX 13-3   WHEN TO SEEK MEDICAL ATTENTION

Severe cramps lasting more than 2 or 3 hours
Deep cut in the stoma
Excessive bleeding from the stoma opening (or a moderate amount in the pouch at several emptyings)
Continuous bleeding at the junction between the stoma and skin
Severe skin irritation or deep ulcers
Unusual change in stoma size and appearance
Severe watery discharge lasting more than 5 or 6 hours
Continuous nausea and vomiting
No stoma output for 4 to 6 hours plus cramping and nausea
Increase in the frequency the pouch requires emptying

Adapted from United Ostomy Associations of America. (2014). *Frequently asked questions.* Retrieved from http://www.ostomy.org/Ostomy_FAQ.html

---

The United Ostomy Associations of America (UOAA) has published recommendations for the patient on when to call his or her doctor or nurse (**Box 13-3**). The person with a urostomy who develops fever, chills, abdominal or retroperitoneal pain, and bloody, cloudy, or foul-smelling urine may have a urinary tract infection and should seek an immediate appointment for follow up. The person with a urinary or fecal diversion needs to be educated on stoma and peristomal complications, management techniques, as well as when to seek medical attention. Peristomal skin problems are frequently encountered, and the patient must be educated on early recognition and treatment of peristomal skin issues. One important patient-focused resource is the WOCN° Peristomal Skin Assessment Guide (2019). This picture-based tool provides a step-by-step guide of peristomal skin assessment, assistance in determining the problem, and suggested interventions. Recommend to patients that they use this tool when they find any peristomal issues; it will help them develop a plan of care or know when to contact their health care team.

LIVING WITH A STOMA

WHERE AND WHEN TO OBTAIN SUPPLIES

The patient may be instructed that many people find it helpful to keep ostomy supplies together on a shelf, in a drawer, or in a box or bag in a dry area away from hot or cold temperatures. An extra ostomy pouching system, a paper towel to wash and dry around the stoma, all accessories used at pouch change, and a bag that can be used for discarding the removed pouch should be carried when leaving home, in case there is a need to change the pouch. Supplies should be ordered in a month's quantity to be sure that the patient does not run out of supplies and to allow time for delivery; the first order placed can take up to 2 weeks to be sent out for delivery.

The WOC nurse should provide the patient written directions on the steps of the pouching system change, the manufacturer's name and product order numbers, and a prescription for all materials used in his or her stoma care. Supplies may be ordered from a durable medical equipment business, either a walk-in store or a mail order company. The WOC nurse should consider developing a list of area suppliers and mail order companies as well as some online companies that the patient can consider using. Many suppliers will bill Medicare or private insurers directly, and the patient should check with his or her health insurance company regarding reimbursement of supply costs, any preferred suppliers, and the allowable amounts of supplies. Some of the manufacturers of ostomy supplies have an assistance program for providing free supplies in case of an emergency. These same companies have a program for patients with no insurance that can help with supplies for a period of time. The patient will need to apply directly to the company (UOAA, 2018).

BATHING

Water is not harmful to the stoma. Patients may take a bath or shower with or without a pouching system in place. Drying the tape or collar of the barrier with a towel or hair dryer can help prevent moisture-associated skin damage. Normal exposure to air or contact with soap and water will not harm the stoma nor will soap irritate it, and water will not flow inward.

Many patients will swim with the pouching system in place as the pouching system is constructed to enable adhesion in water. The pouching system will remain in place and can be dried or replaced after being in the water.

Before swimming, the pouch should be emptied. Many people protect the barrier by taping the edges with waterproof tape. When in the water, a support ostomy belt can be left in place, if commonly used. Females may wear stretch undergarments made especially for swimsuits; consider using a bathing suit with tummy control panel, or a tankini bathing suit with a waist-high stretch bottom or a skirt with a ruffle. Using a swim suit with a lining for a smoother profile in a dark color or a busy pattern can also help disguise the pouching system. Females may want to choose a suit with a well-placed skirt or ruffle. Males may want to wear a swim shirt to conceal a pouch located above the bathing suit waistband, a concealment belt, or bike shorts under their bathing suits.

CLOTHING

Clothing is important, especially to women. Style can influence a better body image and confidence socially when having an ostomy. There are many resources for undergarments and pouch covers for both women and men (see Appendix C). For the most part, most patients can wear the same clothing as they wore before surgery. Pouching systems today are predominately unnoticeable even when wearing the most stylish, form-fitting clothing for men and women, especially when pouches are emptied routinely and not allowed to overfill. If the stoma is placed above the waistline, over blouses, a stretch cami or shirts may be used. In these patients, they may be unable to wear a belt or "tuck in" shirts or blouses, and this does result in a change in clothing style for many people. There are, however, some devices available that act as a shield to protect the stoma and allow patients to wear a belt over their pouching system (see Appendix C). Depending on the activity of the individual, clothing may need to be adjusted, as in swimming or bathing.

SEXUAL CONCERNS

It is recognized that ostomy surgery has an effect on intimacy and sexuality (Albaugh et al., 2017; Merandy, 2016). The ostomy nurse should provide time to ask the patient, regardless of age, if he or she has any sexual concerns. Sexual function in the female may be affected by vaginal dryness or by the vaginal resection (when a cystectomy is done in a woman, the posterior wall of the vagina is removed) that may cause dyspareunia (painful intercourse). Males may experience damage to nerves that control erection and ejaculation (Albaugh et al., 2017; Taylan & Akil, 2019). There is, however, a period of adjustment after surgery, and attitude is a key factor in reestablishing sexual expression and intimacy. Patients should talk to their doctor and/or WOC nurse about any problems or concerns they or their partner might have. (See Chapters 8 and 14 for discussions of sexual counseling.)

The influence of a partner's support on women's psychosocial adjustment to having an ostomy resulting from colorectal cancer is described by Zhou et al. (2017). The demonstration or withdrawal of support is reported to have a considerable impact on the patient's adjustment in both the long term and short term. Geng et al. (2017) reported that in the Chinese person living with an ostomy, social support was found to have a positive effect on quality of life.

Ostomy surgery may present more concerns for single people. When, how, and who to tell about the ostomy is a personal decision, which perhaps could be discussed with an ostomy visitor who has had experience with this issue. However, if a relationship is leading to physical intimacy, it is best the partner is told about the ostomy before discovery is imminent.

DIETARY CONCERNS

The UOAA lists foods that affect the person with an ostomy (**Table 13-1**).

KEY POINT

Patients with a fecal stoma should be instructed to chew food well, especially fibrous foods, to prevent blockage formation.

TABLE 13-1 FOODS THAT AFFECT THE PERSON WITH AN OSTOMY

EFFECT	FOODS
Color changes	Asparagus
	Beets
	Food coloring
	Iron pills
	Licorice
	Red gelatin
	Strawberries
	Tomato sauces
	Colored frosting
Constipation relief	Coffee, warm/hot
	Cooked fruits
	Cooked vegetables
	Fresh fruits
	Fruit juices
	Water
	Any warm or hot beverage
Diarrhea control	Applesauce
	Bananas
	Boiled rice
	Creamy peanut butter
	Pectin supplement (fiber)
	Tapioca
	Toast
Gas-producing	Alcoholic beverages
	Beans
	Soy
	Cabbage
	Carbonated beverages
	Cauliflower
	Chewing gum
	Cucumbers
	Dairy products
	Milk
	Nuts
	Onions
	Radishes
Increased stools	Alcoholic beverages
	Whole grains
	Bran cereals
	Cooked cabbage
	Fresh fruits
	Greens, leafy
	Milk
	Prunes
	Raisins
	Raw vegetables
	Spices
Odor control	Buttermilk
	Cranberry juice
	Orange juice
	Parsley
	Tomato juice
	Yogurt

(Continued)

TABLE 13-1 FOODS THAT AFFECT THE PERSON WITH AN OSTOMY (Continued)

EFFECT	FOODS
Odor-producing	Asparagus
	Baked beans
	Broccoli
	Cabbage
	Cod liver oil
	Eggs
	Fish
	Garlic
	Onions
	Peanut butter
	Some vitamins
	Strong cheese
Stoma obstructive	Apple peels
	Cabbage, raw
	Celery
	Chinese vegetables
	Corn, whole kernel
	Coconuts
	Dried fruit
	Mushrooms
	Oranges
	Nuts
	Pineapple
	Popcorn
	Seeds
	Coleslaw

Adapted from United Ostomy Associations of America Ostomates Food Reference Chart (Pasia, M. (2011). *Diet & nutrition guide.* United Ostomy Associations of America. Retrieved from http://www.ostomy.org, info@ostomy.org). Eating well with an ostomy: A comprehensive nutritional guide for those living with an ostomy (2019) publication of UOAA.

DIETARY CONCERNS

After ostomy surgery, individuals should eat a regular balanced diet that includes the necessary vitamins, minerals, and calories needed for good health (Burgess-Stacks, 2019). When bowels sounds return, first foods may be liquid or a low-fiber/low-residue diet until edema resolves, a regular diet can be resumed. New foods should be added gradually to determine their effect on ostomy management.

Some foods cause gas, such as eggs, cabbage, broccoli, onions, fish, beans, milk, cheese, and alcohol. Food should be taken at regular intervals; skipping meals increase the incidence of watery stools and flatus (gas). Instruct the patient to avoid fasting and skipping meals, smoking, chewing gum, and drinking through a straw. Some people benefit from eating six smaller meals, but these should equal three regular meals.

ILEAL CONDUIT

Maintaining adequate fluid intake in the individual with an ileal conduit is important to prevent infection, since the ileal conduit has almost continuous output without any antireflux properties. Patients need to take in 30 cc/kg/d of fluids (8 to 10, 8 ounces glasses) at regular intervals throughout the day in order to keep a constant one-way urinary flow. Nighttime drainage system should be recommended to keep the pouch empty while sleeping. Patients are instructed to empty the nighttime drainage system (there is an adapter to place between the pouch tap and the night time drainage tubing) and to discard after 14 days. The patient may be discharged with stents placed in the stoma and the ostomy nurse will have demonstrated how to change and apply a pouch system. Shreds of mucus in the urine are normal, as mucus is produced by the bowel segment (ileum).

ILEOSTOMY

Food blockage with an ileostomy can occur when insoluble fiber amasses near the fascia-muscle layer. Signs of blockage are constant spurting of liquid or a watery stool, feeling full or bloated, cramping, swollen stoma, nausea and vomiting, and absence of stoma output. Foods known to cause blockage problems include corn, celery, popcorn, nuts, coleslaw, coconut macaroons, grapefruit, and Chinese vegetables such as bamboo shoots, water chestnuts, and raisins.

Insoluble fiber foods should be eaten in small amounts and chewed thoroughly along with fluid intake to prevent the mass from forming. If it is determined that the patient has a food bolus blockage, the WOC nurse may perform ileal lavage where 30 to 50 mL of warm saline is instilled though a 14- to 16-French soft catheter, which is then removed to allow drainage. This is repeated until the blockage is relieved. The UOAA has described interventions for when a blockage is suspected. (See Chapter 14 for listed recommendations.)

Dehydration and acute renal problems can occur with the high-volume ileostomy that may require a hospital readmission. Normal output for an ileostomy is <1,200 cc/24 hours. More frequent emptying and/or watery effluent may indicate the person is at risk for dehydration. The patient needs to recognize signs of both obstruction and dehydration and when to seek help. (See Chapter 14 for management.)

Colostomy

There is no special diet for a person with a colostomy. The ostomy nurse should instruct the patient to gradually return to his or her normal diet after surgery. Constipation can still occur. Diet that includes whole grains, vegetables, and fruits along with increased fluids can help prevent constipation.

The person with a colostomy may also develop diarrhea that can be caused by foods, medications, chemotherapy, or other medical conditions (WOCN, 2017).

(See **Table 13-1** and Chapter 14 for management of constipation and diarrhea.)

Odor

Many factors, such as foods, normal bacteria in the intestine, illness, certain medicines, and vitamins can cause odor. There should only be odor when the pouch is emptied or changed: pouching systems are odor proof. Some foods can produce odor: eggs, cabbage, cheese, cucumber, onion, garlic, fish, dairy foods, and coffee. Patients need to determine which foods cause odor and decide if they need to avoid those foods (**Table 13-1**). Learning by experience is the only way to discover this; odors may be worse with transverse colostomies. Hints for odor control include the following:

- Use an odor-proof pouch.
- Check to see that the skin barrier is properly adhered.
- Empty the pouch often.
- Place special deodorant liquids, odor eliminators, and/or tablets in the pouch.
- Use medicines that control odor; the physician or ostomy nurse can advise about these products and how to use them. Some things may help with odor are chlorophyll tablets, bismuth subgallate, and bismuth subcarbonate.
- Air deodorizers or spray odor eliminators that can be used before the pouch is emptied and can control odor very well when emptying the pouch.

Pelvic Exenteration

Total pelvic exenteration (PE) is an extensive surgical option for selected patients with the diagnosis of advanced or recurrent cancer of the pelvis. This procedure for women involves removal of all pelvic organs; rectum, distal sigmoid colon, urinary bladder with distal ureters, internal iliac vessels, pelvic node dissection, uterus, ovaries, tubes, and vagina (Rausa et al., 2017). In men, the bladder, prostate, urethra, seminal vessels, vas deferens, rectum, and lower colon are removed along with pelvic node dissection. A urinary diversion and descending colostomy will be created.

- Anterior pelvic exenteration surgical procedure requires removal of female or male reproduction organs, bladder along with pelvic nodes; the colon and rectum remain. A urinary diversion, either continent diversion or ileal conduit will be created.
- Posterior pelvic exenteration surgical procedure requires removal of rectum, sigmoid colon, anus along with pelvic node dissection. The urinary tract is spared. This results in a colostomy.

Postoperative ostomy education will depend on the type of diversion(s) (fecal, urinary or both) that the patient will have. The WOC nurse should plan teaching sessions when the patient's family is available and the patient is able to follow the sessions. If the patient has two diversions, the instructions should first start on the urinary diversion and then the fecal diversion. It is helpful to use one ostomy company's products for both diversions. The supplies should be labeled clearly with the type of the stoma. The urinary pouch system should be changed first, before changing the colostomy pouch system. This will decrease the risk of the urinary system being exposed to stool.

An interdisciplinary team should follow the person who has PE surgery. Providing ongoing support to not only the patient but also the family is important. The hospital stay may be longer, and there is a risk of complications. (See Chapter 14 for more information.)

MEDICATIONS

Absorption may vary with individuals and types of medication. Certain drug problems may arise depending on the type of ostomy and the medications used. Patients inform their pharmacy or pharmacist about the type of ostomy to ensure that they are receiving their medications in the appropriate format. Patients with an ileostomy or ascending colostomy should not take laxatives as it could lead to dehydration. Extended-release medications (i.e., time-released and enteric-coated medications) may only be partially absorbed or not at all absorbed, depending on how much of the small bowel was removed. Many patients in the hospice or palliative care setting take long-acting opioids, which are sustained release and dependent on the amount of small bowel still accessible for absorption. In addition, many of these medications can cause constipation and blockage, diarrhea, or altered fluid and electrolyte balances. (See Chapter 14 for a discussion of medications.)

PHYSICAL ACTIVITIES

There are limited studies on physical exercises to recommend following ostomy surgery. Russell (2019) describes a gentle core and abdominal exercise starting on postoperative days three or four. The ostomy nurse needs to assess the patient first to see if he or she can participate in an exercise program based on age, medical and surgical history, and motivation. A gradual abdominal exercise program can reduce the incidence of peristomal hernias (Russell, 2019).

FOLLOW-UP CARE

Fingren et al. (2018) found that the majority of patients reported it took months to feel comfortable with daily care and diet, and problems may continue for years after surgery. Further, it is suggested that long-term access to a WOC nurse is important in improving and maintaining the quality of life of these patients. Sun et al. (2013) describes persistent ostomy concerns and adaptations in long-term (>5 years) colorectal cancer survivors with an ostomy. Most common concerns were identified as stoma location and pouch problems, activity limitations, leakage, odor, pouch adhesive issues, and skin irritation. The authors suggest the need for long-term supportive care strategies. Cengiz and Bahar (2017) identified a need for follow-up telephone calls and more frequent home visits. Taylan and Akil (2019) study found the effect of preoperative counseling on patient's sexual concerns made a difference in their sexual lives. However, being aware of these specific issues, the WOC nurse should intervene early in the preoperative and postoperative course to teach and inform patients in these specific areas, and provide follow-up with community resources as well as physician and nursing follow-ups. Colwell et al. (2019) identified in the international practice guidelines that the patient's ostomy pouch system should be reassessed 2 weeks after discharge to assure correct fit to avoid any problems.

Listings of ostomy clinics and referral sources for stoma clinics should be given to all ostomy patients at discharge: most ostomy patients will require some measure of lifelong follow-up and must receive advice on where to find these services. Hendren et al. (2015) recommended that all patients with an ostomy should have access to an ostomy nurse. Appendix B lists ostomy support resources, and Appendix C lists suppliers of ostomy products.

SUPPORT GROUPS

Nurses may refer ostomy patients to support groups and to the online UOAA at http://www.uoaa.org/; the site has active discussion boards for various types of incontinent and continent diversions, along with youth, adult, and parent networks (UOAA, 2018). The UOAA can provide information for the patient and family on the closes support group in their area.

 CONCLUSIONS

KEY POINT

Some studies relate the presence of an ostomy to a negative impact on the quality of life of these patients. However a consensus of expert opinion is that this is patient specific; many patients after a period of recovery and adjustment manage to overcome many of the negative effects of living with an ostomy.

Adaptation to a new ostomy requires meeting many challenges that the WOC nurse can help the individual with. Education and training in self-stoma care as well as answering the concerns of the patient will help the patient to cope with these challenges. The WOC nurse can prepare the patient for living with a stoma and to help to arrange follow-up care when the person goes home from the hospital.

REFERENCES

Albaugh, J., Tenfelde, S., & Hayden, D. (2017). Sexual dysfunction and intimacy for ostomates. *Clinics in Colon and Rectal Surgery, 30*(3), 201–206.

Burgess-Stacks, J. (2019). Eating with an ostomy. Retrieved January 5, 2020, from https://www.ostomy.org/wp-content/uploads/2019/10/Eating_with_an_Ostomy.pdf

Cengiz, B., & Bahar, Z. (2017). Perceived barriers and home care needs when adapting to a fecal ostomy. *Journal of Wound, Ostomy, and Continence Nursing, 44*(1), 63–73.

Collado-Boira, E., Machanconcoses, F., & Temprado, M. (2018). Development and validation of an instrument measuring self-care in persons with a fecal ostomy. *Journal of Wound, Ostomy, and Continence Nursing, 46*(4), 335–340.

Colwell, J., Bain, K., Hansen, A., et al. (2019). Development of practice guidelines for assessment of peristomal body and stoma profiles, patient engagement and patient follow-up. *Journal of Wound, Ostomy, and Continence Nursing, 46*(6), 497–504.

Colwell, J. & Beitz, J. (2007). Survey of wound, ostomy and continence (WOC) nurse clinicians on stomal and peristomal complications: A content validation study. *Journal of Wound, Ostomy and Continence Nursing, 34*(1), 57–69.

Fingren, J., Lindholm, E., Lic, M., et al. (2018). A prospective, explorative study to assess adjustment 1 year after ostomy surgery among Swedish patients. *Ostomy/Wound Management, 64*(6), 12–22.

Geng, Z., Howell, D., Honglian, X., et al. (2017). Quality of life in Chinese persons living with an ostomy. *Journal of Wound, Ostomy, and Continence Nursing, 44*(3), 249–256.

Hendren, S., Hammond, K., Glasgow, S., et al. (2015). Clinical practice guidelines for ostomy surgery. *Diseases of the Colon & Rectum, 58*(4), 375–387.

Joint Commission Patient Education Requirements. (2012). Retrieved from http://www.mghpcs.org/eed_portal/Documents/PatientEd/JC_Standards_PatientEd.pdf

Jones, D. (2017). Ready to go home? Patients' experiences of the discharge process in an enhanced recovery after surgery (ERAS) program for colorectal surgery. *Journal of Gastrointestinal Surgery, 21*, 1865–1878.

Merandy, K. (2016). Factors related to adaptation to cystectomy with urinary diversion. *Journal of Wound, Ostomy, and Continence Nursing, 43*(5), 499–508.

Merandy, K., Morgan, M., Lee, R., et al. (2017). Improving self-efficacy and self-care in adult patients with a urinary diversion: A pilot study. *Oncology Nursing Forum, 44*(3), E90–E100.

Pasia, M. (2011). *Diet & Nutrition Guide*. United Ostomy Associations of America. Retrieved from http://www.ostomy.org, info@ostomy.org

Pedziwiatr, M., Mayrilda, J., Witowski, J., et al. (2018). Current status of enhanced recovery after surgery (ERAS) protocol in gastrointestinal surgery. *Medical Oncology, 35*(6), 95–109.

Pouresmail, Z., Nabavi, F., Shakeri, T., et al. (2019). Effect of using a simulation device for ostomy self-care teaching in Iran: A pilot randomized clinical trial. *Wound Management & Prevention, 65*(6), 30–39.

Rausa, E., Kelly, M., Bonavina, L., et al. (2017). A systematic review examining quality of life following pelvic exenteration for locally advanced and recurrent rectal cancer. *Colorectal Disease, 19*, 430–436.

Russell, S. (2019). Exercise after ostomy surgery and peristomal hernia. *Journal of Wound, Ostomy, and Continence Nursing, 46*(3), 215–218.

Sun, V., Grant, M., McMullen, C. K., et al. (2013). Surviving colorectal cancer. Long-term, persistent ostomy-specific concerns and adaptations. *Journal of Wound, Ostomy, and Continence Nursing, 40*(1), 61–72.

Taylan, S., & Akil, Y. (2019). The effect of postoperative telephone counseling on sexual life of patients with a bowel stoma: A randomized controlled study. *Wound Management & Prevention, 65*(6), 14–29.

United Ostomy Association of America, Inc. (2018). Intimacy after ostomy surgery guide. Retrieved from https://www.ostomy.org/wp-content/uploads/2018/03/Intimacy-After-Ostomy-Surgery-Guide.pdf

Washula, L. (2017). *Basic ileostomy care new ostomy patient guide*. UOAA.

WOCN Society Ostomy Consensus Statement. (2007). Skill set for the postoperative ostomy patient. Mt. Laurel, NJ, author.

World Council of Enterostomal Therapist (WCET). (2014). WCET International Guideline Recommendations: 3.2 preoperative education. In K. Zulkowski (Ed.), *WCET international ostomy guideline* (pp. 14–15). Osborne Park, Australia: WCET.

Wound, Ostomy and Continence Nurses Society™. (2017). *Clinical guideline: Management of the adult patient with a fecal or urinary ostomy*. Mt. Laurel, NJ: Author.

Wound, Ostomy and Continence Nurses Society™. (2019). *Peristomal skin assessment guide for consumers*. Mt. Laurel, NJ: Author. Retrieved from htttps://www.wocn.org

Zhou, X., Chen, Y., Tang, X., et al. (2017). Sexual experiences of Chinese patients living with an ostomy. *Journal of Wound, Ostomy, and Continence Nursing, 44*(5), 469–474.

QUESTIONS

1. The WOC nurse is teaching a patient with a new colostomy how to empty the pouch. What is a recommended step in this procedure?
A. Sit on the front edge of the toilet seat to empty the pouch.
B. Hold the pouch up and open to empty into the toilet.
C. Clean the inside and outside end of the pouch with alcohol wipe.
D. Always rinse the pouch with hot water and dry with toilet paper.

2. An elderly gentleman with a new ostomy tells the WOC nurse: "I'll never be able to figure out this system; I don't know where anything goes and I'm going home tomorrow!" What patient teaching strategy would best meet this patient's needs?
A. Provide general written instructions for stoma care and encourage patient describe how he will accomplish this at home.
B. Encourage the patient to develop a care plan independently and follow it step by step in the home environment.
C. Assure the patient that there is no recommended procedure for stoma care and that he should figure out a routine that works as soon as possible.
D. Teach the care plan to the patient's family/caregiver since he is elderly and ask the caregiver to decide if the patient is able to provide self-care.

3. What teaching point would the WOC nurse emphasize as a recommended guideline for emptying and changing an ostomy pouch?
A. Empty pouch after the sensation of urine or stool comes through the stoma.
B. Empty the pouch when it is three-fourths full to avoid strain on the adhesive seal.
C. If a leak occurs outside the edge of the barrier, the barrier can be taped.
D. Routinely change the pouch 2 or 3 times per week or if leakage occurs.

4. A patient with a new ostomy is experiencing skin breakdown under the barrier. What would be the priority intervention for this patient?
A. Schedule a follow-up visit with the WOC nurse.
B. Change to a different ostomy pouching system.
C. Change the size of the stoma opening of the skin barrier.
D. Clean the peristomal skin with a petroleum product.

5. The nurse is teaching a patient with a new ostomy tips for successful stoma care. Which tip meets recommended guidelines for care?
A. Always remove the pouch standing up in the shower.
B. Keep pouching system in place until leakage occurs.
C. Remove the pouching system gently using push–pull technique.
D. Wash the peristomal skin with mild oil-based soap and water.

6. The WOC nurse is teaching stoma care to a patient with a new ileostomy who is being discharged to home care. Under what condition would the nurse tell the patient to seek medical attention?
A. Pouch is being emptied twice daily.
B. If there is a large volume of air in the pouch.
C. If there is copious water discharge lasting more than 5 or 6 hours.
D. If there is no output in 2 hours.

7. A nutritionist is helping a patient with a new ostomy plan a diet. Which food would the nurse recommend to maintain odor control?
A. Eggnog
B. Tomato juice
C. Ginger ale
D. Milk

8. A patient with a new colostomy is complaining of diarrhea. What food would the WOC nurse recommend to help resolve this problem?
   A. Cooked vegetables
   B. Fruit juices
   C. Dairy products
   D. Creamy peanut butter

9. The WOC nurse has a consult to provide stoma siting for a patient scheduled for posterior pelvic exenteration. What type of ostomy will this procedure require?
   A. Colostomy
   B. Ileal conduit
   C. Indiana pouch
   D. Ileal pouch–anal anastomosis

10. A patient with a new ostomy tells the WOC nurse: "I am a bit nervous about having sex with my partner after this surgery." What should be the nurse's response?
   A. "Sexuality is not affected by this surgery."
   B. "You and your partner will need to see if sex is possible."
   C. "What part of thinking about having sex makes you nervous?"
   D. "You need to explore other forms of sexual intimacy besides intercourse."

ANSWERS AND RATIONALES

1. B. Rationale: The drainable pouch needs to be carefully opened and held up to avoid spillage, before directing the pouch to empty into the toilet. Placing toilet paper in the toilet before emptying will also avoid any splashing.

2. A. Rationale: Providing written instructions and reviewing simple survival skills for managing an ostomy at home should be less overwhelming for an elderly person. The caregiver and patient should not be responsible for a care plan.

3. D. Rationale: Guidelines for changing a pouch is 2 to 3 times a week or if leakage or pain under the barrier occurs. If leakage occurs, the pouch system must be changed regardless of when the pouch system had been applied.

4. A. Rationale: A new patient with an ostomy having problems with peristomal skin breakdown should contact a WOC nurse instead of changing size of the barrier opening and ostomy system. This may not address the problem.

5. C. Rationale: One of the best ways to prevent any peristomal skin stripping is removing the barrier from the top down with a "push–pull" technique.

6. C. Rationale: The patient with an ileostomy should seek medical help if there is an increase of ileostomy output that does not subside within 6 hours. The person will become dehydrated requiring medical care.

7. B. Rationale: Tomato juice would be the best recommendation to manage odor control because it is acidic and can kill bacteria that causes odor for some people.

8. D. Rationale: Creamy peanut butter would be the best choice to manage diarrhea because it is a carb and carbs absorb fluid and thicken the stool.

9. A. Rationale: The surgery for a posterior pelvic exenteration will result in a fecal diversion, colostomy. This surgery will remove the sigmoid, colon, rectum, anus, and pelvic nodes.

10. C. Rationale: "What part of thinking about having sex makes you nervous?" will allow the patient to put into words why he or she is nervous so the WOC nurse can start to explore options to address the fears.

CHAPTER 14

ADAPTATIONS, REHABILITATION, AND LONG-TERM CARE MANAGEMENT ISSUES

Jane Carmel and Jody Scardillo

OBJECTIVES

1. Analyze specific management issues related to fecal and urinary diversions.

2. Identify factors that impact adaptation to an ostomy and implement measures to promote full recovery and adaptation.

3. Assess the needs of special populations and incorporate identified needs into the ostomy plan of care.

TOPIC OUTLINE

Introduction   202

Temporary Fecal Diversions   202

Colostomy   203
  Irrigation   203
    Patient Selection   203
  Odor and Flatus Management   204
  Prevention and Management of Constipation   205
  Prevention and Management of Diarrhea   206
  Bowel Prep   206

Ileostomy   206
  Dehydration   206
  High Output and Hospital Readmissions   206
  Food Blockage   207
  Diet   207
  Medications   208
  Bowel Prep   208

Ileal Conduit   208
  Stent Management (Urostomy)   208

Pelvic Exenteration   209

Impact of an Ostomy   209
  Stages of Adaptation Process   210
  Factors Affecting Ability to Adapt   210
    Self-Esteem/Coping Skills   211
    Self-Efficacy   211
    Past Experience with Ostomy/ Expectations   211
    Support Provided by Significant Others   211
    Assistance Provided by Health Care Team/ WOC Nurse   211
    Impact of Ostomy Visitor   211
    Age/Developmental Stage   212

Sexual Function   212
  Potential Impact of Pelvic Dissection on Sexual Function   212
  Potential Impact of the Ostomy on Body Image/ Sexual Relationships   213
  Counseling Models   213
  Pregnancy   213
    Contraception   214
  Morbid Obesity   214
  End of Life   214

Cognitive Deficits   215
Chemotherapy and Radiation Therapy   215
Chemotherapy   215
    Mucositis/Stomatitis   216
Radiation Therapy   216
Physical and Mental Limitations   217
    Visually Impaired   217

Hearing Deficit   217
Spinal Cord Injury   217
Cultural, Religious, and Spirituality Diversity   217
    Language Barriers   218
    Long-Term Issues with an Ostomy   218

Conclusions   219

 ## INTRODUCTION

A fecal and/or urinary diversion presents many concerns for the individual who is adapting and trying to return to his or her previous life style. The wound ostomy continence (WOC) nurse needs to address many issues related to the type of ostomy the person has as well as whether the diversion is temporary or permanent. This chapter discusses areas related to both fecal and urinary diversions to enable the WOC nurse to provide information to help the person to return to his or her former lifestyle. There are many options and interventions to help to manage his or her concerns, and these are addressed in this chapter.

TEMPORARY FECAL DIVERSIONS

Not all fecal diversions are permanent, and this will depend on the patients' diagnosis and prognosis. Types of temporary fecal stomas are an end stoma with a Hartmann's pouch and loop ileostomy or colostomy. Temporary stomas are created to divert the stool from the distal bowel, allowing the bowel to heal. The surgeon can reverse the stoma within 3 to 6 months with minimal loss of intestinal function (Beck, 2017). There are many conditions that can require a temporary diversion (**Box 14-1**).

In the Hartmann's procedure, a resection of the diseased bowel is performed, the rectal stump is closed, and an end ileostomy or colostomy is created (see Chapter 9). This procedure can be performed for emergency conditions, for example perforated diverticular disease or colon cancer or the first step in the ileal anal anastomosis pouch surgery (see Chapter 6). The patient will be taught that he or she may experience passing retained stool or mucus from the anus. Sometimes there is an urge to move the bowels just as if the ostomy is not present. If the bowel was not cleansed before surgery, old stool will pass, and after the bowel is emptied mucus will be passed.

With the loop stoma, a loop of the bowel is brought through the abdominal wall (Fig. 9-4 in Chapter 9). An opening is made in the bowel to allow stool to be expelled. A temporary rod or support bridge can be placed below the loop to prevent retraction of the stoma. There are two openings in a loop stoma, a proximal opening where the stool will pass and a distal opening leading to the defunctionalized intestine. Loop ileostomies are more common than are loop colostomies. Reversal surgery for loop ileostomy is usually an easier recovery as a small incision is made around the loop, and the two ends are brought through the incision and reconnected (Beck, 2017).

Although not commonly created, a mucous fistula can be created during emergency surgery at the same time as the ileostomy or colostomy. The colon is resected (cut apart with or without removal of a section), and the proximal end is matured as the active stoma (will pass stool) and the distal end of the remaining colon or rectum is brought out onto the abdomen as a mucous fistula. It is called a mucous fistula because some mucus will pass from this opening. The purpose of the mucous fistula is to reduce the risk of stump dehiscence, which can occur with active rectal disease and preoperative steroid use. The patient will be taught to cover the mucous fistula with a stoma cap (**Fig. 14-1**), a mini drainable pouch,

BOX 14-1   CONDITIONS REQUIRING TEMPORARY FECAL STOMA

Emergency condition for distal bowel obstruction, perforation or distal trauma
To rest distal segment of the bowel that may have a disease process, fistula, or Crohn's disease
To protect an anastomosis such as after a low anterior resection for rectal cancer or the creation of an ileal pouch–anal anastomosis

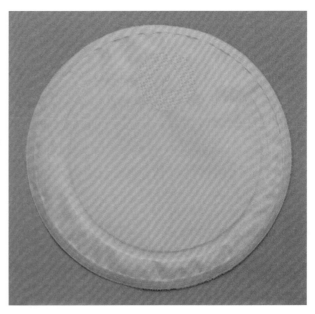

FIGURE 14-1. Stoma Cap.

or in some cases a gauze pad, changed, based on the amount of mucous drainage.

 COLOSTOMY

IRRIGATION

The person with a descending or sigmoid colostomy has the option of managing his or her colostomy with irrigation, and this should be offered as a management method to a person with a left-sided colostomy (**Fig. 14-2**). This is usually recommended for a permanent colostomy. Managing a colostomy by irrigation is for many people a simple, cost-effective procedure. Carlsson et al. (2010) studied the positive and negative aspects of colostomy irrigation (CI) and found that negative aspects reported were time required for CI, less flexibility to plan CI, and more flatulence. Positive aspects reported were feeling secure, an empty pouch, sense of freedom, and fewer pouch changes.

CI can be performed daily or every other day with the goal of being "stool free," that is, no stool passing from the stoma between irrigation. Once the colostomy is regulated, the person can wear a stoma cap, or any type of pouching system since there should be no stool passing (until the next irrigation), but gas can pass from the stoma so some containment system is recommended. Pouching system options include one- or two-piece

systems; some people prefer the two-piece system to use with the irrigation sleeve. Stoma caps are available with a filter to manage gas and absorb mucous discharge.

Patient Selection

Irrigation is not always suitable for all patients with a colostomy. The WOC nurse should evaluate the person's understanding of the irrigation procedure as well as the person's motivation, manual dexterity and eyesight, and the current function of his or her colostomy. Good candidates for a successful outcome with irrigation have one or two semiformed or formed stools in 24 hours. Irrigation is recommended only for descending or sigmoid colostomy as this section of the colon has less peristalsis and can hold stool for several days; there is less frequent output, and the stool is formed unlike the right-sided colostomies.

The WOC nurse should explain to the patient that CI is an option to manage the ostomy. It is not always recommended early postoperatively. If a patient will undergo chemotherapy or has a healing perineal incision, the irrigation procedure can be delayed. The patient should be assured that he or she can always stop the irrigation procedure at any time and resume using a pouching system. See **Box 14-2** for contraindications to CI. Complications associated with irrigation include no return of fluid, vasovagal response, and abdominal cramps.

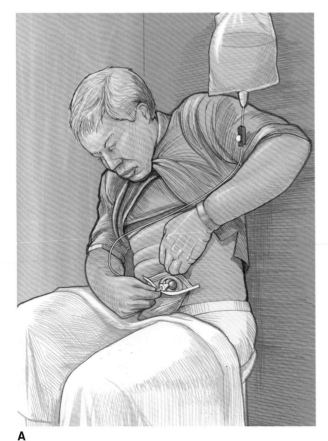

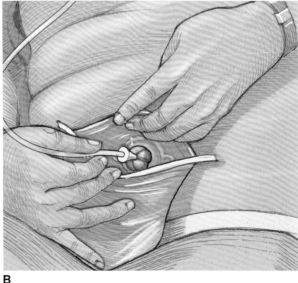

A
B

FIGURE 14-2. Colostomy Irrigation. **A.** Set up for performing colostomy irrigation. **B.** Insertion of cone into the ostomy. (From Pullen, R. L. (2006). Teaching your patient to irrigate a colostomy. *Nursing, 36*(4), 22.)

BOX 14-2   CONTRAINDICATIONS TO COLOSTOMY IRRIGATION

Current chemotherapy/radiotherapy
Stoma stenosis
Large parastomal hernia or stoma prolapse
Crohn's disease
Poor prognosis
Diarrhea

During the learning stage of CI, the person will need encouragement and support while he or she becomes proficient in the procedure. **Box 14-3** explains the CI procedure. Tips on performing this procedure are identified

---

BOX 14-3   COLOSTOMY IRRIGATION PROCEDURE

1. Gather the following equipment*:
   • Irrigation kit: 2-L bag, tubing with flow regulator, soft cone
   • Water-soluble lubricant
   • Irrigation drain sleeve
   • Ostomy belt
   • Warm water
   • Coat hanger or wall hook to hang the irrigation bag from
2. Attach irrigation cone to tubing and fill the bag with 1,000 mL of warm tap water.
3. Hang the irrigation bag from hook at shoulder level when seating on toilet.
4. Open the regulator clamp on the tubing and let the water run through the tube to remove the air. Reclamp the tube.
5. Remove colostomy pouch; if two piece, leave the barrier in place. Place the irrigation sleeve over the stoma or attach to the barrier or secure with an ostomy belt.
6. Lubricate the cone with water-soluble lubricant and gently insert the cone into the stoma until it fits snugly. First, gently insert a lubricated finger to determine the direction to point the cone.
7. While holding the cone in place with one hand, open the clamp on the tubing and let 500 to 1,000 mL of water flow slowly into the colon over 5 to 10 minutes. Regulate the flow of water using the clamp. Note: start with 500 mL of water.
8. Once the amount of water is instilled, clamp the tube and hold the cone in place for about a minute, and then remove the cone from the stoma.
9. Close the top of the irrigation sleeve, and wait for results to flow into the toilet. Most is expelled in the first 5 to 10 minutes; the rest may take up to 30 to 45 minutes.
10. Once returns are complete, remove the sleeve, clean the skin, and apply the pouching system or stoma cap/mini pouch.
11. Wash the equipment with mild soap and warm water, hang to dry, and store in a clean container.

*Supplies can be obtained from ostomy companies that have irrigation sets.

Adapted from Prinz, A. (2013). Irrigation for the colostomate-life without the pouch! Colostomy New Patient Guide. UOAA The Phoenix Magazine; Hayes, D. (2013). Colostomy irrigation: Retraining continence and regaling confidence. *Journal of Stomal Therapy Australia, 33*(2), 18–20.

BOX 14-4   COLOSTOMY IRRIGATION TIPS

Cramping may occur when instilling water; this may be caused by the flow being too fast or the water being too cold or hot. The irrigation should be stopped until cramps subside, and then the procedure should be resumed.
If water does not go in, the cone tip should be repositioned.
If water leaks around the stoma during instillation, clamp the tube and readjust the cone.
If no return, possible cause may be dehydration; discontinue irrigation, increase oral fluids, and wear a drainable pouch.
Complete return of water and stool may take up to 45 minutes.
Irrigation should be done at the same time of day, every 1 to 2 days.
It may take up to 6 to 8 weeks to achieve a predictable bowel pattern with an irrigation procedure.

---

in **Box 14-4**. CIs should be discontinued if a person develops a peristomal hernia. Some other contraindications for CI are Crohn's disease, diverticulitis, current chemotherapy treatment, and radiation damage to the colon (Bauer et al., 2016). Medicare covers four sleeves per month, two cones every 6 months, and two irrigation bags every 6 months.

KEY POINT

The WOC nurse should assess the person with a colostomy to determine if this is an appropriate management plan.

ODOR AND FLATUS MANAGEMENT

Odor is a common fear for the person with a diversion; pouching systems are odor proof, but this is essentially when the pouching system is intact; odor can be a sign of leakage. Teach the person that odor should only occur when emptying and changing the pouching system and taking time to clean the pouch tail prevents odor. If using a pouch clip for open-ended pouch, teach to wash and dry the clip after emptying the pouch to eliminate any risk of odor.

Deodorants/eliminators are available in the form of droplets and liquid that can be added to the inside of the pouch to help eliminate the odor of stool. The liquid deodorant/eliminator is placed into the newly applied pouch, and as the stool drains into the pouch, the deodorant/eliminator mixes with the stool to decrease odor. When the pouch is emptied, the deodorant/eliminator is replaced. A lubricating deodorant can be used to both deodorize the stool and lubricate the inside of the pouch for easy emptying.

There are orally ingested products available to help deodorize the stool internally before it reaches the pouch. Bismuth subgallate (Devrom®) is one option for both odor and flatus, usually recommended in doses

BOX 14-5	FOODS THAT MAY CAUSE GAS AND ODOR

Asparagus
Beans
Beer
Cabbage family
Carbonated drinks
Eggs (hard boiled)
Fish
Melon
Milk products
Onions
Spiced foods

of 200 mg before meals and at bedtime. The patient should be taught that this medication will turn the stool dark. Chlorophyllin 100 mg is another product that is taken orally three times a day. This will turn the stool or urine green and initially can cause loose stools, but this is a temporary side effect. Both of these products can be obtained without a prescription, but the patient should discuss this with his or her health care provider and WOC nurse before trying the product; some feel that the green color can mask blood in the stool, which is an important symptom requiring further investigation.

Other recommendations to help control odor from stool include parsley, buttermilk, cranberry juice, and yogurt. Foods to avoid that can produce odor and gas are listed in **Box 14-5**

In the large intestine, flatus is formed from bacterial activity related to undigested carbohydrates including cellulose in the colon. About 500 mL of flatus may be expelled daily and can increase based on high-carbohydrate foods eaten. Proteins and fats cause little gas. In the small intestine, flatus can occur from swallowing air, chewing gum, eating fast, and using loose-fitting dentures. For flatus management, pouches are available with built-in charcoal filter, vents, and self-sealing filters that can be attached to the outside of the pouch. Integrated pouch charcoal filters are usually placed at the top of the pouch and, in many cases, may only last 24 to 36 hours when the filter becomes plugged or wet from stool. Vents, an external device, are designed without a filter and have a plug that needs to be manually opened to release built-up gas in the pouch. These are an alternative to relieving gas and will last as long as the pouch is in place.

Room sprays can be used to eliminate odor rather than mask it and are best used prior to emptying the pouch rather than afterward.

PREVENTION AND MANAGEMENT OF CONSTIPATION

Constipation can occur in the patient with a sigmoid colostomy; a person with an ileostomy rarely will become constipated as there is little storage capacity in the small bowel. Fiber is recommended for the person with a colostomy to increase bulk to the stool and make it easier to pass. The person being managed with opioid pain medication may also suffer from constipation. Other medications that can contribute to constipation are iron supplements, antidepressants, anticholinergics, antihistamines, and nonsteroidal anti-inflammatory drugs. Mild constipation can be managed by adjusting the diet in the following ways: increase fluids, high-fiber foods, and exercise. It is recommended that fiber be increased in small increments as it may cause bloating, fullness, and gas (Kuczynsha et al., 2017). Stool softeners should also be recommended when taking pain medications. There are four types of laxative to consider: bulk forming, stimulant, osmotic, and stool softeners (**Table 14-1**). The WOC nurse should assess for signs of stoma prolapse, stenosis, or peristomal hernia that may contribute to constipation.

Stimulant laxatives such as senna along with a stool softener may be used in colostomy patient (Tilley, 2012). However, it is not good practice to depend on laxatives. A thorough physical examination and history is important. Digital examination of the stoma needs to be performed by an experienced ostomy nurse, to determine

TABLE 14-1 TYPES OF LAXATIVES

TYPE	ACTION	SIDE EFFECTS
Bulk-forming/fiber Example: psyllium (Metamucil, FiberCon)	Absorb water to form soft bulky stool Slow acting 12 hours to 3 days Adequate fluid intake is necessary for effective fiber therapy	Bloating Cramping Gas
Osmotic Magnesium citrate Magnesium hydroxide (milk of magnesia) Sodium phosphate (Fleet phospho-soda) Polyethylene glycol 3350 (MiraLax®)	Pulls water into the large intestine to soften stool and stimulate peristalsis Rapid onset: 30 minutes to 3 hours Should be used short term, no longer than 3 consecutive days	Bloating Gas Cramping Nausea Dehydration
Stimulant Examples: Senna (Senokot) Phenolphthalein (Ex-Lax) Diphenylmethane (Dulcolax®)	Stimulates the lining of the bowel causing increased peristaltic activity Considered the most powerful of the laxatives	Cramping Nausea Urine discoloration Diarrhea
Stool softener Example: Colace	Retains water within the stool and makes the stool to pass easier	Bloating Cramping Gas Bitter taste

if there is hard stool in the colon. This should be performed by gently inserting a lubricated gloved finger into the stoma lumen to assess for impaction or blockage (Tilley, 2012).

PREVENTION AND MANAGEMENT OF DIARRHEA

A person with a colostomy who experiences loose stools should first consider if this is related to ingestion of certain foods. The WOC nurse should review the patient's history of foods that caused diarrhea before surgery to create a fecal diversion. Causes of diarrhea are osmotic, mechanical, secretory, and pharmacological or a combination of factors (Tilley, 2012). It is also important to review medications and previous history. A person undergoing chemotherapy of 5-fluorouracil and irinotecan can cause diarrhea.

Some foods recommended for managing diarrhea are cheese, bananas, applesauce, marshmallows, pretzels, rice, pasta, and tapioca pudding.

BOWEL PREP

For the patient with a colostomy who is scheduled for a procedure: barium studies or colonoscopy or surgery for ostomy closure, an oral laxative such as Dulcolax®, MiraLAX, or GoLYTELY® will be prescribed (WOCN, 2011). The ostomy nurse should instruct the patient to change to a high-output pouch system or irrigation sleeve, as the patient will have increased liquid stool requiring emptying every 30 to 60 minutes. The person may also experience cramping, nausea, and gas. People with an ileostomy would not receive a bowel prep.

ILEOSTOMY

The person with an ileostomy may have the entire colon, rectum, and anus removed. The WOC nurse needs to explain to the patient that he or she has lost the absorptive function of the colon. Two complications that need to be taught to the patient to recognize are dehydration and obstruction.

DEHYDRATION

The ostomy nurse needs to teach the patient signs of dehydration: increased thirst, lethargy, muscle cramps, dry mouth, abdominal cramps, dark urine, and decreased urine output. Without the colon, electrolyte deficiency can occur. An important aspect of dietary interventions is to maintain electrolyte levels. The average daily fluid loss for ileostomy can be 1,200 mL compared to 100 to 200 mL lost by the average person with an intact colon. Dehydration can occur due to losses of sodium and potassium. The patient may need to increase his or her sodium intake. This can be done by adding high-sodium fluids/foods: broth, canned vegetables, and tomato juice. Potassium is also needed to be added to the diet. Some

foods high in potassium are bananas, potatoes, peppers, chicken, beef, and spinach. (See below for diet modification when encountering high-volume watery stools.) This should be discussed with the person's physician, and blood work should be monitored. It is important to teach the person to increase fluids especially in hot weather, or when participating in sports.

> **KEY POINT**
>
> Close monitoring and collaboration can prevent readmissions in patients with a new ileostomy.

HIGH OUTPUT AND HOSPITAL READMISSIONS

The person with a new ileostomy is at a high risk for hospital readmission for severe dehydration and renal problems. Readmission rates, as high as 20% to 40%, have been identified (Fish et al., 2017; Justiniano et al., 2018; Shaffer et al., 2017; Sy et al., 2018) within 60 days of surgery. Stankiewicz et al. (2019) reported in 6 months, 91% readmissions of patients with acute kidney failure and electrolyte disturbance. Studies have identified a need for more intense education and postoperative follow-up including reporting stoma and urine output, routine laboratory, ileostomy dehydration programs.

Guidelines proposed by Stankiewicz et al. (2019), Villafranca et al. (2015) consisted of a two-stage pathway; initial treatment consisting of restricted fluid intake, intravenous hydration, and loperamide 2 to 4 mg 30 minutes before meals, not prn. Stage two was started if high output continued after 48 to 72 hours. Loperamide was increased to 4 to 16 mg and omeprazole 20 to 40 mg added (Villafranca et al., 2015). Before starting antimotility agents, *Clostridium difficile* should be ruled out (Parrish, 2019; Villafranca et al., 2015). Other protocols have prescribed codeine 15 mg, if no improvement after stage two. Tincture of opium is another medication that can be considered for use. Parrish's (2019) medication protocol supported codeine instead of loperamide. Other recommendations included the following: fluid intake during meals should be avoided, drinks with high sugar content as well as tea, coffee and juices should be avoided, and fluid intake should be restricted to 500 to 1,000 mL/day (Villafranca et al., 2015). Oral rehydration fluids are recommended starting at 500 mL/day. Foods known to thicken stool can be included in the diet such as pretzels, pasta, rice, bananas, and applesauce. Starches and carbohydrates can slow down transit time by absorbing fluid and thicken the stool. Increasing fluids is not recommended as they will increase the volume of ileostomy output, as they are not absorbed in the small bowel. Hypertonic drinks should be avoided as they increase the stool output by pulling water into the small bowel. Bridges et al. (2019) recommend a diet of complex carbohydrates, avoiding simple sugars, drinking small amounts with meals and sipping more between meals, avoiding hypertonic fluids, limiting hypotonic fluids, and increasing salty foods. It is important that the patient is followed carefully and measures both ileostomy and urine output. Electrolytes, and renal function, are closely monitored, along with a strict intake and output. The goal is to maintain ileostomy output below 1,500 mL and a minimum of urine output at 1,200 mL. Hypomagnesemia and vitamin B_{12} absorption deficiency has been noted in long-standing ileostomies (Raju et al., 2018).

An aggressive prevention program should be established before discharge in order to prevent this serious complication. Grahn et al. (2019) studied compliance of an ileostomy education and monitoring program based on the rate of hospital readmissions for dehydration. Unfortunately, readmissions did not decrease; they did observe that weekend discharges had a higher rate of readmissions.

> **KEY POINT**
>
> Lab studies: electrolytes, renal studies and magnesium need to be routinely evaluated.

FOOD BLOCKAGE

Food blockage, or small bowel obstruction, can be partial or complete. A partial blockage can present with abdominal distention, cramping, pain, stoma edema, and watery output. A complete blockage presents with an absence of stoma output with abdominal distention, cramping, pain, and stoma edema. The following instructions can be given: take a warm bath or shower to relax abdominal muscles, a heating pad may be used, and lie on the right side and massage the peristomal area or try the knee–chest position (**Box 14-6**). Fluids can be taken if there is still some stool output; solid foods should be avoided. For most people with a food blockage, the stoma becomes edematous and the pouching system should be changed and the barrier opening made larger to accommodate the swollen stoma. If the blockage is complete, and there is no stoma output, food and fluids should not be taken, and the physician should be called and/or the patient should go to the emergency department. Once a blockage is relieved, the patient should expect that he or she will have a large volume of liquid stool (from the bowel edema) for several days and may experience some abdominal soreness.

Ileal lavage (see **Box 14-6**)—is recommended if the obstruction does not resolve. This procedure is performed by a WOC nurse or physician. A soft rubber catheter (usually a 14 to 16 Fr) is lubricated and gently inserted into the stoma up to or if possible beyond the obstruction, and 30 to 50 mL of saline is gently instilled to move the blockage. The fluid is allowed to drain, and the instillation of the fluid is continued several more times to try and

---

BOX 14-6   TEACHING HOW TO TREAT AN ILEOSTOMY BLOCKAGE

Symptoms: Thin, clear liquid output with foul odor; cramping, nausea, vomiting, abdominal pain near the stoma; decrease in amount of output; abdominal and stomal swelling.

Step One: At home

1. Cut the opening of the skin barrier of your pouching system a little larger than normal because the stoma may swell.
2. If there is some stoma output and you are not nauseated or vomiting, only consume liquids such as soft drinks, sports drinks, or tea.
3. Ambulate as walking can stimulate bowel function.
4. Take a warm bath to relax the abdominal muscles.
5. Try several different body positions, such as a knee–chest position, as it might help move the blockage forward.
6. Massage the abdomen and the area around the stoma as this might increase the pressure behind the blockage and help it to be relieved. Most food blockages occur just inside the stoma.

Step Two: If you are still blocked, are vomiting, or have no stomal output for several hours:

1. Call your doctor or WOC nurse and report what is happening and what you tried at home to alleviate the problem. Your doctor or WOC nurse will give you instructions (e.g., meet at the emergency room, come to the office). If you are told to go to the emergency room, the doctor or WOC nurse can call in orders for your care when you arrive.
2. If you cannot reach your WOC nurse or surgeon and there is **no output** from the stoma, go to the emergency room immediately.

Important: Take all of your pouch supplies (two changes at least) with you (e.g., pouch, skin barrier, accessories).

Adapted from United Ostomy Associations of America. (2020). How to treat ileostomy blockage. https://www.ostomy.org/wp-content/uploads/2020/10/Ileostomy_Blockage_2020.pdf

---

break up the blockage. This is not the same as CI. United Ostomy Associations of America (UOAA) has a card for managing an ileostomy obstruction that the patient can take to the emergency room. See Appendix: Emergency Room Staff: Ileostomy Obstruction Management.

> **KEY POINT**
>
> Ileostomy lavage should not be performed until there is a confirmed obstruction.

DIET

After surgery for an ileostomy, the person can gradually go back to his or her usual diet. Because of postop stoma edema, some patients are instructed to follow a low-residue diet (to prevent cramping or an obstruction) until the edema has subsided. Patients should be instructed to chew food thoroughly and eat slowly. High-fiber foods should be slowly added to the diet in small amounts to prevent the risk of a food blockage.

Obstruction can occur when high-fiber foods have difficulty passing through the small intestine and exiting the stoma. Some foods that can contribute to a blockage include Chinese vegetables, corn, celery, and nuts.

MEDICATIONS

An important consideration when selecting medication for the person with a stoma is the length of the small bowel available for drug absorption. Enteric-coated and sustained-release medications should be avoided by the person with high-output ileostomy or short bowel because of slow dissolution properties. People with an ileostomy are at a higher risk for suboptimal drug absorption than a person with a colostomy. The WOC nurse needs to teach the person with ileostomy to ask his or her pharmacist about medications prescribed, if they will dissolve quickly and be absorbed. Women taking birth control and estrogen replacement medication also need to check with their pharmacist.

BOWEL PREP

Any type of bowel prep that may be ordered for different diagnostic procedures or surgeries should not be given to people with ileostomies. The patient and health care clinicians need to know there is a high risk for electrolyte imbalance and dehydration with bowel prep.

ILEAL CONDUIT

Urinary diversions can have a metabolic effect, hyperchloremic metabolic acidosis along with malabsorption syndromes, such as vitamin B_{12} deficiency. Vitamin B_{12} deficiency may not be clinically apparent until 2 to 5 years after the surgery (Reddy & Kader, 2018). Some patients complain of diarrhea; this can be due to diminished bile salt and fat absorption. See Chapter 8 for more information on complications.

Because a continent urinary diversion uses a longer segment of small bowel, there is a greater chance of metabolic changes when compared to the patient with an ileal conduit. Urinary calculi are another possible complication in the patient with an ileal conduit. Long-term follow-up of individuals with urinary diversions is strongly recommended not only from an oncologic but also from a metabolic perspective (Reddy & Kader, 2018; Stein & Rubenwolf, 2014).

Urine should be kept acidic. The presence of crystals on stoma and/or peristomal skin is caused by urine alkalosis and can lead to pseudoverrucous lesions. See Chapter 16 for management of this condition. Alkaline urine can also cause urinary tract infection (UTI) and renal calculi. The patient should to be taught signs of a UTI odor, discolored urine, back pain, fever, and chills.

There is no specific diet for a person with a urinary diversion. However, it is important to teach the need for adequate fluid intake. Recommended fluid intake is 1,500 to 2,000 mL/day. Unsweetened cranberry juice or capsules can help to keep the urine more acidic, which can decrease crystal formation and may decrease the risk of a UTI. Cranberry juice or capsules have been shown to be beneficial in preventing UTI (Luczak & Swanoski, 2018). Cranberry juice should have no additives. There is no consensus on the dosage of the cranberry tablets or capsules, and further studies are needed.

Orange and grapefruit juice should be avoided as they may cause alkaline urine.

People who are on anticoagulants (warfarin) should avoid cranberry products because of interference with the blood levels of the anticoagulants. Certain foods and medications can discolor urine and produce strong odor. Foods that cause urine odor are fish, broccoli, beer, and asparagus. Antibiotics may cause odor in urine. Foods that may change the color of urine are beets and foods containing dye.

STENT MANAGEMENT (UROSTOMY)

Preoperatively, the WOC nurse should teach the patient that stents will be exiting the urostomy. The purpose of the stents is to maintain patency and to allow the ureteral/conduit anastomosis to heal. Sometimes, the surgeon will identify the right from the left stent in some manner; that is, different color stents or cutting on end of the stent straight across and the other obliquely. These are left in place up to 10 days but may be left in longer depending upon the surgeon's preference and the patient's ability to heal.

Stents may fall out, and the patient is instructed not to consider this an emergency. Care must be taken when changing the pouching system not to pull on the stents, as they can migrate and become longer. As the stents lengthen, they may require coiling the stent to place in the pouch due to antireflux valve. The urologist may agree that the ostomy nurse should trim the stents as they become too long. It is important that they are cut correctly to distinguish the right from the left ureter. A two-piece pouching system may help in managing the stents as it is easier to place in the pouch once the skin barrier is applied and then applying the pouch once the seal is secure. The WOC nurse should explain that it will be normal to have mucus in the urine and on the stoma postoperatively but it will decrease over time.

KEY POINT

Stents are not to be irrigated.

Night drainage systems are recommended so that the patient does not have to have his or her sleep disturbed by having to empty the urostomy pouch during the night. An adapter is placed on the nighttime drainage collector to allow attachment of the collector to the pouch. Each manufacturer has a specific adapter to make the connection. Most pouches have a capacity of

350 mL before they must be emptied, whereas a night drainage system has a capacity of 2,000 mL. However, some people worry about having the tubing become twisted or restricted by the system and prefer not to use the night drainage system. Leg straps can be used to secure the tube to prevent twisting. Placing the night drainage system at the bottom of the bed, rather than on the side, may lessen the chances of twisting of the tube. The nighttime bag should be replaced every 15 days.

KEY POINT

Medicare covers two nighttime urinary drainage systems per month.

A leg bag may also be connected to the end of the pouch; this will provide an extra 500-mL capacity. This is an option for people who are traveling and may not have access to a toilet for long period of time. However, some people who use a leg bag find that the leg bag pulls on the pouch adhesive (in various positions) and may not opt to use it. All the individuals should be given information about leg bags and encouraged to make their own decisions whether or not to use them.

The WOC nurse should review the medications the patient is taking for any side effects that would cause urine discoloration or odor. Some medications can change the color of urine, including the following:

- Cascara: black color
- Doxorubicin: red color
- Metronidazole: initially red and then turns to brown
- Antibiotics: strong odor
- Sulfonamides: greenish-blue color

There may be a need to obtain a urine specimen from the ileal conduit. WOCN® has published a procedure for obtaining urine specimen. (Refer to WOCN Best Practice Obtaining Urine Specimen from Ileal Conduit, Appendix D.)

Urine specimen from an ileal conduit may be obtained by catheterization of the stoma or collected by the urine dripping from the stoma into a sterile specimen container or a clean urostomy pouch (Vaarala, 2018). Ideally the recommendation has been to collect the urine specimen by catheterizing the stoma. However, a catheter may not be available or the nurse is not comfortable in performing this procedure. Vaarala (2018) compared the three methods of collecting a urine specimen from an ileal conduit diversion and found no significant difference in the results.

 PELVIC EXENTERATION

Pelvic exenteration (PE) is a devastating, extensive surgery that will impact both physical, psychological and quality of life (Nelson et al., 2018). Careful selection and

counseling of a patient and family about the risk and long-term issues related to the surgery is important. A multidisciplinary team approach pre- and postoperatively as well as long-term follow-up are indicated. PE is an extensive long surgical procedure with the risk of complications. However, with the advent of robotically assisted laparoscopy, this surgical approach has reduced surgical time, hospital days, and complications (Xuan et al., 2018). Newer surgical techniques can now reduce the incidence of creating diversions. Women identified feeling socially isolated in regard to having ostomies due to the fear of odor and leakage.

Pelvic exenteration is an aggressive, extensive surgery that involves removal of all pelvic organs: reproductive organs, colon, rectum, bladder, distal ureters, and surrounding lymphatics (see Chapter 4). This surgery is a palliative option, more common for women with cervical cancer. Women may choose to have vaginal reconstruction to improve their quality of life. There are various reconstructive surgical techniques for creating a neovagina.

 IMPACT OF AN OSTOMY

The goals of successful adaptation to an ostomy are to restore or improve the lifestyle the person had before the surgery. This process begins in the period before surgery and continues throughout the postoperative period where the person must learn new self-care techniques and adjust to changes and a lack of control of body functions. Level of psychosocial adaptation to the ostomy is known to be a predictor of quality of life in the future (Zhang et al., 2019). In the immediate postoperative period, the patient's ability to learn ostomy care is complicated by the need to accept and integrate the fact that the ostomy is present, recover from surgery, and decrease length of stay (Grant et al., 2013). The WOC nurse can help facilitate transition and adaptation to these changes. Knowledge about self-care is an important factor in adjustment to the ostomy, and the WOC nurse can play a pivotal role in patient education. Issues of social isolation, sleep disturbances, sexual dysfunction, and financial concerns have all been identified (Kenderian et al., 2013) in the postoperative period. It is important to discuss the potential for functional problems, psychosocial needs, and anxiety (Jin et al., 2019) during preoperative counseling to allow the patient to begin to adjust to the changes and to assess for these after surgery to facilitate adaptation.

A preoperative appointment with a WOC nurse is very valuable in addressing any fears, anxiety, and uncertainty the patient and family may have. Providing information on what to expect before and after surgery and the medical diagnosis, education, and encouragement can help decrease uncertainty and facilitate adaptation to the ostomy (Riemenschneider, 2015) (see Chapter 10).

STAGES OF ADAPTATION PROCESS

Borwell (2009) defines some milestones of psychological recovery such as beginning to look at and touch the stoma, then allowing others to look at the stoma, expressing interest, asking questions about care, beginning to take responsibility for aspects of stoma care, and finally, socializing with others. Ostomy patients adjust differently, so an individualized plan of care is vital. Gemmill et al. (2010) found that it took from many months to up to 10 years for patients to adjust and accept their urinary diversions.

The ability to adapt and adjust to an ostomy is a significant factor in how well a person can accept these changes in his or her life. Successful adaption to an ostomy is defined by Thorpe et al. (2016) as the process of recoordination of body, self, and the external world. Care planning to facilitate adaptation to the ostomy can be guided by the use of a theoretical framework such as the Roy Adaptation Model (Roy, 2009) or Orem's Self-Care Model (Orem et al., 2001). According to Roy, the level of adaptation will affect a person's ability to respond positively or negatively to situations. Roy (2009) described people as adaptive systems with biological and physical processes that are used to adjust effectively to changes in the environment. The two processes for individual coping are the cognator and regulator subsystems, which are integrated life processes that are manifested in a person's behavior. The cognator subsystem include four cognitive–emotive channels of perceptual and information processing, learning, judgment, and emotion (Roy, 2009). According to Roy (2009), the process of adaptation is initiated when input or stimuli from the environment (internal or external) provoke a response in the human system. Three classifications of input or stimuli are identified in this model. The first classification is the focal stimulus or stimuli that are immediately affecting the system. Focal stimuli may be internal or external, and the system is aware of their presence. The contextual stimuli are all other stimuli that contribute to the effect of the focal stimulus, including age, gender, race, education level, insurance coverage, diagnosis, and household living situation. The residual stimuli are unknowns related to the presence of having an ostomy (Roy, 2009). The behaviors that result from the control processes of the regulator–cognator subsystem are observed in four adaptive modes (Roy, 2009) that are the physiologic, self-concept, role function, and interdependence modes. Roy defined the physiologic mode as "the physical and chemical processes involved in the function and activities of living organisms" (p. 89). Elimination is one of five physiologic needs in this mode. According to Roy, physiological integrity or the degree of wholeness attained by adapting to changes in elimination is necessary for individual health and functioning.

Roy (2009) describes the self-concept mode as "the composite of beliefs and feelings held about oneself that is formed from perceptions of others' reactions" (p. 95). It is made up of two subsystems, the physical self and personal self. A person views his or her physical self as a physical being with traits that include bodily appearances, bodily functions, sexuality, healthy states, and illness states. Feelings about the physical self may influence adjustment to having a permanent ostomy, so body image should be assessed.

The ability to engage in self-care activities is reflected in the role function mode (Roy, 2009). How individuals relate with others and the quality of one's support systems constitute the interdependence mode. The level of social engagement was measured to reflect effective or ineffective interdependence mode adjustment.

Orem's theory (2001) consists of three interrelated theories described as self-care theory, self-care deficit theory, and nursing system theory. Self-care theory describes why people act to take care of themselves. This is a learned behavior developed by active participation in self-care. Orem et al. (2001) define the ability to participate in self-care as self-care agency. The self-care deficit theory defines when nursing is necessary to assist the patient with self-care. This can be determined by a thorough nursing assessment. Nursing systems theory describes the different relationships between the patient and the nurse to meet self-care needs. Orem et al. (2001) describe nursing agency as meeting the self-care needs of the patient while assisting the patient to develop self-care behaviors. Nursing agency occurs in three systems (Orem et al., 2001). The wholly compensatory system occurs when the patient is unable to perform effective self-care activities, so the nurse performs the care. The partly compensatory system occurs when then the patient participates in self-care but cannot meet all self-care demands. In the supportive-education system, the patient is able to perform self-care, so the nurse promotes this.

Orem's theory (2001) uses a three-step nursing process that directs the nurse to use effective interventions to develop effective solutions. Nursing diagnosis and prescription can be determined by assessing the ostomy patient's self-care demands and self-care agency. Design for regulatory operation involves selecting interventions that promote self-care agency and developing a plan to implement these interventions. This includes encouraging the patient to look at the stoma and verbalize concerns about the ostomy. Production and management of nursing systems includes reassessment and modifying interventions as the patient progresses toward self-care.

FACTORS AFFECTING ABILITY TO ADAPT

There are many factors that impact adaptation to the ostomy. These include the diagnosis that necessitated the ostomy, age, social support, and self-care ability. Zhang et al. (2019) found that ability to take care of the ostomy and absence of leaking and complications had better adaptation to living with an ostomy. Psychosocial needs of ostomy patients can be met by identifying and monitoring those who experience difficulty adjusting to the ostomy and isolating the problem unique to the person (Simmons et al., 2009). The role of religion/spirituality in the ostomy patient's life can be used for support. Li et al. (2012) found that spiritual well-being was associated with psychosocial adjustment to the ostomy.

> **KEY POINT**
>
> The WOC nurse should work with the patient to develop goals for successful adaptation to the ostomy.

There are many tools available to measure adjustment to an ostomy. One example is the Ostomy Adjustment Inventory-23 (OAI-23), a 23-item self-report tool that assesses psychosocial adjustment to an ostomy (Simmons et al., 2009). The Ostomy Adjustment Scale (OAS) is a 34-item tool to measure psychological and social adjustment and another example of a way for the WOC nurse to assess adjustment (Olbrisch, 1983).

Self-Esteem/Coping Skills

Williams (2012) and Salome and Almaida (2014) found that altered body image and low self-esteem were present in people with ostomies. Once the initial stress of the surgery and recovery is resolved, body image, physical appearance, and sexuality become greater concerns. Identification of coping skills used for other life stressors may help the patient with a new ostomy apply these skills to adapting to the ostomy. Gemmill et al. (2010) found gender differences in psychological well-being with women having significantly lower scores than did men and found that over 75% of participants had difficulty adjusting to the ostomy. The average participant had undergone surgery 9 years prior to the study, concluding that many people have long-term difficulties with ostomy adaptation. They also found that mastering self-care was an important part of adjustment to the ostomy.

Self-Efficacy

Self-efficacy, related to the presence of an ostomy, is the person's belief that he or she can accomplish self-care or competent care related to the ostomy (Bandura, 1997). The WOC nurse can help the patient identify and prioritize concerns. Initial goals can then be set to enhance self-management behaviors. Ercolano et al. (2016) found that management of an ostomy is multidimensional and changing. Initial goal setting should be related to physical care and later goals related to social roles such as return to work and travel.

Past Experience with Ostomy/Expectations

Identification of previous experiences with ostomy and exploring expectations of the person anticipating ostomy surgery are needed in a baseline assessment. Preoperative counseling should include an assessment of how the disease has affected his or her functional abilities, lifestyle, and sexuality. Negative previous experiences with an ostomy can result in anxiety and fear in the person facing surgery. Exploration of the details of this and education about current management strategies can help allay fears. Anticipation of the change in body function and body image by forward planning allows the ostomy patient to predict the loss and assume a more positive approach that will promote adjustment (Borwell, 2009). The person who has undergone emergency surgery has not had that opportunity prior to surgery, so this should be considered in the postoperative period.

Support Provided by Significant Others

The WOC nurse should discuss the amount of involvement of family or significant others and determine from the patients if this meets their needs. Including significant caregivers in ostomy teaching can ease transition from hospital to home, ease fears, and facilitate adaptation for the patient with a new ostomy.

Assistance Provided by Health Care Team/WOC Nurse

The WOC nurse and the multidisciplinary team including the surgeon, dietician, nursing, and discharge planners collaborate with the patient to provide education, psychosocial support, physical care, management of complications, and long-term follow-up. Referral to home care agency for visiting nurse care after discharge from acute care is very helpful. Specific product information should be given at discharge from acute care to facilitate transition to other care settings.

Impact of Ostomy Visitor

The support of an ostomy visitor can be invaluable to the patient undergoing a new ostomy procedure. Ostomy visitors are former patients who have an ostomy and have received specialized training, so they can assist the patient's transition to living with an ostomy, and share experiences, although this should not substitute for professional medical advice in any way. Many take advantage of online resources for support and education (see Appendix B).

Ostomy support groups can enhance recovery from surgery and promote adaptation by providing an atmosphere of acceptance and mutual respect and helping to develop coping skills to manage day-to-day life with an ostomy. These groups provide peer support and role modeling for people with ostomies. Many WOC nurses facilitate ostomy support groups or provide support and serve as a resource. The WOC nurse also can encourage patient participation in these groups as they follow the patient through his or her pre- and postoperative course (Cross & Hottenstein, 2010). Evidence shows that participation in an ostomy support group decreases hospital readmissions and emergency department visits (Rojana-sarot, 2018) and positively impacts a person's ability to cope and manage his or her stoma (Perrin, 2019). Social media has also become a presence for support and information for the person with an ostomy.

> **KEY POINT**
>
> The WOC nurse should provide support and be a resource for the ostomy support group.

Age/Developmental Stage

Knowledge about the lifespan, developmental stage, and basic human characteristics assist the nurse to make an accurate assessment of the individual's psychosocial needs (Sirota, 2006a,b). An adolescent with a new ostomy will have different challenges than an adult in a stable married relationship in terms of sexuality, body image, and socialization (Sirota, 2006a,b). Mohr and Hamilton (2016) identified in a small study of adolescents that one of their many concerns was disclosure. They developed an "inner circle" of ostomy friends that was their resource when having any ostomy problems or questions. Nursing care must be individualized to the person's situation for best results. The psychosocial phase of adolescence is described by Erickson as identity versus role confusion where altered body image and appearance are the focus. They may also fear loss of sexual function and inability to have a normal relationship (Cengiz & Bahar, 2017). The WOC nurse must ensure privacy for the patient and consider using a low-profile appliance to ensure that the appliance is concealed under clothing. Elastic-type support garments are available to secure the ostomy system. Facilitating an ostomy visitor who is the same age is often beneficial.

For the young adult, intimacy versus isolation is the focus of this phase. The ostomy patient may fear rejection or commitment at the time when long-term relationships may develop. Support of the patient by family and significant others can facilitate adaptation. Educating and including the significant other can allay fears of both partners. Partners sometimes have fears of hurting the patient or the stoma that can be allayed with open communication.

The focus of the middle-aged adult in Erickson's model is generativity versus stagnation. Fears of loss of occupation or spouse and role changes dominate this phase. Assessment of job role and how care of ostomy will impact this are important in the preoperative phase. Does the patient travel? Is heavy lifting required? What are the bathroom facilities like in the work setting? These discussions will help the patient and nurse determine individualized management strategies to ease the transition back to work.

For the older adult, integrity versus despair is the phase. At this stage, loss of spouse and independence, loneliness, and change in living environment are the primary concerns. Physiologic and psychological changes related to the ostomy are compounded by other medical problems. Maintaining a positive attitude, continuing the usual daily routine, not allowing the ostomy to interfere with normal life, and preventing social isolation are helpful in the elder (Santos et al., 2019). Brief frequent teaching sessions with small amounts of information work well for the elder. Assessing and modifying care for the ostomy patient are important for adaptation. The WOC nurse must assess individual needs, attitudes, ability for self-care, and capacity to identify and manage problems. Does the patient have arthritis or other conditions affecting mobility? Are vision and memory adequate for self-care?

> **KEY POINT**
>
> It is important to include another family member during the teaching sessions.

SEXUAL FUNCTION

POTENTIAL IMPACT OF PELVIC DISSECTION ON SEXUAL FUNCTION

Pelvic surgery, cancer, and radiation therapy can have a short- or long-term impact on sexual health (Saracco et al., 2019). Men can develop erectile dysfunction, retrograde ejaculation, and loss of libido, while women can experience loss of desire, dyspareunia, and vaginal dryness, (Sutsunbuloglu & Vural, 2018) after ostomy surgery. The shape and angle of the vaginal vault change when the rectum is removed. Erectile dysfunction can be temporary or permanent. Men with urinary diversions have a high rate of erectile dysfunction. Pelvic radiation may also cause symptoms of vaginal stenosis and dryness. Vaginal lubricants are helpful for some women as is experimentation with different positions to determine which is most comfortable.

Research shows that many people with ostomies experience sexual dysfunction and that many health care providers don't bring up the topic (Sarocco et al., 2019; Sutsunbuloglu & Vural, 2018). Sarocco et al. (2019) found that 50% of the patients in their study were not informed about the effect of the surgery on sexual activity. This has a negative effect on quality of life that can be prolonged (Saracco et al., 2019; Sutsunbuloglu & Vural, 2018).

The WOC nurse should reassure the patient that giving and receiving sexual pleasure can continue to be a part of his or her life, even if different because of bodily changes after ostomy surgery.

POTENTIAL IMPACT OF THE OSTOMY ON BODY IMAGE/SEXUAL RELATIONSHIPS

Concerns about appearance of the stoma and ostomy system, odor, noise, potential for leakage, physical changes, fatigue, and sexual dysfunction may occur, often after the acute phase of surviving the illness (Gonzalez et al., 2016). Careful assessment, guidance, validation of experiences, education about disease and impact on sexual health, and referrals when indicated form the basis of the WOC nurse role in this area of care (Junkin & Beitz, 2005). A baseline preoperative assessment of sexual functioning will assist the WOC nurse to identify postoperative concerns. Basic suggestions for managing sexual relations should be given to the patient and partner including being prepared for sexual activity by having a clean, secure, and empty pouching system and maintaining open and clear communication between partners (Junkin & Beitz, 2005).

The stoma should never be used for sexual purposes. Firm objects may damage the bowel or mucocutaneous junction, cause bleeding, and cause possible scarring and constriction since the bowel does not distend like the rectum. Stimulation of the stoma will not produce the pleasurable response that may be experienced with stimulation of the anal area as the stoma is not an erogenous area.

COUNSELING MODELS

Permission, Understanding-Limited Information, Specific Suggestions, Intensive Therapy (PLISSIT) (Anon, 1976) provides four levels of response to issues with sexual health and encourages the nurse to intervene at the level he or she is most comfortable with. WOC nurses should be able to function at permission and limited information stage (Junkin & Beitz, 2005). It is important for the WOC nurse to be aware of his or her own personal attitudes and values toward sexuality in order to identify sexual health needs in their patients (Ayaz, 2009; Junkin & Beitz, 2005). Understanding anatomy and physiology of male and female reproductive system and nervous system function will help to teach patients about bodily changes.

The permission stage is a beginning exploratory phase that provides a person an opportunity to share questions or sexual concerns. Active listening and sensitivity are needed to assist the patient to express concerns or questions (Borwell, 2009). The use of open-ended questions, such as asking how the ostomy has affected relationship with the partner or what kind of changes the patient has experienced in his or her sexual life will encourage the patient to discuss and ask questions (Ayaz, 2009). It is important to instruct the patient that other ostomy patients may have the same problems he or she is experiencing.

The understanding-limited information phase allows the nurse to assess if there are any difficulties and if a referral to a WOC nurse is required. A sexual history, identification of problems and goals, and expectations of the patient should be identified so an action plan can be developed (Borwell, 2009). Interventions at this level are geared toward increasing the patient's knowledge level in areas such as treatment side effects, emotional changes, and sexuality (Ayaz, 2009).

The WOC nurse can provide reassurance in the specific suggestion phase. Written information on sexuality can be provided. The United Ostomy Associations of America (UOAA) has many resources including Intimacy after Ostomy Surgery, available on their Web site www.ostomy.org.

Pouch covers, mini-pouches, and specialized underwear are available that can conceal and support the pouching system during intimacy. Internet search or ostomy supply catalogs have many options for undergarments to meet personal preferences. (See Appendix C.)

The intensive therapy stage usually involves WOC nurse involvement to address possible psychological, interpersonal, or physical needs. The WOC nurse should be aware of appropriate resources and refer as needed (Anon, 1976).

The Ex-PLISSIT model (Taylor & Davis, 2006) differs from the PLISSIT model in that permission giving is a key element in each of the stages of the model, so that all interventions begin with permission giving. Reflection and review follows all interventions (Taylor & Davis, 2006). This ensures that patient needs are met and the nurse continues to learn. Self-reflection by the WOC nurse regarding personal attitudes and beliefs may be helpful in determining which stage of the sexuality models he or she is most comfortable in.

PREGNANCY

Women with a fecal or urinary diversion can become pregnant and have a normal pregnancy. The female patient who has had an ileostomy may be advised to wait a year after surgery to consider becoming pregnant. Many women with an ileostomy have successful pregnancy delivered by the vaginal route.

Management of the ostomy during pregnancy must take into consideration the changing abdominal contour and stoma dimensions. The WOC nurse should be available to assess and recommend changes in ostomy system during the person's pregnancy (Seligman et al., 2011). As the abdomen increases in size, it may become too difficult see the stoma. A partner may need to be taught to assist with ostomy care when the person cannot manage stoma care. Stoma prolapse is another possible complication with the changing body contour and increased abdominal pressure.

If iron is prescribed during pregnancy let the patient know that it can change the color of the stool or urine and there is no harm related to this.

Most females who have ulcerative colitis are in the childbearing age and are concerned when having an ileal pouch anal anastomosis (IPAA) whether they can have a safe pregnancy. As the fetus develops, the woman may experience perianal irritation, frequency and urgency, and nocturnal incontinence (Perry-Woodford, 2008). Some of the literature differs on recommendation of vaginal or cesarean delivery. Some surgeons recommend a cesarean section in order to avoid risk of injury to the anal sphincter; however, there is little evidence to support this practice. Studies have found that vaginal delivery appears as safe as cesarean delivery for most females with IPAA. However, there is limited information on long-term function of the pouch in women who have had vaginal deliveries.

Contraception

Women with an ileostomy should be advised that contraceptive pills may be less effective (Oxford University Hospital, 2016). The birth control pills may not be absorbed with loose, ileostomy effluent. It is important for the patient to discuss this with her health care provider, and she may consider another birth control method. It is good practice to advise the patient to check also with her pharmacist.

MORBID OBESITY

The care of the obese patient having ostomy surgery presents a challenge both pre- and postoperatively.

Preoperative stoma siting is a challenge to identify an optimal location for the stoma with the goal of the patient being independent in his or her ostomy care. The ideal site recommended is the upper abdomen above the umbilicus as the patient cannot see his or her lower abdomen. Also the upper abdomen is thinner above the umbilicus making it easier for the surgeon to create a well-vascularized stoma. The surgeon may request that the site be marked at both above and below the umbilicus (Beck, 2011).

Postoperatively, the obese person is at higher risk for complications: mucocutaneous separation, parastomal hernia, stoma retraction, and prolapse (Beck, 2011). Colwell (2014) found that the data were inconsistent on the impact obesity has on surgical risks. Braumann et al. (2019) found that patient with a BMI > 40 had an 88.9% rate of complications after emergency surgery and 66.9% rate with elective procedures and the complications were more severe than those with normal BMI. BMI > 30 was an independent risk factor for stoma retraction, skin irritation, and parastomal hernia.

The WOC nurse should be sensitive to the patient's needs when assessing and teaching the obese person. Time must be taken in having the patient find the best position when performing ostomy care. A floor-length mirror on the back of the bathroom door may work well for the patient at home. The WOC nurse in home care has the advantage of assessing the patient's bathroom to make practical suggestions.

END OF LIFE

One of the goals for a person with a fecal and/or urinary diversion is to be independent in his or her ostomy care. However, if the patient's condition changes due to terminal condition or dementia, the WOC nurse will need to help identify a responsible person who can take over the ostomy care when the patient is no longer able to physically manage his or her care. The person with dementia will demonstrate a loss of memory and cognitive and functional skills by not knowing when and how to empty his or her pouch. The role of the WOC nurse is to develop and teach the caregiver the skills for ostomy care that will not overwhelm him or her by providing simple and clear instructions.

Progressive diseases such as Parkinson's, ALS, multiple sclerosis, and dementia will gradually cause functional impairment and lessening cognitive skills. Motor, sensory, and vision can become impaired resulting in the patient needing assistance in his or her ostomy care.

As the patient's condition deteriorates, there may be weight loss that will change the abdominal plane and stoma. The occurrence of tumors and fungating wounds can create a challenge to provide an ostomy pouching system with a good seal. Where needed, the WOC nurse will need to measure the stoma and recommend a new pouching system that will fit better. Catheterization schedules may need to be adjusted in the person with a continent diversion. In the case of abdominal ascites, the ostomy system will also need to be reevaluated for a different system.

The person with end-stage cancer may encounter metastasis to the liver that can result in peristomal varices. With this condition, the caregivers will need to be aware of the risk of bleeding and how to manage it (see Chapter 16). A two-piece system should not be used that would cause pressure on the varices. The patient or caregiver should be instructed to remove the system very gently to avoid trauma. A liquid skin barrier wipe can be used to provide added protection.

Obstruction and constipation may occur related to the disease process, and the caregiver needs to be aware of these conditions and when to call for help. Pickard et al. (2018) studied the effect of palliative ostomy surgery for nonresectable advanced colorectal cancer. The surgery was offered to help reduce symptoms of bowel obstruction and improve quality of life for short life expectancy.

Many strategies can be implemented to provide a simple procedure for the caregivers to follow: moldable barriers, precut barriers, close end, and/or Velcro pouch closure. The person with ileal conduit or high-output ileostomy can be managed with connecting the pouch to a larger capacity drainage system that will not require frequent emptying of the pouch. Indwelling catheters may need to be considered in the person unable to self-catheterize a continent urinary diversion.

COGNITIVE DEFICITS

Cognitive changes are usually associated with the older adult. The WOC nurse when teaching the older person needs to allow more time for the patient to process and understand the information. The degree of memory impairment should be assessed and the patient's teaching plan tailored to meet his or her needs. It may be necessary to involve a family member. Written material along with prompts should be given to the patient to review at home (Falvo, 2011).

Psychomotor assessment should be conducted before starting ostomy teaching. This would include motor coordination, muscle strength, energy level, and sensory acuity. Resources such as occupational therapy can help with techniques to facilitate ostomy management skills. There may be cognitive changes associated with aging that may affect the speed at which the person can process the information, working memory, and recall.

The person with learning disabilities will need to have short teaching sessions involving repeating and reinforcing the tasks to learn and demonstrate. It is important to set short-term goals and respect the uniqueness of each individual.

The severely mentally ill person may benefit from using the Makaton signs and symbols as a form of communication. This form of communication uses pictures, signs and symbols, real objectives, photographs, and written word. This teaching option is also used in young children. The pictures and symbols are placed on a large ring for the child to use for communication. With the adult, a scrapbook is more appropriate. Many times, recreational therapy or physical therapy departments are excellent resources for teaching repetitive, physical tasks.

CHEMOTHERAPY AND RADIATION THERAPY

Fecal and/or urinary diversion surgery for cancer of colon and/or bladder may not be the only type of treatment. The patient may need to receive chemotherapy and/or radiation therapy, sometimes preoperatively as well as postoperative. It is important that the WOC nurse understands the effects that chemotherapy and/or radiation therapy can have on a patient with a diversion.

Treatment with chemotherapy is designed for cure, control or palliation and is classified as:

- Single agent
- Combination therapy—use of two or more drugs to produce additive or synergistic effects
- Neoadjuvant—given before surgery to provide optimal tumor removal or cosmesis
- Adjuvant—treatment given after surgery aimed at any remaining cancer cells

- Concurrent chemoradiation—chemotherapy sensitizes tumor cells to radiation.
- Systemic chemotherapy—absorbed and distributed by bloodstream, exerts effects widely. Given orally or IV
- Regional chemotherapy—chemotherapy delivered to the site of the tumor

CHEMOTHERAPY

Common side effects associated with chemotherapy are diarrhea, nausea and vomiting, fatigue, mucositis, anemia, peripheral neuropathy, and palmar–plantar syndrome known as "hand and foot syndrome." The patient with a fecal diversion undergoing chemotherapy will need to be taught to expect changes in bowel output. Patients who receive postoperative chemotherapy are more likely to experience peristomal moisture–associated skin damage. Nagano et al. (2019) found this occurred two times more frequently in a postoperative ostomy patient who was receiving chemotherapy than one who wasn't. People with loop ileostomies are more likely to experience leakage, increased night time output, and odor (Oliphant et al., 2015).

The WOC nurse will need to advise patients on the possibility of changing their current pouch system to another one to manage diarrhea in order to avoid risk of leakage and peristomal skin problems. A person who has been using a closed-ended pouch will need to change to a drainable pouch, and the pouch will need to be emptied more often. If the colostomy is being managed with irrigation procedure, the patient needs to be advised to wear a pouch system and may have to discontinue irrigation during chemo and radiation therapy. Stoma edema may occur, and the pouch opening will need to accommodate this change. The person with an ileostomy is at high risk for dehydration from the side effects of nausea, vomiting, and diarrhea. He or she will need to be taught to maintain adequate fluid and food intake. High-calorie, high-protein, low-residue foods should be encouraged and high-fiber and fatty foods avoided while experiencing diarrhea. Antidiarrheals can be given to help manage the volume and thicken the consistency of the stoma output. Education should include contacting the provider immediately for increased output above usual daily parameters.

Medications may be recommended to manage diarrhea, nausea, and vomiting. The person may find that he or she cannot tolerate his or her normal diet and may have difficulty in maintaining an adequate nutrition and hydration. Antiemetic should be given before the chemotherapy begins.

Oxaliplatin, chemotherapy agent for colorectal cancer, can have a side effect of peripheral neuropathy (numbness in hands and feet). Hand and foot syndrome is a side effect of 5-fluorouracil (chemotherapy agent for colorectal cancer). Manual dexterity can be affected by both these side effects, and the person with a stoma may have difficulty changing and emptying the pouch. The WOC nurse will need to recommend another pouch system the patient can manage better or teach a caregiver to assist the patient in his or her care. Drott et al. (2019) studied the neurotoxic side effect of oxaliplatin on patients being treated for colorectal cancer. All patients reported a negative effect on their quality of life and daily activities. Raphael et al. (2017) reported that patients over 65 years receiving oxaliplatin had an increase in toxicity.

Mucositis/Stomatitis

Stomatitis is an oral inflammatory condition related to use of target therapies. Mucositis, also chemotherapy or radiation induced, is painful inflammation and ulceration of the mucosa lining of the GI tract; it can involve the mouth, the small intestine, or the rectal mucosa. The patient needs to be taught to practice gentle care of the stoma, as edema and friability of stoma can be common. Patients undergoing chemotherapy and radiation therapy need to also have assessment of their mouth. Oral hygiene is very important. Teach the patient to use a soft toothbrush and antibacterial mouthwash. Topical protective agents such as orabase, lidocaine, magic mouthwash, frequent mouth rinses, and pain medications may be indicated. Foods that are bland, cool, and softer in consistency may be tolerated better with chemotherapy agents commonly used for bowel and bladder cancer (**Table 14-2**).

RADIATION THERAPY

Common side effects associated with radiation therapy are fatigue and radiation-induced skin changes. Skin damage is classified as erythema, dry desquamation, moist desquamation, and necrosis (rarely occurs). These do not usually appear until 4 to 6 weeks into treatment. Newer techniques of intensity modulation radiation therapy (IMRT) deliver radiation to treatment areas while decreasing the dose to normal tissue resulting in lessened toxicities from the radiation. This has been shown to improve the timely completion of chemoradiation treatments and decrease need for ostomy in a sample of 779 patients (Bryant et al., 2018).

The patient needs to be taught not to use any creams or lotions for 2 hours before treatment. Moisturizing creams containing lanolin or alcohol or petroleum-based creams should be avoided. Cleanse skin with unscented soap and pat dry gently. Use good hand-washing technique to prevent infection. Radiation treatments may need to be temporarily discontinued if marked stoma friability occurs. Ostomy irrigation should be discontinued during radiation therapy to avoid potential mechanical irritation to intestinal and stoma mucosa.

TABLE 14-2 CHEMOTHERAPY AGENTS FOR BLADDER AND COLON CANCER*

AGENT	INDICATION	ADVERSE EFFECTS
5-Fluorouracil	Colorectal cancer Bladder cancer with cisplatin for radiosensitization with RT	Diarrhea, photosensitivity, palmar–plantar erythrodysesthesia, alopecia, mucositis, cardiotoxicity (EKG changes, congestive heart failure, cardiomyopathy, angina, dysrhythmias)
Irinotecan	Colon cancer	Diarrhea, early onset, neutropenia, alopecia
Oxaliplatin	Colon cancer	Diarrhea, peripheral neuropathy, ototoxicity
Mitomycin C	Colon, rectal, and bladder cancer	Fatigue, decreased white blood cells and platelet count, hair loss, pulmonary injury (pneumonitis, pulmonary fibrosis)
Doxorubicin	Bladder cancer	Discolored or red urine, nausea and vomiting, loss of appetite, alopecia, cardiotoxicity, mucositis
Cisplatin	Bladder cancer	Nausea and vomiting, decrease in WBC and platelet count, bleeding, peripheral neuropathy, renal and ototoxicity
Capecitabine	Colon cancer—neoadjuvant	Stomach pain, loss of appetite, fatigue, dizziness, cardiotoxicity
FOLFOX (fluorouracil, oxaliplatin, leucovorin)	Stage III colon cancer—adjuvant	Fatigue, nausea and vomiting, diarrhea, neurotoxicity especially to cold, neuropathy, low RBC Leucovorin can cause oral mucositis.
CAPEOX—oxaliplatin, capecitabine	Colon cancer—adjuvant	Stomach pain, loss of appetite, fatigue, dizziness, cardiotoxicity, diarrhea, peripheral neuropathy, ototoxicity
MVAC (methotrexate, vinblastine, adriamycin, cisplatin)	Presurgery bladder cancer or advanced bladder cancer	Nausea and vomiting, decrease in WBC and platelet count, bleeding, peripheral neuropathy, renal and ototoxicity
Gemcitabine	Advanced bladder cancer with cisplatin	Nausea and vomiting, decrease in WBC and platelet count, bleeding, peripheral neuropathy, renal and ototoxicity

*Not an all-inclusive list.

PHYSICAL AND MENTAL LIMITATIONS

Preoperatively, the WOC nurse should assess the patient and his or her level of understanding about his or her surgery and any physical and mental limitations. The WOC nurse needs expertise and patience in understanding of physical, psychosocial, and emotional needs of this population. Assessment of the person who has some challenges may require some innovative techniques to promote optimal ostomy care. The WOC nurse may have to seek other resources to meet their needs.

Visually Impaired

People with limited to total vision loss are still capable of becoming independent in their ostomy care. Legally blind is defined as a person who cannot read one letter on 20/100 line. Most people who are legally blind can see shadows and shapes. However, there is limited literature on ostomy education for the visually impaired patient.

A two-piece pouching system makes it easier to apply the barrier to the stoma. Some creative techniques have been developed over the years to assist teaching the person who is visually impaired.

Whiteley (2013) describes a method for managing ileostomy output using a 30-mL syringe barrel (slightly smaller than the stoma): the barrel could be filled with cotton balls if the stoma was active. The syringe barrel is placed over the stoma to maintain a clean, dry peristomal skin, while the barrier is placed over the syringe barrel and adhered to the skin. This method can be used for both ileal conduit and colostomy.

Heale (2013) developed a cardboard tube technique for ostomy wafer placement for a stoma with persistent output (ileal conduit, ileostomy). This technique would also be appropriate for a visually impaired person. For a stoma that measured 1 inch, a 5 x 9 cm index card was used to make the tube. The card was wrapped around stoma and secured with tape. Both of these techniques would allow time to treat any peristomal skin conditions. This would also act as a guide to place the barrier for the visually impaired person. However, these techniques can be a challenge for the person with peripheral neuropathy. When developing a teaching plan for the visually impaired, it is important to have all sessions taught by the same WOC nurse and consistently taught exactly the same way.

Hearing Deficit

There are several levels of hearing loss. A person can be born deaf or may start losing his or her hearing after the age of 60. Some people may acquire a hearing aid while others choose not to have an aid. The person who is born deaf may use either sign language or lip reading. The WOC nurse needs to be aware of the person's preference for communicating. When teaching a person who is hard of hearing, face the person directly; speak slowly with short sentences in a normal tone. Use the "teach back method," and have the patient repeat back information. Allow time for the patient to ask questions and provide written instructions/information. It is helpful to have a family member present who will hear all of the education information.

Some facilities may have a sign language interpreter that can be arranged when the WOC nurse is teaching ostomy care. Another communication method available at some facilities is a live video service with sign language interpreters, called MARTTI, which stands for My Accessible Real-Time Trusted Interpreter (Sattinger, 2007). This on-demand video interpreting service is not only for the deaf or hard of hearing person but also for the person who has English as his or her second language. Over 150 languages are provided.

Spinal Cord Injury

Colostomy is many times offered to the person with a spinal cord injury (SCI) for a bowel management program or as a part of a surgical management plan for pressure injury repair or flap procedures. Boucher (2016) states that this option should be offered early after the injury to increase independence in their care. Xu et al. (2016) reported that an elective colostomy improved the quality of life for the SCI person. There was less time spent with colostomy management than with the previous bowel management program. The WOC nurse will be instrumental in providing both preoperative and postoperative education with the goal of obtaining independence in ostomy care. Important areas to assess and discuss are baseline functional status related to level of injury, dexterity, and support systems for ostomy care. The placement of the stoma should be in a location that the patient can change and empty the pouch independently if at all possible.

CULTURAL, RELIGIOUS, AND SPIRITUALITY DIVERSITY

The ostomy nurse needs to recognize different beliefs, values, and health care practices of different cultures in order to provide appropriate care for people from many multicultural backgrounds. Ayik et al. (2019) identified that spirituality is usually not identified by nursing when conducting a holistic assessment of the person's quality of life and adjustment to an ostomy. Culture and religion play an important role in psychosocial adjustment. In Jewish, Muslim, Hindu, and certain other orthodox Christian religions, an intact body and cleanliness are a requirement to perform obligatory religious rituals. It is not unusual for people from these backgrounds to initially refuse stoma surgery even when dispensations have been granted. Iqbal et al. (2016) recommended the presence of a spiritual leader along with family members for the Muslim patients, for both the preoperative and postoperative sessions. Hibbert (2016) identified a high risk for peristomal hernia formation and stoma prolapse in the Muslim person with an ostomy. This was found to be related to frequent bending (elbow knee position) during prayer. Muslim practice involves prayer ritual five times a day.

Altuntas et al. (2013) conducted a prospective study to analyze the effects of Ramadan fasting on people with a fecal stoma. Ramadan fasting is an Islamic ritual where they fast from sunrise to sunset for 30 days; this occurs in the 9th month of the Islamic calendar. Fasting can last up to 18 hours, with no food or drink. Altuntas et al. (2013) studied the effects of fasting on nutritional, metabolic status, and quality of life on people with ileostomy and colostomy. Fasting did decrease prealbumin levels, but there was no influence on quality of life. Some noted improvement in flatulence and fecal incontinence during this time period. Results of this study recommend that the decision to fast should be the patient's and the patient should not be prohibited from fasting but close follow-up may be necessary.

Some cultures and religious beliefs may view bodily excretions as polluting them and would not be willing to participate in ostomy care. The Muslim and South Asian cultures view the left hand for cleaning and hygiene and the right hand for eating and touching things (McGrath & Fulham, 2005). Only using the left hand to change the pouching system would be very difficult, and it can be suggested that they wear gloves when changing the pouch (WCET International Ostomy Guideline, 2014). Pouresmail et al. (2019) conducted a pilot study in Iran using a wearable stoma simulator for the patients with religious concerns of touching the stoma and stool output. The simulator was worn on the abdomen, over the patient's ostomy, to facilitate the patient practicing ostomy pouch change without the fear of having to touch any stool discharge. This study was conducted with Muslim patients, who believe that stool is untouchable. Once the person was comfortable with the skill, they were able to perform pouch changing on their stoma. This teaching method was found to improve the patient's adjustment and confidence in becoming independent in ostomy care. Further studies are recommended to evaluate patient's satisfaction with the simulator teaching method.

Language Barriers

Effective communication is needed for the non–English-speaking patient, or the patient will feel frustrated, angry, and isolated. Selecting a translator is important; family members should not be interpreters. Trained interpreters are usually available through organizations or arrangements within the health care setting. Some ostomy manufacturers provide education materials in languages other than English on their Web sites and upon request. More communication tools are needed to eliminate these barriers for the limited English speaking person.

The World Council of Enterostomal Therapists (WCET) International Ostomy Guidelines (2014) cites 10 countries with description of cultural and religious belief that can impact ostomy care and adjustment. Vegetarian diets used in the Hindu and Sikh religion can affect stoma output; there may be increase in output and flatus, so the patient should be advised of this effect.

Long-Term Issues with an Ostomy

The person with a fecal or urinary diversion should be seen by a health care provider and the WOC nurse yearly to assess for any problems and evaluate blood work if indicated. The WOC nurse should assess the person for any stomal and peristomal problems, discuss pouching system wear time and describe any issues they might be encountering living with a stoma. The pouching system should be removed, and the peristomal skin and stoma should be assessed. A person with an ileostomy or ileal conduit should have his or her B_{12} levels checked annually. Appliance leakage and peristomal skin complications that impact adaptation can be addressed to improve quality of life (Zhang et al., 2019). The stoma can change over time, so problems experienced may differ and need to be evaluated on an individual basis (Vonk-Klaassen et al., 2016). Weight changes and normal effects of aging may cause changes in stoma size requiring WOC nurse assessment and modification. Some patients have long-term effects of rectal cancer treatment including fatigue, neuropathy, and problems with the ostomy or sexual function (Sanoff et al., 2015), so long-term follow-up is indicated. Sun et al. (2020) found that 11% of cancer survivors with ostomies had significant challenges with ostomy management, regardless of the length of time since surgery, and recommended that support should continue from the perioperative period through long-term survivorship.

KEY POINT

It is important to ask the patient and family about cultural practices and the potential impact it may have on ostomy care, so that an effective culturally sensitive plan of care is developed.

KEY POINT

The WOC nurse should address sexuality pre- and postoperatively and refer to those with additional expertise as needed.

CONCLUSIONS

Both fecal and urinary diversions present with specific management issues that the WOC nurse needs to address when teaching the patient. The patient may have many concerns and fears related to odor, flatus, and returning to former ADLs/social life. The WOC nurse needs to provide positive support along with specific education.

Management of the ostomy patient includes ongoing assessment and teaching with the main goal of the patient becoming independent in his or her ostomy care. Factors such as adjustment, depression, anxiety, sleep difficulties, return to activities of daily living, and sexuality are major issues for the person. The WOC nurse needs to be aware of resources available in order to provide the person with different teaching and communication options to meet individual needs. Care needs to be individualized in those with special needs to promote adaptation and good quality of life. All patients deserve the best quality of life possible.

REFERENCES

Altuntas, Y. E., Gezen, F. C., Sahoniz, T., et al. (2013). Ramadan fasting in patients with a stoma: A prospective study of quality of life and nutritional structure. *Ostomy/Wound Management, 29*(5), 26–32.

Anon, J. S. (1976). The PLISSIT model: A proposed conceptual scheme for the behavioral treatment of sexual problems. *Journal of Sex Education Therapy, 2*(2), 1–15.

Ayaz, S. (2009). Approach to sexual problems of patients with stoma by PLISSIT model: An alternative. *Sexual Disability, 27*, 72–81.

Ayik, C., Ozden, D. & Cenan, D. (2019). Relationships among spiritual well-being, adjustments, and quality of life in patients with a stoma: A cross-sectional, descriptive study. *Wound Management & Prevention, 65*(5), 40–47.

Bandura, A. (1997). *Self-efficacy: The exercise of control.* New York, NY: Freeman.

Bauer, C., Arnold-Long, M., & Kent, D. (2016). Colostomy irrigation to maintain continence: An old method revived. *Nursing, 46*(8), 59–62.

Beck, D. (2017). *Temporary ostomies.* New Patient Ostomy Guideline, UOAA.

Beck, S. (2011). Stoma issues in the obese patient. *Clinics in Colon and Rectal Surgery, 24*(4), 259–262.

Borwell, B. (2009). Rehabilitation and stoma care: Addressing the psychological needs. *British Journal of Nursing, 18*(4), S20–S25.

Boucher, M. (2016). Early elective colostomy following spinal cord injury. *British Journal of Nursing, 25*(5) (Stoma Supplement), S4–S10.

Braumann, C., Muller, V., Knies, M., et al. (2019). Complications after ostomy surgery: Emergencies and obese patients are at risk—Data from the Berlin Ostomy Study (BOSS). *World Journal of Surgery, 43*, 751–757.

Bridges, M., Nasser, R., & Parrish, C. (2019). High output ileostomies: The stakes are higher than the output. *Practical Gastroenterology, XLIII*, 20–33.

Bryant, A., Huynh-Le, M., Simpson, D., et al. (2018). Intensity modulated radiation therapy versus conventional radiation for anal cancer in the veteran's affairs system. *International Journal of Radiation Oncology, Biology, Physics, 102*(1), 109–115.

Carlsson, E., Gylin, M., Nilsson, L., et al. (2010). Positive and negative aspects of colostomy irrigation. A patient and WOC Nurse perspective. *Journal of Wound, Ostomy, and Continence Nursing, 37*(5), 511–516.

Cengiz, B., & Bahar, Z. (2017). Perceived barriers and home care needs when adapting to a fecal stoma. *Journal of Wound, Ostomy, and Continence Nursing, 44*(1), 63–73.

Colwell, J. (2014). The role of obesity in the patient undergoing colorectal surgery and fecal diversion: A review of the literature. *Ostomy/Wound Management, 60*(1), 24–28.

Cross, H., & Hottenstein, P. (2010). Starting and maintaining a hospital-based support group. *Journal of Wound, Ostomy, and Continence Nursing, 37*(4), 393–396.

Drott, J., Fomichov, V., Starkhammar, H., et al. (2019). Oxaliplatin-Induced neurotoxic side effects and their impact on daily activities: A longitudinal study among patients with colorectal cancer. *Cancer Nursing, 22*(6), E40–E48.

Ercolano, E., Grant, M., McCorkle, R., et al. (2016). Applying the chronic care model to support ostomy self-management: Implications for oncology nurse practice. *Clinical Journal of Oncology Nursing, 20*(3), 269–274.

Falvo, D. (2011). *Effective patient education* (4th ed.). Sudbury: Jones and Bartlett.

Fish, D., Mancuso, C., Garcia-Aguilar, J., et al. (2017). Readmission after ileostomy creation: Retrospective review of a common and significant event. *Annals of Surgery, 265*(2), 379–387.

Gemmill, R., Sun, V., Ferrell, B., et al. (2010). Going with the flow quality of life outcomes of cancer survivors with urinary diversion. *Journal of Wound, Ostomy, and Continence Nursing, 37*(1), 65–72.

Gonzalez, E., Holm, K., Wennstrom, B., et al. (2016). Self-reported well-being and body image after abdominoperineal excision for rectal cancer. *International Journal of Colorectal Disease, 31*(10), 1711–1717.

Grahn, S., Lowry, A., Osborne, M., et al. (2019). System-wide improvement for transitions after ileostomy surgery: Can intensive monitoring of protocol compliance decrease readmissions? A randomized trial. *Diseases of the Colon & Rectum, 62*(3), 363–370.

Grant, M., McCorckle, R., Hornbrook, C., et al. (2013). Development of a chronic care ostomy self-management program. *Journal of Cancer Education, 28*(1), 70–78.

Heale, M. (2013). Cardboard tube technique for ostomy wafer placement and management of peristomal skin with persistent output. *Journal of Wound, Ostomy, and Continence Nursing, 40*(4), 424–426.

Hibbert, D. (2016). Caring for persons with ostomies in Saudi Arabia. *Journal of Wound, Ostomy, and Continence Nursing, 43*(4), 398–399.

Iqbal, F., Kujan, O., Bowely, D., et al. (2016). Quality of life after ostomy surgery in Muslim patients. *Journal of Wound, Ostomy, and Continence Nursing, 43*(4), 385–391.

Jin, Y., Zhang, J., Zheng, M., et al. (2019). Psychosocial behavior reactions, psychosocial needs, anxiety and depressions among patients with rectal cancer before and after colostomy surgery: A longitudinal study. *Journal of Clinical Nursing, 28*, 3547–3555.

Junkin, J., & Beitz, J. (2005). Sexuality and the person with a stoma implications for comprehensive WOC nursing practice. *Journal of Wound, Ostomy, and Continence Nursing, 32*(2), 121–128.

Justiniano, C., Temple, L., Swanger, A., et al. (2018). Readmissions with dehydration after ileostomy creation: Rethinking risk factors. *Diseases of the Colon & Rectum, 61*, 1297–1305.

Kenderian, S., Stephens, E. K., & Jatoi, A. (2013). Ostomies in rectal cancer patients: What is their psychosocial impact? *European Journal of Cancer Care, 23*, 328–332.

Kuczynsha, B., Bobkiewicz, A., Studniarek, A., et al. (2017). Conservative measures for managing constipation in patients living with a colostomy. *Journal of Wound, Ostomy, and Continence Nursing, 44*(2), 160–164.

Li, C., Rew, L., & Hwang, S. (2012). The relationship between spiritual well-being and psychosocial adjustment in Taiwanese patients with colorectal cancer and a colostomy. *Journal of Wound, Ostomy, and Continence Nursing, 39*(2), 161–169.

Luczak, T., & Swanoski, M. (2018). A review of cranberry use for preventing urinary tract infections in older adults. *The Consultant Pharmacist, 33*(8), 450–453.

McGrath, A., & Fulham, J. (2005). Understanding chemotherapy and radiotherapy for a person with a stoma. In T. Porrett & A. McGrath (Eds.), *Stoma care.* Oxford, UK: Blackwell.

Mohr, L., & Hamilton, R. (2016). Adolescent perspectives following ostomy surgery. *Journal of Wound, Ostomy, and Continence Nursing, 43*(5), 494–498.

Nagano, M., Ogata, Y., Ikeda, M. K., et al. (2019). Peristomal moisture-associated skin damage and independence in pouching system changes in persons with new fecal ostomies. *Journal of Wound, Ostomy, and Continence Nursing, 46*(2), 137–142.

Nelson, A., Albizu-Jacob, A., Fenech, A., et al. (2018). Quality of life after pelvic exenteration for gynecologic cancer: Findings from a qualitative study. *Psycho-oncology, 27*, 2357–2362.

Olbrisch, M. E. (1983). Development and validation of the ostomy adjustment scale. *Rehabilitation Psychology, 28*(1), 3–12.

Oliphant, R., Czerniewski, A., Robertson, I., et al. (2015). The effect of adjuvant chemotherapy on stoma-related complications after surgery for colorectal cancer a retrospective analysis. *Journal of Wound, Ostomy, and Continence Nursing, 42*(5), 494–498.

Orem, D., Taylor, S., & McLaughlin, K. (2001). *Nursing concepts of practice* (5th ed.). St Louis, MO: Mosby Year Book.

Oxford University Hospitals, Colorectal Nursing Department. (2016). Contraception and pregnancy: Information for women with a stoma. Review June, 2019. Author.

Parrish, C. (2019). High output ostomies: New evidence and best practice. Presentation at WOCN® conference, Nashville, TN.

Perrin, A. (2019). Exploring individuals' perceptions of living with a stoma. *British Journal of Nursing, 28*(16), S18–S22. doi: 10.12968/bjon.2019.29.16.S18.

Perry-Woodford, Z. (2008). Intestinal pouches. In J. Burch (Ed.), *Stoma care* (pp. 149–150). West Sussex: John Wiley & Sons Ltd.

Pickard, C., Thomas, R., Robertson, I., et al. (2018). Ostomy creation for palliative care of patients with nonresectable colorectal cancer and bowel obstruction. *Journal of Wound, Ostomy, and Continence Nursing, 45*(3), 239–241.

Pouresmail, Z., Nabavi, F., Abbdollahi, A., et al. (2019). Effect of using a simulation device for ostomy self-care teaching in Iran: A pilot randomized clinical trial. *Wound Management & Prevention, 65*(6), 30–39.

Raju, D., Sheshagiri, N., Kadarapura, S., et al. (2018). A systematic approach in the management of a high output ileostomy resulting in a favorable clinical outcome. *Anesthesiology Case Reports, 1*(1), 1–3.

Raphael, M., Fischer, H., Austin, P., et al. (2017). Neurotoxicity outcomes in population-based cohort of elderly patients treated with adjuvant oxaliplatin for colorectal cancer. *Clinical Colorectal Cancer, 16*(4), 397–404.

Reddy, M., & Kader, K. (2018). Follow-up management of cystectomy patients. *The Urologic Clinics of North America, 45*(2), 241–247.

Riemenschneider, K. (2015). Uncertainty and adaptation among adults living with incontinent ostomies. *Journal of Wound, Ostomy, and Continence Nursing, 42*(4), 361–367.

Rojanasarot, S. (2018). The impact of early involvement in a post discharge support program for ostomy surgery patients on preventable healthcare utilization. *Journal of Wound, Ostomy, and Continence Nursing, 45*(1), 43–49.

Roy, C. (2009). *The Roy adaptation model* (3rd ed.). Stamford, CT: Appleton & Lange.

Salome, G., & Almaida, S. (2014). Association of sociodemographic and clinical factors with the self-image and self-esteem of individuals with intestinal stoma. *Journal of Coloproctology, 34*, 159–166.

Sanoff, H., Morris, W., Mitcheltree, A., et al. (2015). Lack of support and information regarding long-term negative effects in survivors of rectal cancer. *Clinical Journal of Oncology Nursing, 19*(4), 444–448.

Santos, R., Silvana, M., & Dazio, E. (2019). Self-care of elderly people with ostomy by colorectal cancer. *Journal of Coloproctology, 39*(3), 265–273.

Saracco, C., Rastelli, G., Roveron, G., et al. (2019). Sexual function in patients with stoma and its consideration among their caregivers: A cross-sectional study. *Sexuality & Disability, 37*(3), 415–427.

Sattinger, A. (November 2007). Video interpreters help hospitals, patient connect. *The Hospitalist*.

Seligman, N. S., Sbar, W., & Berghella, V. (2011). Pouch function and gastrointestinal complications during pregnancy after ileal pouch-anal anastomosis. *Journal of Maternal-Fetal and Neonatal Medicine, 24*(3), 525–530.

Shaffer, V., Owi, T., Kumarusamy, M., et al. (2017). Decreasing hospital readmission in ileostomy patients: Results of novel pilot program. *Journal of the American Chemical Society, 224*(4), 425–430.

Simmons, K. L., Smith, J., & Maekawa, A. (2009). Development and psychometric evaluation of the ostomy adjustment inventory-23. *Journal of Wound, Ostomy, and Continence Nursing, 36*(1), 69–75.

Sirota, T. (2006a). Meeting the psychosocial needs of ostomy patients through therapeutic interaction. *World Council of Enterostomal Therapist Journal, 26*(2), 24–26.

Sirota, T. (2006b). Meeting the psychosocial needs of the ostomy patients through therapeutic interaction. Part II: Effective uses of nurses possessional competencies. *World Council of Enterostomal Therapist Journal, 26*(2), 5–15.

Stankiewicz, M., Gordon, J., Rivera, J., et al. (2019). Clinical management of ileostomy high-output stomas to prevent electrolyte disturbance, dehydration and acute kidney injury: A quality improvement activity. *Journal of Stomal Therapy Australia, 39*(1), 8–10.

Stein, R., & Rubenwolf, P. (2014). Metabolic consequences after urinary diversion. *Frontiers in Pediatrics, 2*, 15.

Sun, V., Bojorquez, O., Grat, M., et al. (2020). Cancer survivors' challenges with ostomy appliances and self-management: A qualitative analysis. *Supportive Care in Cancer, 28*, 1551–1554. doi: 10.007/s00520-019-05156-7. Accessed November 24, 2019.

Sutsunbuloglu, E., & Vural, F. (2018). Evaluation of sexual satisfaction and function in patients following stoma surgery: A descriptive study. *Sexuality & Disability, 36*, 349–361.

Sy, C., Stem, C., Cerullo, M., et al. (2018). Predicting the risk of readmission from dehydration after ileostomy formation: The dehydration readmission after ileostomy prediction score. *Diseases of the Colon & Rectum, 61*(12), 1410–1417.

Taylor, B., & Davis, S. (2006). Using the extended PLISSIT model to address sexual health care needs. *Nursing Standard, 21*(11), 35–40.

Thorpe, G., Arthur, A., & McArthur, M. (2016). Adjusting to bodily change following stoma formation: A phenomenological study. *Disability & Rehabilitation, 38*(18), 1791–1802.

Tilley, C. (2012). Caring for the patient with a fecal or urinary diversion in palliative and hospice settings: A literature review. *Ostomy/Wound Management, 58*(1), 24–34.

Vaarala, M. (2018). Urinary sample collection methods in ileal conduit urinary diversion patients: A randomized control study. *Journal of Wound, Ostomy, and Continence Nursing, 45*(1), 59–62.

Villafranca, J., Lopez-Rodriguez, C., Abiles, J., et al. (2015). Protocol for the detection and nutritional management of high-output stomas. *Nutritional Journal, 14*(45), 1–7.

Vonk-Klaassen, S., de Vocht, H., den Ouden, M., et al. (2016). Ostomy-related problems and their impact on quality of life of colorectal cancer ostomates: A systematic review. *Quality of Life Research, 25*, 125–133.

Whiteley, I. (2013). Educating a blind person with ileostomy; enabling self-care and independence. *Journal of Stomal Therapy Australia, 33*(3), 6–10.

Williams, J. (2012). Stoma care: Intimacy and body image issues. *Practice Nursing, 23*(2), 91–93.

World Council of Enterostomal Therapists. (2014). In K. Zulkowski, E. A. Ayello, & D. Stelton (Eds.), *WCET international ostomy guideline*. Perth, Australia: WCET.

Wound Ostomy and Continence Nurses Society™. (2011). *Bowel Prep for Patients with a Colostomy*. Mt. Laurel, NJ: Author.

Xu, J., Dharmarajan, S., & Johnson, F. (2016). Optimal colostomy placement in spinal cord injury patients. *The American Surgeon, 82*(3), 278–280.

Xuan, H., Delomenie, M., Nqo, C., et al. (2018). Pelvic exenteration by robotically-assisted laparoscopy: A feasibility series of 6 cases. *Gynecologic Oncology Reports, 25*, 56–59.

Zhang, Y., Xian, H., Yang, Y., et al. (2019). Relationship between psychosocial adaptation and health-related quality of life of patients with stoma: A descriptive, cross-sectional study. *Journal of Clinical Nursing, 28*, 2880–2888.

QUESTIONS

1. Which strategy for teaching a patient about a new stoma would the WOC nurse find most appropriate for a 12-year-old?
   A. Teach the parents or guardian the procedure first.
   B. Discuss any limitations in activities or work.
   C. Use brief, frequent teaching sessions with small amounts of information.
   D. Ensure privacy, and use a low-profile appliance.

2. A WOC nurse is using the PLISSIT model to counsel patients with new ostomies. Which level of response to issues with sexual health would be appropriate for this nurse?
   A. Permission and specific suggestions
   B. Permission and understanding-limited information
   C. Understanding-limited information and specific suggestions
   D. Specific suggestion and intensive therapy

3. A patient with colon cancer is receiving chemotherapy as a neoadjuvant treatment. The WOC nurse explains to the patient that this treatment is:
   A. The primary treatment for the cancer.
   B. The treatment given after surgery to eradicate remaining cancer cells.
   C. The treatment before surgery.
   D. The treatment is aimed at limiting effects of a cancer that cannot be cured.

4. The WOC nurse is caring for a patient who is receiving mitomycin C for rectal cancer. For which common side effects should the nurse alert the patient?
   A. Fatigue, decreased white blood cells and platelet count, hair loss
   B. Diarrhea, photosensitivity, palmar–plantar erythrodysesthesia, alopecia
   C. Stomach pain, loss of appetite, fatigue, dizziness
   D. Discolor urine red, nausea and vomiting, loss of appetite, alopecia

5. The WOC nurse would recommend colostomy irrigation (CI) as an appropriate therapy for the patient?
   A. A patient who is undergoing radiotherapy
   B. A patient with Crohn's disease
   C. A patient with a sigmoid colostomy
   D. A patient with an ileostomy

6. The WOC nurse is teaching a patient with a new colostomy how to perform colostomy irrigation (CI). Which of the following should be included in the teaching plan?
   A. Irrigation bag should be hung at waist level.
   B. Cramping is normal, and the procedure should be continued if this occurs.
   C. Irrigation should be done daily at the same time each day.
   D. Complete return of water and stool may take up to 2 hours.

7. A patient calls the WOC nurse with signs and symptoms of an ileostomy blockage. What would the nurse suggest the patient try first to move the blockage forward?
   A. Cut a new skin barrier that is a little smaller than normal to stimulate the stoma.
   B. Take a warm bath to relax the abdominal muscles.
   C. Consume foods high in fiber for a day.
   D. Remain in a knee–chest position for 20 minutes to try to move the blockage.

8. A patient with an ileostomy reports the following symptoms: no stomal output, cramping abdominal pain, nausea, and abdominal distention. The emergency room (ED) nurse notes no bowel sounds on auscultation. After contacting the patient's surgeon or WOC nurse, the ED staff should:
   A. Give patient small sips of warm water
   B. Start IV antibiotics
   C. Obtain an abdominal x-ray
   D. Force fluids

9. Which food would the WOC nurse recommend for a patient with an ileostomy who is experiencing high watery stoma output?
   A. Fresh fruits
   B. Prunes
   C. Leafy vegetables
   D. Pasta

10. A potential complication of an ileal conduit is
   A. Hyperchloremic metabolic alkalosis
   B. Vitamin B_{12} deficiency
   C. Kidney failure
   D. Edema

ANSWERS AND RATIONALES

1. D. Rationale: Altered body image and appearance are the focus of the psychosocial phase of adolescence according to Erickson.

2. B. Rationale: A WOC nurse should be minimally comfortable with addressing this stage, and should refer as needed.

3. C. Rationale: Chemotherapy prior to surgery for colon cancer is a common management plan for cancer patients.

4. A. Rationale: These are common side effects of chemotherapies used in colorectal cancers.

5. C. Rationale: A person with a sigmoid colostomy should be an appropriate candidate for irrigation as the sigmoid colon has the ability to retain stool for 24 hours. Radiation therapy, chemotherapy, liquid stools, and Crohn's disease are all contraindications to ostomy irrigation.

6. C. Rationale: Regular irrigation helps train the bowel more effectively.

7. B. Rationale: A warm bath or shower can relax the abdominal muscles and may help loosen the blockage.

8. C. Rationale: The first step is to determine the exact nature of the patient's problem; a radiology study can provide this information.

9. D. Rationale: Starches can absorb fluid and thicken output and slow down transit time.

10. B. Rationale: Vitamin B_{12} deficiency can occur due to resection of small bowel for the procedure. The terminal ileum absorbs vitamin B_{12} and bile salts.

CHAPTER 15

ASSESSMENT AND MANAGEMENT OF THE PEDIATRIC PATIENT

Christine Baker, Laura Ann Phearman, and Kimberly McIltrot

OBJECTIVE

Describe the assessment and management of the pediatric and neonatal patient undergoing fecal and/or urinary diversions.

TOPIC OUTLINE

◉ Introduction **224**

◉ **Pathology and Management Conditions 224**
　　Intestinal Atresia and Stenosis 224
　　Duodenal Atresia and Stenosis 224
　　　Incidence 225
　　　Presentation 225
　　　Assessment 226
　　　Management 226
　　Jejunoileal Atresia and Stenosis 226
　　　Incidence 226
　　　Presentation 226
　　　Assessment 227
　　　Management 227
　　Colonic Atresia 227
　　　Incidence 227
　　　Presentation 227
　　　Assessment 227
　　　Management 227
　　Malrotation and Volvulus 227
　　　Incidence 228
　　　Presentation 228
　　　Assessment 228
　　　Management 228
　　Anorectal Malformations 229
　　　Incidence 229
　　　Presentation 229
　　　Assessment 230
　　　Management 230
　　　Perineal Fistulas and Rectovestibular
　　　　Fistulas 230

　　　Rectourethral Fistulas or Cloaca 230
　　Necrotizing Enterocolitis 231
　　　Incidence 231
　　　Presentation 231
　　　Assessment 231
　　　Management 231
　　Hirschsprung Disease 233
　　　Incidence 233
　　　Presentation 233
　　　Assessment 233
　　　Management 235
　　　Duhamel Technique (1960) 235
　　　Swenson Technique (1964) 235
　　　Soave Endorectal Pull-Through (1964) 235
　　Meconium Ileus 236
　　　Incidence 236
　　　Presentation 237
　　　Assessment 237
　　　Management 237
　　Inflammatory Bowel Disease 238
　　　Incidence 238
　　Crohn's Disease 238
　　　Incidence 238
　　　Presentation 238
　　　Assessment 238
　　　Management 238
　　Ulcerative Colitis 239
　　　Incidence 239
　　　Presentation 239
　　　Assessment 239

Management   239
Familial Polyposis Syndromes   239
    Incidence   239
    Presentation   240
    Assessment   240
    Management   240
Pediatric Trauma   240
    Incidence   240
    Presentation   240
    Assessment   240
    Management   240

Management of Fecal Diversions   240
    Techniques and Indications for Pediatric
        Pouching   240
    Refeeding Ostomy Output   241

Pathology and Management Conditions Leading to Urinary Diversion   241
    Prune Belly Syndrome   241
        Incidence   241
        Presentation   242
        Assessment   242
        Management   242

Myelomeningocele   242
    Incidence   242
    Presentation   242
    Assessment   242
    Management   242

Construction and Management of Pediatric Urinary Diversions   243
    Vesicostomy   243
    Ileovesicostomy   244
    Appendicovesicostomy   244

Rehabilitative Issues   244
    Support and Education for the Child and
        Family   244
    Developmental Phase and Implications for Care
        and Education (Age Specific)   245
    Premature Infant/Full-Term Infant   245
    Toddler (12 Months to 3 Years) and Preschool
        (3 to 5 Years)   245
    School Age (6 to 12 Years)   245
    Adolescent (13 to 18 Years)   246

Conclusions   246

INTRODUCTION

It is important for the wound, ostomy, and continence (WOC) nurse to understand the assessment and management of the neonatal and pediatric patient who may undergo surgery for fecal and/or urinary diversion to assist in decreasing the morbidity and mortality of these often-fragile patients. More than half of all stomas are placed in the neonatal period and another one-fourth in infants younger than 1 year of age (Gauderer, 2012).

The use and management of gastrointestinal (GI) stomas in children has evolved with improved surgical techniques, better understanding of the physiologic and psychological consequences of intestinal stomas, and advances in stoma care that have contributed to more rational use of ostomies by pediatric surgeons. The exact frequency of intestinal stomas in the pediatric population is difficult to determine (Minkes et al., 2019).

Most decompressing intestinal stomas in the pediatric age group are temporary, and after correcting the underlying problem, the diverting stoma is taken down (Gauderer, 2012).

An ileostomy or colostomy may be essential in the management of neonates and children with a variety of conditions that include necrotizing enterocolitis (NEC) Hirschsprung disease (HD), complex meconium ileus (MI), imperforate anus, complex hindgut anomalies, malrotation with volvulus, intestinal atresias, trauma, and inflammatory bowel disease (IBD). The type of stoma created is determined by the specific condition (Minkes et al., 2019).

Urostomies involve a portion of externalized ileum or colon that are used as conduits and are less common today with catheterizable stomas. In children, the appendix is often mobilized and used as a catheterizable stoma to the urinary bladder (Gauderer, 2012).

PATHOLOGY AND MANAGEMENT CONDITIONS

INTESTINAL ATRESIA AND STENOSIS

Atresia and stenosis are congenital defects of a hollow viscus that result in complete obstruction (atresia) or narrowing (stenosis) of the lumen. Intestinal atresia is one of the most frequent causes of bowel obstruction in the newborn and can occur at any point in the GI tract with approximately 50% of cases involving the duodenum. The outcome of intestinal atresia following surgical repair is very good. In general, morbidity and mortality depend upon associated medical conditions such as prematurity or cystic fibrosis (CF), other congenital anomalies, the complexity of the lesion, and surgical complications (Wesson, 2018).

The reported incidence of intestinal atresia ranges from 1.3 to 3.5 per 10,000 live births with approximately 20% associated with a chromosomal anomaly. The incidence and associated anomalies vary by anatomical site. Interruption of the normal development of the GI tract may result in intestinal atresia, and the mechanism varies with the segment of bowel affected (Wesson, 2018).

DUODENAL ATRESIA AND STENOSIS

The duodenum is derived partly from the embryonic foregut and partly from the midgut. During the 6th to 7th week of gestation, portions of the intestinal tract become

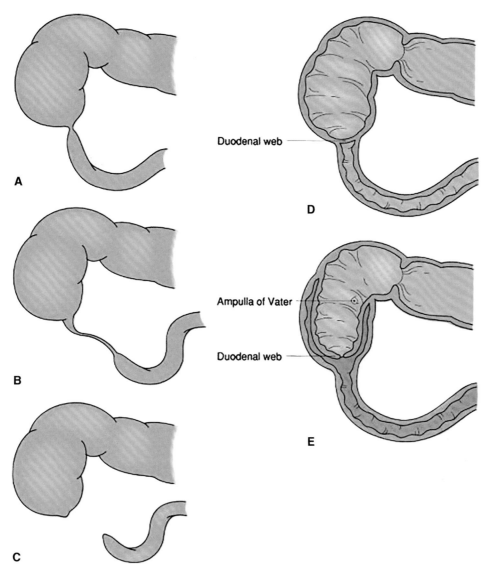

Duodenal web

Ampulla of Vater

Duodenal web

FIGURE 15-1. Duodenal Atresia (types I, II, and III): Classification of Intestinal Atresia.

occluded as the endodermal epithelium proliferates. During the 8th to 10th week, patency is restored as recanalization occurs. Duodenal atresia is thought to result from failure of the bowel to recanalize (formation of new canals or paths) during this period (Wesson, 2018). Duodenal obstructions are classified as atresias (complete obstruction) or stenosis (incomplete obstruction due to web or diaphragm). Atresias are then classified into three types: types I (most common), II, and III (**Fig. 15-1**).

Incidence

Duodenal atresia occurs in 1 in 5,000 to 10,000 live births and represents up to 60% of small intestinal atresias (Gossman et al., 2019). It is often associated with other anomalies, including trisomy 21 and cardiac malformations. Approximately 30% of children with duodenal atresia have Down syndrome. There is a 3% prevalence of congenital duodenal atresia among patients with trisomy 21. There is also an association with VACTERL (vertebral

defects, anal atresia, cardiac defects, tracheoesophageal fistula, renal anomalies, and limb abnormalities), annular pancreas, and other bowel atresias including jejunal, ileal, and rectal atresias (Gossman et al., 2019). No difference in prevalence between genders and genetic predisposition has been found; however, it is reported among siblings and generations of families.

Presentation

> **KEY POINT**
>
> Intestinal atresia may present with suspicious findings on prenatal ultrasound (US) or with clinical symptoms that develop shortly after birth.

Prenatal findings—Less than one-half of infants with intestinal atresias are identified by prenatal US examination, based on signs of intestinal obstruction. If an abnormality is detected in prenatal US, this knowledge enhances clinical care, and the infants can be treated promptly after birth reducing the risk of complications that include vomiting, poor feeding, volume depletion, electrolyte imbalance, and aspiration pneumonia. However, there is a low sensitivity in detecting GI atresias with routine prenatal ultrasound in part because sonographic signs of obstruction may not become evident until the late second trimester, after the typical time of a fetal anatomic survey. The sensitivity tends to decrease for more distal lesions (Wesson, 2018).

Duodenal atresia usually has a characteristic "double bubble" appearance on prenatal ultrasound, similar to the postnatal abdominal radiograph. This finding is due to dilation of the stomach and the first part of the duodenum and appears as two air-filled bubbles in the abdomen, representing two discontiguous loops of bowel. Polyhydramnios, excessive accumulation of amniotic fluid in the uterus during pregnancy, develops in up to 50% of cases. These findings typically develop in the mid to late second trimester. Duodenal atresia is particularly difficult to distinguish from choledochal cyst by antenatal US (Wesson, 2018).

Assessment

Postnatal findings—Duodenal atresia is typically characterized by the onset of vomiting within hours of birth. While this is most often bilious, it may be nonbilious because 15% of defects occur proximal to the ampulla of Vater. It should be assumed that any child with bilious vomiting has a proximal GI obstruction until proven otherwise, and further workup should begin expeditiously (Karrer et al., 2016). The abdomen is usually distended due to the dilated stomach and proximal duodenum but becomes scaphoid or sunken when the contents are aspirated (Glasseer & Springer, 2016). Passing meconium within the first 24 hours of life is not usually altered. Fluid and electrolyte losses should be adequately replaced to avoid dehydration, weight loss, and electrolyte imbalance. An orogastric (OG) tube in an infant with suspected duodenal obstruction typically yields a significant amount of bile-stained fluid. Occasionally, infants with duodenal stenosis escape detection of an abnormality and proceed into childhood or, rarely, into adulthood before a partial obstruction is noted (Karrer et al., 2016).

A plain abdominal x-ray is used for diagnosis of duodenal atresia revealing gas in the stomach and the proximal duodenum but an absence of gas distally in the small or large bowel. The double-bubble sign is considered a reliable indicator of duodenal atresia although other causes of intestinal obstruction may simulate the double-bubble sign. Annular pancreas is the second most common cause of duodenal atresia. Annular pancreas is a condition where the second part of the duodenum is surrounded by a ring of pancreatic tissue continuous with the head of the pancreas. This portion of the pancreas can constrict the duodenum and block or impair the

flow. Jejunal or more distal obstruction may have dilation more distally or more than two bubbles may be present (Wesson, 2018). The radiographic appearance of the double-bubble sign should prompt immediate surgical consultation. For cases of suspected duodenal atresia not identified antenatally, barium fluoroscopy may be used to assess the GI tract. If necessary, further evaluation with US or upper gastrointestinal series (UGI) may be performed. The main purpose of the UGI is to differentiate between duodenal atresia and midgut volvulus; an important distinction, because midgut volvulus requires emergency surgery, whereas duodenal atresia can be managed on an urgent basis (Wesson, 2018).

Management

Treatment involves NG suction to decompress the stomach, IV resuscitation, and surgery to correct the obstructing lesion. Duodenoduodenostomy is the most common surgery performed as an open or laparoscopic procedure (Gossman et al., 2019). A diamond-shaped anastomosis is constructed to join the areas of the intestine, bypassing the obstruction or stenosed section. If this is unable to be done due to size or anatomy, then a duodenojejunostomy is performed (Aguayo & Ostlie, 2010). Possible complications of duodenoduodenostomy include gastroesophageal reflux, megaduodenum, and impaired duodenal motility. A complete operative evaluation includes looking for additional areas of intestinal obstruction (Gossman et al., 2019).

JEJUNOILEAL ATRESIA AND STENOSIS

Jejunal and/or ileal atresia is typically an acquired lesion thought to result from vascular disruption leading to ischemic necrosis of the fetal intestine. In general, the more proximal the vascular disruption, the more extensive the defect in the bowel. Because the fetal bowel is sterile, the necrotic tissue is resorbed, leaving blind proximal and distal ends, often with a gap in the mesentery. Causes of the vascular disruption in the human fetus include segmental or midgut volvulus, intussusception, internal hernia, and interruption of the segmental mesenteric blood supply (Wesson, 2018).

Jejunoileal atresia has been classified into four types (**Fig. 15-2**) based upon anatomic characteristics. Type III is the most common, and type I is the least common form (Wesson, 2018).

Incidence

Jejunal or ileal atresia occurs in approximately 0.7 per 10,000 births, each representing about 20% of small intestinal atresias (Wesson, 2018).

Presentation

The jejunoileal atresia defect may be noted on prenatal ultrasound. Affected infants typically develop abdominal distension and vomiting, usually bilious, within the first 2 days of life. While most infants with bowel obstruction fail to pass meconium, it may remain in the distal bowel

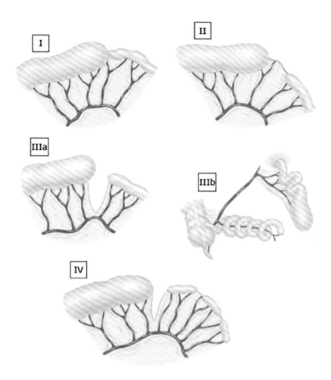

FIGURE 15-2. Classification of Intestinal Atresia Type I, Muscular Continuity with a Complete Web. Type II, mesentery intact, fibrous cord. Type IIIa, muscular and mesenteric discontinuous. Type IIIb, apple-peel deformity. Type IV, multiple atresias. (Adapted with permission from Grosfeld, J. L. (1998). Jejunoileal atresia and stenosis. In J. A. O'Neill Jr, M. I. Rowe, J. L. Grosfeld, et al. (Eds.), *Pediatric surgery* (5th ed., pp. 114–118). St. Louis, MO: Mosby.)

beyond the obstruction and as a result the newborns with this type of atresia may pass meconium (Wesson, 2018).

Less than 5% of infants with jejunal or ileal atresia have associated chromosomal anomalies. Jejunal atresia is sometimes associated with other major malformations (e.g., cardiac malformations 10% to 20%, and other GI malformations such as gastroschisis), but this is rare in ileal atresia. Jejunal or ileal atresia is also associated with CF due to inspissated, or compacted, meconium and volvulus during fetal life (Wesson, 2018).

Assessment

Diagnosis is usually made by radiographic study of the abdomen showing proximal loops of bowel with gas and fluid, and the gasless abdomen beyond the defect.

Management

An NG tube is placed for decompression, antibiotics are started with concern for perforation or sepsis, and fluids are given for hydration and electrolyte resuscitation. The most common surgical approach is resection of the dilated and hypertrophied proximal bowel with end-to-end anastomosis, with or without tapering of the proximal bowel. Normal small bowel length in neonates is 250 cm, 160 to 240 cm in premature infants,

with approximately 100 cm of intestines needed for normal intestinal function (Aguayo & Ostlie, 2010). Parenteral nutrition will be required until the infant is able to begin oral feeds and longer if feeding intolerance is present. Bowel lengthening procedures may be performed later in life.

COLONIC ATRESIA

Colonic atresia occurs due to vascular compromise in utero, similar to jejunoileal atresia.

Incidence

Colonic atresia is the least common type; the incidence is approximately 0.25 per 10,000 births, or 7% to 10% of cases (Wesson, 2018).

Presentation

Like other types of bowel obstruction, colonic atresia presents with marked abdominal distension, failure to pass meconium, and bilious vomiting. Because the obstruction is distal, symptoms may appear later than those with more proximal lesions, but still usually within the first 3 days of life.

Colonic atresia typically affects otherwise normal newborns. In rare cases, it may be associated with gastroschisis, skeletal abnormalities, other intestinal atresias, and HD.

In infants with partial intestinal obstruction (stenosis or web), the presentation may be more insidious, with obstructive symptoms developing days or weeks after birth. In some cases, the symptoms are intermittent, which cause further delay in diagnosis (Wesson, 2018).

Assessment

Dilated loops of bowel with a cutoff point showing an abrupt end to the intestinal gas pattern can be seen on a plain abdominal film. A contrast enema shows a microcolon with a discontinuation of contrast at the atretic point.

Management

Colonic atresia management is similar to duodenal and jejunoileal atresia and is dependent on the specific anatomy of the defect. An NG tube is placed for intestinal decompression, and fluids are given to maintain hydration and provide electrolyte resuscitation. Surgery is done to promote the continuity of the intestines (Stellar & Widmer, 2013).

MALROTATION AND VOLVULUS

The alimentary tract develops from the embryologic foregut, midgut, and hindgut. Due to rapid midgut growth and the inability of the abdominal cavity to house all of the intestines during normal development, a portion of the intestines herniate out of the abdominal cavity where they then undergo a 270-degree counterclockwise rotation around the superior mesenteric artery (SMA). Following this rotation, the intestine returns to the abdominal cavity, with fixation of the duodenojejunal loop to the left of the midline and the cecum in the right lower quadrant (Bensard et al., 2018).

Malrotation, also known as intestinal nonrotation or incomplete rotation, refers to any variation in this rotation and fixation during fetal development. Interruption of this expected pathway of intestinal rotation and fixation can occur at any location, leading to various acute and chronic presentations. Without the normal 270-degree rotation, the intestines are not fixed, stable, or in proper position (Bensard et al., 2018).

The most common type of alteration in rotation found in pediatric patients is incomplete rotation, predisposing the child to midgut volvulus which requires emergent operative intervention (Bensard et al., 2018). A volvulus occurs when the intestines twist upon themselves with at least a 360-degree twisting, causing the vascular obstruction. This can occur at any age but is more frequent in children and infants. Intestinal malrotation can make an infant more likely to develop a midgut volvulus and often occurs in the first few weeks of life. A volvulus can also occur in any part of the intestine without malrotation present (Coste & Waheed, 2019) (**Fig. 15-3**).

Incidence

Intestinal malrotation occurs in between 1 in 200 to 500 live births. Most patients with malrotation are asymptomatic, with symptomatic malrotation occurring in only 1 in 6,000 live births. Male predominance is observed in neonatal presentations at a ratio of 2:1 with no sexual predilection observed in patients older than 1 year. Symptoms and diagnosis may occur at any age, with some reports of prenatal diagnosis of intestinal malrotation (Bensard et al., 2018). Patients with omphalocele, gastroschisis, and congenital diaphragmatic hernia (CDH) may have a higher incidence of malrotation. Additional related defects seen are intestinal atresias, HD, and Meckel diverticulum (McIltrot & Wilson, 2014).

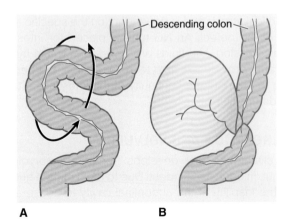

FIGURE 15-3. Volvulus of the Sigmoid Colon. **A.** Clockwise rotation of colon. **B.** Twistings of colon with obstruction. (Moore, K. L., Agur, A. M. R., & Dalley, A. F. (2013). *Clinically oriented anatomy*. Philadelphia, PA: Wolters Kluwer.)

Presentation

Midgut volvulus can happen at any age, but most commonly occurs during the first few weeks of life with bilious emesis as the first sign. Infants that present with bilious emesis, acute duodenal obstruction, or abdominal tenderness associated with hemodynamic deterioration must be rapidly evaluated to ensure that they do not have intestinal malrotation along with volvulus. Left untreated, vascular compromise of the midgut initially causes bloody stools but may progress to circulatory collapse. Physical examination findings for the advanced disease will show signs of peritonitis suggestive of intestinal ischemia with erythema and edema of the abdominal wall. This will lead to shock and death if left untreated. Plain abdominal x-rays show a paucity of gas throughout the intestine with a few scattered air-fluid levels. Fluid resuscitation should be implemented immediately to ensure adequate perfusion and urine output followed by prompt exploratory laparotomy. In cases where the child is stable, laparoscopy may be considered.

In older children and adults, abdominal pain is the most common symptom and may present with abrupt onset over hours or days or as chronic intermittent pain over weeks, months, or years. Additional presenting symptoms include intermittent vomiting, chronic diarrhea, malabsorption, or failure to thrive (Coste & Waheed, 2019).

Assessment

Plain abdominal films may suggest partial duodenal obstruction. An UGI that shows incomplete rotation with the duodenojejunal junction displaced to the right is the best indication of obstruction. The duodenum may show a corkscrew effect, diagnosing volvulus or complete duodenal obstruction, with the small bowel looping entirely on the right side of the abdomen. A barium enema may show a displaced cecum, but this sign is unreliable, especially in a small infant in whom the cecum is normally in a somewhat higher position than in an older child (Coste & Waheed, 2019).

Management

When volvulus is suspected, early surgical intervention is mandatory if the ischemic process is to be prevented or reversed. Volvulus occurs clockwise and is therefore untwisted counterclockwise follow by a Ladd procedure, named after William Edward Ladd, the pediatrician who first performed the procedure in 1936. This operation does not correct the malrotation but helps to open the narrow mesenteric pedicle to prevent volvulus from recurring. The Ladd procedure is performed by lysing the band formed between the cecum and the lateral abdominal wall as well as duodenum and terminal ileum. This allows the SMA to relax, the duodenum to relax into the right lower quadrant and the cecum into the left lower quadrant; these structures do not need to be secured with a suture. An appendectomy is also done to circumvent errors in the event the patient has diagnostic imaging (Coste & Waheed, 2019).

When a patient presents with advanced ischemia, a simple reduction of the volvulus without the Ladd procedure should be performed followed by a "second-look" laparotomy 24 to 36 hours later to evaluate the vascular integrity of the small intestines.

A transparent plastic silo may be placed over the intestine to facilitate constant evaluation and to plan the timing of reexploration. If a necrotic bowel is present, the surgeon can conservatively resect it to ensure adequate length for feeding and prevention of short-gut syndrome. With early diagnosis and correction, the prognosis is excellent. Delay can lead to mortality or short-gut syndrome (Coste & Waheed, 2019).

Postoperative care is determined by the extent of the surgery and damage to the intestines. Management of fluid and electrolytes and pain is crucial. An NG tube is used to decompress the stomach until bowel function returns. Depending upon the amount of necrotic bowel removed, there may be a central line and gastrostomy tube (GT) for feedings as well as a potential for ostomy creation.

ANORECTAL MALFORMATIONS

Anorectal malformation (ARM) includes a spectrum of congenital defects that may occur in the bowel, urinary, and reproductive systems. They range from a low imperforate anus that requires a simple anoplasty within the first few days of life (as seen in **Fig. 15-4A**) to a cloacal exstrophy with involvement of all three systems and a high lesion requiring a three-stage repair with (1) diverting colostomy, (2) posterior sagittal anorectoplasty (PSARP), and (3) colostomy closure. The colostomy decompresses the bowel and prevents infection until surgical site healing is complete (Guardino & Pieper, 2013). The timing between each procedure is individualized and

TABLE 15-1 VACTERL ASSOCIATION	
V	**V**ertebral anomalies
A	Imperforate **A**nus
C	**C**ardiac anomalies
T	**T**racheoesophageal fistula
E	**E**sophageal atresia
R	**R**enal anomalies
L	**L**imb anomalies, particularly radical agenesis

dependent in part on the size and age of the child (some may get the diverting colostomy first to allow the child time to grow), the degree of their anomaly and the surgical repair, and approach required for repair (Rosen, 2019).

Incidence
One in 5,000 births worldwide has an ARM and approximately 60% of those patients will have an associated anomaly. There is a correlation of ARMs with the VACTERL defects (vertebral, anorectal, cardiac, tracheoesophageal fistula/esophageal atresia, renal, and limb). ARMs are slightly more common in males (1.2 to 1) and approximately 70% of male patients have some form of connection to the urinary system, or a rectourethral fistula. The most common type of ARM in female patients is a rectovestibular fistula (Smith & Avansino, 2019 May 27).

Table 15-1 shows VACTERL association and commonly seen defects with ARMs.

Presentation
The diagnosis of ARM is often made in the delivery room upon examination of the newborn or when the nurse attempts to take a rectal temperature and no anus is present. The infant may have an absent or displaced anal opening yet meconium may be seen in the genitalia of the female or on the perineum of the male, away from the anus. Anteriorly displaced anus is common where the

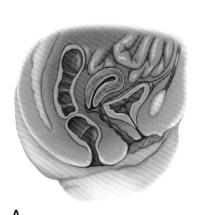

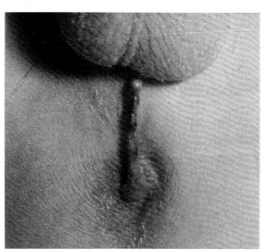

A   **B**

FIGURE 15-4. Anorectal Malformation. Imperforate anus, in which the rectum ends in a blind pouch.

anus is not in the correct location, halfway between the coccyx and the base of the scrotum or vagina. Although the term imperforate anus may accurately describe a child's outward appearance, it often belies the true complexity of the malformation beneath as the muscles and nerves associated with the anus often have a similar degree of malformation. The spine and urogenital tract may also be involved (Rosen, 2019).

Assessment

A complete physical examination to check anatomy should be done when all infants are born, paying close attention to the genitalia and perianal area. A normal-sized anus for a full-term infant is equivalent to a 10 to 12 Hegar dilator (see below for further information). The anal opening should be in the center of the anal muscle complex which cannot always be discerned solely on examination and may require an examination under anesthesia (EUA). The perineum should be evaluated with close attention to features such as the development of the buttocks, presence of a gluteal fold, and examination for any type of opening or orifice on the perineum. Females should have a thorough vaginal examination, noting the number of openings on the perineum. These physical examination findings can give clues as to the type of ARM present. In addition, the heart should be assessed for a murmur, the limbs for anatomic abnormality, and a full genitourinary examination should be completed (Smith & Avansino, 2019).

Management

General supportive medical care should be established followed by a full workup to rule out other congenital malformations and determine the severity of the ARM. Because of the known VACTERL association, the following radiographic studies are necessary; plain abdominal and chest films to rule out the presence of esophageal atresia with or without tracheoesophageal fistula, spine radiographs to rule out vertebral anomalies, echocardiogram to rule out congenital heart issues, and a spinal US to screen for tethered spinal cord. The sacral ratio should also be calculated from anteroposterior and lateral films as this helps give prognostic information about bowel control for the child as they grow and develop. For female patients with a single perineal orifice and a cloaca diagnosis, an abdominal US should be obtained to evaluate for both hydrocolpos (vaginal distension due to obstruction and resulting fluid accumulation) and hydronephrosis (Levitt, 2007; Smith & Avansino, 2019).

The exact diagnosis guides the surgical plan. It is important to have an experienced pediatric surgeon who has training in PSARP perineal nerve sparing to have the best outcome for fecal continence.

Perineal Fistulas and Rectovestibular Fistulas

For perineal fistulas, a repair can be performed in the neonatal period if there are no other anomalies that would preclude anesthesia such as a cardiac defect. The repair may be delayed if the fistulous tract is large enough to perform dilations with a Hegar dilator and stool evacuation can be reliable. The same dilation strategy works for a female patient with a rectovestibular fistula as the anatomy can be challenging in the neonatal period, and dilating can allow the child time to grow and improve the ease of surgical intervention (Smith & Avansino, 2019).

If dilation management is chosen, an instrument called a Hegar dilator (developed by Alfred Hegar in 1879) is used. The dilators are a set of plastic or metal rods that are round, slightly curved, have a conal tip, and come in gradually increasing sizes. Once the appropriate size is identified, the dilator is lubricated and inserted into the opening on a scheduled basis, usually twice per day, to ensure patency. It is crucial that stool is decompressing well with dilation management to avoid distension. If being managed with dilations, the surgical repair should occur at approximately 3 months of age allowing the defect to be corrected before the child transitions to solid food and reducing the risk of developing constipation which will impact future bowel function (Smith & Avansino, 2019).

Rectourethral Fistulas or Cloaca

Male patients with a urinary fistula should undergo diversion in the neonatal period with a diverting descending sigmoid colostomy and a mucus fistula. This allows the child to grow before surgical intervention and to evacuate stool from the distal limb of the bowel that connects to the urinary system. Preoperatively a distal colostogram via the mucus fistula will be performed to determine the exact type of rectourethral fistula and assist with preoperative planning and operative strategy for repair (Smith & Avansino, 2019).

Patients with a single perineal orifice consistent with a diagnosis of cloaca will also undergo a diverting ostomy and mucous fistula in the neonatal period. Cloacal anomalies involve failure of the urogenital septum to separate resulting in a single common channel and occur in about 1 in 50,000 live births, involving the urogenital sinus and anorectum. These anomalies require a multidisciplinary team experienced in these complex congenital malformations requiring multiple procedures involving the urological, GI, and gynecological systems (Fernando et al., 2015).

With severe congenital defects such as cloacal defects, pouching may be difficult due to an open, draining bladder on the abdominal wall in close proximity to the stoma. Good skin care and prevention of yeast infection and denuded skin is a priority to preserve the skin for upcoming surgical repairs. This is a huge adjustment for the family, who will be bringing their child to the hospital for many visits and extended hospital stays following surgery, in addition to the complex care of the child. The WOC nurse is an integral member of the interdisciplinary team and plays an important role in skin care assessment and recommendations for preventive care as well as ostomy teaching for families. The WOC nurse is most familiar with available products and methods to best manage stomas that are in close proximity, including vesicostomies, or set adjacent to or within a wound making the WOC nurse an invaluable resource to families and staff. This process can be challenging and being available to support the family and teach them independence is reassuring. The neonatologist, gastroenterologist, surgeon, case manager, and social worker are additional members of the interdisciplinary team.

The timing of the definitive repair of high malformations depends on the exact type of malformation and other associated anomalies, especially cardiac defects. Typically, surgical repair occurs sometime around 3 months of age. Repair of an ARM requires a meticulous, delicate technique and a surgeon with experience in treating these defects. The PSARP is ideal for defining and repairing anorectal anomalies (Levitt & Wood, 2019).

In 90% of newborn boys, ARMs may be repaired with a posterior sagittal approach alone, whereas 10% require an additional abdominal component (laparotomy or laparoscopy to mobilize a very high rectum). The posterior sagittal approach is used to repair ARMs in newborn girls with the exception of approximately 30% of cloacas. In this 30%, the rectum or vagina is high enough to also require an abdominal approach.

Postoperatively nothing is placed in the rectum for 2 weeks. Anal dilatations are started after 2 weeks to avoid a skin-level stricture. Dilations are performed twice daily with the dilator size gradually increased until the rectum reaches the desired size at which time the colostomy may be closed. The dilations are continued postoperatively to avoid stricture and are gradually tapered over the subsequent 3 to 4 months. These are general guidelines and individual surgeon preference may vary. After colostomy closure, severe diaper rash or IAD (incontinence-associated skin damage) is common due to the perineal skin's initial exposure to stool. Prevention is key with use of moisture barriers immediately postoperatively to protect the skin (Levitt & Wood, 2019).

NECROTIZING ENTEROCOLITIS

NEC is a life-threatening illness almost exclusively affecting neonates with a mortality rate as high as 50%. The pathophysiology of NEC is inflammation of the intestine leading to bacterial invasion causing cellular damage and death and leads to necrosis of the mucosal and submucosal layers of the colon and intestine. As NEC progresses, it can lead to intestinal perforation causing peritonitis, sepsis, and death.

The specific mechanism and cause of this bacterial invasion are not yet fully understood. In premature neonates, GI tract immaturity is believed to play a role and typically occurs in the 2nd to 3rd week of life. Sev-

eral risk factors have been identified, but prematurity, low birth weight, and formula feeding have been identified as primary risks. Specifically, high osmotic strength formula feeding has been implicated as a risk factor. Genetic factors may also play a role (Ginglen & Butki, 2019).

While NEC primarily occurs in premature infants, it has been documented in full-term infants. In this population, onset is typically in the first few days of life and is usually associated with a hypoxic event, such as a cyanotic congenital heart defect (**Fig. 15-5**).

Incidence

In the United States, incidence is approximately 1 to 3 per 1,000 births (Kim, 2019). Incidence worldwide varies between 0.3 and 2.4 infants per 1,000 live births. Nearly 70% of reported cases occur in premature infants born before 36 weeks gestation, affecting 2% to 5% of all premature infants and responsible for nearly 8% of all NICU admissions. Overall, mortality ranges from 10% to 50%. In the most severe cases, involving perforation, peritonitis, and sepsis, mortality approaches 100% (Ginglen & Butki, 2019).

Presentation

Early recognition is key, but initial symptoms can be highly variable, nonspecific, and subtle. The clinician should be suspicious of infants that exhibit poor feeding, vomiting (usually bilious), diarrhea, blood in the stool, and lethargy (Ginglen & Butki, 2019; Kim, 2019a,b).

Physical examination findings may include abdominal distention and tenderness to palpation, visible intestinal loops, decreased bowel sounds, palpable abdominal mass, and erythema of the abdominal wall. As the disease progresses, systemic signs related to respiratory failure and circulatory collapse such as cyanosis and unresponsiveness may occur (Ginglen & Butki, 2019).

Assessment

The single most important diagnostic tool is an abdominal plain film series including anterior–posterior and left lateral decubitus views. Findings of dilated loops of bowel, pneumatosis intestinalis, and portal venous air is diagnostic. Pneumatosis intestinalis is the visualization of small amounts of air within the bowel wall and is specifically characteristic for NEC. Portal venous air is not universally present but is a poor prognostic sign when found. Free air in the abdomen may be seen when perforation has occurred.

The abdominal radiograph is a valuable tool for tracking the progression of the disease as well and is repeated serially every 6 hours until definitive treatment has occurred (Ginglen & Butki, 2019).

Management

The medical and surgical teams are notified, and the infant is placed on NEC watch. Many NICUs have a NEC protocol that includes making the child NPO, placing an OG or NG tube to decompress the stomach and intestines, starting IV antibiotics, and ordering serial

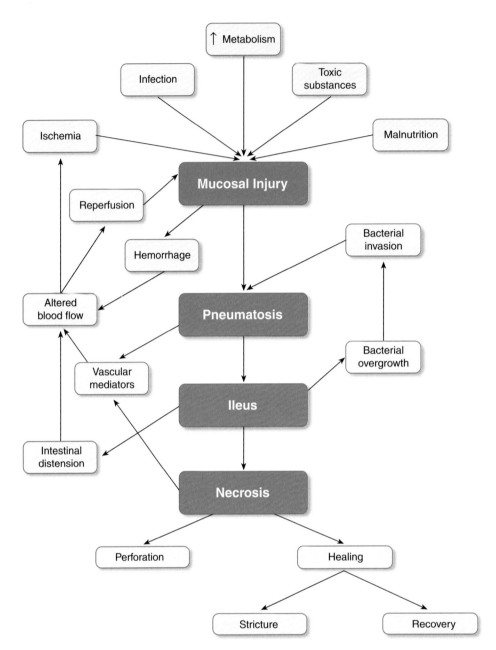

FIGURE 15-5. Necrotizing Enterocolitis (NEC). This schematic is a composite of the theories about factors thought to be involved in the pathogenesis of NEC. The progression of this disease is denoted in large type. The factors thought to initiate or propagate the disease process are in smaller type. (Adapted with permission from Crouse, D. T. (1993). Necrotizing enterocolitis. In J. J. Pomerance & C. J. Richardson (Eds.), *Neonatology for the clinician* (p. 364). Norwalk, CT: Appleton & Lange.)

radiographs. Depending upon the infant's condition, ventilator support may be warranted. A surgical consult is placed to assess the infant and monitor for worsening symptoms and radiographs. In cases of bowel perforation or worsening condition, surgery will be performed.

KEY POINT

If the child is too sick to travel to the operating room (OR), surgery may be done at the bedside in the NICU.

Bowel length preservation is the goal of surgery, and only fully necrotic bowel is surgically removed. There may be patchy areas of necrosis, but the surgery team may be conservative and reluctant to remove sections that may improve. The fully necrotic areas may be resected and anastomosed, and often, the patient has an ileostomy with mucus fistulas. The surgeon removes as little bowel as possible to help prevent short bowel syndrome. In very-low-birth weight infants or hemodynamically unstable infants who will not tolerate surgery, the infant may have a peritoneal drain placed to decompress the area until the infant is older, stable, and able to tolerate surgery (Rapoport & Nishii, 2013).

In review, it is vital that the nurse recognize the symptoms and initiate a NEC protocol in an effort to stop the progression of bowel injury. If the damage progresses and surgical intervention and ostomy creation is necessary, education for the family should begin as soon as possible. The ostomy is usually reversible and will remain in place for at least 6 weeks. Depending on the patient's condition and length of stay in the NICU, the ostomy takedown may occur prior to being discharged home. The parents should be educated in the child's care while continuing to bond and feel a part of the infant's care during the hospital stay

HIRSCHSPRUNG DISEASE

HD or congenital aganglionic megacolon is a motor disorder of the gut, caused by the failure of neural crest cells, the precursors of enteric ganglion cells, to migrate completely during intestinal development. The resulting aganglionic segment of the colon fails to relax, causing a functional obstruction. In approximately 80% of patients, HD affects the rectosigmoid colon, known as short-segment disease. In 20% of patients, the aganglionosis extends proximal to the sigmoid colon, known as long-segment disease. In approximately 5%, the entire colon is affected, known as total colonic aganglionosis (TCA), and in rare cases, the small bowel may also be involved. Outcomes are generally worse for patients with long-segment as compared with short-segment disease (Wesson & Experanza-Lopez, 2019).

Incidence

HD occurs in approximately 1 in 5,000 live births with an overall male:female ratio of 3:1 to 4:1; when the entire colon is involved, the gender ratio more nearly approaches 1 to 2:1. There is familial clustering for nonsyndromic HD, with an overall recurrence risk of approximately 3% in siblings for short-segment disease or up to 17% if the proband (first identified family member with a genetic disorder) has long-segment disease. This sibling recurrence risk is higher if the proband is a female and is also higher if multiple family members are affected (Wesson & Experanza-Lopez, 2019). HD affects all races; however, it is roughly 3 times more common among Asian-Americans (Wagner, 2020).

Presentation

The age at which HD is diagnosed has progressively decreased over the past century. In the early 1900s, the median age at diagnosis was 2 to 3 years and from the 1950s to 1970s, the median age was 2 to 6 months. Currently, approximately 90% of patients with HD are diagnosed in the first several days of life with failure to pass meconium within 48 hours after birth. The child may develop a distended abdomen, emesis, sepsis, and occasionally perforation (Wagner, 2020).

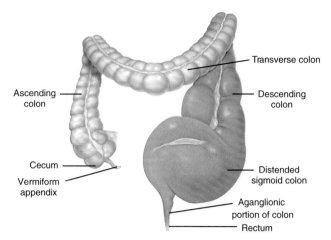

FIGURE 15-6. Hirschsprung Disease: Bowel Dilation. (Anatomical Chart Company.)

HD is confined to the rectosigmoid region in about 75% of cases. Approximately 60% of infants with HD have an associated condition, ranging from subtle to severe. Ophthalmologic problems affect 43% of infants, 20% have congenital anomalies of the genitourinary tract, 5% have congenital heart disease, 5% have hearing impairment, and 2% have central nervous system anomalies.

HD is associated with chromosomal abnormalities or syndromes in approximately 9% of cases, including trisomy 21 (Wagner, 2020).

If not diagnosed in infancy, the child may have patterns of severe constipation, abdominal distension, and megacolon (**Fig. 15-6**).

Assessment

A plain radiograph may be obtained showing distended loops of bowel; if the presence of free air is noted, this is an emergency and denotes perforation. A water-soluble contrast enema should be done to determine if there is a transition zone (TZN) between possible aganglionic and ganglionic intestine. The ganglionic portion is usually the enlarged colon where the stool has backed up, and the aganglionic portion is narrow and nonfunctioning. If the study is done on a newborn, or on a child with total colonic HD, the film may not show a TZN because of the lack of dilated intestine (**Fig. 15-7**).

Anorectal manometry is not widely used in the United States but reportedly is done more often in Europe. This study involves pressure-measuring balloon catheters placed into the anus and rectum to determine the absence of the relaxation reflex of the internal sphincter (Holder & Jackson, 2013). The "gold standard" for diagnosing HD is the suction rectal biopsy. This may be performed in the OR or at the bedside. Two to three rectal specimens are taken at 2 and 5 cm above the dentate line for the pathologist to determine if ganglion cells are present. If an inadequate biopsy is done or the patient is an older child

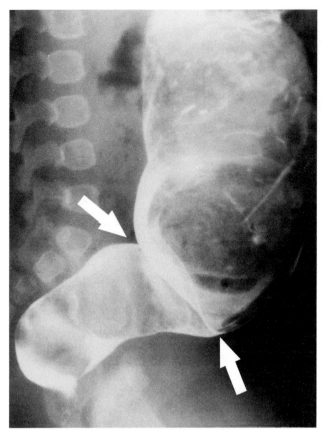

A

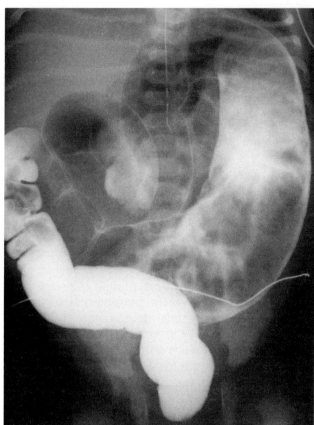

B

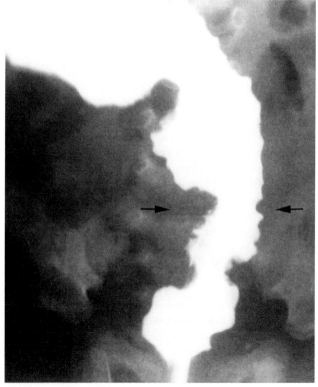

C

FIGURE 15-7. Hirschsprung Disease. **A.** Characteristic TZN (*arrows*) is seen between the dilated, feces-filled colon above and the relatively narrowed rectum below. **B.** The rectum in this newborn infant is smaller than the sigmoid and descending colon, but a well-defined TZN is not present. **C.** A contrast enema in another infant shows spasm and irregularity of the aganglionic segment (*arrows*). (From Brant, W. E., & Helms, C. A. (2006). *Brant and Helms solution*. Philadelphia, PA: Wolters Kluwer.)

who requires sedation, a full-thickness biopsy may be done in the OR with anesthesia.

Management

Treatment of HD is surgical resection of aganglionic bowel and anastomosis of ganglionic bowel to the distal rectum. If diagnosed in the neonatal period, a possible primary pull-through procedure may be performed. If the child has distended bowel, which occurs after multiple feedings and buildup of stool, a colostomy should be done to decompress the bowel, and a two- or three-stage surgical repair is performed. There are three classic pull-through procedures, with additional modifications performed per surgeon preference, all of which are modifications based on Dr. Swenson's original surgery in 1964. In addition, there is a single-stage pull-through for HD that is laparoscopic-assisted transanal endorectal pull-through (LATEP) with abdominal exploration and laparoscopic biopsies (Georgeson, 2010).

KEY POINT

The goal in surgery is to avoid injury to the pelvic nerves to conserve continence and function.

Duhamel Technique (1960)

Combined abdominoperineal approach of a retrorectal pull-through of ganglionated segment to the posterior aspect of the aganglionated rectum and sewn to the anus. The septum between the two is then divided using a stapler. This creates a neorectum with an aganglionic anterior wall and ganglionic posterior wall (**Fig. 15-8**).

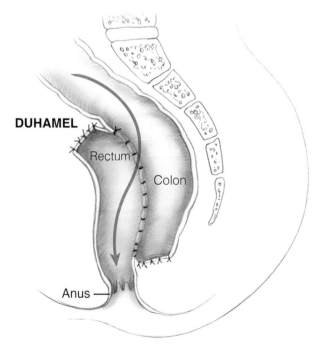

FIGURE 15-8. Duhamel Procedure.

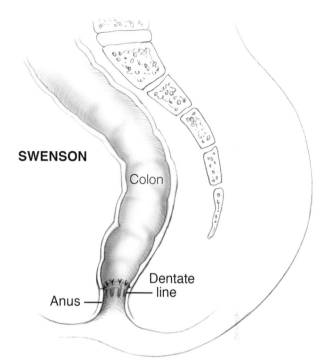

FIGURE 15-9. Swenson Procedure.

Swenson Technique (1964)

Resection of aganglionic bowel will leave a small portion of aganglionic segment at just above the dentate line. The ganglionic and aganglionic are anastomosed at an angle to prevent stricture development. The surgery is done with an abdominal incision and the end-to-end anastomosis done by prolapsing the rectum and pulled through ganglionic bowel through the anus to avoid injury to pelvic nerves (**Fig. 15-9**).

Soave Endorectal Pull-Through (1964)

Dissection of the mucosal layer from the muscular layer of the aganglionic segment and pulling the ganglionic portion down through the dissected aganglionic muscular cuff (**Fig. 15-10**) (Georgeson, 2010; Holder & Jackson, 2013).

Postoperative care consists of an NG tube and IV fluid maintenance until the return of bowel function, followed with clear liquids and advance as tolerated diet. Nothing may go in the rectum, including thermometers or medications (suppositories), due to the potential for injury to the anastomotic site. Pain medication is given IV until tolerating a PO diet, when meds are transitioned to PO. If the patient has a new ostomy, the stoma is assessed for color, size, shape, and output (see Table 11-1 in Chapter 11). Ostomy care teaching begins immediately with the child and family. If a pull-through procedure was done, care of the perineum is taught. There is frequent stooling after surgery, approximately 6 to 12 times per day. Contact dermatitis often develops in the diaper area, and the skin can become severely denuded.

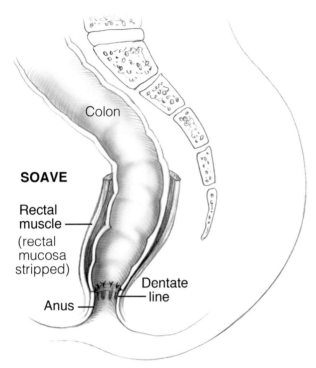

SOAVE

Colon

Rectal muscle (rectal mucosa stripped)

Anus

Dentate line

FIGURE 15-10. Soave Procedure.

KEY POINT

A moisture barrier containing petrolatum or zinc oxide is recommended to protect the perineal area. Many NICUs have a skin care algorithm based on AWHONN (Association of Women's Health, Obstetric and Neonatal Nurses) guidelines that will guide practice. Current recommendation is for 40% zinc oxide as initial protection (AWHONN, 2013).

With diaper changes, gently wipe the stool away with recommended cleansing agent and warm water, reapplying moisture barrier. If red satellite lesions are noted, this can be indicative of a *Candida* (yeast) skin infection and an antifungal barrier cream or ointment may be applied. Alternately, an antifungal powder can be sprinkled on the skin and sealed with a nonalcohol liquid skin barrier. Institutions' protocols for skin protection may vary. Two to three weeks after surgery, the surgical team will begin teaching the family rectal dilations and possibly, rectal irrigations. Surgical dilators are passed into the anus to keep the anastomosis from becoming stenotic and to remain open for the passing of stool (see **Table 15-2** for appropriate-size dilators for patient age). The patient should pass at least one soft, formed stool daily and diet should be adjusted to prevent constipation or frequent stooling. Toilet training may be delayed; however, bowel management is highly successful, and incontinence rates are low. Reviewing the signs and symptoms of enterocolitis (**Box 15-1**) is important with each visit to reduce mortality and morbidity.

TABLE 15-2 RECTAL DILATOR CHART

AGE	DILATOR NUMBER
1–4 mo	12
4–12 mo	13
8–12 mo	14
1–3 y	15
3–12 y	16
>12 y	17

MECONIUM ILEUS

MI is a disorder of the neonate caused by an obstruction of the small intestine at the level of the terminal ileum with inspissated meconium. Approximately 10% of patients with CF present as neonates with MI. In most cases, these patients have CF transmembrane conductance regulator gene (*CFTR*) variants associated with inadequate CFTR production (Katkin, 2019). This reduced production causes abnormal changes in the chloride, sodium, and water transport that occurs across the apical membrane of epithelial cells affecting the respiratory, GI, biliary, pancreatic, and reproductive systems. MI was considered fatal until 1948, when the first enterotomy was done by Hiatt and Wilson. In 1969, Dr. Helen Noblett discovered a nonoperative treatment with a hyperosmolar enema to remove the abnormal stool (Stellar & Widmer, 2013).

Incidence

MI is strongly correlated with CF as 80% to 90% of infants with MI have CF. Due to this correlation, all patients with MI should be tested for CF through sweat chloride and genetic testing. A sweat test may be done after 48 hours of age, but it may be difficult to collect sweat in an infant under approximately 2.5 kg, infants who are stressed, or in a warmer bed. If the sweat test cannot be completed, genetic testing may be considered. MI can occur

---

BOX 15-1   ENTEROCOLITIS SIGNS AND SYMPTOMS

Enterocolitis: Life-threatening acute inflammation of the mucosa of the small intestinal or colonic epithelium. Enterocolitis may occur preoperatively or postoperatively. If enterocolitis is suspected, instruct the family to report immediately to the closest emergency department for assessment and management of sepsis and shock.

Distended abdomen
Hyperactive bowel sounds
Signs and symptoms of sepsis
Darker green or gray stool
Explosive foul-smelling stool
Lethargy
Fever

in patients with a variety of CFTR variants. A high familial recurrence rate suggests that other genetic modifiers predispose to the development of MI. In approximately 40% of cases, there is associated perforation, or jejunal or ileal atresia. Premature and low birth weight infants are more likely to have MI without CF (Katkin, 2019).

Presentation

Infants with MI generally present during the first 3 days of life with abdominal distension and failure to pass meconium, with or without vomiting. Meconium is normally thick, tarry, and green, but with MI, it becomes firm, gray, and pellet-like which causes the obstruction due to its failure to pass through the intestine. MI is divided into two categories that guide management.

Complex MI is complicated by GI pathology that may include tenderness, abdominal wall erythema, intestinal perforation, atresia, or volvulus. Prenatal perforation may cause meconium peritonitis, which can lead to adhesions, calcifications, and meconium cysts. Approximately 40% of MI in newborns with CF is complex (Katkin, 2019).

Simple MI is indicated when there is no associated GI pathology.

The widespread use of prenatal carrier testing and prenatal detection of MI by US affords clinicians the ability to counsel patients and plan proactive management.

Assessment

An abdominal plain film is obtained to assess for dilated loops of bowel, perforation, calcifications, or other abnormalities (**Fig. 15-11A**). If there is no evidence of perforation, hyperosmotic contrast enema radiography is performed to confirm the diagnosis using a water-soluble agent. This will usually identify a small-caliber or microcolon of disuse and meconium pellets in the terminal ileum. The ileum proximal to the obstruction is dilated (**Fig. 15-11B**) (Katkin, 2019).

Management

Due to concern for obstruction, an NG or OG is placed for decompression and hydration, and electrolyte management with IV fluids is initiated. Prophylactic antibiotics may be administered.

Simple MI—managed by administration of hyperosmolar enema (typically, diluted sodium meglumine diatrizoate, Gastrografin), closely monitored by fluoroscopy. The hyperosmolar contrast often breaks up the meconium mass and clears the obstruction. This approach is successful in 20% to 40% of neonates with simple MI. Complications including intestinal perforation and fluid shifts with hypotension and shock occur with 2% to 10% of these procedures.

Complex MI (or if enema is not successful in clearing meconium from the bowel)—Surgical intervention is

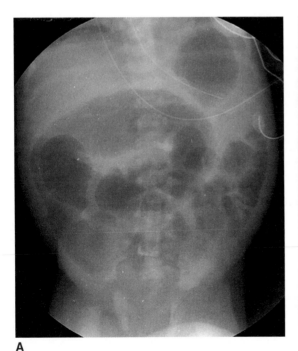
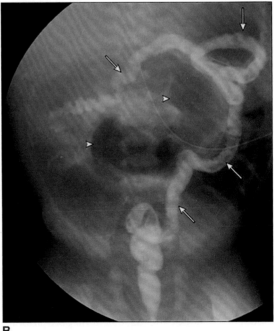

A   **B**

FIGURE 15-11. A, B. The frontal radiograph in supine position shows dilated loops of bowel, indicating intestinal obstruction. The 9-hour-old male infant had a known prenatal diagnosis of intestinal obstruction. (**A** from Courtesy of Michael Callahan, MD. Graphic 100556 Version 2.0. **B** from https://www.uptodate.com/contents/image?imageKey=RADIOL%2F100557&topicKey=PEDS %2F5858&search=meconium+ileus&rank=1%7E23&source=see_link. Reproduced with permission from Sabharwal, S., & Schwarzenberg, S. J. Cystic fibrosis: Overview of gastrointestinal disease. In T. W. Post (Ed.), *UpToDate*. Waltham, MA: UpToDate. (Accessed on [Date].) Copyright © 2020 UpToDate, Inc. For more information visit www.uptodate.com.)

indicated. This may include enterotomy with lavage, double enterostomy, and/or resection of dilated, perforated, or atretic bowel, with a diverting ileostomy. The surgeon will use the most conservative option that relives the obstruction as loss of intestine in a patient with CF has consequences related to future nutrition that are out of proportion to what is seen in children without CF.

Infants with MI are at an increased risk for developing cholestasis, but because this is considered transient in most cases and does not appear to predict clinically significant hepatobiliary disease (Katkin, 2019).

INFLAMMATORY BOWEL DISEASE

IBD is a chronic inflammatory disorder of the GI tract of unknown etiology. IBD includes ulcerative colitis (UC) and Crohn's disease (CD) which are differentiated by their location and depth of involvement in the bowel wall. There is a relationship to heredity, environmental factors, and immunologic responses.

Ulcerative colitis involves diffuse inflammation of the colonic mucosa that most often affects the rectum (proctitis) but may extend into the sigmoid (proctosigmoiditis), beyond the sigmoid (distal UC), or include the entire colon into the cecum (pancolitis).

Crohn's disease results in transmural ulceration of any portion of the GI tract most often affecting the terminal ileum and colon.

Both diseases are classified by the extent of involvement (mild, moderate, or severe) and the location. CD is also classified by phenotype; inflammatory, structuring, or penetrating. In approximately 10% of patients, the diagnosis of CD versus UC may be difficult to distinguish due to similar features (McDowell & Haseeb, 2019).

Although there is an in-depth review of IBD in Chapter 5, it is mentioned again in the pediatric chapter because approximately 25% of patients with IBD present before the age of 20, with peak incidence between the ages of 15 and 30 years. Adults and children with IBD may present with similar clinical features but children demonstrate unique complications including growth failure and delayed puberty. Management of the pediatric patient with IBD includes treating the underlying disease with medical and/or surgical management, while carefully monitoring growth and development (Higuchi & Bousvaros, 2020).

Suspicion of IBD typically arises from a combination of symptoms including screening and laboratory data (that are described under the assessment paragraph). The diagnosis is established by radiographic studies and endoscopy with biopsies. These studies also help to localize the disease and differentiate between UC and CD (Higuchi & Bousvaros, 2020).

Incidence

The incidence of pediatric IBD is approximately 10 per 100,000 children in the United States and Canada. The prevalence is reported as 100 to 200 per 100,000 children in the United States with an estimated total of 70,000 cases. Among children with IBD, 4% present before age 5 years and 18% before age 10 years, with the peak onset in adolescence. IBD is generally a disorder of developed countries and colder climates (Rosen et al., 2015).

CROHN'S DISEASE

CD (also known as regional enteritis) is an immune-mediated inflammatory disease that can affect any portion of the intestinal tract from the mouth to the anus (Setty et al., 2018).

Incidence

The incidence of CD is approximately 5 to 10 new cases per 100,000 individuals per year and appears to be rising (Setty et al., 2018) with 20% of patients developing their disease before the age of 20. It occurs more often in the Northern hemisphere and is slightly more common in females than males (McDowell & Haseeb, 2019).

Presentation

Children with CD may present with the following symptoms, which are dependent on disease progression; abdominal pain, diarrhea, weight loss, rectal bleeding, fever, fatigue, perianal disease, poor growth, joint pain, vomiting, or mouth sores. Younger children (<6 years) presenting with CD are more likely to present with rectal bleeding. In both age groups, growth failure is frequently present at the time of diagnosis. The earliest and most subtle form of growth failure is a decrease in height velocity, which may progress to short stature for age, delayed bone age, and/or pubertal delay (Setty et al., 2018).

Assessment

A thorough history and physical growth evaluation and a rectal examination is done to assess for perirectal disease. An EUA may be scheduled for the anxious child or for a more complete examination, including an anorectal endoscopic examination. Blood work including a complete blood count (CBC), erythrocyte sedimentation rate (ESR), C-reactive protein (CRP), baseline nutritional laboratory tests, stool cultures, and IgA and IgG anti-*Saccharomyces cerevisiae* antibody (ASCA) should be performed (Adibe & Georgeson, 2012).

Management

CD therapy includes medical management to achieve remission of the disease and appropriate nutrition to delay surgical procedures as long as possible. Within 10 years of diagnosis, most patients will require surgery and 50% of patients who have had surgery require a second surgery. Surgical procedures are usually due to obstruction from strictures and require a resection or strictureplasty. There is an increased risk of malignancy due to the inflammatory process, and CD patients should follow the recommended guidelines for surveillance

(Adibe & Georgeson, 2012). Multiple studies have shown that endoscopic surveillance improves CRC-related survival in IBD patients at increased risk for colon cancer. It is widely recommended by GI societies for early detection and resection of dysplasia. While there is agreement about the necessity of surveillance, the recommendation of frequency varies by organization and ranges from every 1 to 5 years, based on a number of risk factors (Clarke & Feuerstein, 2019).

ULCERATIVE COLITIS

UC is a chronic inflammatory disease of the large intestine that affects the lining of the colon and causes ulcerations to form. The ulcerations may produce pus, mucous, abdominal discomfort, and an urgent sense to empty the bowels.

Incidence

The North American incidence of IBD ranges from 2.2 to 19.2 cases per 100,000 individuals per year for UC with 12% of patients developing the disease before the age of 20. UC appears to be equally present in both genders and is thought to be a disorder of developed countries and colder climates (McDowell & Haseeb, 2019).

Presentation

UC in children principally occurs in teenagers but can also occur earlier in life with presentation similar to that in adults. Affected patients usually present with a subacute illness characterized by frequently bloody diarrhea, weakness, anemia, abdominal pain, and often weight loss. Those with a more advanced presentation may exhibit severe abdominal pain, frankly bloody diarrhea, tenesmus, fever, leukocytosis, and hypoalbuminemia. Symptoms may be less severe initially, with nonbloody diarrhea and sometimes poor weight gain prior to developing the more overt symptoms noted above. Osteopenia, weight loss, and anorexia with growth retardation are a concern as well, and nutrition becomes crucial with these patients. Fistulas and abscesses are rare and if noted may be suggestive of CD (Bousvaros et al., 2019).

Assessment

There are no specific diagnostic criteria for IBD, and therefore, the diagnosis is primarily established by the combination of clinical features, laboratory findings including stool specimens for enteric pathogens, characteristic findings on imaging, and endoscopy and colonoscopy with biopsies. Small bowel imaging may be done with abdominal magnetic resonance enterography (MRE) computed tomography enterography (CTE) or UGI series with SBFT. MRE has emerged as the preferred small bowel imaging modality for evaluation of IBD in children, if available, due to the lack of radiation exposure. The technology for CTE has also improved so that it now has less radiation than conventional fluoroscopy. Because of this, conventional fluoroscopy (UGI/SBFT) is being used

less frequently in many centers. It is suggested that a child suspected of IBD be referred to a pediatric gastroenterologist (Higuchi & Bousvaros, 2020).

Management

Management of UC includes medication to promote suppression of the disease and possible surgery that may have side effects but can be curative, avoids a permanent stoma, and helps maintain bowel continence. The surgery of choice (open or laparoscopic) is the ileoanal reservoir or ileal pouch–anal anastomosis (IPAA) with pouch construction to create a reservoir to assist in reducing stool frequency and urgency. A protective loop ileostomy is created to help prevent an anastomotic leak and is left in place for several months. UC patients are often undernourished and on high-dose steroids and have rectal inflammation that causes complications with healing (Adler et al., 2012). Many of these UC patients are very sick and have been hospitalized and receiving medical management prior to surgery. Patients will often report feeling significantly better after the ostomy surgery.

The WOC nurse can provide preoperative education and stoma siting followed by postoperative teaching for the ileostomy. Pouchitis, a nonspecific mucosal inflammation in the IPAA with increased stooling, nighttime fecal incontinence, pain, and bleeding, may occur, and the WOC nurse can be invaluable in navigating best management (see Chapters 6 to 8). It is not life threatening but is life altering with the child feeling ill. There is usually an adequate response with antibiotics or long-term low-dose alternating antibiotics. Patients should be followed long term by the pediatric GI service to monitor symptoms, medications, and surveillance of disease.

KEY POINT

Children can present with the classic symptoms of weight loss, abdominal pain, and bloody diarrhea, and many present with nonclassic symptoms of isolated poor growth, anemia, or other extraintestinal manifestations.

FAMILIAL POLYPOSIS SYNDROMES

Incidence

Intestinal cancers in children are rare, and surgical procedures are often preventative as in familial adenomatous polyposis (FAP), an autosomal dominant inherited syndrome characterized by multiple adenomatous polyps, predisposing to colorectal cancer development, and numerous extracolonic manifestations. FAP is the most common polyposis syndrome, affecting 1 in 10,000 children. The classic and attenuated forms of FAP are caused by mutations in the APC (adenomatous polyposis coli) gene (Campos, 2014).

Presentation

FAP is usually noted as mucus in the stool, blood per rectum, and a change in bowel habits that often includes frequency.

Assessment

A family history of FAP, genetic testing, and endoscopic surveillance yearly starting by age 10.

Management

With FAP, a proctocolectomy and IPAA are usually performed. The surgery is done prophylactically to prevent the increased likelihood of developing cancer rather than related to the severity of symptoms. The risk of cancer helps to determine the timing of surgery but is often done during the early teenage years. Reasons are unclear, but there are fewer complications in FAP patients than in UC patients with regard to pouchitis, nighttime soiling, and incontinence (Moir, 2010). Polyposis syndromes are discussed further in Chapter 7.

PEDIATRIC TRAUMA

Incidence

Unintentional injuries are the leading cause of death and disability for children ≥1 year of age, adolescents, and young adults in the United States (Gill & Kelly, 2019). There are numerous reliable sources that provide injury statistics; however, Gill and Kelly (2019) reports unintentional injuries resulted in the deaths of more than 17,000 children, adolescents, and young adults ages 0 to 24 years in 2017.

Presentation

The primary mechanisms of injury are development and age dependent (Gill & Kelly, 2019). In 2017, more than 6 million children under the age of 19 years old were injured seriously enough to require a visit to a hospital emergency department. The most common injuries were open wounds, superficial injuries and contusions, dislocations and sprains, followed by upper-limb fractures, intracranial injury, foreign body, burns, and poisoning. Unintentional falls are the leading cause of nonfatal injury in children presenting to hospital emergency departments in the United States, followed by being struck by or against an object (Centers for disease control and prevention WISQARS, 2017).

Assessment

A full head-to-toe assessment should always be done on the child in addition to obtaining a history from the child and family member or guardian.

Management

Although most children treated for injuries do not require surgery, and even more rarely, an ostomy, it is worth mentioning. Traumas are usually unexpected and if requiring an ostomy, the event is even more stressful and involves comprehensive teaching. Family education and support is necessary. Examples of traumas that may require surgery for an ostomy are blunt abdominal trauma from an MVA with perforation to the intestines, child and sexual abuse such as rectal injury from objects, severe perineal burns requiring diverting ostomy for burn care, and gunshot wounds (GSW) whether accidental or related to gang violence.

Gun-related deaths are the third leading cause of death among U.S. children, killing 1,297 each year, according to a new study from the Centers for Disease Control and Prevention (2014) based on data analyzed from 2002 to 2014. Of the children who died from gun-related injuries, 53% were homicides, 38% were suicides, and 6% were unintentional. On average, 5,790 children each year received medical treatment in an emergency department for a gun-related injury, and nationally, gun-related injuries account for 2% to 7% of injuries in pediatric trauma centers (Fowler et al., 2017).

The WOC nurse provides ostomy education and helps the multidisciplinary team provide psychosocial adjustment to children experiencing a traumatic event. Additional members of the multidisciplinary team include the primary physician, surgeon, child life support, and social services. When violence is involved in the traumatic event, safety of the staff is of utmost importance when dealing with potentially violent patients and/or families. Refer to WOCN® (2011), Surgical indications for fecal diversions (pediatric ostomy care best practice for clinicians).

 MANAGEMENT OF FECAL DIVERSIONS

TECHNIQUES AND INDICATIONS FOR PEDIATRIC POUCHING

Stool output should be contained, and the peristomal skin should be kept clear of rashes, denuded skin, and infection. Most often, stool output is contained in a pouching system; however, depending on the age of the child, stool may be contained in a diaper with good skin care to prevent the output from irritating the peristomal skin. If a stoma has a mucous fistula, they may be pouched together or separately. Some infants have more than 1 or 2 stomas, may have an open wound or additional potential pouching issues on their abdomen, such as an open wound or a vesicostomy. These children will benefit from the experience and resourcefulness of the WOC nurse as pouching systems will need to be adapted to incorporate more than one stoma, wound dressings may be applied with ostomy appliances layered on top, and waterproof tape may be incorporated to separate pouching systems from vesicostomy drainage. Fecal stomas and urostomies should not be pouched together due to the risk of infection. The peristomal skin may be washed with water, a mild soap, stomal wipes or "baby wipes" specifically without additives to avoid irritating the skin or leaving residual lotions on the skin that would repel the barrier and prevent it from adhering.

Younger children are active and frequently dislodge their pouches. They may wear any clothing; however, clothing with snaps between the legs or "onesies" can help to hold the pouch in place. Adaptive clothing is now readily available for older children as well on the Internet, addressing the needs of those with special needs that may still attempt to dislodge their appliances. Pediatric ostomy belts for securing pouches for the toddler and older child may be beneficial; in addition, there are versions of abdominal binders and netting available. Pouches may be secured inside or outside of the diaper per family preference. Children with fragile skin are at risk for developing pressure injury and must be monitored to prevent medical device–related pressure injuries such as lying on a pouch, spout, or clamp for an extended period of time. Infants may be excessively gassy from crying, sucking, and swallowing air and pouches with filters can help easily release the gas.

Older children are embarrassed by smells and sounds. It can be reinforced that if there is a good seal with the pouching system, and no leakage, there should be no odor. Using a deodorizer in the pouch and room atomizers to neutralize the odor when emptying and changing pouches works well. Dropping toilet paper into the toilet bowl will help prevent splashing when emptying pouch contents into the bowl. Before a quiet time in class such as an examination, avoiding foods that cause excessive gas will lessen the likelihood of audible bowel sounds. The older child will quickly learn what foods affect the stool output. Encourage school-aged children to have an emergency kit with all supplies needed for a pouching system change to be kept at school. Being prepared ahead of time can boost confidence in their ability to self-manage. For liquid high output stomas, crystals placed in the pouch to turn the stool into gel are effective. Typical pouch wear time is anywhere from 24 hours to 5 days. Children may bathe with or without their pouch on depending upon personal preference. Children may participate in all sports and can use ostomy belts or spandex compression garments to help hold their ostomy pouch in place, and a stoma dome or protector can be used for contact sports.

REFEEDING OSTOMY OUTPUT

Children with resection of the small bowel causing feeding problems related to bowel length or stomas with high-volume output causing poor growth, long-term total parenteral nutrition, dehydration, and electrolyte imbalance may require refeeding of ostomy output. Refeeding is thought to help intestinal adaptation and improve peristalsis and mucosal growth (Richardson et al., 2006). Refeeding is often done in the premature and full-term infant for short bowel symptoms and occasionally adolescents for rare events such as severe trauma to the intestines (Stellar & Widmer, 2013). To refeed via the stoma, the child must have a patent distal intestinal limb. The patient is on strict intake and output, and the stool output is collected from the ostomy pouch and refed via a pump and catheter. Strict labeling is imperative to avoid accidental administration of stool in intravenous catheters and central lines.

A catheter is placed into the distal stoma and threaded through an opening created in the ostomy pouch. Initial catheter placement may be done by the surgical team and possibly under radiograph to determine position and length and to closely monitor to prevent intestinal trauma and perforation. Anatomically, if it is possible to pouch the stomas separately, it may be easier to collect stool in one pouch and instill the stool through the second pouch into the mucous fistula. When instilling stool, there may be leakage and frequent catheter displacement. If leakage occurs, attempt to quantify the amount to determine how much needs to be replaced. Refeeding requires a WOC nurse consult, good team communication, and patience and creativity for pouching and tube securement.

PATHOLOGY AND MANAGEMENT CONDITIONS LEADING TO URINARY DIVERSION

PRUNE BELLY SYNDROME

Prune belly (Eagle-Barrett) syndrome (PBS) is a congenital disorder defined by a characteristic clinical triad of abdominal muscle deficiency with characteristic wrinkled appearance due to partial or complete absence of the abdominal wall muscles, severe urinary tract abnormalities, and bilateral cryptorchidism in males. PBS is multisystem disease with patients displaying concomitant cardiopulmonary, GI, and musculoskeletal anomalies in varying degrees. The etiology is unknown (Wallner & Kramar, 2019) (**Fig. 15-12A and B**).

Incidence

Based upon data from the Kids' Inpatient Database (KID) from 2002, 2003, and 2006, the incidence of PBS in the United States was approximately 3.8 cases per 100,000 live births. Approximately 50% of affected patients were white, 30% black, and 10% Hispanic. PBS primarily occurs in males, although there are rare case reports of this disorder in females without noted gonadal abnormalities found in males (Wallner & Kramar, 2019).

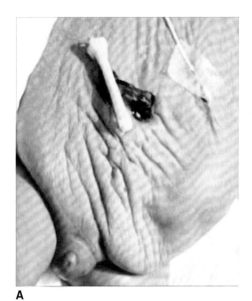 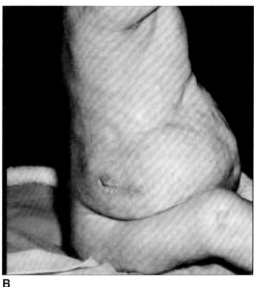

A   **B**

FIGURE 15-12. A, B. Prune belly syndrome. (Courtesy of Karen M. Polise, MSN, RN, Division of Nephrology, The Children's Hospital of Philadelphia.)

Presentation

PBS may be noted on prenatal ultrasound, noted at birth, or in early childhood with the identification of the characteristic features of abdominal muscle deficiency, severe urinary tract abnormalities identified by US, and bilateral cryptorchidism in males.

Assessment

Once diagnosed, further testing may be done to rule out other anomalies. Radiographs are done to assess the internal anatomy of the genitourinary tract. The upper urinary tract with the ureters and kidneys may be severely torturous.

Management

The appropriate therapy of PBS in early childhood remains controversial. Severely affected patients require early surgery such as a supravesical diversion or primary reconstruction, with a goal of adequate urinary drainage and avoidance of recurrent infections. Additional surgical options may include the insertions of a cystostomy button, a temporary vesicostomy, or ureterostomies to facilitate bladder drainage and avoid backup of urine that will damage the urinary system (Wallner & Kramar, 2019).

MYELOMENINGOCELE

Neural tube defects (NTDs) are the most common congenital central nervous system (CNS) anomalies, and myelomeningocele or "spina bifida" is the most common NTD. It is characterized by a cleft in the vertebral column with a corresponding defect in the skin exposing the meninges and spinal cord. Children may experience weakness or absence of sensation that affects the lower extremities and includes bowel/bladder dysfunction, dependent upon the level of the spinal lesion (Bowman, 2020) (**Fig. 15-13A–C**).

The etiology is unclear, but genetic factors and environmental factors including folic acid deficiency play a role in NTDs (Rosenblum, 2014).

Incidence

The incidence of spina bifida has decreased with the recommendation of daily folic acid for pregnant women and with antenatal testing procedures that detect NTD. Testing facilitates prenatal counseling with the parents that should include information on myelomeningocele and the prenatal management decisions, including pursuit of additional prenatal testing, choice of delivery setting, the possibility of fetal surgery, and termination of the pregnancy (Bowman, 2020).

Presentation

Prenatal diagnosis of spina bifida is with US fetal amniotic fluid assays, or elevated maternal alpha-fetoprotein. When a child is born with spina bifida, there may be varying degrees of lesions, which correlate to the level of dysfunction.

Assessment

A complete physical examination with emphasis on the defect size, level, tissue covering, and if there is, any cerebral spinal fluid (CSF) leakage. The most common lesion is in the lumbosacral area, which may leave the child able to walk. Neurologic symptoms should be assessed as well as fontanelles on the newborn to examine for hydrocephalus (Rosenblum, 2014).

Management

Management decisions will be made by the parents and the medical team after the parents have been fully advised and are able to verbalize understanding of

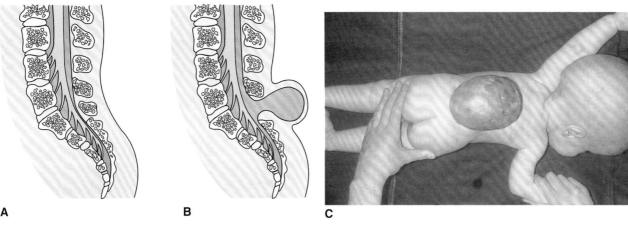

A   **B**   **C**

FIGURE 15-13. Myelomeningocele. Spina bifida is incomplete closure of the spinal cord.
A. Normal spinal cord. **B.** Spina bifida with protrusion of the meninges (meningocele). **C.** Protrusion
of the spinal cord and meninges (myelomeningocele). (Reprinted with permission from Pillitteri, A.
(2008). *Maternal and child health nursing* (5th ed.). Philadelphia, PA: Wolters Kluwer.)

proposed management and expected outcomes. Fetal surgery may arrest leakage of spinal fluid from the back and may be able to prevent or reverse herniation of the hindbrain (Chiari II malformation) and hydrocephalus. The recommendation of the American College of Obstetricians and Gynecologists (ACOG) is that fetal surgery only be performed at facilities with the special expertise, multidisciplinary teams, and facilities able to provide the intensive care required for these patients (Bowman, 2020).

When a child is born with spina bifida, the lesion should be assessed for CSF leakage and covered with sterile gauze or the infant should be evaluated by a team of specialists including a thorough neurologic examination to define the baseline neuropathy of the child and identify the level of spinal cord defect, associated anomalies, signs of hydrocephalus, and evidence of brainstem compression (Chiari II malformation). Prophylactic antibiotics are given to reduce the risk of infection of the CNS, and surgery to close the lesion is done within 72 hours of birth. Hydrocephalus is common postoperatively and may require placement of a ventriculoperitoneal shunt. These children are prone to a host of neurological issues and should be followed closely (Bowman, 2020).

Nearly all patients with myelomeningoccle have bladder dysfunction (neurogenic bladder), affecting urinary continence and quality of life, and may lead to progressive deterioration of the upper urinary tract and chronic renal disease. Some degree of renal dysfunction is present in 30% to 40% of children with myelomeningocele (Baskin, 2019).

The management goal for neurogenic bladder patients with myelomeningocele is to preserve renal function and establish independent continence of bowel and bladder at a developmentally appropriate age. Management is based on US, symptoms, and urodynamic findings, as well as psychosocial assessment of readiness. Clean intermittent catheterization (CIC) is recommended for all patients with neurogenic bladder along with close

monitoring for changes in bladder function which may indicate a neurologic complication (shunt malfunction or tethered cord). Young children can be taught self-catheterization once they show an interest and are able to learn the procedure. They may begin by assisting their parent or caregiver until they become independent. Medical management may include the use of anticholinergics or prophylactic antibiotics (Baskin, 2019). Surgical interventions may include vesicostomy, ileovesicostomy, or appendicovesicostomy (APV) (Bowman, 2020).

Innervation of the bowel and anus are affected in most children born with myelomeningocele that may lead to dysmotility, poor sphincter control, and fecal incontinence (which occurs in 60% to 70% of cases). An effective bowel management program will be prescribed and may include oral laxatives, suppositories, and/or enemas. If these first-line options are not effective, transanal irrigation and antegrade continence enema (ACE) may be warranted. The ACE procedure (Malone antegrade continence enema) uses the appendix and cecum to create a catheterizable stoma. An irrigation is instilled through the stoma to clean out the colon. The irrigation is usually performed on a schedule and may be combined with medications with a goal of achieving bowel continence. If none of these methods is effective, surgical creation of a stoma may be indicated (Bowman, 2020).

 CONSTRUCTION AND MANAGEMENT OF PEDIATRIC URINARY DIVERSIONS (FIG. 15-14)

VESICOSTOMY

Vesicostomy is a procedure that provides an outlet for urine, protects the upper urinary tract, decreases hydronephrosis, and improves kidney function. The bladder is externalized to the abdominal wall so that urine can drain, avoiding the back up of urine (Rouzrokh et al., 2013).

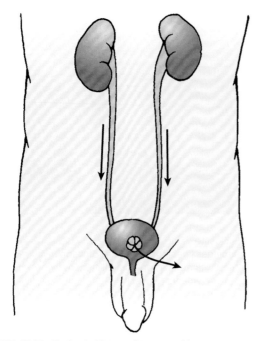

FIGURE 15-14. Pediatric Urinary Diversion. Vesicostomy.

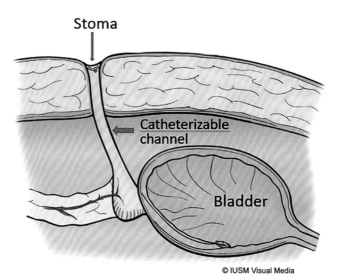

FIGURE 15-15. Mitrofanoff Procedure.

Surgery can be performed soon after birth and the vesicostomy may be left in place until the child is of school age and better equipped to manage a catheterizable continent stoma. The family will require teaching for peristomal skin care to prevent skin breakdown from the constant drainage of urine. A diaper that is large enough to cover the vesicostomy can be used to collect the urine with frequent application of a skin barrier cream for protection.

ILEOVESICOSTOMY

Ileovesicostomy is an effective surgical treatment for patients with neurogenic bladder dysfunction who are unable to perform clean intermittent self-catheterization. A small section of the ileum is removed and the remaining intestines are anastomosed or sewn back together. The piece of ileum is used as a "conduit" to attach the bladder out to the abdominal wall for the diversion of urine. Outcomes for ileovesicostomy show improved bladder compliance, reduction of urethral incontinence, and improved quality of life after a successful procedure. Ileovesicostomy surgery is associated with possible complications including high rates of wound infection (34%), urethral incontinence (28%), and extended hospital length of stay (Vanni et al., 2009). Ileovesicostomy surgery may be done in open, laparoscopic, or robotic methods. Refer to WOCN (2011), surgical indication for urinary diversions (pediatric ostomy care best practice for clinicians).

APPENDICOVESICOSTOMY

An APV (Mitrofanoff procedure) is a surgical procedure similar to the ileovesicostomy). The Mitrofanoff procedure, developed in 1980 by Paul Mitrofanoff, creates a continent catheterizable stoma on the abdominal wall at the level of the umbilicus or on the lower abdomen. For patients who are unable to catheterize their own urethra, this procedure offers an alternative method to achieve independence by creating an abdominal catheterizable channel constructed between the bladder and the skin utilizing appendix or bowel as a conduit. The diversion is continent because of the valve arrangement, which prevents urinary leakage. The most common complication is stenosis or leaking of the stoma at the skin, which may require dilation or surgical revision. An APV is achieved with the Mitrofanoff procedure and an ileovesicostomy is performed with the Monti procedure.

If the appendix is short in length or the patient is heavy-set, then the appendix will not reach the belly-button and is instead sewn to the right lower part of the abdomen.

The other end of the narrow tube is connected to the bladder (reservoir) using a tunneling technique to create a flap-valve (see **Fig. 15-15**).

The bladder should have a large capacity (usually 500 mL) and will need to store urine at low pressures. If the bladder is small, then the capacity of the bladder will have to be increased by patching the bladder with a piece of bowel. This bladder patching surgery is done at the same time as creation of the Mitrofanoff.

KEY POINT

Spina bifida requires a team approach and lifelong monitoring, and many large medical centers or children's hospitals have a multidisciplinary spina bifida clinic.

REHABILITATIVE ISSUES

SUPPORT AND EDUCATION FOR THE CHILD AND FAMILY

It is imperative with pediatrics to provide family-centered care, and the WOC nurse is an invaluable resource for the child and family, as well as other members of the health care team. Whenever possible, the WOC nurse should meet the family preoperatively and then follow the child closely after surgery. From assisting the parents to bonding with their new premature infant with an ostomy, to educating the school nurse of an adolescent with a new and unexpected ostomy, the psychosocial and educational opportunities are limitless. In the age of the Internet and social media, there are multiple ways to obtain information. A Google search for "pediatric ostomy management" provides more than 600,000 links ranging from scholarly articles, university and hospital Web sites, ostomy organizations and support groups such as UOAA and the Pull Through Network, ostomy appliance suppliers, Facebook groups, and the professional organizations such as the Wound Ostomy Continence Nurses Society™. The Wound Ostomy Continence Nurses Society™ Pediatric Ostomy Care: Best Practice for Clinicians (2011) and The Wound, Ostomy, and Continence Nurses Society™ Pediatric Ostomy Complications: Best Practice for Clinicians (2016) are invaluable resource for the health care team and are located on the WOCN Web site, www.wocn.org. The American College of Surgeons (2012) also has a pediatric ostomy skills kit that can be ordered to assist patients to prepare for home ostomy management. The information comes in written, CD, and online formats (www.facs.org/patienteducation). Appendix B lists many support groups focused on ostomies and children.

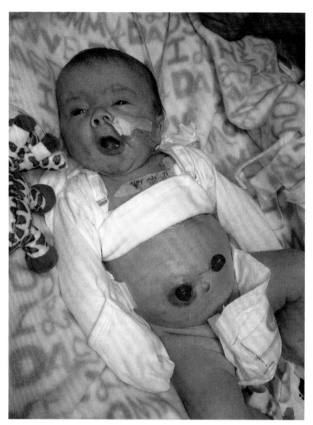

FIGURE 15-16. An Infant with Stoma. (Bowden, V., & Greenberg, C. S. (2013). *Bowden children and their families*. Philadelphia, PA: Wolters Kluwer.)

DEVELOPMENTAL PHASE AND IMPLICATIONS FOR CARE AND EDUCATION (AGE SPECIFIC)

Premature Infant/Full-Term Infant

Developmentally, the epidermal barrier is immature and leads to trans epidermal water loss and absorption of topical agents through the skin. Premature infants have a weak epidermal and dermal bond and are more prone to friction injury and blistering of the skin. There is increased toxicity to chemicals due to immature organs, and nutritional deficiencies should be accounted for due to the immature GI tract. The acid mantle is not developed until day 4 of life, so, younger infants are more prone to invasion of microbes. Fragile skin should be protected, and friction should be minimized. Many of the infant ostomies are temporary and may be closed prior to discharge. For the infant going home with an ostomy, a caregiver should be able to fully demonstrate emptying, removing, and applying an ostomy pouch and be able to verbalize the signs and symptoms of complications. The infant will not remember having an ostomy but does experience pain, and the parents need a lot of support bonding and reviewing stoma care. **Figure 15-16** shows an infant with stoma, and **Figure 15-17** shows an infant with an ostomy pouch. Minimal products should be used on the skin, and manufacturer's guidelines should be followed in relation to age.

Toddler (12 Months to 3 Years) and Preschool (3 to 5 Years)

This age group has a busy and fun time with exploration of the environment, and play time is a big part of the child's day. Teaching for toddlers and preschoolers is primarily focused on the parent but should also include the child. Teaching should be age appropriate and may be enhanced with the use of ostomy dolls, stuffed animals, story books, and coloring books, often available from the ostomy product manufacturers. Short attention spans should be considered when teaching. They are rapidly growing and will have increased improvement with gross motor and fine motor skills, and as their dexterity improves, they can help with more difficult things. Children like to participate and be autonomous. Although the parent or health care provider should change the ostomy pouch, the child can help organize supplies, remove adhesives, and assist per their comfort level. Normal toilet training should take place for urine and stool if not diverted.

School Age (6 to 12 Years)

Advances in cognitive and physical ability should promote independence and support maturity as they grow. They learn readily and enjoy "jobs" as their confidence increases. The older school-aged child can become

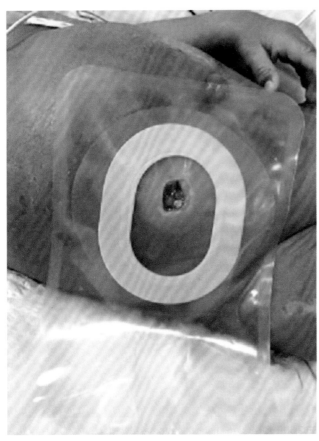

FIGURE 15-17. An Infant with an Ostomy Pouch. (Courtesy Christine Carter.)

independent in ostomy care and should participate in overnight sleepovers and camps. Nutrition should be discussed, and the child should participate in meal planning and preparation to help eat nutritious foods for his or her health. They should drink plenty of water and chew food well to prevent blockages.

Adolescent (13 to 18 Years)
Hormonal changes and rapid brain growth during the adolescent years may produce emotional lability and often influence their ability to learn and comply with management recommendations. Extra sensitivity and understanding may be necessary when dealing with this age group. Adolescents can receive full education and should be their own caregivers when dealing with their ostomy with the parents as backup support. Adolescents are very concerned about hygiene, social situations, and sexuality. All these aspects should be addressed in addition to overall good health, exercise, and nutrition. They may not fully understand their disease process and may rebel or be fearful with this situation. They may participate in risky behaviors at this age and may not plan to take supplies on an outing or order more supplies when running low.

Ostomy camps such as the Youth Rally can be a place for sharing, and meeting peers with similar situations. Camp promotes independence, self-esteem, learning, friendship, and fun. The Youth Rally Web site and the Internet allow these teens to remain in contact throughout the year. Teenagers appreciate choices and should participate in choosing which supplies they will use. This age group may seek out their peers instead of their parents or health care professions for medical advice (Mohr, 2012), which is why attending camps that are staffed with WOC nurses and Web sites that are monitored by professionals are important for these teens. It is important that the WOC nurse recognize that children and their families need time to form a relationship with their WOC nurse and be comfortable asking questions. WOCN® Society & UOAA publications, Teen Chat: You and Your Ostomy (2013), and camps are valuable resources. Whenever possible, meeting with the child and family prior to surgery can alleviate some anxiety and be a time to begin education. Stoma siting can be extremely helpful to place the stoma in an appropriate place for anatomical differences and types of clothing the child wears.

CONCLUSIONS

There has been a decrease in the number of ostomies performed in childhood with advances in surgical techniques and single-stage procedures. The majority of pediatric stomas are placed during infancy and are not usually permanent with stoma takedown normally done within 6 weeks to 12 months from the original surgery. This group can be challenging due to the lack of products designed for infants and children to meet the needs of high-output stomas, convexity, belts, and extended wear materials. While there has been an explosion in the types of ostomy pouching systems and products to meet the needs of teens and young adults with stomas from swimwear, sports guards, support belts, pouch covers, and undergarments to help them achieve an active lifestyle, the same cannot be said for babies, toddlers, and preschoolers. There are only a handful of companies that have pediatric specific products, and the options within those pediatric lines are limited. The WOC nurse is instrumental in developing a management plan to address the unique needs and stomal management complications of this age group. These families require a large amount of information, education, and emotional support and follow-up to help them deal with their challenges.

REFERENCES

Adibe, O., & Georgeson, K. (2012). Chapter 95: Crohn's disease. In A. G. Coran, N. S. Adzick, T. M. Krummel, et al. (Eds.), *Pediatric surgery* (7th ed., Vol. 1 & 2, pp. 1209–1215). Philadelphia, PA: Elsevier/Saunders.

Adler, J., Coran, A., & Teitelbaum, D. (2012). Chapter 96: Ulcerative colitis. In: A. G. Coran, N. S. Adzick, T. M. Krummel, et al. (Eds.), *Pediatric* surgery (7th ed., Vol. 1 & 2, pp. 1217–1229). Philadelphia, PA: Elsevier/Saunders.

Aguayo, P., & Ostlie, D. (2010). Chapter 31: Duodenal and intestinal atresia and stenosis. In G. Holcomb & J. Murphy (Eds.), *Ashcraft's pediatric surgery* (5th ed., pp. 400–415). Philadelphia, PA: Saunders/Elsevier.

American College of Surgeons Division of Education Pediatric. (2012). Pediatric Ostomy Home Skills Kit ASCRS. Retrieved from: https://www.facs.org/education/patient-education/skills-programs/ostomy-program/pediatric-colostomy-ileostomy

Association of Women's health, Obstetrics and Neonatal Nurses (AWHONN). (2013). New Neonatal Skin Care Evidence-Based Practice Guideline. *Nursing for Women's Health, 17*(6), 545–546. https://doi.org/10.1111/1751-486X.12085

Baskin, L. S. (Updated October 28, 2019). Urinary tract complications of myelomeningocele (spina bifida). In *UptoDate*. Retrieved from https://www.uptodate

Bensard, D., Acker, S., & Kulungowski, A. (Updated December 19, 2018). Intestinal malrotation. Retrieved from https://emedicine.medscape.com/article/930313

Bousvaros, A., Setty, M., & Kaplan, J. L. (Updated June 3, 2019). Management of mild to moderate ulcerative colitis in children and adolescents. In *UptoDate*. Retrieved from https://www.uptodate.com

Bowman, R. M. (Updated January 2, 2020). Overview of the management of myelomeningocele (spina bifida). In *UptoDate*. Retrieved from https://www.uptodate.com

Campos, F. G. (2014). Surgical treatment of familial adenomatous polyposis: Dilemmas and current recommendations. *World Journal of Gastroenterology, 20*(44), 16620–16629. doi: 10.3748/wjg.v20.i44.16620.

Centers for Disease Prevention and Control. (2017). Injury prevention & control. Retrieved from https://cdc.gov/injury/wisqars/nonfatal.html

Centers for Disease Prevention and Control. (2014). Pediatric injury prevention: Epidemiology, history, and application. Retrieved from https://cdc.gov/nchs/data/hus/2014/089.pdf

Centers for Disease Control and Prevention. (2017). WISQARS leading causes of nonfatal injury reports, 2000-2017. Retrieved from https://webapp.cdc.gov/sasweb/ncipc/nfilead.html

Clarke, W. T., & Feuerstein, J. D. (2019). Colorectal cancer surveillance in inflammatory bowel disease: Practice guidelines and recent developments. *World Journal of Gastroenterology, 25*(30), 4148–4157. doi: 10.3748/wjg.v25.i30.4148.

Coste, A. H., Waheed, A., & Ahmad, H. (Updated May 5, 2019). Midgut volvulus. In *StatPearls [Internet]*. Treasure Island, FL: StatPearls Publishing. Retrieved from https://www.ncbi.nlm.nih.gov/books/NBK441962

Fernando, M., Creighton, S., & Wood, D. (2015). The Long-term management and outcomes of cloacal anomalies. *Pediatric Nephrology, 30*(5), 759–765.

Fowler, K. A., Dahlberg, L. L., Haileyesus, T., et al. (2017). Childhood firearm injuries in the United States. *Pediatrics, 140*(1), e20163486. doi: https://doi.org/10.1542/peds.2016-3486.

Gauderer, M. (2012). Chapter 98: Stomas of the small and large intestine. In A. G. Coran, N. S. Adzick, T. M. Krummel, et al. (Eds.), *Pediatric surgery* (7th ed., Vol. 1 & 2, pp. 1058–1061). Philadelphia, PA: Elsevier/Saunders.

Georgeson, K. (2010). Chapter 35: Hirschsprung's disease. In G. W. Holcomb & J. P. Murphy (Eds.), *Ashcraft's pediatric surgery* (5th ed., pp. 456–467). Philadelphia, PA: Saunders/Elsevier.

Gill, A. C., & Kelly, N. R. (Updated September 1, 2019). Pediatric injury prevention: Epidemiology, history, and application. In *UptoDate*. Retrieved from https://www.uptodate.com

Ginglen, J. G., & Butki, N. (Updated July 18, 2019). Necrotizing enterocolitis. In *StatPearls [Internet]*. Treasure Island, FL: StatPearls Publishing. Retrieved from https://www.ncbi.nlm.nih.gov/books/NBK513357/

Glasseer, J. G., & Springer, S. C. (Updated March 17, 2016). Intestinal obstruction in the newborn clinical presentation. Retrieved from https://emedicine.medscape.com/article/2066380

Gossman, W., Eovaldi, B. J., & Cohen, H. L. (Updated May 19, 2019). Duodenal atresia and stenosis. In *StatPearls [Internet]*. Treasure Island, FL: StatPearls Publishing. Retrieved from https://www.ncbi.nlm.nih.gov/books/NBK470548/

Guardino, K., & Pieper, P. (2013). Chapter 20: Anorectal malformations in children. In N. Browne, L. Flanigan, C. McComiskey, et al. (Eds.), *Nursing care of the pediatric surgical patient* (3rd ed., pp. 359–372). Burlington, MA: Jones & Bartlett Learning.

Higuchi, L. M., & Bousvaros, A. (Updated January 20, 2020). Clinical presentation and diagnosis of inflammatory bowel disease in children. In *Up-to-Date*. Retrieved from https://www.uptodate.com

Holder, M., & Jackson, L. (2013). Chapter 19: Hirschsprung's disease. In N. Browne, L. Flanigan, C. McComiskey, et al. (Eds.), *Nursing care of the pediatric surgical patient* (3rd ed., pp. 347–356). Burlington, MA: Jones & Bartlett Learning.

Karrer, F. M., Potter, D. D., & Calkins, C. M. (Updated August 9, 2016). Pediatric duodenal atresia. Retrieved from https://emedicine.medscape.com/article/932917

Katkin, J. P. (Updated October 23, 2019). Cystic fibrosis clinical manifestations and diagnosis. In *UptoDate*. Retrieved from https://www.uptodate.com

Kim, J. H. (Updated June 21, 2019a). Neonatal necrotizing enterocolitis: Clinical features and diagnosis. In *UptoDate*. Retrieved from https://www.uptodate.com

Kim, J. H. (Updated June 12, 2019b). Neonatal necrotizing enterocolitis: Management. In *UptoDate*. Retrieved from https://www.uptodate.com

Levitt, M. A., & Peña, A. (July 26, 2007). Anorectal malformations. *Orphanet Journal of Rare Diseases, 2*, 33.

Levitt, M. A., & Wood, R. J. (Updated April 2, 2019). Surgery for pediatric anorectal malformation (Imperforate Anus) treatment & management. Retrieved from https://emedicine.medscape.com/article/933524-treatment#d10

McDowell, C., & Haseeb, M. (Updated December 29, 2019). Inflammatory bowel disease (IBD). In *StatPearls [Internet]*. Treasure Island, FL: StatPearls Publishing. Retrieved from https://www.ncbi.nlm.nih.gov/books/NBK470312/

McIltrot, K., & Wilson, L. (2014). Chapter 18: The child with altered gastrointestinal status. In V. Bowden & C. Greenberg (Eds.), *Children and their families: The continuum of nursing care* (pp. 783–874). Philadelphia, PA: Lippincott Williams & Wilkins.

Minkes, R., Grewal, H., McHard, K., et al. (2019). Medscape. Retrieved from https://emedicine.medscape.com/article/939455

Mohr, L. (2012). Growth and development issues in adolescents with ostomies: A primer of the WOC nurse. *Journal of Wound, Ostomy, and Continence Nursing, 39*(5), 515–521.

Moir, C. (2010). Chapter 42: Inflammatory bowel disease and intestinal cancer. In G. Holcomb & J. Murphy (Eds.), *Ashcraft's pediatric surgery* (5th ed., pp. 532–548). Philadelphia, PA: Saunders/Elsevier.

Rapoport, K., & Nishii, F. K. (2013). Chapter 16: Necrotizing enterocolitis. In N. Browne, L. Flanigan, C. McComiskey, et al. (Eds.), *Nursing care of the pediatric surgical patient* (3rd ed., pp. 295–311). Burlington, MA: Jones & Bartlett Learning.

Richardson, L., Banerjee, S., & Heike, R. (2006). What is the evidence in the practice of mucous fistula re-feeding in neonates with short bowel syndrome. *Journal of Pediatric Gastroenterology and Nutrition, 43*(2), 267–270.

Rosen, M. J., Dhawan, A., & Saeed, S. A. (2015). Inflammatory bowel disease in children and adolescents. *JAMA Pediatrics, 169*(11), 1053–1060. doi: 10.1001/jamapediatrics.2015.1982

Rosen, N. G. (Updated December 30, 2019). Pediatric imperforate anus (anorectal malformation). Retrieved from https://emedicine.medscape.com/article/929904-overview

Rosenblum, R. (2014). The child with altered neurologic status. In V. Bowden & C. Greenberg (Eds.), *Children and their families: The continuum of nursing care* (pp. 1021–1103). Philadelphia, PA: Lippincott Williams & Wilkins.

Rouzrokh, M., Mirshemirani, A., Khaleghnejah-Tabaii, A., et al. (2013). Protective temporary vesicostomy for upper urinary tract problems in children. *Iranian Journal of Pediatrics, 23*(6), 648–652.

Setty, M., Russel, G. H., & Bousvaros, A. (Updated April 23, 2018). Clinical manifestations of Crohn's disease in children and adolescents. In *UptoDate*. Retrieved from https://www.uptodate.com

Smith, C. A., & Avansino, J. (Updated May 27, 2019). Anorectal malformations. In *StatPearls [Internet]*. Treasure Island, FL: StatPearls Publishing.

Stellar, J., & Widmer, T. (2013). Chapter 17: Intestinal atresia, duplications and meconium ileus. In N. Browne, L. Flanigan, C. McComiskey, et al. (Eds.), *Nursing care of the pediatric surgical patient* (3rd ed., pp. 313–329). Burlington, MA: Jones & Bartlett Learning.

Vanni, A., Cohen, M., & Stoffel, J. (2009). Robotic-assisted ileovesicostomy. *Urology, 74*(4), 814–818.

Wagner, J. P. (Updated September 9, 2020). *Hirschsprung disease.* Retrieved April 29, 2019, from http://emedicine.medscape.com/article/178493-overview.

Wallner, M., Kramar, R. (Updated October 30, 2019). Prune-belly syndrome. In *UptoDate*. Retrieved from https://www.uptodate.com

Wesson D. (Updated May 17, 2018). Intestinal atresia. In *UptoDate*. Retrieved from https://www.uptodate.com

Wesson, D., Experanza-Lopez, M. (Updated July 8, 2019). Congenital aganglionic megacolon (Hirschsprung's disease). In *UptoDate*. Retrieved from https://www.uptodate.com

WOCN. (2011). *Pediatric ostomy care: Best practice for clinicians.* Mount Laurel, NJ: Author.

WOCN. (2013). *Teen chat: You and your ostomy.* Mount Laurel, NJ: Author.

WOCN. (2016). *Pediatric ostomy complications: Best practice for clinicians.* Mount Laurel, NJ: Author.

QUESTIONS

1. What neonatal condition generally necessitates the creation of an ileostomy?
   A. Necrotizing enterocolitis
   B. Colonic atresia
   C. Severe perineal trauma
   D. Pelvic malformation

2. What finding would alert the WOC nurse of a possible intestinal obstruction in an infant?
   A. Gastroesophageal reflux disease
   B. Hypoxemia of the bowel
   C. Thrombocytopenia
   D. Bilious emesis

3. A neonate is diagnosed with malrotation. What life-threatening complication of malrotation may occur where torsion occurs?
   A. Necrotizing enterocolitis
   B. Meconium ileus
   C. Prune belly syndrome
   D. Volvulus

4. A neonate is diagnosed with imperforate anus. For what surgical intervention would the WOC nurse prepare the parents?
   A. Urologic surgery
   B. Anoplasty
   C. General surgery
   D. Creation of an ostomy

5. The nurse is caring for a neonate who failed to pass meconium in the first 48 hours after birth. Upon assessment, the nurse notes a distended abdomen, emesis, and sepsis. What condition would the nurse suspect?
   A. Necrotizing enterocolitis
   B. Hirschsprung disease
   C. Volvulus
   D. Inflammatory ileus

6. An 8-year-old female patient is diagnosed with Crohn's disease following symptoms of weight loss, bloody diarrhea, abdominal pain, and perianal disease. What should be the priority management goal for this patient?
   A. Surgical resection of the bowel
   B. Medical therapy to achieve remission of the disease
   C. Immediate strictureplasty
   D. Radiation therapy

7. A 10-year-old male patient presents with the following symptoms: intermittent abdominal cramping, pain, tenesmus, fatigue, and anemia. Osteopenia, weight loss, and anorexia with growth retardation are also noted. What condition would the WOC nurse suspect?
   A. Ulcerative colitis
   B. Familial polyposis syndrome
   C. Crohn's disease
   D. Inflammatory bowel disease

8. An infant diagnosed with prune belly syndrome would be managed by
   A. Vesicostomy
   B. Ileal conduit
   C. ACE procedure
   D. Mitrofanoff procedure

9. Which of the following would be the best to recommend for an active toddler to prevent dislodgement of the pouch?
A. Use one-piece pouch system.
B. Use a diaper instead of a pouch.
C. Dress in clothing that has snap crotch.
D. Restrict active playtime.

10. An infant is diagnosed with myelomeningocele (spina bifida). For what surgery would the WOC nurse prepare the family of this patient?
A. Colostomy
B. Appendicovesicostomy
C. Vesicostomy
D. Ileal or colon conduit

ANSWERS AND RATIONALES

1. A. Rationale: Ileostomy is performed as a surgical emergency in neonates that present with necrotizing enterocolitis. Ileostomy is performed to remove necrotic bowel, and care is taken to remove as little bowel as indicated to prevent short bowel syndrome.

2. D. Rationale: Bilious emesis is an indication of a possible intestinal obstruction in an infant. This can present with midgut volvulus.

3. D. Rationale: Volvulus is a life threatening complication of malrotation. This occurs when the intestine twist 380 degrees on itself, causing vascular obstruction.

4. B. Rationale: Anoplasty is performed for a low imperforate anus.

5. B. Rationale: Meconium ileus presents failure to pas meconium in the first 48 hours after birth. Cystic fibrosis is common with this condition.

6. B. Rationale: Management of Crohn's disease is medical therapy with the goal of achieving remission.

7. A. Rationale: Ulcerative colitis.

8. A. Rationale: Prune belly syndrome presents with severe urinary tract abnormalities. A temporary vesicostomy is performed to provide adequate urinary drainage and prevent back up of urine.

9. C. Rationale: Clothing with a snap crotch ("onesies") can prevent an active toddler from dislodging their colostomy pouch.

10. C. Rationale: Vesicostomy is an initial surgical intervention for an infant with myelomeningocele (spina bifida). The goal is to preserve renal function. The child may be a candidate for clean intermittent catheterization (CIC).

CHAPTER 16

PERISTOMAL SKIN COMPLICATIONS

Ginger Dawn Salvadalena and Virginia Hanchett

OBJECTIVE

Distinguish between peristomal skin complications and select the associated management strategies.

TOPIC OUTLINE

Introduction **250**

Scope of the Problem **250**

Assessment Guidelines **251**

Guidelines for Management of Peristomal Skin Complications **252**

Specific Peristomal Skin Complications **252**
Peristomal Moisture–Associated Skin Damage **252**
Maceration **254**
Pseudoverrucous Lesions **254**
Mechanical Damage **255**
Pressure Injuries **256**
Allergic Contact Dermatitis **256**
Fungal/Candidiasis Infection **257**
Folliculitis **258**
Varices **259**

Granuloma **259**
Peristomal Abscess **260**

Peristomal Fistula **261**

Mucosal Transplantation **261**
Peristomal Pyoderma Gangrenosum **262**

Autoimmune and Atypical Presentations **263**
Peristomal Psoriasis **263**

Less Common Autoimmune Presentations **264**
Bullous Pemphigoid **264**
Pemphigus Vulgaris **264**
Epidermolysis Bullosa Acquisita **265**
Familial Benign Chronic Pemphigus (Hailey-Hailey Disease) **265**
Malignancy **265**

Conclusions **266**

INTRODUCTION

The focus of this chapter is complications affecting the peristomal skin. Presented first is information about the scope of the problem, followed by general guidelines for assessment and management of patients who present with peristomal skin problems. The remainder of the chapter covers specific types of complications, including their etiology, clinical presentation, assessment, and management.

SCOPE OF THE PROBLEM

Peristomal skin problems are common, and they are clinically challenging to prevent and to manage. In prospective studies, the incidence of peristomal skin complications ranged from 11% to 63% (Carlsson et al., 2016; Colwell et al., 2018; Lindholm et al., 2013; Malik et al., 2018; Persson et al., 2010; Salvadalena, 2013). Although individuals with stomas are often unaware that they have a skin problem (Herlufsen et al., 2006; Nybaek et al., 2009), peristomal skin issues were shown to be the cause of over 30% of the visits to an outpatient stoma clinic (Jemec & Nybaek, 2008). Skin problems cause pain, contribute to higher product usage, adversely affect life satisfaction, and may raise health care costs (Meisner et al., 2012; Nichols & Riemer, 2011; Pittman et al., 2008; Taneja et al., 2017, 2019). Clearly, maintaining and restoring the integrity of the peristomal skin has important implications.

KEY POINT

Peristomal complications consist of skin inflammation, injury, or damage in the area covered by the adhesive of the pouching system, typically within a 4-inch area.

The peristomal skin is exposed to mechanical, chemical, and microbial threats on an ongoing basis (Lyon, 2010). Mechanical threats include abrasion, skin stripping, and pressure injury that can occur due to the use of ostomy skin barriers, tapes, and accessories. The physical forces involved in repeated removal of adhesive products can strip away varying amounts of stratum corneum, pull away hair, and even change the architecture of the skin. Peristomal skin becomes thicker and has higher transepidermal water loss compared to healthy contralateral skin (Nybaek et al., 2010); characteristic changes in the structure of the skin have been identified and vary by the type of skin barrier used for stoma care (Omura et al., 2010). Skin stripping and occlusion can predispose the peristomal area to the development of peristomal skin complications (Cressey et al., 2016; Williams & Lyon, 2010). Best practice for care of people with stomas includes early identification and timely intervention for peristomal skin complications (WCET, 2014; WOCN, 2017a).

While there are a number of chemical threats to the peristomal skin, the most noxious is the effluent draining from the stoma; it provides a constant source of moisture, can cause inflammation, and, in the case of an ileostomy, contains enzymes that can damage the skin. Difficulty obtaining the proper fit or size of the skin barrier can allow the effluent from the stoma to drain between the skin barrier and the skin, underscoring the importance of carefully selection of an appropriate stoma site, construction of a protruding stoma on a flat surface, and providing thorough postoperative instruction about ostomy care (Murken & Bleier, 2019). Even appropriately selected and applied topical products carry some risk. The repeated skin stripping with product removal and the use of occlusive barriers increases the risk of irritation and sensitization (Williams & Lyon, 2010). Products used for stoma care contain a variety of ingredients that may be sensitizing or contribute to skin irritation, and their selection and application should be done with attention to their intended use and a clear understanding of the patient's individual needs, history, and risk factors.

Peristomal skin is warm and may be moist, increasing its vulnerability to pathogens (Lyon, 2010). Pathogens normally present on the skin can proliferate producing infection; the ones that most commonly occur are fungal or bacterial. Moist skin is more susceptible than dry skin to pressure-induced skin damage and reductions in regional blood flow (Woo et al., 2017); thus, the risks for skin problems are intensified in the presence of leakage. Complicating the mechanical, chemical, and microbial threats are the influences of the host environment: the health conditions of the individual who has the stoma, his or her age, self-care status, and other individual factors impacting his or her risk of illness.

ASSESSMENT GUIDELINES

The general approach to peristomal skin assessment includes taking a patient history and completing an examination. Begin the assessment by taking a problem-focused history. Include the following: when and how the problem started, description of the problem, signs and symptoms, prior treatment, and any prior episodes of similar problems. Ask about pouching system wear time (usual and current), presence of any leakage (usual and current), peristomal pain, pruritus, and any other sensations in the area of the skin condition. Review the patient's general health history, allergies, and medications. Ask the patient to describe or list each of the products he or she is using for ostomy care, method of use, and the duration of use.

Begin the physical examination *before* removing the pouching system if possible. Note how the pouching system has been applied, its security, and any areas of leakage, tension, channeling, or pressure. After removing the skin barrier and *before* discarding, look at the adhesive/skin side of the barrier. Under good lighting, look at the barrier for any signs of erosion, noting its location and any evidence of leakage. The barrier provides important clues about the location of leakage of effluent onto the peristomal skin. When the pouching system is off, examine the peristomal skin in the presence of good lighting. For the purposes of this discussion, the peristomal skin is defined as the area of skin surrounding the stoma that had contact with the skin barrier of the pouching system. For adults, this area is typically 4 inches or less in diameter. Cleanse the skin to allow a thorough evaluation and note the color and condition of the skin. Normal peristomal skin is free of any damage, that is, the skin is unbroken and rash-free. Variations in pigmentation may occur, particularly in individuals with resolving dermatitis and those with darker skin tones (Williams & Lyon, 2010). Lift the stoma to allow visualization of the skin beneath the lower edge of the mucosa, if needed. Palpate any bumps or nodules. Note any areas of localized redness or warmth in the peristomal skin. If wounds are present, measure their size and depth and note location in relationship to the stoma. If a rash is present, note the type and distribution. A photograph may be useful for documentation and for future comparison purposes.

If the fit of the pouching system is in question, assess the stoma, peristomal skin, and peristomal contours in lying, sitting, and standing positions. Look for incisions or scars in the area of the stoma or beneath the skin barrier as these can cause irregular pouching surface and contribute to skin creases and leakage. New incisions may produce drainage that undermines adhesive skin barriers. Measure the size of the stoma. Compare the result to the size the patient has been using to determine whether the opening is appropriately sized for the stoma. Is the shape of the pouching system or barrier (flat or convex) appropriate for the contour of the peristomal skin and the height of the stoma? Is the pouching system flexible enough to move with the contours and/or firm enough to keep creases or folds from forming? A careful evaluation and critical appraisal of the patient's situation are important at each encounter.

A consistent approach to skin assessment helps ensure clear documentation and communication about changes in the skin. A number of validated measurement instruments are available for research and clinical use including the Peristomal Lesion Scale (Menin et al., 2019), Ostomy Skin Tool (Jemec et al., 2011), and the Peristomal Skin Lesions Assessment Instrument (Bosio et al., 2007). The Wound, Ostomy Continence Nurse Association provides a mobile tool to guide clinicians needing basic guidance on how to identify and treat peristomal skin complications, including instructions for patient care (WOCN, 2017b). A companion peristomal assessment guide is available for consumers.

GUIDELINES FOR MANAGEMENT OF PERISTOMAL SKIN COMPLICATIONS

The general guideline for managing peristomal skin complications is to first identify and treat the cause of the peristomal skin condition and address any possible contributing factors. For example, the patient may need to use a different-sized barrier opening or change the barrier more or less frequently. The patient may also require a specific type of topical therapy to treat the underlying disorder, manage moisture, or protect healing skin. Generally, products applied for topical therapy of peristomal skin problems should be used for a limited period of time, until the condition resolves. Provide patient education about the management plan, including the suspected etiology of the skin

condition and how it is managed, how to apply and use any new products, when to discontinue the treatments, and when to return for follow-up care. Finally, consider whether consultations with other health care providers and specialists are needed. Multidisciplinary care is important in the management of patients with unusual peristomal skin complications and ones that fail to improve with usual care. Referrals may include surgeons, dermatologists, gastroenterologists, general practitioners, oncologists, and other advanced practice providers depending on the type of complications present.

The overall goal with any peristomal skin complication is to promote healing while maintaining adequate wear time of the pouching system. When the cause of the skin problem is unclear, optimize the pouching system, refer the patient for further diagnosis and treatment, and provide patient education about self-care and completing the next steps in the management plan. The following sections will cover additional information about specific peristomal skin complications, beginning with the most common, those associated with moisture-related skin damage.

SPECIFIC PERISTOMAL SKIN COMPLICATIONS

PERISTOMAL MOISTURE–ASSOCIATED SKIN DAMAGE

Peristomal moisture–associated skin damage (PMASD) is a broad category of skin complication that includes several conditions (irritant contact dermatitis [ICD], maceration, and pseudoverrucous lesions). PMASD is defined as inflammation and erosion of the skin adjacent to the stoma, associated with exposure to effluent such as urine or stool (Colwell et al., 2011; Gray et al., 2013). The affected area typically begins at the stoma–skin junction and can extend outward. Other terms used to describe this type of skin problem include irritant dermatitis, irritant contact dermatitis, and peristomal dermatitis. Contact dermatitis (CD) is a common skin condition among adults, reported to occur in 20% of individuals in the general population (Alinaghi et al., 2019). CD consists of two types, ICD and allergic CD (ACD) with the most common of these being ICD. The signs of ICD include redness, swelling, a burning or itching sensation, and/or peeling. It can occur in response to ingredients in lotions, creams, and skin care products as well as contact with stoma effluent. PMASD can develop quickly, particularly in patients who have highly corrosive alkaline effluent, such as with an ileostomy. While the principal cause is prolonged exposure to stoma effluent, other sources of moisture (perspiration, swimming, use of hot tubs, etc.) can also contribute to the development of PMASD.

PMASD presents as an area of erythema adjacent to the stoma (red hues in light-skinned individuals or discoloration in darker skin), which may be accompanied

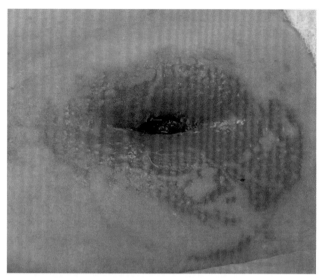

FIGURE 16-1. PMASD Around a Retracted Ileostomy Stoma Where Leakage Had Undermined the Skin Barrier. (Courtesy of Laura Vadman, RN, CWOCN.)

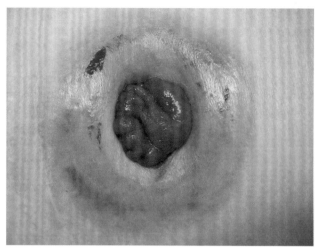

FIGURE 16-3. Irritant Dermatitis with Patchy Areas of Skin Loss. (Courtesy of Janice Colwell, MS, RN, CWOCN, FAAN.)

by superficial skin loss. The skin loss may be uniform or patchy, and the edges may be well defined or irregular. The affected area mirrors the pattern of exposure of the skin to stoma effluent. Moist skin is vulnerable to adhesive-related skin injury associated with the removal of adhesive pouching systems, further complicating the skin condition (Zulkowski, 2017). If chronic, moisture-associated hyperkeratosis and scarring can contribute to stoma stenosis at the skin level, particularly with a urostomy (Szymanski et al., 2010). **Figures 16-1 through 16-4** display PMASD associated with leakage. In extreme cases where leaking pouching systems have gone unchanged for a long time, the effluent can track

into skin folds or dependent areas leaving erythema and skin loss over a large area. The patient with PMASD often reports stinging pain, especially when anything touches the area, including stoma effluent. The patient may also report itching (pruritus) and often has difficulty getting the pouching system to adhere.

Management of PMASD includes identifying and correcting the cause of the leakage; this may include resizing the skin barrier, modifying the pouching system (e.g., changing from flat to convex), and selecting accessories that can improve the seal of the pouching system to the contours of the patient's abdomen. Manage contributing factors such as excess perspiration and external sources of moisture as appropriate; keep nearby skin folds clean and dry; and dry all aspects of the pouching system after exposure to water from baths, showers, and water sports. Topical care of the affected area usually consists

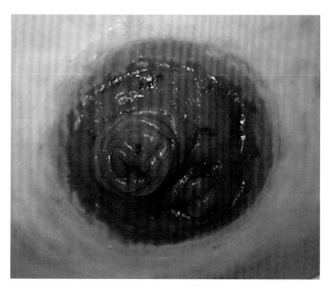

FIGURE 16-2. PMASD Around a Loop Stoma Where the Skin Barrier Opening Was Too Large. (Courtesy of Laura Vadman, RN, CWOCN.)

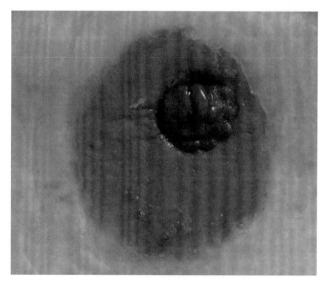

FIGURE 16-4. Irritant Dermatitis with Even Area of Partial-Thickness Skin Loss. (Courtesy of Laura Vadman, RN, CWOCN.)

of applying skin barrier powder to help absorb excess moisture from the areas of damaged skin and provide a dry surface on which the barrier can adhere. The skin barrier powder is sprinkled over the irritated skin gently rubbed into the skin and the excess brushed off. A liquid barrier film may be applied over the powder and allowed to dry before the pouching system is applied; multiple layers may be added in a process known as "crusting" (Doughty, 2005; Seungmi et al., 2011). If the area of skin damage is large or highly exuding, it may be helpful to apply a thin hydrocolloid skin barrier before applying the pouching system.

Provide the patient with information about the etiology and contributing factors for PMASD, and directions about how to use products. Provide guidance about the frequency of pouch changes, which may be needed more frequently until the skin has healed. Remind the patient that normal peristomal skin is intact and free of redness and to seek care if skin problems do not resolve quickly.

MACERATION

Maceration presents as soft moist skin that appears waterlogged; it may be whiter or lighter in color than is the skin next to it. The softening of tissue results in increased susceptibility to the damaging effects of friction and irritants (McNichol et al., 2013). Macerated peristomal skin (**Fig. 16-5**) is most common with urostomy stomas, but it can also occur with other stoma types. The patient may present with complaints of pouch leakage or short wear time or may report that the skin around the stoma appears unusual. This finding is also consistent with patients who are cutting the opening on the skin

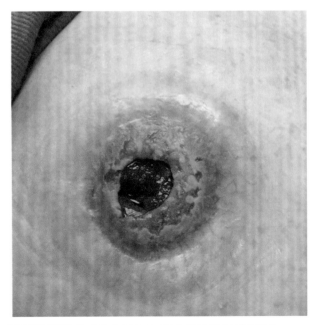

FIGURE 16-5. Peristomal Maceration. (Courtesy of Janice Colwell MS, RN, CWOCN, FAAN.)

barrier larger than the stoma size, which allows urine to pool against the peristomal skin.

Management techniques are directed toward reducing moisture where it is causing the skin to be overhydrated. If urine is pooling around the stoma ensure that the skin barrier opening is properly sized and that the shape of the barrier is preventing urine from getting between the barrier and the skin. Addition of convexity or accessory products (barrier strips, rings, or a stoma belt) may improve fit and help prevent leakage. Consider using a night drainage bag to help reduce pooling of urine around the stoma during sleep. A liquid barrier film can help prevent external moisture from hydrating the skin. If the macerated area is beneath the entire barrier, simply changing the pouching system more often may suffice, or consider use of an extended wear type of skin barrier. Maceration at the outside edges of the skin barrier or under the tape borders can be reduced by drying the pouching system after swimming and bathing to keep moisture from pooling against the skin and by applying a liquid barrier film to the skin before applying the pouching system. Use of a hair dryer on a low setting, or blotting with an absorbent towel can assist in drying tape borders after swimming or bathing. Identify the cause and contributing factors for the maceration; discuss options with the patient, and provide instructions about how to implement the solutions.

PSEUDOVERRUCOUS LESIONS

The term pseudoverrucous lesion refers to an exuberant growth of benign papules that occurs around a stoma when urine or stool irritates the skin. This condition is a type of chronic irritant contact dermatitis that is thought to develop from prolonged exposure to liquid stool and/or urine (Steinhagen et al., 2017); it is also sometimes seen in the diaper area during childhood (Fernández et al., 2010). The inflammatory response to the irritant causes thickening and elevation of skin layers next to the stoma. Other terms used to describe this condition are chronic papillomatous dermatitis (CPD), peristomal epitheliomatous hyperplasia (PEH), and pseudoverrucous papules and nodules (PPN). The lesions are often wart-like in appearance, and when biopsied, the lesions have a papillomatous histological appearance with acanthosis, lengthened rete ridges, hyperkeratosis, and dermal inflammation (Williams & Lyon, 2010). One example is shown in **Figure 16-6**. Another condition associated with urostomy and often found in the presence of pseudoverrucous lesions is the development of grainy crystals adhering to the peristomal skin (Szymanski et al., 2010; Zhou et al., 2019). Crystal deposition occurs when the urine is alkaline and concentrated, and it may be associated with urinary tract infections and renal calculi.

The patient with pseudoverrucous lesions presents with a thickened, bumpy, or irregular area that may be higher than the rest of the skin around it and may appear

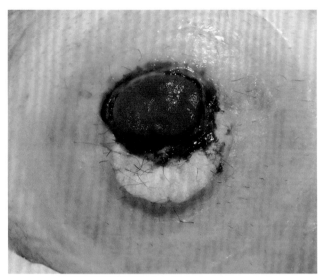

FIGURE 16-6. Pseudoverrucous Lesions Beneath a Urostomy Stoma. (Courtesy of Laura Vadman, RN, CWOCN.)

different in color than the surrounding skin (white, gray, brown, or dark red). The affected area is next to the stoma, where effluent has been in contact with the skin. The patient may report that the lesions itch or that bleeding is seen. Pseudoverrucous lesions often become eroded and tender. Assess the location, distribution, and appearance of the affected area. Gently probe the lesions. Encrustations will feel hard or gritty. Inquire about the product wear time and leakage and confirm appropriate sizing of the skin barrier. Inspect the skin barrier for indications of leakage. If a urostomy, ask the patient about the pattern and volume of fluid intake and determine whether the pouching system has an antireflux feature to help stop urine from pooling around the stoma.

Management consists of preventing contact of the stoma effluent with the affected area, which will lead to resolution of the condition. Ensure appropriate skin barrier opening size, modify the pouching system to provide a leak-free fit, and change the pouching system frequently enough to prevent leakage or pooling of urine on the skin. Confirm that the urostomy pouch has an antireflux feature and that the patient is emptying the pouch before the fluid level reaches the level of the stoma (even at night). If urostomy, discuss using a night drainage bag.

If the lesions are elevated and they interfere with getting a good seal between skin barrier and skin, cautery with silver nitrate may be helpful (Steinhagen et al., 2017). Several weekly applications may be required. Apply skin barrier powder to the lesions to absorb excess moisture and to provide a dry adhesion surface. If urostomy, recommend ways to lower the pH of the urine (increase fluid intake; consider adding cranberry juice or cranberry tablets to the diet or use of acidic skin barrier such as Colly–Seal. See chapter 14). If urine encrustations are also present, discuss increasing fluid intake, acidifying the urine, and applying dilute (30% to 50%) vinegar solution to the affected area for

20 minutes when the skin barrier is off for pouching system changes. Refer the patient if there is no improvement with usual care or in cases where the etiology of the lesions is unclear. Additional diagnostics may include microbiological culture and skin biopsy.

MECHANICAL DAMAGE

Mechanical damage can result from a variety of causes. When the peristomal skin is injured due to mechanical damage, it often presents as a defined area of skin loss or skin discoloration in a distinct area inconsistent with leakage of stoma effluent. The most common types of mechanical damage seen in the peristomal area are medical adhesive–related skin injuries and pressure injuries.

Medical adhesive–related skin injuries are common and can occur with any medical product that sticks to the skin; this includes ostomy pouching systems and accessories (McNichol et al., 2013; Yates et al., 2017). Removal of ostomy skin barriers is associated with increased transepidermal water loss, a measure of the integrity of the skin (Grove et al., 2019; Nichols et al., 2019). Peristomal medical adhesive–related skin injuries are defined as: "an alteration in skin integrity with erythema and/or other skin alterations such as skin tears, erosion, bulla, or vesicle that is apparent after removal of an adhesive ostomy pouching system" (LeBlanc et al., 2019). Some of the causes of this condition are preventable, such overuse of tackifiers and bonding agents, improper application of tapes, wrong type of tapes, and repeated application and removal of adhesive products in a short period of time. Patient teaching should include how to remove adhesive barriers using both hands, removing the barrier slowly at a low angle parallel to the skin while supporting the surrounding skin (LeBlanc et al., 2019). Risk factors include extremes in ages, preexisting health conditions (diabetes mellitus, dermatologic conditions, use of immunosuppressive medications, and treatments, etc.), malnutrition, and dry or damaged skin. **Figure 16-7** displays peristomal skin with an area of mechanical damage associated with improper removal of a tape bordered skin barrier.

The patient with a peristomal medical adhesive–related skin injury presents with a defined area of skin damage beneath the adhesive portion of the pouching system; it may be adjacent to the stoma or found further away from the stoma. The patient often reports that the area is painful, and moisture from the wound causes the barrier or tape to lift from the skin.

Inquire about the history of the injury and how it occurred. Ask about prior management of the wound and response to date. Gently remove the pouching system to examine the skin. Generally, these types of wounds can be assessed and categorized as partial or full thickness, and measured for length and width. Note the location of the wound relative to the stoma.

Management consists of identifying the cause of the injury and providing patient teaching about how to

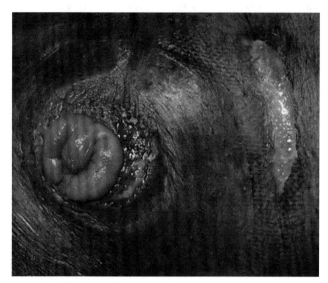

FIGURE 16-7. Peristomal Skin Tear Is Shown Several Inches from the Stoma. (Courtesy of Laura Vadman, RN, CWOCN.)

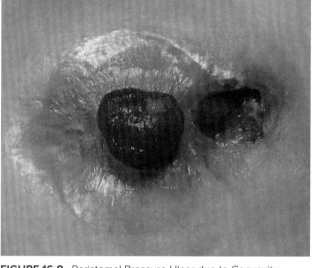

FIGURE 16-8. Peristomal Pressure Ulcer due to Convexity. (Courtesy of Laura Vadman, RN, CWOCN.)

prevent it from occurring in the future. Modify the pouching system as indicated, and apply a topical product that absorbs exudate and allows the pouching system to adhere while the wound heals. Use products such as adhesive removers/releasers, skin barrier sheets, and alcohol-free liquid skin film to ease the application and removal of topical products to the affected area. See Appendix C.

PRESSURE INJURIES

Detection of medical device–related pressure injuries has increased over the past several years, in part due to increased awareness of the risks of skin injury (Black & Kalowes, 2016; Fletcher, 2012). In ostomy care, pressure injuries can occur when belts, binders, and firm convex flanges are pressing against the skin for a prolonged period of time. Peristomal pressure injuries are thought to be more common among patients who have peristomal hernias, perhaps due to the use of convexity and other products that hold products firmly against the body. The clinical presentation of a peristomal pressure injury is a partial- or full-thickness wound in an area where there is product-related pressure or friction. The shape of the wound may closely resemble the shape of the item causing the pressure. A pressure injury caused by convexity is shown in **Figure 16-8**. The patient with a peristomal pressure injury may complain of pain and may report that drainage from the wound is interfering with the adherence of the skin barrier and pouching system.

KEY POINT

Note changes in color and integrity, and measure the length, width, and depth of wounds.

Assessment consists of evaluation of the patient in sitting, standing, and reclining positions in order to determine the forces present between the skin, the pouching products, and any accessories such as belt and closures.

Management of peristomal pressure injuries consists of identifying and removing the cause of the pressure, treating the wound while it heals, and providing an alternative pouching system for the patient if appropriate. Teach the patient how to care for the wound while it is healing, and how to use the new pouching system. Describe the cause of the injury and why it is important to avoid use of the type of product that created the pressure (or how to use it differently so it won't create injury).

ALLERGIC CONTACT DERMATITIS

Expert WOC Nurses define peristomal ACD as an inflammatory skin response resulting from hypersensitivity to direct contact with chemical elements (Colwell & Beitz, 2007; Owen et al., 2018). When peristomal skin irritation occurs, patients and clinicians often suspect allergy; however, ACD in the literature is estimated to be very low at 0.5% to 4.7% (Caroppo et al., 2019; Cressey et al., 2016). Allergens found to have been involved with peristomal ACD are components of adhesive pastes containing Gantrez® copolymers, tapes, skin barriers, skin wipe preparations, adhesive removers, dyes, perfumes, preservatives, soaps, and lotions (Caroppo et al., 2019; Cressey et al., 2016).

ACD presents as erythema that may be accompanied by blisters, which are unroofed when the pouching system is removed. **Figures 16-9 and 16-10** provide examples of peristomal ACD. Typically, the affected area at first mirrors the area of contact with the allergen, but as the inflammation progresses, the area enlarges, making the original contact area hard to discern. The patient

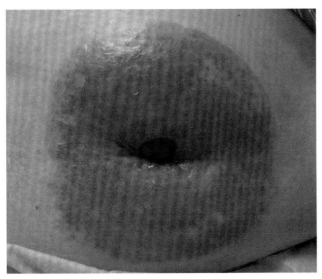

FIGURE 16-9. Allergic Contact Dermatitis. (Courtesy of Laura Vadman, RN, CWOCN.)

often complains of intense pruritus and may report difficulty with pouch adherence because of the moisture coming from the blistering dermatitis. Ask about all products used on the skin (including soaps, lotions, wipes, and stoma products) and in the pouching system (e.g., lubricants and deodorizers). Ask about prior history of contact allergies, atopic dermatitis, and product sensitivities. Assess the affected area, noting the distribution and characteristics of the condition such as rash, peeling, blisters, fissures, etc. Note any signs of secondary infection. Identify whether the affected area is associated with one or more specific product application areas.

Management of ACD consists primarily of identifying and removing the allergen. In some cases, a simple

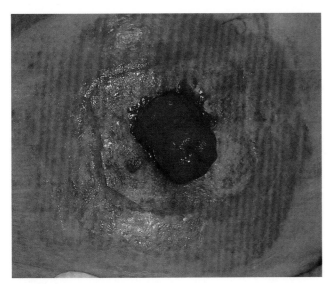

FIGURE 16-10. Allergic Contact Dermatitis. (Courtesy of Laura Vadman, RN, CWOCN.)

product change can be made without a full workup, such as using barrier-only products if tape sensitivity is reported. Patch testing using standard dermatologic skin test kits and the patient's products is useful to identify allergens as are customized testing panels reflecting the patient's current products and stoma series panels that test for the most frequent allergens in stoma products (Caroppo et al., 2019; Cressey et al., 2016). Ostomy product manufacturers may provide information about product components upon specific request for assistance in identification of options for patients with specific needs and a list of chemical ingredients for stoma products.

Until the dermatitis resolves, consider use of triamcinolone available in an aerosol or liquid spray, although not a first-line therapy, lotion or cream may be suggested, and if used should be rubbed into the skin thoroughly as lotions/creams can interfere with the pouch seal. Antihistamines are often needed to reduce inflammation and provide symptomatic relief. Overuse of topical steroids under occlusion can cause skin atrophy and so caution must be exercised. Treat secondary infection, if present. If the affected area must be covered by the pouching system, manage excess moisture by applying skin barrier powder to provide a dry pouching surface. Check skin barrier opening size, modify the pouching system if needed, and alter the frequency of pouching system changes to ensure that the affected area does not become exposed to stoma effluent.

Refer the patient to a dermatologist if standard patch testing is needed, if the source of the skin problem is unclear, or if it persists. Collaborate with consulting providers and specialists about appropriate forms of topical medication to ensure that the prescriptive products will be compatible with use of adhesive barrier products changed once or twice a week. Teach the patient about the source of the problem, avoidance of the allergen, how to use any new topical medications, and when to discontinue their use.

FUNGAL/CANDIDIASIS INFECTION

Candida albicans is one of the many opportunistic fungal pathogens that are part of the normal microflora in the digestive tract and on the skin; this species accounts for up to 75% of all *Candida* skin infections (Almutairi et al., 2018; Morales-Mendoza et al., 2014). Patients who have had recent treatment with antibiotics are at higher risk to develop cutaneous candidiasis, as are those who are immunosuppressed, who have diabetes mellitus, and who have had corticosteroid therapy or chemotherapy. The infection presents as erythema with a maculopapular rash accompanied by satellite lesions. A typical presentation is shown in **Figure 16-11**. Fungal rashes start in moist areas; thus, they tend to occur beneath the skin barrier and sometimes beneath tape-bordered products and pouches if moisture accumulates after showers

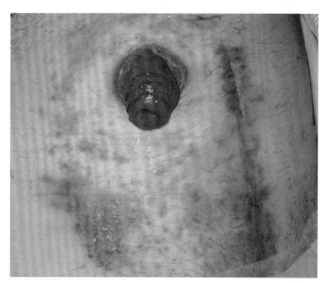

FIGURE 16-11. Peristomal Candidiasis. (Courtesy of Laura Vadman, RN, CWOCN.)

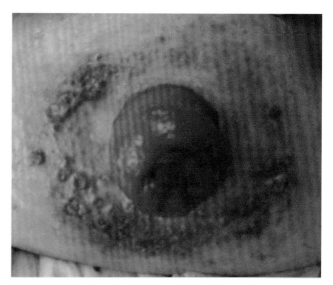

FIGURE 16-12. Complex Peristomal Skin Infection Requiring Microbial Cultures and Antibiotics. (Courtesy of Laura Vadman, RN, CWOCN.)

and baths. As the condition worsens, the inflammation causes extensive redness, the lesions coalesce, and the rash extends to a broader area. The patient usually complains of intense pruritus, a desire to scratch and sometimes to want to remove his or her pouching system. Patients with peristomal candidiasis may have it in other locations, particularly skin folds or creases. Inquire about recent use of antibiotics or immunosuppressive medications that are known to increase risk. Assess the location and extent of the rash, and look at the back of the skin barrier for signs of leakage.

Treatment for peristomal candidiasis includes gentle cleansing of the affected area, drying the skin, and applying a topical antifungal agent. Antifungal powders are dusted onto the affected area; this may be followed by the application of a liquid barrier film. After the film dries, the pouching system is applied. Powder is discontinued when rash resolves. Optimize the size of the opening and the fit of the pouching system to prevent leakage of stoma effluent onto the skin to reduce any sources of moisture that contribute to growth of pathogens.

Teach the patient to thoroughly dry the pouching system and any tape borders after showers and/or bathing to reduce moisture against the skin. Patients with complicated infections and those with immunosuppression or failure to respond to usual care should be referred for further diagnostics and treatment. An example of a polymicrobial infection of the peristomal skin that required referral is shown in **Figure 16-12**.

FOLLICULITIS

Defined as hair follicle inflammation; folliculitis typically develops when there is inflammation due to injury or infection (Napierkowski, 2013). **Figure 16-13** displays mild folliculitis. In the case of peristomal skin, the mech-

anism of injury may be multidirectional shaving or pulling of hair when the adhesive skin barrier is removed, followed by secondary infection with gram-positive bacteria such as *Staphylococcus* and *Streptococcus*. The clinical presentation is redness and pustules around the hair follicles under the skin barrier of the pouching system, as shown in **Figure 16-14**. The patient may report that the area is tender to touch, and skin barrier removal is painful. Instruct the patient to clip hair in the direction of hair growth, decrease the frequency of clipping, or use an electric shaver. Dusting skin barrier powder on the skin prior to shaving can also assist with the hair removal. Topical treatment for folliculitis consists of cleansing with antibacterial soap after barrier removal. Cultures may help to differentiate the cause of the infection if it is unclear whether fungal rash or folliculitis is involved. In

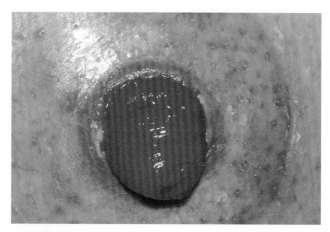

FIGURE 16-13. Peristomal Folliculitis. (From Corman, M., Nicholls, R. J., Fazio, V. W., et al. (2012). *Corman's colon and rectal surgery*. Philadelphia, PA: Wolters Kluwer.)

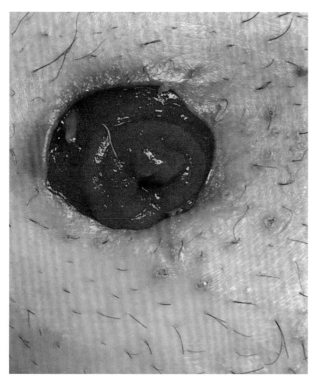

FIGURE 16-14. Peristomal Folliculitis. (Courtesy of Virginia Hanchett, FNP, APRN-CB, DCNP, COCN, CWCN.)

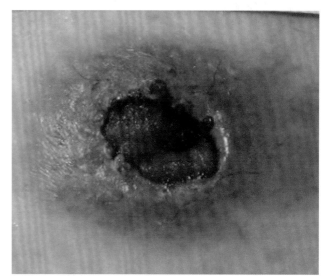

FIGURE 16-15. Peristomal Varices. (Courtesy of Laura Vadman, RN, CWOCN.)

cases that do not resolve with topical care, an oral antibiotic may be required.

VARICES

Peristomal varices, also referred to as caput medusae, are caused by portal hypertension that leads to enlarged venous channels at locations where the high-pressure portal and low-pressure systemic venous systems meet (Pennick & Artioukh, 2013). The most common causes of portal hypertension are liver cirrhosis and primary sclerosing cholangitis. Peristomal varices occur in up to 5% of individuals with a stoma. These varices may be visible as dilated veins in the submucosal area (bluish discoloration of the skin in the stoma area (**Fig. 16-15**) and/or a raspberry-like appearing stoma (Strauss et al., 2014). Varices may also present as spontaneous bleeding from the stoma or mucocutaneous junction without any visible skin changes. The patient may report that the skin bleeds when the pouching system is removed from the skin and/or that there are spontaneous episodes of bleeding from the stoma. Parastomal bleeding is a potentially serious complication in patients with varices, requiring treatment to stop the bleeding and treat the underlying cause.

Assessment includes inspection of the skin around the stoma, a problem-focused history, and a review of available laboratory test results. Local conservative measures are initiated with acute bleeding including pressure to the parastomal area, surgical suturing or ligation, and/or cautery. Severe bleeds may require transfusion

and hospitalization. To reduce the risk of bleeding when removing the pouching system, use adhesive removers/releasers to ease the product from the skin. Use a liquid barrier film on the skin to help reduce skin trauma (Beitz & Colwell, 2016) and use a one-piece pouching system, (a two-piece pouching system can have a plastic ring that could press on the peristomal area causing bleeding) with a standard-wear skin barrier rather than extended-wear skin barriers. Ensure that the opening in the skin barrier does not rub against the mucocutaneous junction, and avoid products that apply pressure to the peristomal skin and mucocutaneous junction, such as convex systems and belts.

Teach the patient how to gently remove the pouching system and gently cleanse the peristomal skin to prevent trauma during self-care. Rebleeding is common and serious; thus, the patient should be referred for further diagnosis and definitive treatment. The transjugular intrahepatic portosystemic shunt (TIPS) procedure has the highest rate of success in preventing recurrent hemorrhage (Pennick & Artioukh, 2013), but other treatments may be discussed (e.g., propranolol, endovascular embolization, sclerotherapy) (Romano et al., 2019).

GRANULOMA

Granulomas are described as erythematous soft to firm papules that bleed easy and may or may not be tender depending on their precise location. These tend to be located at the juncture of the stoma and the peristomal skin (**Figs. 16-16 and 16-17**) but can also occur on the stoma. They develop when there is an immunologic response to foreign material such as retained sutures or friction and rubbing from the pouch system in the presence of a moist environment from urine or stool (Steinhagen et al., 2017; WOCN, 2016). Refer to the

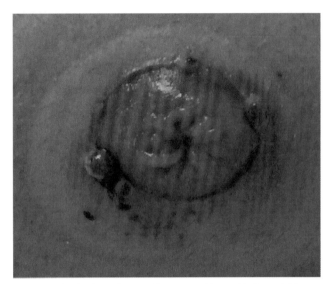

FIGURE 16-16. Granulomas. (Courtesy of Laura Vadman, RN, CWOCN.)

atypical parastomal lesion section for more rare diseases that can resemble the common granuloma. The patient may report having problems with pouch leakage caused by the moisture from the lesions. The patient may also be concerned by the appearance of the new lesions.

Treatment includes the following: Probe each lesion to determine whether loose suture material is present and remove it if possible. Apply topical silver nitrate to the areas of elevated tissue and repeat twice weekly if needed. Apply stoma powder and liquid barrier film to help absorb moisture and protect tender areas during healing. If the affected area is large and moisture is excessive, consider using a foam dressing and convex skin barrier to provide gentle pressure to the area, which may reduce the growth of new lesions. Patients

with peristomal granulomas that do not resolve with topical treatment, or who have enlarging granulomas require referral to an advanced practice provider or dermatologist for definitive diagnosis, biopsy, and more aggressive treatment with electric cautery via hyfrecator or excision (Steinhagen et al., 2017; WOCN, 2016).

PERISTOMAL ABSCESS

Peristomal abscesses can occur at any time; however, acute abscesses are typically seen within 2 weeks after stoma creation. WOC nurse experts define peristomal abscess as a collection of purulent material beneath the skin, most typically associated with a foreign body (such as a suture) or a disease process (Colwell & Beitz, 2007). Other causes include preoperative colonization of the peristomal skin, infected hematoma, and infected suture granulomas (Kann, 2008). Peristomal abscess occurring near an established stoma may also develop due to underlying disease such as inflammatory bowel disease or pyoderma gangrenosum (PG) (Aboulian, 2019). Abscesses present as areas of localized redness, swelling, and tenderness in the peristomal area, which may be accompanied by systemic signs of infection. **Figure 16-18** displays a peristomal abscess.

Patient assessment includes inspection and palpation of the peristomal skin and abdomen, and assessment for signs of systemic infection. If an abscess is suspected, consultation is indicated. Management of a peristomal abscess often requires drainage of the fluid collection, which may include placement of a temporary drain, local wound care with absorbent dressings, and treatment with systemic antibiotics. The affected area not only needs protection from stoma effluent but also may require more frequent observation and access for dressing changes; thus, the pouching system changes may need to be more frequent. Provide the patient with

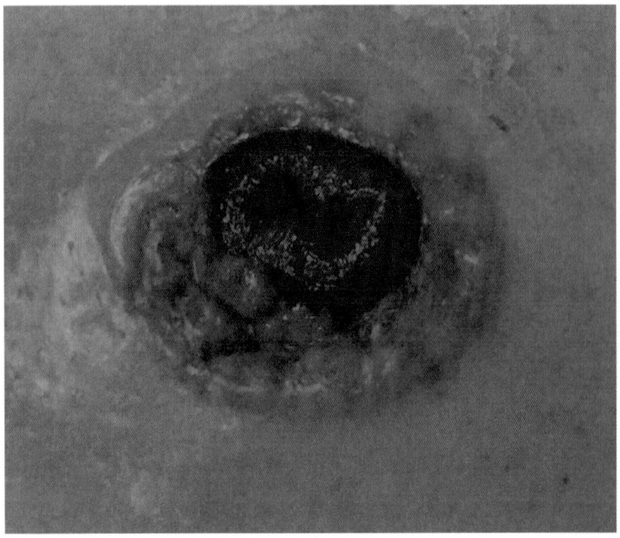

FIGURE 16-17. Granulomas. (Courtesy of Laura Vadman, RN, CWOCN.)

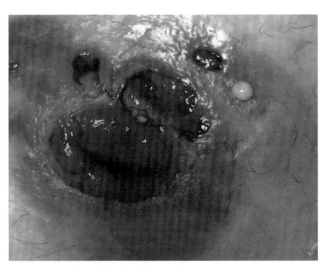

FIGURE 16-18. Peristomal Abscess. (Courtesy of Virginia Hanchett, FNP, APRN-CB, DCNP, COCN, CWCN.)

information about self-care and completing the next steps in the management plan.

PERISTOMAL FISTULA

An enterocutaneous (EC) fistula is an abnormal connection between the intestine and the skin. EC fistulas can occur on the skin of the abdomen, and they are particularly challenging when the opening is on the peristomal skin undermining the adherence of the pouching system and putting skin integrity at risk. Appearance of a fistula may be indicative of active pathology such as Crohn's disease (Aboulian, 2019; Hoentjen et al., 2012) or ulcerative colitis or occur as a complication of intestinal surgery in patients with malnutrition, infection, and other risk factors.

A patient with a fistula may present with complaints of difficulty maintaining adherence of his or her pouching system, leakage, and peristomal skin irritation accompanied by pain. The patient may notice the fistula is draining fecal effluent or simply describe it as a new open wound. Components of the patient history include onset and duration of symptoms, prior history of fistulas, health history, and medication history. Inquire about a decrease in the amount of effluent draining from the stoma since the fistula was first noticed.

Assessment includes examination of the stoma and peristomal skin, including the mucocutaneous juncture where fistulas may be present but easily overlooked, as shown in **Figure 16-19**. Evaluate draining areas for evidence of warmth, swelling, and fluctuance that may indicate infection or abscess. Evaluate the patient for signs and symptoms of systemic infection. Note the size of the fistula and its location in relationship to the stoma. Note the characteristics and amount of any drainage.

Peristomal fistulas are managed symptomatically, while medical evaluation is completed and treatment options are pursued. The initial goal is to protect the peristomal skin from the fistula drainage while also providing a secure pouching system to collect stoma effluent. With a fistula that is close to the stoma, the best option may be to adjust the opening of the skin barrier to simply accommodate the fistula within the same pouching system. Use accessories such as skin barrier rings, strips, paste, or liquid skin barriers to customize the opening and protect healthy skin from further damage. Select a two-piece pouching system to allow easy access for subsequent medical evaluations. Fistulas that cannot be pouched with the stoma may be managed by using a wound dressing with adequate skin protection on the surrounding skin or accommodated by a separate pouching system. Appropriate options depend on the location of the peristomal fistula, the volume and type of effluent, the method used to treat the fistula, and the patient's preferences and capabilities. See Chapter 18 for Fistula management.

Refer the patient for evaluation and treatment. Procedures may include radiologic examinations such as fistulogram, CT scan, and insertion of drainage tube. Patients with high-volume drainage or complicated presentations may require hospitalization. Provide the patient with instruction about the next steps in the plan of care, and how to manage stoma care needs until the condition is resolved.

MUCOSAL TRANSPLANTATION

Often misdiagnosed as hypergranulation tissue, mucosal transplantation or implantation is thought to occur as a sequelae of suturing the bowel to the epidermis instead of the dermis during stoma creation (WOCN®, 2016). The peristomal presentation is typically several bright red erythematous moist papules, similar to the stoma mucosal tissue, see **Figure 16-20**. They can be friable and

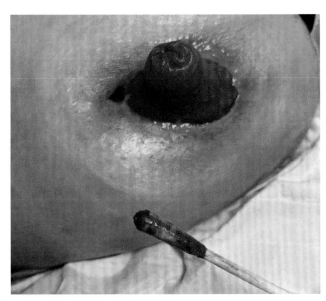

FIGURE 16-19. Peristomal Fistula. (Courtesy of Virginia Hanchett, FNP, APRN-CB, DCNP, COCN, CWCN.)

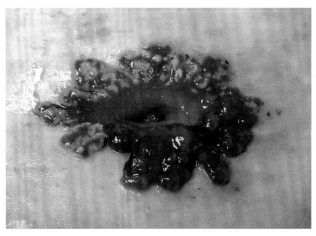

FIGURE 16-20. Biopsy-Proven Mucosal Implantation. (Courtesy of Virginia Hanchett, FNP, APRN-CB, DCNP, COCN, CWCN.)

impair the pouching ability of the skin barrier. Treatment recommended through quantitative data collection from ostomy experts (Beitz & Colwell, 2016) includes the use of skin barrier powder to manage moisture, refitting of the pouching system, use of silver nitrate to retard the growth of the bowel mucosa, and if needed, referral to an ostomy specialist advanced practice provider or dermatologist for use of electrocautery. In rare instances, the patient can be referred back to the surgeon for stoma resiting or excision of the lesions (WOCN®, 2016).

PERISTOMAL PYODERMA GANGRENOSUM

PG is a neutrophilic dermatosis characterized by recurrent, painful ulcerations. PG classically appears on the lower extremities, most frequently on the tibial areas, but it can also occur in other parts of the body, including the peristomal area. Peristomal pyoderma granulosum (PPG) is often associated with the presence of systemic disease such as inflammatory bowel disease, arthritis, or hematologic disorders; however, the cause is idiopathic up to 50% of the time (George et al., 2019; Shavit et al., 2017). The etiology is not fully understood; however, pathergy, caused by fecal exposure, mechanical stripping, and surgical excision, exists in up to 30% of individuals with the disorder (George et al., 2019).

PPG presents as pustules that enlarge and open into partial- or full-thickness wounds, sometimes with darkcolored (purple), irregular borders and purulent exudate as shown in **Figures 16-21 and 16-22**. These painful undermined ulcerations progress rapidly and fail to heal with usual treatment. In addition to reports of painful lesions, the patient may complain of difficulty with adherence of the pouching system due to the excessive drainage from the wounds. Application of topical anesthetic

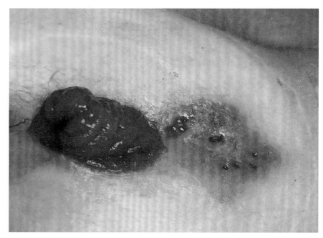

FIGURE 16-22. Peristomal Pyoderma Gangrenosum. (Courtesy of Virginia Hanchett, FNP, APRN-CB, DCNP, COCN, CWCN.)

such as lidocaine may allow the patient some pain relief during the examination. Assessment includes appearance, size, depth, and location of the wounds, prior history of PG, and evaluation of possible contributing factors. It can be difficult to determine whether a wound is caused by pressure (such as convexity) or PPG by visual assessment and history; the use of convexity may be a precipitating factor for PPG. Assess the patient for signs and symptoms of local and deep wound infection, and obtain a wound culture if indicated.

PPG is a diagnosis of exclusion, which means all other potential causes of the ulcer are ruled out. A Delphi consensus of international experts established guidelines for diagnosing ulcerative PG (Maverakis et al., 2018). The single major criteria that must exist is a biopsy-proven neutrophilic infiltrate and four of eight of the following: exclusion of infection; evidence of pathergy; a history of IBD or arthritis; a history of a papule, pustule, or vesicle ulcerating within four days of appearing; peripheral erythema, undermining border and tenderness at the ulceration site; multiple ulcerations, at least one on the anterior lower leg; cribriform or "wrinkled paper" scars at healed ulcer sites; and decreased ulcer size within one month of initiating immunosuppressive medications (Maverakis et al., 2018, p. 461).

Medical management of PPG involves advanced wound care to manage exudate and reducing the inflammatory process via topical steroids, topical tacrolimus preparations, and injection of the erythematous periphery of the lesion with triamcinolone (George et al., 2019). In a comprehensive review, Shavit et al. (2017) reported that oral prednisone therapy at a dose of 0.5 to 1 mg/kg/d has been effective in controlling PPG, or the use of Cyclosporine 2.5 to 5 mg/kg/d in combination with prednisone or as a second-line therapy is recommended (George et al., 2019). Additionally, in mild cases or in combination with systemic treatment, the use of dapsone, minocycline, apremilast, methotrexate,

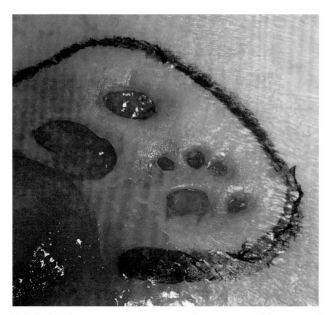

FIGURE 16-21. Peristomal Pyoderma Gangrenosum. (Courtesy of Virginia Hanchett, FNP, APRN-CB, DCNP, COCN, CWCN.)

colchicine, azathioprine, and cyclophosphamide provide anti-inflammatory effects. IVIG has also been used as an immune modulator (George et al., 2019). Anti-TNF-α medications biologic agents may also be effective in refractory cases; however, there is no agreed-upon consensus for the treatment of PG with biologics. Infliximab has the most research showing success in treating PG; however, there are more biologics on the market none of which are FDA approved for the treatment of PG (George et al., 2019; Shavit et al., 2017).

Local management of PPG lesions includes efforts to remove sources of pressure and friction; thus, a critical evaluation of all pouching products is required. For example, convex products and belts should be avoided or replaced with options that are soft or padded to prevent trauma and pressure to peristomal skin and open wounds. Topical wound management requires absorptive products such as alginates and foam dressings secured by a thin hydrocolloid sheets to absorb excess wound exudate and provide a dry pouching surface for a predictable period of time between dressing changes. Use standard-wear skin barriers rather than extended-wear skin barriers to prevent damage to peristomal skin due to frequent removal of the pouching system for dressing changes, and consider use of adhesive remover wipes and no-sting liquid skin barriers to protect the fragile peristomal skin. Nonadhesive pouching systems are also an appropriate option. Debridement should be discouraged due to the 30% likelihood of pathergy and resultant exacerbation of the wounds (Maverakis et al., 2018).

Referral to dermatology is indicated for patients presenting with suspected PPG, as medical workup will include evaluation for underlying pathology with lab work to rule out autoimmune disease, drug-induced vasculitis, coagulopathies, and malignancies. A tissue culture of lesions and skin biopsy are recommended (George et al., 2019). Biopsies taken from the edge of the lesions in PG will show a dense neutrophilic infiltration; however, the primary objective of biopsy in PPG is to rule out other causes of ulceration such as infection and thrombosis of small vessels as in vasculitis (George et al., 2019; Shavit et al., 2017). Instruct the patient about the next steps in the treatment plan and when to return for follow-up care.

AUTOIMMUNE AND ATYPICAL PRESENTATIONS

The majority of this chapter is dedicated to the recognition of the most common complications of the peristomal skin. As a clinician however, there are less common autoimmune skin diseases which while not part of the core curriculum are of interest to the WOC nurse. Atypical lesions that should always be included in the differential diagnosis and may require the involvement of an advanced practice provider or dermatologist to do a skin biopsy with or without direct immunofluorescence (DIF).

Examples of autoimmune diseases are psoriasis, bullous pemphigoid, pemphigus vulgaris, epidermolysis bullosa, and familial benign chronic pemphigus (Hailey-Hailey disease [HHD]). All of these diseases have a bullous variant and may be difficult to discern by physical examination alone. Individual atypical lesions should be biopsied to rule out malignancy or more benign findings such as colonic mucosal implantation.

PERISTOMAL PSORIASIS

Psoriasis is a chronic inflammatory and autoimmune disorder with many clinical variants (Brandon et al., 2019). Psoriasis affects 1% to 3% of the population in the United States and Europe. In two separate studies of patients with a stoma, the incidence of peristomal psoriasis was 4.7% to 7%, and in one of these studies, 68% of those with peristomal psoriasis also had widespread disease (Lyon et al., 2000; Marshall et al., 2017). Psoriasis most commonly occurs on the extensor surfaces of the extremities but psoriasis can occur for the first time on the peristomal skin (Marshall et al., 2017). See **Figure 16-23** which displays psoriasis in the peristomal area. Peristomal and periwound skin is particularly vulnerable for patients with psoriasis because of the Koebner Phenomenon (**Fig. 16-24**), in which a flare of the disorder occurs in an area of localized skin trauma. This often becomes evident 1 to 2 weeks after a minor skin trauma (Brandon et al., 2019).

The clinical presentation of peristomal psoriasis is typically an erythematous plaque with or without excessive flakiness of the skin, which may be shiny or silvery in appearance (**Fig. 16-24**). Inquire about a history of psoriasis, eczema, or other skin diseases, and obtain a complete history of medications (including topical products).

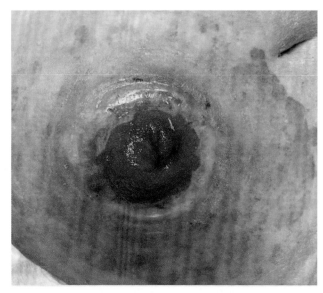

FIGURE 16-23. Peristomal Psoriasis. (Courtesy of Virginia Hanchett, FNP, APRN-CB, DCNP, COCN, CWCN.)

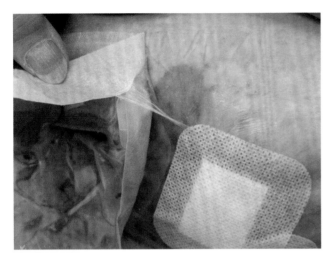

FIGURE 16-24. Nail Changes of Psoriasis, and Koebnerization Occurring When Adhesive Was Removed. (Courtesy of Virginia Hanchett, FNP, APRN-CB, DCNP, COCN, CWCN.)

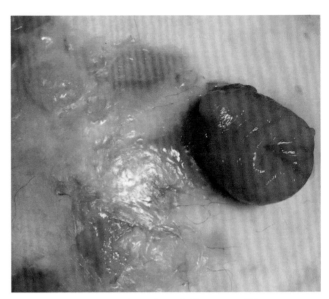

FIGURE 16-25. Bullous Pemphigoid. (Courtesy of Virginia Hanchett, FNP, APRN-CB, DCNP, COCN, CWCN.)

Examine the affected area, noting the color, texture, and integrity of the skin.

Management of peristomal psoriasis is directed at reducing inflammation by use of adhesive removers/releasers, hydrocolloid barriers without tape edges to reduce trauma to the skin, and application of topical or intralesional corticosteroids. Topical creams, ointments, and petrolatum-based medications used for psoriasis elsewhere on the body may not be appropriate for use under skin barriers due to their occlusive and antiadhesive properties; thus, collaboration with the prescribing provider is necessary to ensure a successful treatment plan. Use of corticosteroid sprays and lotions and products with low alcohol content are recommended to reduce burning (Marshall et al., 2019). Topical steroid potency is enhanced when used under occlusion and therefore should be used with caution or skin atrophy will occur. Patients who have systemic disease should be referred to a dermatologist for consideration of biologics, immunotherapy, or phototherapy (Marshall et al., 2017).

Teach the patient the importance of using a properly sized skin barrier, wearing products that prevent leakage, and changing the pouching system before stoma effluent leaks onto the skin. Prevention of peristomal trauma and irritation may reduce peristomal psoriasis occurrence.

LESS COMMON AUTOIMMUNE PRESENTATIONS

BULLOUS PEMPHIGOID

Bullous pemphigoid (BP) is typically an autoimmune disease of the elderly affecting 2 to 23 cases per million among those <80 years of age and affects 190 to 312 cases per million over the age of 80 (Kridin & Ludwig, 2018). The dramatic increase is thought to be related to our increased life expectancy and the growing evidence of a high association between neurological disorders and BP (Kridin & Ludwig, 2018). BP occurs when the host develops an autoantibody response to hemidesmosomal proteins BP180 and BP230 (Genovese et al., 2019; Kridin & Ludwig, 2018). It is thought that the incidence of peristomal BP is under reported as it is steroid responsive and often not biopsied or sent for DIF if it is localized to the peristomal area (Felton et al., 2012). The literature on peristomal BP is sparse.

Clinical findings in nursing assessment will reveal vesicles, bullae, or decompressed blisters of the peristomal area as shown in **Figure 16-25**. The majority of patients will have additional blisters elsewhere on the torso or extremities. **Table 16-1** lists management pearls, which are conservative in nature.

PEMPHIGUS VULGARIS

Pemphigus vulgaris (PV) is also an autoimmune disease of middle ages 40 to 60 years with an incidence of 2 cases per million in Europe and up to 32 cases per million in the US Jewish populations (Kasperkiewicz et al., 2018; Porro et al., 2019). It is more common in women than men. PV is the presence of antigens desmoglein 1 and 3, which affect the adhesion of the squamous epithelium resulting in blister formation (Porro et al., 2019).

There are three main types of PV, which include mucosal, mucocutaneous, and cutaneous variants (Kasperkiewicz et al., 2018). There are only rare case reports of peristomal PV in the literature (Bhange et al., 2019), again as it is likely under reported. **Figure 16-26** displays an example of peristomal skin in a patient with PV. Clinical findings in nursing assessment will reveal dark beefy red papules

TABLE 16-1 WOC NURSING MANAGEMENT PRINCIPLES OF AUTOIMMUNE DISEASES

- Refer to an advanced ostomy practice provider or dermatologist for biopsy with direct immunofluorescence (DIF) as well as topical and systemic treatment recommendations
- Reduce trauma and koebnerization (A process in which injury to the skin causes further formation of psoriasis.) by using adhesive removers at every pouching system change
- Switch the patient to all barrier products (no tape) and reassess the stoma to make recommendations to get a better seal and reduce leaking
- Isolate blisters, wounds with nonadherent advanced wound care products
- Look for signs of secondary infection such as pain, erythema, honey-colored crusting
- Educate the patient on their disease, the importance of diligent skin care and how to apply topical agents if recommended by a provider

Courtesy of Virginia Hanchett, FNP, APRN-CB, DCNP, COCN, CWCN.

at the mucocutaneous junction. **Table 16-1** lists management pearls, which are conservative in nature.

EPIDERMOLYSIS BULLOSA ACQUISITA

Epidermolysis bullosa acquisita (EBA) is a rare blistering disorder described as an autoimmune presence of auto-antibodies to collagen VII which results in a blistering at the basement membrane zone of the epidermal dermal junction (Kridin et al., 2019). The type of EBA patients with stomas would have would be the mechanobullous type common at sites of mechanical trauma such as removing the wafer. According to Kridin et al. (2019), 38% of all EBA have the mechanobullous variant, and the incidence is <0.5% per million per year and affects males and females equally, with the peak onset being under the age of 30 and age 70s to 80s. EBA is associated with Crohn's disease in case reports and literature review (Kridin et al.,

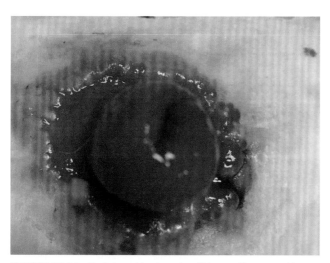

FIGURE 16-26. Peristomal Lesions in a Woman Known to Have PV. (Courtesy of Virginia Hanchett, FNP, APRN-CB, DCNP, COCN, CWCN.)

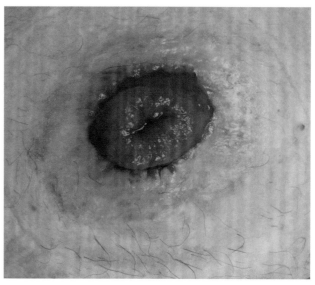

FIGURE 16-27. Peristomal HHD. (Courtesy of Virginia Hanchett, FNP, APRN-CB, DCNP, COCN, CWCN.)

2019; Ormaechea-Perez et al., 2014). Clinical findings include vesicles or bullae in the peristomal region and can resemble bullous pemphigoid. **Table 16-1** lists management pearls, which are conservative in nature.

FAMILIAL BENIGN CHRONIC PEMPHIGUS (HAILEY-HAILEY DISEASE)

Familial benign chronic pemphigus is also known as HHD. It is an autosomal dominant inherited ATP2C1 mutation that causes either vesicular or erythematous plaque formation most common in sites where there is friction, heat, or moisture. The eruption is usually in intertriginous skin folds. It is commonly bilateral in areas such as the groin, axillae, and inframammary regions. There is no predominant gender affected, and HHD most commonly occurs in the third decade of life with an incidence of 1 to 4 per 100,000 people. Sites with HHD become chronic and place patients at risk for a velvety and thick plaque, which becomes a holding source for secondary bacterial infections (Patel et al., 2019). Clinical findings in nursing assessment include accentuated and thickened skin in the peristomal region, as shown in **Figure 16-27**. **Table 16-1** lists management pearls, which are conservative in nature.

MALIGNANCY

Malignancy of the skin can occur in the peristomal area. The precise incidence is unknown but is thought to be rare (Al-Niaimi & Lyon, 2014; Chang et al., 2014), and it has been reported more often with fecal stomas than urinary stomas. Ileostomy-associated lymphoma, squamous cell carcinoma, and adenocarcinoma have been reported (Chang et al., 2014). Squamous cell cancer (SCC) is the most prevalent of the cancers and occurs in 2 to 4 of every 1,000 patients who have long standing stomas (Almutairi et al., 2018). The underlying predisposition to developing SCC is thought to be chronic inflammation, exposure to caustic effluent, and recurring infection (Almutairi et al., 2018). The clinical findings and nursing assessment will reveal a papule, plaque, nodule or nonhealing wound in the peristomal area, stoma, or mucocutaneous junction that does not resolve with usual treatment. For this reason, individuals with peristomal lesions unresponsive to therapy should be referred for biopsy to an advanced practice ostomy provider or a dermatologist (Almutairi et al., 2018). Diagnostic tests and treatments depend on the type of malignancy and the stage of the disease. Peristomal metastasis of colorectal cancer may be diagnosed with dermoscopy and subsequent biopsy of suspicious tissue (Ito et al., 2014). Treatment options may include excision of the affected area, stoma relocation, and novel approaches such as electrochemotherapy (Campana et al., 2013).

 ## CONCLUSIONS

A variety of conditions can affect the peristomal skin; most of them are related to exposure to leakage from the stoma. Some are due to mechanical, chemical, or infectious causes and fewer are immunologically mediated or related to systemic disease. Moisture-associated skin damage with irritant dermatitis is the most prevalent, and it is often associated with leakage of stoma effluent under the skin barrier. Because of the high incidence of peristomal skin problems, it is vital that health care providers routinely ask about the condition of the peristomal skin when caring for an individual with a stoma. Ask about the patient's usual skin condition and how the skin appeared at the time of the last pouch change. To evaluate the skin completely, remove the pouching system and examine the skin, the stoma, and the adhesive side of the barrier. Evaluate the appropriateness of the sizing and fit of the pouching products, and determine the etiology of any skin complications. Treatment of the underlying cause of the disorder, identification and management of any contributing factors, and appropriate topical care for open wounds are key steps to restoring and sustaining peristomal skin integrity.

REFERENCES

Aboulian, A. (2019). Ostomy complications in Crohn's disease. *Clinics in Colon and Rectal Surgery, 32*, 314–322.

Alinaghi, F., Bennike, N. H., Egeberg, A., et al. (2019). Prevalence of contact allergy in the general population: A systematic review and meta-analysis. *Contact Dermatitis, 80*(2), 77–85.

Almutairi, D., Le Blanc, K., & Alavi, A. (2018). Peristomal skin complications: What dermatologists need to know. *International Journal of Dermatology, 57*, 257–264.

Al-Niaimi, F., & Lyon, C. C. (2014). Primary adenocarcinoma in peristomal skin: A case study. *Ostomy/Wound Management, 60*(5), 45–47.

Beitz, J., & Colwell, J. (2016). Management approaches to stomal and peristomal complications: A narrative descriptive study. *Journal of Wound, Ostomy, and Continence Nursing, 43*(3), 263–268.

Bhange, S., Bhansali, M., Shaikh, T., et al. (2019). Rare case of peristomal pemphigus vulgaris in an operated case of carcinoma of the rectum. *British Medical Journal, 12*(11), e230956.

Black, J. M., & Kalowes, P. (2016). Medical device-related pressure ulcers. *Chronic Wound Care Management and Research, 3*, 91–99.

Brandon, A., Mufti, A., & Sibbald, R. (2019). Diagnosis and management of cutaneous psoriasis: A review. *Advances in Skin & Wound Care, 32*(2), 58–69.

Bosio, G., Pisani, F., Lucibello, L., et al. (2007). A proposal for classifying peristomal skin disorders: Results of a multicenter observational study. *Ostomy/Wound Management, 53*(9), 38–43.

Campana, L. G., Scarpa, M., Sommariva, A., et al. (2013). Minimally invasive treatment of peristomal metastases from gastric cancer at an ileostomy site by electrochemotherapy. *Radiology and Oncology, 47*(4), 370–375.

Carlsson, E., Fingren, J., Hallén, A. M., et al (2016). The prevalence of ostomy-related complications 1 year after ostomy surgery: A prospective, descriptive, clinical study. *Ostomy/Wound Management, 62*(10), 34–48.

Caroppo, F., Brumana, M., Biolo, G., et al. (2019). Peristomal allergic contact dermatitis caused by ostomy pastes and the role of Gantrez ES 425. *Giornale Italiano De Dermatolgia E Venereologia, 154*(1), 1–5.

Chang, A., Davis, B., Snyder, J., et al. (2014). Considerations for diagnosis and management of ileostomy-related malignancy: A report of two cases. *Ostomy/Wound Management, 60*(5), 38–40, 42–43.

Colwell, J. C., & Beitz, J. (2007). Survey of wound, ostomy and continence (WOC) nurse clinicians on stomal and peristomal complications: A content validation study. *Journal of Wound, Ostomy, and Continence Nursing, 34*(1), 57–69.

Colwell, J. C., Pittman, J., Raizman, R., et al. (2018). A randomized controlled trial determining variances in ostomy skin conditions and the economic impact (ADVOCATE Trial). *Journal of Wound, Ostomy, and Continence Nursing, 45*(1), 37–42.

Colwell, J. C., Ratliff, C. R., Goldberg, M., et al. (2011). MASD part 3: Peristomal moisture-associated dermatitis and periwound moisture-associated dermatitis. A consensus. *Journal of Wound, Ostomy, and Continence Nursing, 38*(5), 541–553.

Cressey, B., Belum, V. R., Scheinman, P., et al. (2016). Stoma care products represent a common and previously underreported source of peristomal contact dermatitis. *Contact Dermatitis, 76*(1), 27–33.

Doughty, D. (2005). Principles of ostomy management in the oncology patient. *Journal of Supportive Oncology, 3*, 59–69.

Felton, S., Al-Niaimi, F., Lyon, C. (2012). Peristomal and generalized bullous pemphigoid in patients with underlying inflammatory bowel disease: Is plectin the missing link? *Ostomy/Wound Management, 58*(12), 34–38.

Fernández, I. S., Moreno, C., Vano-Galvan, S., et al. (2010). Pseudoverrucous irritant peristomal dermatitis with an histological pattern of nutritional deficiency dermatitis. *Dermatology Online Journal, 16*(9), 16. Retrieved from http://escholarship.org/uc/item/5sg6m25r

Fletcher, J. (2012). Device related pressure ulcers made easy. *Wounds UK, 8*(2). Retrieved June 25, 2014, from http://www.wounds-uk.com

Genovese, G., DiZenzo, G., Cozzani, E., et al. (2019). New insights into the pathogenesis of bullous pemphigoid: 2019 update. *Frontiers in Immunology, 10*(1506), 1–8.

George, C., Deroide, F., & Rustin, M. (2019). Pyoderma gangrenosum—A guide to diagnosis and management. *Clinical Medicine, 19*(3), 224–228.

Gray, M., Colwell, J. C., Doughty, D., et al. (2013). Peristomal moisture-associated skin damage in adults with fecal ostomies: A comprehensive review and consensus. *Journal of Wound, Ostomy, and Continence Nursing, 40*(4), 389–399.

Grove, G., Houser, T., Sibbald, R. G., et al. (2019). Measuring epidermal effects of ostomy skin barriers. *Skin Research and Technology, 25*, 179–186.

Herlufsen, P., Olsen, A. G., Carlsen, B., et al. (2006). Study of peristomal skin disorders in patients with permanent stomas. *British Journal of Nursing, 15*, 854–862.

Hoentjen, F., Colwell, J. C., & Hanauer, S. B. (2012). Complications of peristomal recurrence of Crohn's disease. *Journal of Wound, Ostomy, and Continence Nursing, 39*(3), 297–301.

Ito, T., Yoshid, Y., Yamada, N., et al. (2014). Dermoscopy of peristomal polyps and metastasis of colon cancer. *Acta Dermato-Venereologica, 94*, 96–97.

Jemec, G. B., Martins, G., Claessens, IL, et al. (2011). Assessing peristomal skin changes in ostomy patients: Validation of the ostomy skin tool. *British Journal of Dermatology, 164*, 330–335.

Jemec, G. B., & Nybaek, H. (2008). Peristomal skin problems account for more than one in three visits to ostomy nurses. *British Journal of Dermatology, 159*, 1211–1212.

Kann, B. R. (2008). Early stomal complications. *Clinics in Colon and Rectal Surgery, 21*, 23–30.

Kasperkiewicz, M., Ellebrecht, C., Takahashi, H., et al. (2018). Pemphigus. *Nature Reviews. Disease Primers, 3*, 17026. doi: 10.1038/nrdp.2017.26.

Kridin, K., Kneiber, D., Kowalski, E., et al. (2019). Epidermolysis bullosa acquisita: A comprehensive review. *Autoimmunity Reviews, 18*, 786–795.

Kridin, K., & Ludwig, R. L. (2018). The growing incidence of bullous pemphigoid: overview and potential explanations. *Frontiers in Medicine (Lausanne), 5*, 220.

LeBlanc, K., Whiteley, I., McNichol, L., et al. (2019). Peristomal medical adhesive-related skin injury: Results of an international consensus meeting. *Journal of Wound, Ostomy, and Continence Nursing, 46*(2), 125–136.

Lindholm, E., Persson, E., Carlsson, E., et al (2013). Ostomy-related complications after emergent abdominal surgery: A 2-year follow-up study. *Journal of Wound, Ostomy, and Continence Nursing, 40*(6), 603–610.

Lyon, C. C. (2010). Infections. In C. C. Lyon & A. Smith (Eds.), *Abdominal stomas and their skin disorders: An atlas of diagnosis and management* (2nd ed., pp. 105–131). London, UK: Informa Healthcare.

Lyon, C. C., Smith, A. J., Griffiths, C. E. M., et al. (2000). The spectrum of skin disorders in abdominal stoma patients. *British Journal of Dermatology, 143*, 1248–1260.

Malik T., Lee, M. J., & Harikrishnan, A. B. (2018). The incidence of stoma related morbidity—A systematic review of randomised controlled trials. *Annals of the Royal College of Surgeons of England, 100*(7), 501–508.

Marshall, C., Woodmansey, S., Lyon, C. (2017). Peristomal psoriasis. *Clinical and Experimental Dermatology, 42*(3), 282–286. doi: 10.1111/ced.13041.

Maverakis, E., Ma, C., Shinkai, K., et al. (2018). Diagnostic criteria of ulcerative pyoderma gangrenosum: A delphi consensus of international experts. *JAMA Dermatology, 154*(4), 461–466.

McNichol, L., Lund, C., Rosen, T., et al. (2013). Medical adhesives and patient safety: State of the science. *Journal of Wound, Ostomy, and Continence Nursing, 40*(4), 365–380.

Meisner, S., Lehur, P. A., Moran, B., et al. (2012). Peristomal skin complications are common, expensive and difficult to manage: A population based cost modeling study. *PLoS One, 7*(5), e37813. doi: 10.1371/journal.pone.0037813.

Menin, G., Roeron, G., Barbierato, M., et al (2019). Design and validation of a "Peristomal Lesion Scale" for peristomal skin assessment. *International Wound Journal, 16*, 433–441.

Morales-Mendoza, Y., Fernández-Martínez, R., Fabián-Victoriano, M. R., et al. (2014). Candida species isolation in peristomal skin in patients with abdominal stomas and correlation to clinical signs: A descriptive study. *Advances in Skin & Wound Care, 27*(11), 500–504.

Murken, D. R., & Bleier, J. I. S. (2019). Ostomy-related complications. *Clinics in Colon and Rectal Surgery, 32*, 176–182.

Napierkowski, D. (2013). Uncovering common bacterial skin infections. *Nurse Practitioner, 38*(3), 30–37.

Nichols, T., Houser, T., & Grove, G. (2019). Comparing the skin stripping effects of three ostomy skin barriers infused with ceramide, honey or aloe. *Journal of Stomal Therapy Australia, 39*(2), 1–5.

Nichols, T., & Riemer, M. (2011). Body image perception, the stoma and peristomal skin condition. *Gastrointestinal Nursing, 9*(1), 22–27.

Nybaek, H., Knudsen, D. B., Laursen, T. N., et al. (2009). Skin problems in ostomy patients: A case–control study of risk factors. *Acta Dermato-Venereologica, 89*, 64–67. doi: 10.2340/00015555-0536.

Nybaek, H., Lophagen, S., Karlsmark, T., et al. (2010). Stratum corneum integrity as a predictor for peristomal skin problems in ostomates. *British Journal of Dermatology, 162*(2), 357–361.

Omura, Y., Yamabe, M., & Anazawa, S. (2010). Peristomal skin disorders in patients with intestinal and urinary ostomies: Influence of adhesive forces of various hydrocolloid wafer skin barriers. *Journal of Wound, Ostomy, and Continence Nursing, 37*(3), 289–298.

Ormaechea-Perez, N., Tuneu-Valls, A. Borja-Consigliere, H., et al. (2014). Peristomal epidermolysis bullosa acquisita in a patient with Crohn's disease. *Acta Dermato-Venereologica, 94*, 489–490.

Owen, J., Vakharia, P., & Silverberg, J. (2018). The role and diagnosis of allergic contact dermatitis in patients with atopic dermatitis. *American Journal of Clinical Dermatology, 19*(3), 293–302.

Patel, V., Rubins, S., Schwartz, R., et al. (2019). Hailey-hailey disease: A diagnostic challenge. *Cutis, 103*(3) 157–159.

Pennick, M. O., & Artioukh, D. Y. (2013). Management of parastomal varices: Who re-bleeds and who does not? A systematic review of the literature. *Techniques in Coloproctology, 17*, 163–170.

Persson, E., Berndtsson, I., Carlsson, E., et al. (2010). Stomal related complications and stoma size—A two year follow up. *Colorectal Disease, 12*, 971–976.

Pittman, J., Rawl, S. M., Schmidt, C. M., et al. (2008). Demographic and clinical factors related to ostomy complications and quality of life in veterans with an ostomy. *Journal of Wound, Ostomy, and Continence Nursing, 35*, 493–503.

Porro, A., Seque, C., Corsi-Ferreira, M., et al. (2019). Pemphigus vulgaris. *Anais Brasileiros de Dermatologia, 94*(3), 264–268.

Romano, J., Welden, C. V., Orr, J., et al. (2019). Case series regarding parastomal variceal bleeding: Presentation and management. *Annals of Hepatology, 18*(1), 250–257.

Salvadalena, G. D. (2013). The incidence of stoma and peristomal complications during the first 3 months after ostomy creation. *Journal of Wound, Ostomy, and Continence Nursing, 40*(4), 400–406.

Seungmi, P., Lee, Y. J., Oh, D. N., et al. (2011). Comparison of standardized peristomal skin care and crusting technique in prevention of peristomal skin problems in ostomy patients. *Journal of Korean Academy of Nursing, 41*(6), 814–820.

Shavit, E., Alavi, A., & Sibbald, R. (2017). Pyoderma gangrenosum: A critical review. *Advances in Skin & Wound Care, 30*(12), 534–542.

Steinhagen, E., Colwell, J., & Cannon, L. (2017). Intestinal stomas—Postoperative stoma care and peristomal skin complications. *Clinics in Colon and Rectal Surgery, 30*, 184–192.

Strauss, C., Sivakkolunthuand, M., & Ayantunde, A. A. (2014). Recurrent and troublesome variceal bleeding from parastomal caput medusa. *Korean Journal of Gastroenterology, 64*(5), 290–293.

Szymanski, K. M., St-Cyr, D., Alam, T., et al. (2010). External stoma and peristomal complications following radical cystectomy and ileal conduit diversion: A systematic review. *Ostomy/Wound Management, 56*(1), 28–35.

Taneja, C., Netsch, D., Rolstad, B. S., et al. (2017). Clinical and economic burden of peristomal skin complications in patients with recent ostomies. *Journal of Wound, Ostomy, and Continence Nursing, 44*(4), 350–357.

Taneja, C., Netsch, D., Rolstad, B. S., et al. (2019). Risk and economic burden of peristomal skin complications following ostomy surgery. *Journal of Wound, Ostomy, and Continence Nursing, 46*(2), 143–149.

WCET. (2014). World Council of enterostomal therapy. In K. Zulkowski, E. A. Ayello, & S. Stelton (Eds.), *WCET International ostomy guideline*. Perth, Australia: Author.

Williams, J. D. L., & Lyon, C. C. (2010). Dermatitis: Contact irritation and contact allergy. In C. C. Lyon, & A. Smith (Eds.), *Abdominal stomas and their skin disorders: An atlas of diagnosis and management* (2nd ed., pp. 52–104). UK: Informa Healthcare.

Woo, K. Y., Beeckman, D., & Chakravarthy, D. (2017). Management of moisture-associated skin damage: A scoping review. *Advances in Skin & Wound Care, 30*(11), 494–501.

Wound, Ostomy and Continence Nurses Society. (2016). *Peristomal skin complications: Clinical resource guide.* Mt. Laurel, NJ: Author.

Wound, Ostomy and Continence Nurses Society. (2017a). *Clinical guideline: Management of the adult patient with a fecal or urinary ostomy.* Mt. Laurel, NJ: Author.

Wound, Ostomy, and Continence Nurses Society. (2017b). Peristomal skin assessment guide for clinicians. Retrieved on June 1, 2020, from https://psag.wocn.org/index.html#home

Yates, S., McNichol, L., Heinecke, S. B., et al (2017). Embracing the concept, defining the practice, and changing the outcome: Setting the standard for medical adhesive-related skin injury interventions in WOC nursing practice. *Journal of Wound, Ostomy, and Continence Nursing, 44*(1), 13–17.

Zhou, H., Ye, Y., Qu, H., et al. (2019). Effect of ostomy care team intervention on patients with ileal conduit. *Journal of Wound, Ostomy, and Continence Nursing, 46*(5), 413–417.

Zulkowski, K. (2017). Understanding moisture-associated skin damage, medical adhesive-related skin injuries, and skin tears. *Advances in Skin & Wound Care, 30*(8), 372–381.

QUESTIONS

1. At a postoperative follow-up visit 2 weeks after hospital discharge, your patient with an ileostomy complains of burning and itching of the peristomal skin. She usually changes her pouching system twice a week, but often experiences leakage at night resulting in extra pouch changes. Her peristomal skin is erythematous and weeping around the stoma, and there is partial thickness skin loss extending 3 inches below the stoma. Which of the following complications is most likely?
A. Peristomal medical adhesive-related skin injury
B. Peristomal moisture-associated skin damage
C. Pyoderma gangrenosum
D. Peristomal candidiasis

2. Your patient with a colostomy changes his pouching system every 3 to 4 days and has not experienced leakage between pouch changes. When you remove the pouching system, you note a linear area of stripped skin at the upper edge of the skin barrier. What aspect of his self-care may be contributing to this complication?
A. Routine use of liquid skin protectant
B. Shaving the abdominal hair
C. Cutting the barrier opening too large
D. Removing the skin barrier incorrectly

3. A 48-year-old man with an ileostomy created 15 years prior reports multiple episodes of bleeding near his stoma. He has purple discoloration of the peristomal skin and small defects at the stoma edge oozing blood. His medical history includes ulcerative colitis and primary sclerosing cholangitis resulting in cirrhosis. What is the most likely cause of the bleeding?
A. Peristomal moisture-associated skin damage
B. Peristomal varices
C. Peristomal pyoderma gangrenosum
D. Peristomal granulomas

4. One of your patients with a colostomy and history of colorectal cancer has scattered peristomal erythematous papules at the mucocutaneous junction. The patient is getting a good fit with a presized convex barrier pouch and skin barrier rings. You have followed the patient three times over the past 2 months, and you have applied silver nitrate to the lesions at during each visit. Despite treatment, there has been no significant improvement. Which of the following interventions are indicated?
A. Referral to an advanced ostomy practice provider or dermatologist
B. Changing the pouching system to a flat barrier product
C. Patient teaching about how to use silver nitrate at home
D. Instruct the patient about use of an ostomy belt

5. A patient you do not know well has called you complaining of pruritus around his urostomy. He has a clinic appointment the following week and wants some ideas about managing the itch today. What additional information is essential to ask before making recommendations?
A. Onset of the itching, type of pouching products being used
B. Intensity of the itching, appearance of the skin
C. History of skin diseases, use of antifungal powder
D. Stoma size, barrier opening size, presence or absence of leakage

6. The urostomy is more likely than other ostomy types to be associated with which peristomal skin complications?
A. PMASD, pseudoverrucous lesions
B. Granuloma, pyoderma gangrenosum
C. Allergic contact dermatitis
D. PMARSI, pemphigus vulgaris

7. Your patient has painful nonhealing peristomal wounds you suspect may be due to pyoderma gangrenosum and you are providing her with a referral to dermatology. What interim stoma/skin care is recommended for this patient?
   A. Conservative sharp débridement and absorbent dressing
   B. Extended wear skin barrier and ostomy belt for security
   C. Absorbent wound products and a flat pouching system
   D. Antimicrobial wound dressing and convex pouching system

8. Your patient with a loop ileostomy for Crohn's disease has a flush oval stoma in a skin fold. He uses a presized soft convex product with an ostomy belt. He reports tenderness and bleeding around the stoma. When you remove the pouching system, you notice erythematous firm papules in a crescent shape just below the stoma. Given this history, what do you suspect is the cause?
   A. Granulomas due to moisture exposure from effluent
   B. Bullous pemphigus related to his Crohn's disease
   C. Pressure injury from use of soft convexity and the belt
   D. Mucosal implantation resulting from surgery

9. What principles apply to the management of patients with a stoma and autoimmune diseases?
   A. Select nonadherent wound dressings when needed, and use adhesive removers at every pouching system change, collaborate with a dermatology specialist
   B. Use the same topical steroid and immune modulator products on the peristomal skin as the patient uses for the rest of the body
   C. Enlarge the skin barrier opening to permit better visualization of the peristomal skin
   D. Use extended wear products with tape borders for a larger surface area of adhesive

10. What do patients need to know about preventing and managing peristomal skin complications?
    A. Prevent leakage, look at the skin, and apply an antifungal powder routinely
    B. Look at the skin and take action if it is persistently red or no longer intact
    C. Make an appointment with a dermatologist at the first sign of skin problems
    D. Watch the area for several pouch changes before seeking assistance

ANSWERS AND RATIONALES

1. **A. Rationale:** This describes the most common form of peristomal skin complication occurring with leakage; peristomal moisture-associated skin damage.

2. **D. Rationale:** The patient without leakage and with a defined area of skin injury away from the stoma is likely to have peristomal medical adhesive-related skin injury.

3. **B. Rationale:** The patient's history and examination are consistent with parastomal varices.

4. **A. Rationale:** Patients with peristomal lesions unresponsive to usual treatment should be referred.

5. **D. Rationale:** All of the listed items are helpful, but leakage and skin condition will allow you to decide whether simply adjusting the fit or barrier sizing may help alleviate the problem temporarily.

6. **A. Rationale:** Moisture around a urostomy commonly results in macerated skin and development of elevated lesions: PMASD, pseudoverrucous lesions.

7. **C. Rationale:** Use of flat products are recommended rather than convex to avoid trauma and worsen pathergy associated with PPG.

8. **A. Rationale:** The area just below the oval stoma is exposed to stoma effluent when using a presized opening; this may contribute to granuloma formation. Mucosal implantation is not painful.

9. **A. Rationale:** As described in **Table 16-1**, select nonadherent wound dressings when needed, use adhesive removers at every pouching system change, and collaborate with a dermatology specialist.

10. **B. Rationale:** Awareness of normal skin appearance is the most important.

CHAPTER 17

STOMA COMPLICATIONS

Joyce Pittman

OBJECTIVE

Distinguish between stoma complications and select the associated management strategies.

TOPIC OUTLINE

Introduction **270**

Early Complications **272**
Mucocutaneous Separation   272
Etiology/Incidence   272
Presentation   272
Assessment   272
Management   272
Stomal Necrosis   272
Etiology/Incidence   272
Presentation   272
Assessment   273
Management   273
Stomal Retraction   273
Etiology/Incidence   273
Presentation   274
Assessment   274
Management   274

Late Complications **274**
Stomal Stenosis   274

Etiology/Incidence   274
Presentation   274
Assessment   275
Management   275
Stomal Prolapse   275
Etiology/Incidence   275
Presentation   275
Assessment   276
Management   276
Stomal Trauma   276
Etiology/Incidence   276
Presentation   277
Assessment   277
Management   277
Parastomal Hernia   277
Etiology/Incidence   277
Presentation   278
Assessment   278
Management   278

Conclusions **279**

INTRODUCTION

Complications following the surgical creation of an ostomy are a significant problem for many individuals. These complications are often multifaceted involving both physiologic and psychosocial aspects (Pittman et al., 2017). The physiologic aspect of ostomy complications involves changes of the stoma and peristomal skin (WOCN, 2017). This chapter will discuss the physiologic aspect of ostomy complications involving the stoma.

Ostomy complications are a significant problem for individuals with an ostomy, yet, definitions and terminology are often not consistent in the literature, making it difficult to accurately measure ostomy complication incidence (Salvadalena, 2013). In addition, differentiating research findings between stomal and peristomal complications can be difficult (see Chapter 16, Peristomal skin complications).

Overall incidence rates of ostomy complications have been reported in the literature, although the ranges vary and are very broad for the above reasons. Three systematic reviews of the literature on ostomy complications indicated that 18% to 55% of individuals with an ostomy experienced peristomal skin irritation, up to 50% experienced parastomal herniation, up to 25% experienced stomal prolapse, 10% experienced stenosis, and 11% experienced retraction of the stoma (Jones et al., 2018; Salvadalena, 2008). Researchers report that up to 80% of individuals with an ostomy develop ostomy complications (Pittman, 2011b; Pittman et al., 2014, 2017).

Various patient characteristics have been identified as being associated with ostomy complications, but studies with predictive analysis models are limited. Several studies have identified that higher body mass index (BMI), older age, emergent surgery, inflammatory bowel disease, having an ileostomy (vs. colostomy), a diverting "loop" procedure, poor bowel quality, ischemic colitis, stomal retraction, lack of preoperative education, and involvement of a wound, ostomy, and continence

(WOC) nurse influence the development of ostomy complications (Bass et al., 1997; Colwell et al., 2001; Duchesne et al., 2002; Hendren et al., 2015; Pittman et al., 2008). In the landmark retrospective study conducted by Bass et al. (1997), complication rates were compared between patients who received preoperative education and stoma site marking by an enterostomal therapist (now known as WOC nurse) and those who did not. They found among those who received preoperative education and stoma site marking by an enterostomal therapist (WOC nurse), 32.5% developed complications compared to 43.5% of those who did not receive these clinical interventions ($p = 0.05$). However, in a small study ($n = 43$) by Salvadalena (2013), no demographic or clinical factors such as age, stoma type, gender, wear time, number of days since surgery, use of steroids, anticoagulants and nonsteroidal medications, frequency of pouch change, or reason for surgery were found to be associated with the development of ostomy complications. The Ostomy Complication Conceptual Model (**Fig. 17-1**) provides a framework for exploring ostomy complications and the risk factors that contribute to their occurrence (Pittman et al., 2014).

One method that has been used to classify ostomy complications is to categorize them into early, within 30 days following surgery, and late complications, >30 days following surgery (Kim & Kumar, 2006; Kwiatt & Kawata, 2013; Salvadalena, 2013; Shabbir & Britton, 2010). This chapter has been organized using the classification of

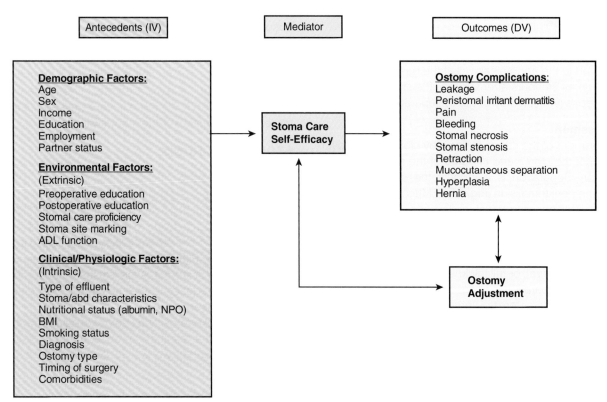

FIGURE 17-1. Pittman Ostomy Complication Conceptual Model.

early and late complications, recognizing that some complications can occur in both early and late time frames. The following stoma complications will be addressed; mucocutaneous separation, stomal retraction, stenosis, necrosis, prolapse, stomal fistula, stomal trauma, and peristomal hernia.

🜚 EARLY COMPLICATIONS

Early stomal complications are those that commonly occur within 30 days following surgery and include mucocutaneous separation, stomal necrosis, and stomal retraction.

MUCOCUTANEOUS SEPARATION

Etiology/Incidence

Mucocutaneous separation is the detachment of stomal tissue from the surrounding peristomal skin (Colwell & Beitz, 2007, 2014; Pittman et al., 2014, 2017). Mucocutaneous separation may be a result of poor healing, tension, or infection. Salvadalena (2013) reported that 2.7% patients (*n* = 37) experienced mucocutaneous separation within 21 days of surgery. Park et al. (1999) reported that 4% of patients had mucocutaneous separation in their review of 1,616 stoma patients. In a prospective study of 3,970 stomas, Cottam et al. (2007) reported that 24% had mucocutaneous separation. In another study of 71 subjects, 13% had mucocutaneous separation (Pittman et al., 2014). Parmar and colleagues (2011) reported 25.2% in their study of 192 patients with an ostomy.

Presentation

Healthy stomas will have a closely approximated and intact mucocutaneous junction (where the stoma is attached to the abdominal wall at the base of the stoma). As soon as 24 hours after surgery, the stoma and mucocutaneous junction may begin to separate.

Assessment

Assessment of the stoma is done by close visual observation of the stoma and integrity of the mucocutaneous junction. Separation is evident if the stoma detaches from the peristomal skin (**Fig. 17-2**). Mucocutaneous separation can occur in variable degrees of severity: partial—if it is only a portion of the stomal circumference, or complete if the entire circumference is involved (Pittman et al., 2014). The separation can also be either superficial, only the skin level, or full thickness. Close observation of the area of separation is necessary noting depth, wound base tissue characteristics (necrotic, granular), and type of drainage (serosanguinous, purulent, fecal).

KEY POINT

Use a cotton tip applicator to gently assess the extent and depth of the mucocutaneous separation.

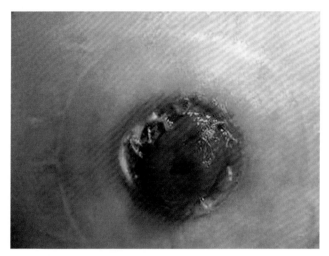

FIGURE 17-2. Mucocutaneous Separation. (Courtesy of Janice Colwell, APRN CWOCN, FAAN.)

Management

Management of mucocutaneous separation depends on the degree of the separation. If the separation is partial and superficial, the subcutaneous defect may be small and able to be managed conservatively. The subcutaneous defect may be treated like a wound and filled with an advanced wound product such as skin barrier powder, hydrofiber, or calcium alginate. The skin barrier of the pouching system is fitted over the peristomal skin and defect to provide protection from the stomal effluent. The pouching system is changed as warranted to manage the drainage, assess healing, and reapply the absorbent filler material.

If the defect is large, then fecal contamination of the peristomal subcutaneous defect is likely and infection may occur. If risk of infection is suspected, an antimicrobial dressing and systemic treatment should be considered (WOCN, 2017). The more severe the separation, the more likely retraction of the stoma will occur.

STOMAL NECROSIS

Etiology/Incidence

Stomal necrosis is defined as death of the stomal tissue resulting from impaired blood flow (Colwell & Beitz, 2007, 2014) and has been identified as one of the most common early complications (Duchesne et al., 2002; Kim & Kumar, 2006; Pittman et al., 2014; Shabbir & Britton, 2010). Ischemia of stomal tissue is usually caused by tension on or inadequacy of the mesenteric vasculature. It can also be caused by trauma to the stomal tissue during creation. Stomal necrosis has been associated with obesity and is often a result of the traction that is placed on the mesentery and bowel wall (Colwell & Fichera, 2005).

Presentation

Impending stomal necrosis is evidenced by a progression of discoloration of the stomal tissue from pink to black. The stoma will usually appear dusky and dry within hours to days of surgery progressing to black and flaccid. The degree of necrosis and amount of stomal tissue involved may vary depending on the degree of ischemia. The whole stoma may be involved or only a portion of the stoma. Stomal ischemia may extend from surface to below the fascia, or only a portion of the stoma, and above skin level. The amount of stomal necrosis determines the severity and treatment.

Assessment

Assessment of stomal necrosis is done by close visual observation. Within 24 hours of surgery, color changes of the stoma are usually visible. Color of the stoma progresses from dusky red to black (**Fig. 17-3**) depending on the degree of vascular compromise (Pittman et al., 2014). A method commonly used to determine the degree or level of ischemia and stomal necrosis is the insertion of a clear, lubricated tube (i.e., lab collection vial) gently inserted into the stoma. Using a penlight directed into the tube, a change in the color of the inner stoma lumen may be detected thus indicating the level of ischemia.

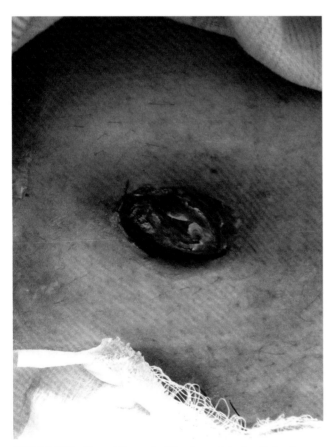

FIGURE 17-3. Stomal Necrosis. (Courtesy of Janice Colwell, APRN CWOCN, FAAN.)

> ### KEY POINT
>
> It is advisable to use a transparent ostomy pouch in the immediate postoperative period to allow for assessment of the stoma color.

An innovative method of evaluating tissue perfusion is the intraoperative laser angiography using indocyanine green. This vascular imaging technology provides real-time assessment of tissue perfusion that correlates with clinical outcomes and can be used to guide surgical decision-making (Gurtner et al., 2013; Ris et al., 2018; Santi et al., 2019). This method is primarily used intraoperatively to assess perfusion of the stoma and intestine at the time of resection.

Management

Stomal necrosis is often a watch-and-wait situation. If the ischemia and necrosis are above the fascial level, observation may be adequate. Often, if the ischemia and necrosis are superficial, the top layer of the stoma may slough off, leaving a red viable stoma. If the stomal ischemia and necrosis are below skin level but still above the fascial level, the necrotic stomal tissue will become malodorous and flaccid. Débridement is often indicated. After the necrotic tissue is removed or sloughs off, usually there is mucocutaneous separation. As the mucocutaneous separation heals, stenosis may occur. In addition, the level of the stoma above the skin is diminished, and this often leads to pouching challenges. If the ischemia and necrosis extend deeper than the fascial level, urgent surgical intervention may be indicated (WOCN, 2017).

STOMAL RETRACTION

Etiology/Incidence

Retraction is the disappearance of stoma tissue protrusion in line with or below skin level (Colwell & Beitz, 2007, 2014; Pittman et al., 2017). Retraction is usually caused by tension on the stoma from a variety of reasons: short mesentery, thickened abdominal wall, excessive adhesions or scar formation, increased BMI, inadequate initial stoma length, or improper skin excision, stomal necrosis, and mucocutaneous separation (Colwell, 2004; Colwell & Beitz, 2007; Kwiatt & Kawata, 2013). Anecdotal evidence suggests that retraction occurs frequently in overweight patients with larger adipose layers. A shortened and fatty mesentery makes adequate mobilization of the bowel difficult, thus producing tension on the stoma (Cottam, 2005; Shabbir & Britton, 2010). The height of the stoma above skin level has been associated with the ability of the patient to successfully care for their stoma (Parmar et al., 2011).

Ratliff and Donovan (2001) found that 4% of 220 ostomy patients had flush or retracted stomas. In a prospective study of 3,970 stomas, Cottam et al. (2007)

reported that 40.1% had retraction. In Pittman's prospective study of 71 participants with an ostomy, 39% had retraction (Pittman et al., 2014). Pittman (2011a,b) (*n* = 144) found the stoma flush or below skin level in 22% of those with a colostomy, 41% (*n* = 19) of those with an ileostomy, and 20% (*n* = 2) in those with an urostomy (Pittman, 2011a). In a 3-year retrospective study of 164 patients who underwent ostomy surgery, retraction occurred in 5% of those patients (Duchesne et al., 2002). Salvadalena (2013) found 5.4% (*n* = 37) incidence of retraction. In a study of 192 ostomy patients, 32.3% had stomal retraction (Parmar et al., 2011). Another study of 97 patients with an ostomy found BMI to be associated with retraction (*p* = 0.003) (Arumugam et al., 2003). The incidence of retraction seems to be increasing. Cottam et al. (2007) reported that the incidence of stomal retraction (stoma below the skin level) is more than doubled between 1996 and 2004 (22% vs. 51%) (Colwell & Beitz, 2007). In a systematic review of the literature, stoma retraction occurred in 9% to 15% of ileal conduits and 1% to 11% of all stomas (Szymanski et al., 2010). In Pittman's study, patients who did not have their stoma site preoperatively marked by a WOC nurse experienced greater severity of ostomy complications, specifically stomal retraction (*r* = 0.32, *p* = 0.01) (Pittman et al., 2014).

Presentation

A healthy stoma should be above the level of the surrounding skin, 2 cm above skin surface for ileostomies, and 1 cm above skin surface for colostomies, according to the American Society of Colon and Rectal Surgeon's Clinical Practice Guidelines for Ostomy (Hendren et al., 2015). In Cottam's study of 1,329 problematic stomas, if the stoma height was <1 cm, the probability of having a problematic stoma was at least 35% (*p* < 0.0001) (Cottam et al., 2007). Parmar et al. (2011) found that those with shorter stomas (less protrusion above skin) had more complications.

Assessment

The stoma needs to be observed without the pouching system in place and in a variety of positions—sitting, supine, and standing. The level of the stoma and the surrounding skin needs to be closely noted. The stoma may disappear in a skin fold or crease when sitting or may become flush or even retracted with position changes and with peristalsis.

Management

In order to achieve successful pouching of the stoma, a flat pouching surface is preferable. When retraction is present, the goal is to augment the level of the stoma above the skin. This may sometimes be achieved using a convex pouching system and/or belt (see Chapter 12). If a predictable wear time is not achieved and complications continue, surgical intervention may be necessary to revise the stoma. Local revision may be possible if there is adequate intestine to mobilize above the skin level; if not, a more invasive surgery may be necessary to create a new stoma (WOCN, 2017).

 ## LATE COMPLICATIONS

Late stomal complications are those that occur at least 30 days after surgery and often include stomal stenosis, prolapse, and parastomal herniation (Duchesne et al., 2002; Kim & Kumar, 2006; Kwiatt & Kawata, 2013; Shabbir & Britton, 2010; Steel & Wu, 2002). Various surgical techniques are being explored to minimize the risk of developing long-term complications such as extraperitoneal versus intraperitoneal technique, intraoperative laser angiography, minimally invasive surgical alternatives, and extraperitoneal tunneling of end colostomies (Gurtner et al., 2013; Heiying et al., 2014; Hendren et al., 2015).

STOMAL STENOSIS

Etiology/Incidence

Stomal stenosis is the impairment of effluent drainage due to narrowing or contracting of the stomal tissue at the skin or fascial level (Colwell & Beitz, 2007; Pittman et al., 2017). In the past, stenosis typically occurred early in the postoperative period due to inadequate surgical technique (at fascial level or at skin) or if not matured properly (Hampton, 1992). Due to the improvement in surgical technique, stomal stenosis is rarely seen early but rather late in the recovery process, >30 days following surgery, usually as a result of mucocutaneous separation, stoma necrosis, or retraction of the stoma or recurrence of disease such as Crohn's disease with stricturing near the stoma (Hoentjen et al., 2012). As healing occurs, formation of granulation tissue around the stoma constricts the lumen. Other causes of stomal stenosis include presence of a tumor, excessive scar formation due to instrumentation (dilatation), or chronic inflammation (peristomal irritant dermatitis or hyperplasia) (Colwell, 2004; Hampton, 1992; WOCN, 2014).

The incidence of stomal stenosis seems to be decreasing over time. Earlier studies report rates as high as 23% (Leong, 1994). However, more recent studies indicate incidence in the range of 2% to 17% (Duchesne et al., 2002; Pittman et al., 2014; Robertson et al., 2005).

Presentation

The appearance of a stenotic stoma opening appears smaller than the usual appearance of a stoma (**Fig. 17-4**). Often the patient with a fecal stoma may report pain with stoma evacuation, small ribbon-like stool, or conversely, constipation followed by large explosive evacuations, loud with excessive gas. Patients with urostomies may report frequent urinary tract infections, projectile urine stream, and/or flank pain (Colwell, 2004; WOCN®, 2014).

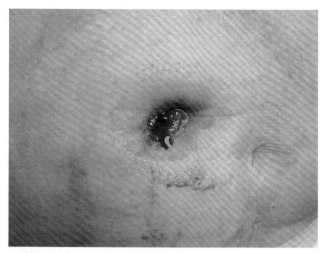

FIGURE 17-4. Stomal Stenosis. (Courtesy of Janice Colwell, APRN CWOCN, FAAN.)

Assessment

Assessment of a stenotic stoma is best performed by a knowledgeable practitioner with a gloved lubricated digit in order to assess the size and mobility of the skin and fascial rings. The Ostomy Complication Severity Index (OCSI) provides an objective assessment of the severity of stomal stenosis. Using the Complication Severity Index (OCSI), stomal stenosis is measured as: stoma less than 5th digit diameter, with no discomfort; less than 5th digit with occasional discomfort or as unable to insert 5th digit with no output (Pittman, et al., 2014). If the digit cannot be inserted into the stomal opening due to severe stricture, a retrograde contrast study through a small rubber catheter may be performed (Colwell, 2004; WOCN, 2017).

KEY POINT

When assessing the stoma with a digital examination, explain to the patient that the stoma does not contain nerves to cause pain, but if they feel pressure to let you know so the examination can be stopped.

Management

Management of mild stenosis of a fecal ostomy may include low-residue diet, stool softeners, or high liquid intake (Beitz & Colwell, 2016) to facilitate thinner/softer fecal consistency. Stoma dilation by gradually and incrementally introducing a dilator or digit into the stoma has been a common practice in the past and is still reported as an available intervention when performed by trained clinicians (Beitz & Colwell, 2016). Stomal dilation can be used to temporarily aid in evacuation but is not recommended as a long-term practice (Pittman et al., 2017). Moreover, chronic dilation has been reported to potentially cause stomal stenosis (Hampton, 1992;

Pittman et al., 2017). For the most severe cases, surgery is warranted. This may involve freeing the stoma from the peristomal skin locally or by performing a laparotomy and resiting the stoma.

STOMAL PROLAPSE

Etiology/Incidence

Stomal prolapse is the telescoping of the intestine through the stoma (Colwell & Beitz, 2007). Prolapse of the stoma can occur for a number of reasons: increased abdominal pressure, obesity, the stomal opening in the abdominal wall is too large, or the stoma was created outside the rectus muscle (Weideman et al., 2012).

All stomas are subject to prolapse, and incidence reports vary. Stoma prolapse is often seen in loop colostomies (Kwiatt & Kawata, 2013; Shabbir & Britton, 2010), and the distal limb is predominantly involved. Incidence ranges from 2% to 22% (Kwiatt & Kawata, 2013). Stomal prolapse is often seen in children. In a study of 144 infants with anorectal malformations, the incidence of stomal prolapse was higher in those with loop versus divided colostomies, 17.8% and 2.8%, respectively ($p = 0.005$) (Oda et al., 2014). Chen et al. (2013) performed a meta-analysis including five randomized controlled trials and seven nonrandomized studies with 1,687 patients in total comparing outcomes in temporary ileostomies versus temporary colostomies. They found a lower incidence of stoma prolapse in temporary ileostomy patients compared to temporary colostomy patients in both randomized control trials and nonrandomized trials (Chen et al., 2013). In a systematic review of the literature related to stoma complications following radical cystectomy and ileal conduit diversions, stomal prolapse was identified in 1.5% to 8% at a mean of 2 years following surgery (Szymanski et al., 2010). It has been reported that up to 50% of patients with prolapsed colostomy also had a parastomal hernia (Kim & Kumar, 2006). Salvadalena (2013) reported 2% experienced stomal prolapse on postoperative day 35 in her prospective study of 43 ostomy participants. There is little evidence of stomal prolapse in urinary diversions.

Presentation

A prolapsed stoma can present in a variety of degrees of severity and length of stomal protrusion (**Fig. 17-5**). The length of the prolapsed stoma will guide management. The greater the length of the prolapse, the greater the likelihood of stomal edema, trauma, and ischemia. As the stoma becomes edematous and dependent, it becomes a deep red color (vasodilation) (WOCN®, 2017). With a very prominent (5 to 13 inches) prolapse, the stoma is susceptible to trauma (WOCN®, 2014). Care needs to include avoiding friction, laceration, or pressure to the stoma. In extreme situations, blood supply to the stoma may become compromised and stomal ischemia may occur.

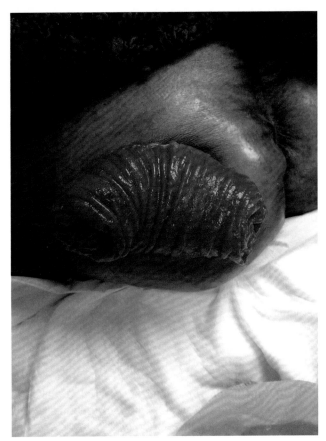

FIGURE 17-5. Stomal Prolapse. (Courtesy of Janice Colwell, APRN CWOCN, FAAN.)

Assessment

Assessment of the prolapsed stoma is performed by observation and palpation. It is recommended to perform the assessment in a variety of patient positions—standing, sitting, and supine. Close observation must be done to determine the degree of the prolapse, viability of the stoma (color of the stoma), output characteristics, presence of stomal and peristomal pain, peristomal skin, presence of parastomal hernia, and fit of the pouching system (WOCN®, 2014, 2017). Palpation is accomplished with the patient in a supine position and attempting to reduce the prolapse with gentle pressure.

Management

Conservative management of the stomal prolapse is usually recommended. It is frequently best to apply the pouching system when the prolapsed is reduced. Have the patient lie flat for at least 10 minutes and apply gentle pressure over the stoma to reduce the prolapse portion (Beitz & Collwell, 2016). Reduction of the prolapse can be augmented by the application of cold (ice packs) to the stoma (over the pouch) for several minutes (Colwell, 2004). The use of sprinkling sugar over an edematous prolapsed stoma has been

reported to be effective to reduce the prolapse (Fligelstone et al., 1997); however, there is little evidence to support this practice. The sugar provides osmotic therapy or causes a fluid shift across the stoma mucosa and reduces edema. Use of moldable skin barrier technology around the stoma, cutting radial slits in the solid skin barrier to accommodate the stomal prolapse, and use of barrier rings may prove helpful (Beitz & Colwell, 2016).

The pouching system should be adapted to fit the size of the prolapsed stoma. The pouch needs to accommodate the length of the stoma and be flexible to avoid stomal trauma. A lubricant may be used on the inside of the pouch to minimize stoma trauma. Large pouching systems (irrigation sleeves or wound managers) should be considered if necessary (Beitz & Colwell, 2016). Education must be provided to the patient to observe the stoma for color changes and to seek immediate attention if the stoma becomes ischemic as surgery may be indicated (Colwell, 2004; WOCN®, 2017).

KEY POINT

If there is significant length to the prolapse, it may be advisable to instruct the patient not to use a two-piece pouching system as the stoma may be injured (pinched) by the plastic flange (the stoma can protrude over the flange and be harmed). A one-piece pouching system may be more advisable (WOCN®, 2017).

STOMAL TRAUMA

Etiology/Incidence

Stomal trauma has been defined as an injury to the stomal mucosa often related to pressure or physical force (Colwell & Beitz, 2007; Pittman et al., 2017). An external force that may cause stomal trauma includes pressure, friction, or physical force of some kind exerted on the stomal mucosal tissue. WOC nurses (n = 281) reported that pouching systems may often be the cause of stomal trauma (Beitz & Colwell, 2016). Stomal trauma terminology is not used in the WOCN® Stoma Complications: Best Practice for Clinicians but rather the term *laceration* (WOCN, 2014). However, the description is congruent with stomal trauma and states that a laceration to the stoma may occur as a result of trauma (car accident, shaving, etc.). Regardless of terminology, there are few studies reporting incidence of stoma trauma. However, in a study of 71 adult participants with an ostomy, 32% of participants reported stomal bleeding. The cause of the bleeding was not specified (Pittman et al., 2014). In another study of 330 patients with an end colostomy, the investigators reported that 34.5% had mucosal bleeding (Mahjoubi et al., 2005). Again, the cause of the bleeding was not specified.

Presentation

Stomal trauma presents differently depending on the type of trauma, but it is usually localized to the area where the trauma occurred. It could present as a linear injury with minimal depth due to a laceration or the stomal mucosa could appear denuded with a deep red/dusky friable area that bleeds easily as a result of an abrasive injury (**Fig. 17-6**). The stoma could appear bruised or dusky if there was trauma as a result of pressure such as a seat belt. The appearance of the stomal injury depends on the type of trauma that occurred.

Assessment

A complete history and physical must include information regarding any recent trauma to the stoma. Removal of the pouch and direct visual observation of the stoma must occur in order to assess the stoma for integrity, color, hydration, and bleeding. Any changes in the stoma characteristics warrant further investigation.

Management

There are three things to consider when managing stomal trauma, elimination of the cause, managing bleeding, and close observation (Beitz & Colwell, 2016). In order to treat the stomal trauma injury, the cause of the trauma must be determined and corrected. Stomal trauma inju-

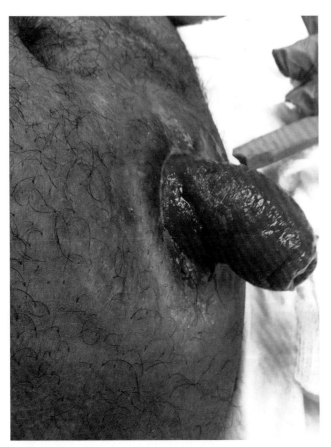

FIGURE 17-6. Stomal Trauma. (Courtesy of Janice Colwell, APRN CWOCN, FAAN.)

ries usually heal spontaneously once the source of the trauma is eliminated. If the injury was due to a seat belt rubbing across the stoma mucosa, padding the seat belt or shifting seat belt position may be adequate. Additional commercially available ostomy accessory products may be considered to protect the stoma (see Appendix K). If the two-piece pouching system flange is too small causing pinching of the stoma, adjusting the size of the pouching system may suffice. Bleeding may be managed by calcium alginate, hemostatic agents (Gelfoam, Surgicel, etc.), skin barrier powder, and silver nitrate (Beitz & Colwell, 2016). Management of stomal trauma includes close observation and assessment of the stoma with each pouch change for indications of healing (Colwell, 2004). Education must be provided to the patient to promptly report to their provider any persistent bleeding or bleeding that comes from inside the stoma in order to rule out other disease-related causes (WOCN®, 2017).

PARASTOMAL HERNIA

Etiology/Incidence

Parastomal (peristomal) hernia is defined as a defect in abdominal fascia that allows the intestine to bulge into the parastomal area (Colwell & Beitz, 2007). When the stoma is surgically created, an opening (or defect) in the abdominal fascia is created intentionally to bring the bowel to skin level. In many patients, the defect enlarges over time and allows the intestines to bulge into the area. The most common abdominal hernias develop at sites where the abdominal wall has natural openings such as the internal inguinal ring, the umbilicus, and the esophageal hiatus. Previous surgical entry sites (incisional hernia and stoma) are also common areas where hernias develop. Factors that increase the pressure in the abdominal cavity, such as obesity, heavy lifting, coughing with chronic lung disease, straining during a bowel movement or urination (prostatism), chronic lung disease, and ascites, have traditionally been considered important in the etiology of a hernia, especially at these natural openings.

Parastomal hernia is one of the most common ostomy complications with incidence reported from 14% to 78% (De Raet et al., 2008; Hendren et al., 2015; Israelsson, 2008; Janes et al., 2011; Temple et al., 2016). De Raet et al. (2008) reported that 46% of 42 open and lap abdominal–perineal resections developed hernias. These investigators found that when the waist circumference exceeded the calculated threshold of 100 cm, there was a 75% probability to develop a parastomal hernia (De Raet et al., 2008). These findings were confirmed in the study by Temple and colleagues (2016) where they identified an association of parastomal hernia and increased abdominal girth. Temple et al. also reported that 50% of those with a parastomal hernia developed their hernia less than a year after stoma surgery.

Janes et al. (2011) reported that the rate of parastomal hernia was 50% after 1 year and 80% after 5 years. In a study comparing complications in 77 patients with laparoscopy surgery versus open surgery, 18% of laparoscopic compared with 2% after open procedures ($p = 0.04$) developed parastomal hernias (Randall et al., 2012).

Poor site selection or technical errors, such as making the fascial opening too large or placing a stoma in an incision, account for some of these hernias. Placing a stoma lateral to the rectus sheath is widely touted as a cause (WOCN, 2014), but this is sometimes challenged (Israelsson, 2008). Obesity, malnutrition, advanced age, collagen abnormalities, postoperative sepsis, abdominal distention, constipation, obstructive uropathy, steroid use, and chronic lung disease also are contributing factors (WOCN, 2014). Following laparoscopic surgery, removal of the intestinal specimen through the site that was later used to create the stoma may also contribute to the development of parastomal hernia (Randall et al., 2012).

Surgical techniques for stomal construction, such as extraperitoneal tunneling, use of prophylactic mesh, three-dimensional mesh, or bioprosthetic material, and trephine (cylindrically shaped opening) ostomy creation show promise for minimizing parastomal hernia development, but continued research is needed to examine long-term advantages (Hendren et al., 2015; Köhler et al., 2015). In a promising study of 100 participants with varied types of ostomies, a program of abdominal exercise, avoidance of heavy lifting, and use of a support binder in the first 6 to 12 months after surgery was associated with a reduced incidence of parastomal hernia (North, 2014).

Presentation

The individual with a parastomal hernia presents with a bulging around or beside the stoma, depending on the size of the defect in the abdominal wall, when abdominal pressure is increased (cough or bears down; **Fig. 17-7**). The individual may not be aware that he or she has a hernia but may report difficulty maintaining the seal of the pouching system, thus experiencing leakage and

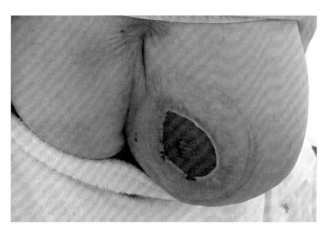

FIGURE 17-7. Peristomal Hernia. (Courtesy of Jane Fellows, MSN, RN, CWOCN.)

irritated peristomal skin. This often occurs because of the change in the abdominal skin in contact with the pouching surface causing a shifting of the skin barrier and breakdown of the seal.

Assessment

Assessment of a parastomal hernia includes close visual observation of the patient in a sitting or standing position. An asymmetric bulge is identified next to the stoma and extending outward. Assessment can also be done with the patient in a lying position and asking the patient to cough, bear down, or lift his or her head. Palpate around the stoma as the patient raises his or her head or coughs to feel the extent of the hernia. The size or extent of the hernia varies according to the size of the defect in the abdominal wall. The defect may encompass the entire parastomal area or only a portion. Assessment may also include insertion of a digit into the stoma, feeling for fascial defect around the intestine. An incomplete fascial ring will be felt in the area of the hernia. Radiographic testing can be done to confirm the presence of the parastomal hernia; upper gastrointestinal x-ray with small bowel contrast, retrograde contrast study through the stoma, or computed tomography scan with oral contrast will identify bowel loops around the stoma and above the abdominal wall (Colwell, 2004; WOCN, 2014).

Management

Conservative management and no surgical intervention is the treatment of choice for the asymptomatic patient. Conservative management options include using a flexible pouching system. A firm convex pouching system should be avoided since firm convexity may cause pressure injury to the peristomal skin. Soft convexity may offer a solution but should be used cautiously. Other management options include hernia support belt, support garments, regular diet/fluids to ensure soft stool and to prevent constipation, and routine follow-up with a WOC nurse (WOCN, 2014, 2017).

A flexible pouching system is recommended in order to accommodate a changing stoma and pouching surface. The pouching system may be either a one-piece or a two-piece system with a floating flange. The stoma should be assessed in both the supine and standing position as the stoma size may enlarge when the hernia is protruding. Individuals who irrigate their colostomy should be informed to stop irrigating if it becomes difficult to introduce water or experience incomplete evacuation.

Hernia support belts are elastic binders or garments with an opening for the pouch and usually are custom-fit according to the size and location of the hernia and the type of pouching system used. Hernia support belts/garments provide support to the area around the stoma, decreasing the hernia protrusion and stabilizing the parastomal plane thus improving the pouching system seal. Effectiveness of the hernia support belt/garment varies widely, but it is an option for the individual who is not

TABLE 17-1 HERNIA SUPPORT BELT ORDERING INFORMATION TO DETERMINE APPROPRIATE BELT

Belt style	Original panel: for prevention and small bulge flattening
	Nu-Form style: for support of nonreducible hernia
Belt fabric	Ventilated fabric
	Solid elastic
Belt size	Measurement of girth standing and lying
Belt width	Varies according to the area needing support (3"–9" or more)
Stoma location	Right or left side of the abdomen
Belt opening	Pouch manufacture product number
Custom options	Auxiliary belt example

Adapted from Nu-Hope Hernia/Ostomy Belt Worksheet (Nu-Hope).

a surgical candidate. Hernia support belts are available in different styles, sizes, and materials, and a thorough assessment should be done prior to ordering the correct belt. Follow the manufacturer instructions for correct fitting of the support belt/garment (see **Table 17-1** Hernia support belt ordering information).

KEY POINT

Once a hernia support belt/garment is obtained, the patient must be instructed how to apply the belt/garment.

Manufacturer instructions should be followed in applying the hernia belt. It is advisable to reduce the hernia if possible before belt/garment application. Usually the patient should be supine and the belt/garment should be placed around the pouch and over the parastomal hernia. Individuals with a parastomal hernia need to be informed of the importance of a diet and fluids to ensure soft stool and to prevent constipation. Education should also include the necessity of seeking immediate medical attention if the stoma darkens in color or if unremitting pain occurs (WOCN®, 2017). In addition, it is important for routine scheduled follow-up with a WOC nurse to monitor the hernia status and condition.

Surgical repair is the next option when conservative measures fail. Indications for surgical repair of the parastomal hernia depend on degree of severity and include obstruction, incarceration with/without strangulation, stenosis, intractable dermatitis, pouching management failure, large size of hernia, cosmesis, and pain. Clinical practice guidelines for ostomy surgery (Hendren et al., 2015) recommend using mesh reinforcement or stomal relocation for parastomal hernia

surgical repair. There are three general types of parastomal hernia repair (Colwell, 2004):

1. Primary fascial repair—an incision is made over the herniated area and the peristomal fascia is reapproximated. There is a high incidence of hernia reoccurrence with this method.
2. Local repair with prosthetic material such as mesh. There is high potential of erosion of the prosthetic material into the intestinal stoma with this method.
3. Stomal relocation to the opposite side of the abdomen. The hernia is repaired and the fascia reapproximated. This is the preferred method.

CONCLUSIONS

Research has shown that ostomy complications (stomal and peristomal) negatively affect the quality of life for individuals living with an ostomy and often result in physical and psychosocial limitations for these individuals and their families (Nichols & Inglese, 2018; Nichols et al., 2019; North, 2014; Pittman et al., 2008). Not only does the person with an ostomy have to cope with a serious and often life-threatening diagnosis but the placement of an ostomy requires significant changes to one's lifestyle.

As we consider how to prevent and/or decrease stomal complications, focus should be on the modifiable risk factors that contribute to their development. The WOC nurse should incorporate preoperative stoma site marking for all individuals undergoing ostomy surgery, weight management education, healthy lifestyle promotion, and evidence-based ostomy management instruction.

REFERENCES

Arumugam, P., Bevan, L., MacDonald, L., et al. (2003). A prospective audit of stomas—Analysis of risk factors and complications and their management. *Colorectal Disease, 5*(1), 49–52.

Bass, E., Del Pino, A., Tan, A., et al. (1997). Does preoperative stomal marking and education by the enterostomal therapist affect outcome? *Diseases of the Colon & Rectum, 40*(4), 440–442.

Beitz, J., & Colwell, J. (2016). Management approaches to stomal and peristomal complications. *Journal of Wound, Ostomy, and Continence Nursing, 43*(3), 263–268.

Chen, J. W., Zhang, D. R., Li, J. R., et al. (2013). Meta-analysis of temporary ileostomy versus colostomy for colorectal anastomoses. *Acta Chirurgica Belgica, 113*(5), 330–339.

Colwell, J. C. (2004). Stomal and peristomal complications. In J. Colwell, M. Goldberg, & J. Carmel (Eds.), *Fecal and urinary diversions: Management principles*. Philadelphia, PA: Mosby Inc.

Colwell, J. C., & Beitz, J. (2007). Survey of wound, ostomy and continence (WOC) nurse clinicians on stomal and peristomal complications: A content validation study. *Journal of Wound, Ostomy, and Continence Nursing, 34*(1), 57–69.

Colwell, J. C., & Beitz, J. (2014). Stomal and peristomal complications prioritizing management approaches in adults. *Journal of Wound, Ostomy, and Continence Nursing, 41*(5), 445–454.

Colwell, J. C., & Fichera, A. (2005). Care of the obese patient with an ostomy. *Journal of Wound, Ostomy, and Continence Nursing, 32*(6), 378–385.

Colwell, J. C., Goldberg, M., & Carmel, J. (2001). The state of the standard diversion. *Journal of Wound, Ostomy, and Continence Nursing, 28*, 6–17.

Cottam, J. (2005). Audit of stoma complications within three weeks of surgery. *Gastrointestinal Nursing, 3*(1), 19–23.

Cottam, J., Richards, K., Hasted, A., et al. (2007). Results of a nationwide prospective audit of stoma complications within 3 weeks of surgery. *Colorectal Disease, 9*, 834–838.

De Raet, J., Delvaux, G., Haentjens, P., et al. (2008). Waist circumference is an independent risk factor for the development of parastomal hernia after permanent colostomy. *Diseases of the Colon & Rectum, 51*, 1806–1809.

Duchesne, J., Wang, Y., Weintraub, S., et al. (2002). Stoma complications: A multivariate analysis. *American Surgeon, 66*(11), 961.

Fligelstone, L. J., Wanendeya, N., & Palmer, B. V. (1997). Osmotic therapy for acute irreducible stomal prolapse. *British Journal of Surgery, 84*(3), 390. doi: 10.1046/j.1365-2168.1997.02594.x.

Gurtner, G. J., Neligan, P., Newman, M., et al. (2013). Intraoperative laser angiography using the SPY system: Review of the literature and recommendations for use. *Annals of Surgical Innovation and Research, 7*(1), 1–14.

Hampton, B. (1992). Peristomal and stomal complications. In B. Hampton, & R. Bryant (Eds.), *Ostomies and continent diversions: Nursing management.* St. Louis, MO: Mosby Year Book.

Heiying, J., Yonghong, D., Xiaofeng, W., et al. (2014). A study of laparoscopic extraperitoneal sigmoid colostomy after abdomino-perineal resection for rectal cancer. *Gastroenterology Report, 2*(1), 58–62.

Hendren, S., Hammond, K., Glascow, S., et al. (2015). Clinical practice guidelines for ostomy surgery. *Diseases of the Colon & Rectum, 58*, 375–387.

Hoentjen, F., Colwell, J. C., & Hanauer, S. B. (2012) Complications of peristomal recurrence of Crohn's disease: A case report and a review of literature. *Journal of Wound, Ostomy, and Continence Nursing, 39*, 297–301. doi: 10.1097/WOCN.0b013e3182487189.

Israelsson, L. (2008). Parastomal hernias. *Surgical Clinics of North America, 88*, 113–125.

Janes, A., Weisby, L., & Israelsson, L. A. (2011). Parastomal hernia: Clinical and radiological definitions. *Hernia, 15*, 189–192. doi: 10.1007/s10029-010-0769-6.

Jones, H. G., Rees, M., Aboumarzouk, O. M., et al. (2018). Prosthetic mesh placement for the prevention of parastomal herniation. *Cochrane Database of Systematic Reviews, 7*(7), CD008905. doi: 10.1002/14651858.CD008905.pub3.

Kim, J., & Kumar, R. (2006). Reoperation for stoma-related complications. *Clinics in Colon and Rectal Surgery, 19*(4), 207–212.

Köhler, G., Mayer, F., Wundsam, H., et al. (2015). Changes in the surgical management of parastomal hernias over 15 years: Results of 135 cases. *World Journal of Surgery, 39*(11), 2795–2804. http://dx.doi.org/10.1007/s00268-015-3187-1

Kwiatt, M., Kawata, M. (2013). Avoidance and management of stomal complications. *Clinics in Colon and Rectal Surgery, 26*, 112–121.

Leong, A. P., Londono-Schimmer, E. E., & Phillips R. K. (1994). Life-table analysis of stomal complications following ileostomy. *British Journal of Surgery, 81*, 727–729.

Mahjoubi, B., Moghimi, A., Mirzaeli, R., et al. (2005). Evaluation of the end colostomy complications and the risk factors influencing them in Iranian patients. *Colorectal Disease, 7*(6), 582–587.

Nichols, T., Goldstine, J., & Inglese, G. (2019). A multinational evaluation assessing the relationship between peristomal skin health and health utility. *British Journal of Nursing, 28*(5), S14–S19.

Nichols, T., & Inglese, G. (2018). The burden of peristomal skin complications on an ostomy population as assessed by health utility and the physical component summary of the SF-36v2®. *Value in Health, 21*, 89–94.

North, J. (2014). Early intervention, parastomal hernia and quality of life: A research study. *British Journal of Nursing, 23*(5), S11–S14.

Oda, O., Davies, D., Colapinto, K., et al. (2014). Loop versus divided colostomy for the management of anorectal malformations. *Journal of Pediatric Surgery, 49*(1), 87–90.

Parmar, K. L., Zammit, M., Smith, A., et al. (2011). A prospective audit of early stoma complications in colorectal cancer treatment throughout the Greater Manchester and Cheshire colorectal cancer network. *Colorectal Disease, 13*(8), 935–938. doi: 10.1111/j.1463-1318.2010.02325.x.

Park, J., Del Pino, A., Orsay, C., et al. (1999). Stoma complications. *Diseases of the Colon & Rectum, 42*(12), 1575–1580.

Pittman, J. (2011a). Characteristics of the patient with an ostomy. *Journal of Wound, Ostomy, and Continence Nursing, 38*(3), 271–279.

Pittman, J. (2011b). Ostomy complications and associated risk factors: Development and testing of two instruments. (Dissertation PhD). Indiana University Purdue University Indianapolis Library.

Pittman, J., Bakas, T., Ellett, M., et al. (2014). Psychometric evaluation of the Ostomy Complication Severity Index. *Journal of Wound, Ostomy, and Continence Nursing, 41*(2), 1–11.

Pittman, J., Nichols, T., & Rawl, S. (2017). Evaluation of web-based ostomy patient support resources. *Journal of Wound, Ostomy, and Continence Nursing, 44*(6), 550–556.

Pittman, J., Rawl, S. M., Schmidt, C. M., et al. (2008). Demographic and clinical factors related to ostomy complications and quality of life in veterans with an ostomy. *Journal of Wound, Ostomy, and Continence Nursing, 35*(5), 493–503.

Randall, J., Lord, B., Fulham, J., et al. (2012). Parastomal hernias as the predominant stoma complication after laparoscopic colorectal surgery. *Surgical Laparoscopy, Endoscopy & Percutaneous Techniques, 22*(5), 420–423.

Ratliff, C., & Donovan, A. (2001). Frequency of peristomal complications. *Ostomy/Wound Management, 47*(8), 26–29.

Ris, F., Liot, E., Buchs, N. C., et al. (2018). Multicentre phase II trial of near-infrared imaging in elective colorectal surgery. *British Journal of Surgery, 105*(10), 1359–1367. doi: 10.1002/bjs.10844.

Robertson, I., Leung, E., Hughes, D., et al. (2005). Prospective analysis of stoma-related complications. *Colorectal Disease, 7*(3), 279–285.

Salvadalena, G. (2008). Incidence of complications of the stoma and peristomal skin among individuals with colostomy, ileostomy, and urostomy: A systematic review. *Journal of Wound, Ostomy, and Continence Nursing, 35*(6), 596–607.

Salvadalena, G. (2013). The Incidence of stoma and peristomal complications during the first 3 months after ostomy creation. *Journal of Wound, Ostomy, and Continence Nursing, 40*(4), 400–406.

Santi, C., Casali, L., Franzini, C., et al. (2019). Applications of indocyanine green-enhanced fluorescence in laparoscopic colorectal resections. *Updates in Surgery, 71*(1), 83–88.

Shabbir, J. B., & Britton, D. C. (2010). Stoma complications: A literature overview. *Colorectal Disease, 12*(10), 958–964.

Steel, M., & Wu, J. (2002). Late stomal complications. *Clinics in Colon and Rectal Surgery, 15*(3), 199–207.

Szymanski, K., St-Cyr, D., Alam, T., et al. (2010). External stoma and peristomal complications following radical cystectomy and ileal conduit diversion: A systematic review. *Ostomy/Wound Management, 56*(1), 28–35.

Temple, B., Farley, K., Popik, K., et al. (2016). Prevalence of parastomal hernia and factors associated with its development. *Journal of Wound, Ostomy, and Continence Nursing, 43*(5), 489–493.

Weideman, Y., Dunn, D., & Culleiton, A. (2012). *Ostomy management.* Brockton, MA: Western Schools Inc.

WOCN®. (2014). *Stoma complications: Best practice for clinicians.* Mt. Laurel NJ: Author.

WOCN®. (2017). *Clinical guideline: Management of the adult patient with a fecal or urinary ostomy.* Mt Laurel, NJ: Author.

QUESTIONS

1. Which patient with an ostomy would be considered at higher risk for developing ostomy complications?
   A. A patient who has a low body mass index (BMI)
   B. A patient whose age is >40 years
   C. A patient who has a colostomy versus an ileostomy
   D. A patient who has a diverting loop procedure performed

2. Which patient would the nurse recognize as having an *early* stomal complication?
   A. A patient experiencing death of the stoma tissue resulting from impaired blood flow
   B. A patient with impairment of effluent drainage due to narrowing or contracting of the stoma tissue at the skin or fascial level
   C. A patient who presents with telescoping of the intestines through the stoma
   D. A patient who has injury to the stomal mucosa related to physical force or pressure

3. Which assessment by the nurse confirms a diagnosis of stomal retraction?
   A. The stoma height is >10 mm.
   B. The stomal tissue turns from pink to black.
   C. The stoma disappears in line with or below skin level.
   D. There is a gap between the stoma and the skin.

4. A patient is diagnosed with stomal retraction. What is *not* a goal of management for this patient?
   A. Use stomal dilation to temporarily aid in evacuation.
   B. Use a convex pouching system to augment level of stoma above skin.
   C. Surgically create a new stoma in a new location.
   D. Revise the stoma with available intestine to mobilize above skin level.

5. The nurse is managing the care of a patient who has a stomal prolapse and the stoma is edematous. Which intervention is most appropriate for this patient?
   A. Sprinkle sugar over the prolapsed stoma.
   B. Apply warm compresses to the stoma over the pouch for several minutes.

C. Apply the pouching system when the prolapse is maximized.
   D. Reduce the prolapse by applying firm pressure to the stoma.

6. A patient with a new stoma complains to the nurse: "I can't always get the pouching system sealed tightly, and then it leaks!" The nurse notes bulging of the peristomal area. What condition would the ostomy nurse suspect is occurring?
   A. Stomal stenosis
   B. Parastomal hernia
   C. Stomal trauma
   D. Stomal prolapse

7. What is a treatment choice for a patient with parastomal hernia who is asymptomatic?
   A. Loosely fitting garments
   B. Surgical intervention
   C. Convex pouching system
   D. Hernia support belt/garment

8. A patient with a stoma reports pain with stoma evacuation and small, ribbon-like stools. What stomal complication may be present?
   A. Stoma trauma
   B. Stoma prolapse
   C. Stoma stenosis
   D. Parastomal hernia

9. A patient with a new stoma is diagnosed with a large mucocutaneous separation. What condition is likely to occur due to this defect?
   A. Retraction of the stoma
   B. Stomal prolapse
   C. Parastomal hernia
   D. Stomal trauma

10. A patient with a parastomal hernia is scheduled for surgical repair. What type of repair is the preferred method?
   A. Primary fascial repair.
   B. Local repair with prosthetic material such as mesh.
   C. Stomal relocation to the opposite side of the abdomen.
   D. Surgical repair is not an option to correct a parastomal hernia.

ANSWERS AND RATIONALES

1. D. Rationale: Loop ileostomies are created in such a way that the lumen of the stoma may not be pointing the effluent into the pouch and could cause peristomal skin.

2. A. Rationale: Stoma necrosis is the death of stoma tissue occurring from impaired blood flow which develops soon after the stoma is created, caused by tension on or inadequacy of the mesenteric vasculature to the intestinal. It can also be caused by trauma to the stomal tissue during creation.

3. C. Rationale: Stoma retraction is defined as disappearance of stoma tissue protrusion in line with or below skin level.

4. A. Rationale: If the stoma is retracted (disappearing below or at the skin level), dilation (making the stoma larger) is not a management intervention as this does not address the problem.

5. A. Rationale: The sugar provides osmotic therapy or causes a fluid shift across the stoma mucosa and may reduce the edema.

6. B. Rationale: A hernia is defined as a defect in abdominal fascia that allows the intestine to bulge into the parastomal area and cause a bulge.

7. D. Rationale: Conservative treatment in an asymptomatic patient is the choice of therapy and the use of a hernia support belt/garment is a noninvasive appropriate treatment.

8. C. Rationale: Stomal stenosis is the impairment of effluent drainage due to narrowing or contracting of the stomal tissue at the skin or fascial level. When the stoma lumen is narrowed, the stool will become ribbon thin to pass through the narrowed intestine segment.

9. A. Rationale: A mucocutaneous separation is a detachment of the stomal tissue from the surrounding peristomal skin leaving a defect. Because the stoma is not attached to the skin at the area of the mucocutaneous separation, it is possible that as healing takes place the stoma may heal below the skin resulting in stoma retraction.

10. C. Rationale: Stomal relocation is for many patients the preference since a new opening can be made in an intact abdominal muscle, and this location should be less likely to develop a peristomal hernia than in a muscle that has previously had a peristomal hernia.

CHAPTER 18

FISTULA MANAGEMENT

Denise Nix and Ruth A. Bryant

OBJECTIVES

1. Describe causative and contributing factors to fistula development.
2. Describe management of the patient with an enterocutaneous fistula.
3. Describe management of the patient with an enteroatmospheric fistula.
4. Outline criteria and guidelines for promotion of spontaneous fistula closure.
5. Explain the significance of pseudostoma formation in the patient with a fistula.
6. Discuss indications for surgical closure of a fistula.
7. Develop and implement individualized management plan for the fistula patient that provides for containment of drainage and odor while protecting perifistular skin.

TOPIC OUTLINE

Introduction **284**

Clinical Presentation and Classification **284**

Etiologic Factors **284**

Medical Management **285**
Definition of the Fistula Tract 286
Control of Infection 286
Maintenance of Fluid and Electrolyte Balance 286
Nutritional Support 287
Measures to Minimize Fistula Output 287
Skin Protection and Containment 288

Fistula Management for the WOC Nurse **288**
Assessment 288
Progress Toward and Impediments to Spontaneous Closure 288

Abdominal Contours and Fistula Opening 289
Effluent Characteristics 290
Interventions and Containment Strategies 290
Skin Protectants and Barriers 290
Pectin-Based Barrier Products 292
Absorptive Dressings and Moisture Barriers 292
Closed Suction 292
Negative Pressure Wound Therapy 293
Pouching Systems 294
Pouching System Adaptations 296
Education and Emotional Support 298

Surgical Closure **298**

Vesicovaginal, Rectovaginal, or Enterovaginal Fistulas **299**

Conclusions **299**

INTRODUCTION

A *fistula (plural fistulas or fistulae)* is an abnormal passage between two or more epithelialized surfaces that results in communication between one body cavity or hollow organ and another hollow organ or the skin (Bryant & Best, 2015). An *enterocutaneous fistula (ECF)* is an abnormal connection between the gastrointestinal (GI) tract and the skin. An *enteroatmospheric fistula (EAF)* is an abnormal connection between the GI tract and the atmosphere (e.g., a fistula that develops in an open surgical wound; Nurses Specialized in Wound, Ostomy and Continence Canada [NSWOCC] [formerly CAET], 2018). ECF and EAF are difficult complications that most often arise after abdominal surgical procedures. Although fistulas *can* be located *within* a wound, they should not be confused with a draining wound, surgically placed drain site, or wound dehiscence.

The mortality rates for patients with a fistula range from 5.5% to 30% (Parli et al., 2018; Quinn et al., 2017; Willcutts et al., 2015). Death is most often due to not only sepsis but also malnutrition, fluid and electrolyte imbalance, and multiorgan failure (Juárez-Oropeza & Román-Ramos, 2012; Wercka et al., 2016). Cost impact is significant. Teixeira and colleagues (2019) compared outcome data of patients with and without an ECF among level 1 trauma center patients who required acute trauma laparotomies. During the 9-year period, 36 of 2,373 (1.5%) patients undergoing a laparotomy developed an ECF. After matching age, gender, and severity scores of patients with ECF to patients without ECF, results showed a statistically significant increase in ICU length of stay and hospital length of stay in patients with ECFs ($p < 0.001$). Hospital charges for patients with an ECF averaged $539,309 as compared to $126,996 in similar patients without an ECF.

An interprofessional approach is needed to meet the needs of the patient with a fistula. Essential team members often include the wound, ostomy, and continence (WOC) nurse, dietitian, pharmacist, clinical nurse, social worker, surgeon, provider, radiologist, physiotherapist, occupational therapist, spiritual advisor, radiation therapist, and interventional radiologist (Heimroth et al., 2018; NSWOCC, 2018; Rahman & Stavas, 2015). Management for this patient population requires a clear understanding of the underlying pathophysiology, astute assessment skills, knowledge about management alternatives and options, competent technical skills, diligent follow-up, and persistence (Bryant & Best, 2015).

CLINICAL PRESENTATION AND CLASSIFICATION

Clinical indications for potential ECF or EAF formation include postoperative abdominal pain, tenderness, distention, prolonged ileus, disruption in intestinal peristalsis, and wound infection. The definitive indicator of an ECF or EAF is the passage of GI secretions into an open wound bed or through an unintentional opening onto the skin. Associated complications in patients with a fistula include fever, tachycardia, increased respiratory rate, fluid and electrolyte imbalance, perifistular skin breakdown, malnutrition, and sepsis (NSWOCC, 2018; Whelan & Ivatury, 2011).

Manifestations of a fistula tract terminating in the vagina include passage of urine (vesicovaginal fistula) or passage of gas, feces, and/or purulent and extremely malodorous drainage (rectovaginal or enterovaginal fistula). Irradiation-induced rectovaginal fistulas often are preceded by diarrhea, passage of mucus and blood rectally, a sensation of rectal pressure, and a constant urge to defecate (Zelga et al., 2017). Fistulas between the intestinal tract and the urinary bladder (e.g., colovesical fistula) present with passage of gas or stool-stained urine through the urethra. Diagnostic tests to confirm the presence of a fistula include computed tomography (CT) scan, contrast radiography of the GI tract, fistulogram, ultrasonography, and plain radiography (NSWOCC, 2018; Whelan & Ivatury, 2011).

KEY POINT

The definitive indicator of an ECF or EAF is the passage of GI secretions into an open wound bed or through an unintentional opening onto the skin.

Most clinicians describe and classify fistulas according to location, involved structures, and volume of effluent. Although less frequently used, fistulas may also be classified by complexity (see **Table 18-1**). Mucous fistulas are intentionally created surgical openings in which a defunctionalized section of bowel is secured to the abdomen. These produce mucus only and are managed with dressings or pouches; the mucous fistula does not increase morbidity or mortality (Bryant & Best, 2015). The mucous fistula is not further discussed in this chapter (see Chapter 9).

KEY POINT

Fistulas are typically "named" for the organ of origin and the organ of termination; for example, an ECF is one from the bowel to the skin, and a colovesical fistula is one from the colon to the bladder.

ETIOLOGIC FACTORS

Approximately 25% of fistulas develop spontaneously and are associated with an intrinsic intestinal disease such as inflammatory bowel disease (most common), cancer, radiation enteritis, ischemic bowel, diverticulitis, appendicitis, perforated duodenal ulcers, or external trauma (Haack

TABLE 18-1   FISTULA CLASSIFICATION

	DESIGNATION	CHARACTERISTICS
Location	Internal	Tract contained within body
	External	Tract exits through skin
Involved structures (not inclusive)	Colon to vagina	Colovaginal
	Intestine to skin	Enterocutaneous
	Bladder to vagina	Vesicovaginal
	Colon to skin	Colocutaneous
	Rectum to vagina	Rectovaginal
Volume	High output	>500 mL/24 h
	Moderate output	200–500 mL/24 h
	Low output	<200 mL/24 h
Complexity	Simple	Short direct tract, no abscess, no other organ involvement
	Complex	Type 1—abscess, multiple organ involvement
Type 2—opens into the base of a wound

Modified from Bryant, R., & Best, M. (2015). Management of draining wounds and fistulas. In R. Bryant & D. Nix (Eds.), *Acute and chronic wounds: Current management concepts* (5th ed.). St. Louis, MO: Mosby.

et al., 2014). Spontaneous fistulas are generally resistant to spontaneous closure. Patients treated for a pelvic cancer are particularly vulnerable to ECFs due to radiation damage; the fistula may develop immediately following radiation or years later (Heimroth et al., 2018; Tran & Thorson, 2008). Irradiation-induced ECFs are more likely to occur in patients who receive higher radiation doses (>5,000 cGy), smoke cigarettes, or have atherosclerosis, hypertension, diabetes mellitus, advanced age, pelvic inflammatory disease, or previous pelvic surgery (Hollington et al., 2004; Tran & Thorson, 2008).

KEY POINT

Most ECF and EAFs occur postoperatively as a result of anastomotic breakdown; however, fistulas may also develop spontaneously as a result of inflammatory bowel disease (e.g., diverticulitis, Crohn's disease, radiation enteritis) or trauma.

The majority of ECF and EAFs (75% to 85%) are iatrogenic (inadvertently induced from a medical procedure); these fistulas develop postoperatively due to anastomotic breakdown (Gribovskaja-Rupp & Melton, 2016; Heimroth et al., 2018; Nussbaum & Fischer, 2006). With respect to postoperative small bowel fistulae, about half are from an anastomotic leak, with the other half occurring from inadvertent injury to the small bowel during dissection (Gribovskaja-Rupp & Melton, 2016). Surgery-related risk factors include poor nutrition, inadequate blood supply, poor suture

technique, inadequate bowel prep (e.g., emergency surgery), extensive lysis of adhesions, and trauma surgery (Kassis & Makary, 2008; Nussbaum & Fischer, 2006; Telem et al., 2010; Wong et al., 2004).

Systemic reviews continue to indicate that the method of anastomosis (stapled or hand-sewn) is not a predictor of ECF following surgery for trauma (Neutzling et al., 2017).

Patients scheduled for elective surgical procedures should have risk factors addressed to minimize the risk of anastomotic breakdown. When emergency surgery is necessary, prevention strategies include adequate intravenous fluids, circulatory support, keeping the patient warm, and broad-spectrum antibiotics (Causey et al., 2012; Kassis & Makary, 2008). Historically, a diverting temporary stoma was commonly performed following bowel resection and anastomosis in trauma patients. However, studies indicate that diversion following colonic anastomosis for penetrating colonic injury did not reduce the incidence of septic complications, including abscess and fistula, and this practice is no longer standard of care (Causey et al., 2012; Chamieh et al., 2018).

MEDICAL MANAGEMENT

Spontaneous closure of a fistula is defined as closing with medical management within 6 to 8 weeks (Teixeira et al., 2009). Spontaneous closure rates in the era of advanced wound care and parenteral nutrition vary considerably with most studies demonstrating closure rates in the 20% to 40% range when sepsis is controlled and appropriate nutritional support is provided (Gribovskaja-Rupp & Melton, 2016; Kassis & Makary, 2008; Nussbaum & Fischer, 2006). According to Wong et al. (2004), 90% of simple fistulas close spontaneously, whereas <10% of complex fistulas close spontaneously.

Historically, 90% of spontaneous closure has been reported to occur in the first month after sepsis resolution, with an additional 10% closing in the 2nd month. More recently, case studies report fistulae closure in the 2nd and 3rd month with use of negative pressure wound therapy (NPWT) to promote wound healing (Gribovskaja-Rupp & Melton, 2016). The use of NPWT in fistula management will be discussed later in this chapter.

Favorable conditions for spontaneous closure (Gribovskaja-Rupp & Melton, 2016) include the following:

- Transferrin >200 mg/dL
- No obstruction, bowel in continuity
- No inflamed intestine, infection, or sepsis
- Balanced electrolytes
- Timely referral to tertiary care center and subspecialty care
- Output <200 mL/24 h

Reducing fistula output has been shown to positively impact fluid and electrolyte balance; similarly, nutritional needs are more easily met as fistula output decreases (Polk & Schwab, 2012). However, there is no statistical evidence to support the concept of an inverse relationship between spontaneous closure and fistula output (Davis & Johnson, 2013; NSWOCC, 2018).

KEY POINT

Reducing fistula output has been shown to positively impact fluid and electrolyte balance and allow for nutrition needs to be more easily met. However, an association between increased rate of spontaneous fistula closure and decreased fistula output and has not been proven.

Objectives of fistula management are described below and include (1) definition of the fistula tract, (2) maintenance of fluid and electrolyte balance, (3) nutritional support, (4) measures to minimize fistula output, (5) control of infection, and (6) skin protection and containment of effluent (Bryant & Best, 2015). The literature sometimes refers to a protocol called "SNAP," which stands for management of *s*kin and *s*epsis, *n*utrition, definition of fistula *a*natomy, and *p*roposing a procedure to address the fistula (Kaushal & Carlson, 2004; Samad et al., 2015). An interdisciplinary team implements the SNAP protocol by early identification and treatment of the sepsis, oral and parenteral nutrition, identification of the type of fistula, and optimal management.

DEFINITION OF THE FISTULA TRACT

Once the patient is stabilized, definition of the fistula tract should be undertaken. The fistula should be assessed for point of origin, condition of adjacent bowel, presence of abscess, and any distal obstruction or bowel discontinuity. This can be accomplished with a range of radiological examinations: fistulagram, ultrasonography, and plain radiography, magnetic resonance imaging (MRI), positive emission tomography (PET) scan, or computerized tomography (Arebi & Forbes, 2004; NSWOCC, 2018; Schecter et al., 2009; Whelan & Ivatury, 2011). During diagnostic workup, it is important that the patient receive nothing by mouth for the first couple of days in order to accurately quantify the fistula output and complete diagnostic testing to determine the origin of the fistula (Kumpf et al., 2017; Willcutts, 2015).

CONTROL OF INFECTION

Uncontrolled sepsis and sepsis-associated malnutrition have been shown to be important determinants of mortality in the patient with a fistula (Dubose & Lundy, 2010; Lynch et al., 2004; NSWOCC, 2018). Patients with an intra-abdominal abscess may present with abdominal pain, fever, anorexia, tachycardia, or prolonged ileus. A palpable mass may or may not be present. Abdominal abscess may be difficult to detect in postoperative

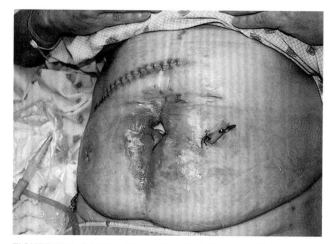

FIGURE 18-1. ECF (Small Bowel to Skin); Extensive Skin Damage Due to Enzymatic Drainage; Drain in Place for Abscess Management. (Reproduced with permission from Davis, M., Dere, K., & Hadley, G. (2000). Options for managing an open wound with draining enterocutaneous fistula. *Journal of Wound, Ostomy & Continence Nursing, 27*(2), 118–123.)

patients as analgesia and antibiotics may mask signs of infection (Mehta & Copelin, 2019).

Blood work is not specific for an intra-abdominal abscess but may reveal signs of infection such as leukocytosis, abnormal liver function, anemia, or thrombocytopenia. CT scan remains the most definitive test to rule out an intra-abdominal abscess. A CT scan can reveal the location, size, and presence of bowel thickening, thumb printing, and ileus. Intra-abdominal abscess almost always requires intravenous (IV) antibiotics. If the abscess is localized, CT-guided aspiration can be performed to drain the abscess (Li et al., 2018). This can obviate the need for early operative intervention. As seen in **Figure 18-1**, if a fistula develops, a definitive procedure can be deferred with the drain left in place to control further abscess formation (Davis et al., 2000; Lynch et al., 2004). Abscess contents should be cultured following percutaneous or surgical drainage, to assure appropriate antibiotic therapy (Wong et al., 2004).

MAINTENANCE OF FLUID AND ELECTROLYTE BALANCE

Fluid and electrolyte imbalance increases mortality and morbidity in patients with ECF/EAF (NSWOCC, 2018). Each day, 8 to 10 L of fluid flows through the jejunum, depending on oral intake. In the intact functioning intestine, 98% of this fluid is (re) absorbed, leaving only 100 to 200 mL of fluid to be excreted in the stool. Development of a fistula permits abnormal fluid losses, with volume of loss determined in part by size of the fistulous opening and in part by anatomic location within the bowel. For example, fistulas located in the proximal small bowel are generally high output, while fistulas occurring in the colon are typically low output.

When providing fluid replacement, the provider must consider both the volume and the composition of the fistulous drainage, both of which are impacted by fistula location within the GI tract. Severe metabolic disturbances have been noted with fistula output >200 mL/day due to loss of hydrogen, chloride, sodium, and potassium ions (Arebi & Forbes, 2004; Makhdoom et al., 2000). Careful monitoring of tissue perfusion, weight, urine, and fistula output is necessary to evaluate fluid balance. Adequate fluid and electrolyte replacement is critical to prevent hypovolemia and circulatory failure in the patient with a high-output fistula (Makhdoom et al., 2000). As previously mentioned, while fluids need to be replaced during diagnostic workup, oral ingestion should be curtailed until tests are completed so that quantification of fistula output is as accurate as possible (Kumpf et al., 2017; Willcutts, 2015).

NUTRITIONAL SUPPORT

Once fluid levels and electrolyte balance have been stabilized and sepsis is managed, nutritional support is required. The goals of nutrition management are to provide adequate nutrition, maintain fluid levels and electrolyte balance, and support spontaneous closure of the ECF whenever possible (Kumpf et al., 2017). The route of nutritional support depends on the patient's ability to ingest sufficient quantities, the location of the fistula tract, the absorptive capacity of the bowel mucosa, and the patient's tolerance.

In the past, the use of total parenteral nutrition (TPN), accompanied by simultaneous "bowel rest," revolutionized the care of the patient with a fistula (Dubose & Lundy, 2010). However, TPN is associated with an appreciable rate of bacteremia and line sepsis. In one study conducted by Wong and colleagues (2004), positive blood cultures were obtained from 24.6% of 88 catheters utilized to deliver TPN to patients undergoing nonoperative management of enteric fistulas. Additionally, there is insufficient evidence to demonstrate that parenteral nutrition is associated with improved spontaneous closure rates (David & Johnson, 2013; NSWOCC, 2018).

Today, there has been a return to enteral nutrition (utilizing the GI tract for direct nutritional support) for prevention and management of fistulas. Enteral intake maintains the health and integrity of the intestinal mucosa, prevents translocation of bacteria, and maintains the normal structural, immunologic, and hormonal integrity of the GI tract. In addition, enteral nutrition can be provided at a lower cost as compared to TPN (Dubose & Lundy, 2010). During a small retrospective study, Collier and colleagues (2007) noted that early postoperative initiation of enteral nutrition (≤4 days) resulted in a lower fistula formation rate than did nutritional approaches involving later initiation of enteral feedings (9% vs. 26%, respectively). Researchers also noted that the use of early enteral nutrition resulted

in earlier primary abdominal closure and lower hospital charges (Collier et al., 2007; Dubose & Lundy, 2010).

Four feet of healthy small intestine (in the adult) are needed to meet nutritional needs via the enteral route (Knechtges & Zimmermann, 2009). Therefore, enteral nutrition may be feasible for the patient whose fistula is located in the most proximal or distal portion of a functional GI tract. When the fistula is located in the most proximal segment of the bowel, the enteral feeding must be administered distal to the fistula. Many types of enteral solutions are available, and a dietician should be consulted to recommend the most appropriate solution and administration procedure so that GI intolerance (e.g., diarrhea, abdominal distention) can be avoided.

Fistuloclysis refers to the infusion of enteral nutrition via the distal stoma of an ECF or EAF with or without reinfusion of the output. The distal opening of the fistula is used for access for a catheter or tube, and enteral nutrition or fistula output is infused (Kumpf et al., 2017). Effective fistuloclysis requires effective pouching and catheter stabilization (Polk & Schwab, 2012). Refeeding enteroclysis is the reinfusion of fistula output (also known as chyme). Refeeding enteroclysis is usually performed in conjunction with enteral nutrition. In select patients with a proximal enteric fistula, however, water, electrolyte, and nutritional requirements can be met by simple refeeding without supplementary enteral nutrition. This technique has not gained widespread popularity (Coetzee et al., 2014).

Depending on the location of the fistula tract, the absorptive capacity of the bowel mucosa, and the patient's tolerance, parenteral nutrition remains an important option for prevention and management of fistulas. Many patients continue to be successfully treated exclusively through bowel rest and parenteral nutrition. In most cases, however, it is an important bridge to, or supplement for, enteral feeds (Polk & Schwab, 2012). A dietician is vital to the prevention and treatment of fistulas and may also recommend vitamins and trace minerals often deficient in malnourished patients with ECF/EAF (NSWOCC, 2018).

MEASURES TO MINIMIZE FISTULA OUTPUT

Reducing fistula output has been shown to reduce the loss of fluids, electrolytes, and nutrients and protect the perifistula skin (NSWOCC, 2018). This may be done with medications or by limiting oral and/or enteral intake to the amount needed to keep the intestinal mucosa healthy. Significantly reduced oral/enteral intake minimizes fistula output by decreasing luminal contents, GI stimulation, and pancreaticobiliary secretion. Medications used to decrease fistula output include antidiarrheals, antimotility agents, and proton pump inhibitors (Bailey & Glasgow, 2016; de Vries et al., 2017; Haack et al., 2014; Polk & Schwab, 2012; Williams et al., 2010). Consultation with a pharmacist is beneficial to understand their risk and benefits of these medications.

The relationship between medications and closure of nonmatured fistulas is not known. However, three separate meta-analyses reported the effectiveness of somatostatin and its analog, octreotide, in reducing closing time and increasing the number of fistulas closed without surgery (Coughlin et al., 2012; Rahbour et al., 2012; Stevens et al., 2011). Mortality, however, was not reduced. Finally, the odds of spontaneous closure and time till closure were improved in patients who received continuous infusion of somatostatin. Somatostatin is administered through continuous intravenous infusion due to its short half-life of 1 to 2 minutes. Octreotide's half-life is almost 2 hours, and it is administered three times daily subcutaneously (Makhdoom et al., 2000). Octreotide is not recommended for routine use due to reports of precipitated villous atrophy, interruption of intestinal adaptation, and acute cholecystitis. Some authors recommend a 5- to 8-day trial, with discontinuation of the octreotide if there is no significant reduction in fistula output within that time frame (Draus et al., 2006).

SKIN PROTECTION AND CONTAINMENT

Establishing and maintaining skin protection and containment of the fistula effluent can be a challenging and yet rewarding experience. When managing a patient with a fistula, it is beneficial to be guided by four general principles presented by Rolstad & Wong (2004).

1. Assess the pouching system and seal frequently; expect to make changes in the management system.
2. Build flexibility into the care plan.
3. Innovate, using the easiest, most practical approach first.
4. Recognize that inexperienced caregivers frequently provide care of the patient.

Skin protection and effluent containment should be initiated as soon as the fistula develops and is not contingent upon medical diagnosis. Goals for topical management of a fistula are listed in **Box 18-1** (Bryant & Best, 2015). Methods and techniques for skin protection and containment will be described in the Interventions and Containment Strategies section of the chapter.

BOX 18-1   GOALS FOR TOPICAL MANAGEMENT OF THE ECF

- Perifistular skin protection
- Containment of effluent
- Odor control
- Patient comfort
- Accurate measurement of effluent
- Patient mobility
- Ease of care
- Cost containment

KEY POINT

Skin protection and effluent containment should be initiated as soon as the fistula develops and is not contingent upon medical diagnosis or the medical plan of care.

FISTULA MANAGEMENT FOR THE WOC NURSE

Methods and strategies for fistula management are guided by a thorough assessment; the parameters first described by Irrgang and Bryant (1984) remain the standard for fistula assessment today (Bryant & Best, 2015).

ASSESSMENT

In addition to determining the type of fistula, assessment must include abdominal contours, fistula opening, effluent characteristics, and the condition of the perifistular skin. Each dressing or pouch change represents an opportunity to reevaluate the fistula and to modify the care plan accordingly. All assessments, reassessments, interventions, responses to interventions, and management and follow-up plans should be documented (see **Box 18-2**).

Progress Toward and Impediments to Spontaneous Closure

A critical aspect of assessment is evaluation of progress toward and impediments to spontaneous closure (see **Box 18-3**). Progress in closure is evidenced by reduced output through the fistula tract along with increased fecal output through the distal bowel (rectum or stoma); thus, fistula output should be monitored, as should the output from any stoma, and the patient with an intact distal bowel should be routinely queried regarding bowel movements. Any indicators of abscess formation (e.g., increasing abdominal tenderness, fever, or purulent drainage mixed with the fecal output) must be promptly reported so that intervention can be initiated. The nurse must also be alert to development of a stomatized fistula, also known as a pseudostoma or an epithelialized stoma; this occurs when the anterior wall of the bowel becomes adherent to the abdominal wall and the fistula tract undergoes mucosal eversion. The end result is a permanent opening into the bowel that must be closed surgically; thus, the surgeon or provider should be made aware when a "stoma" is observed in the wound bed (see **Fig. 18-2**).

KEY POINT

Assessment of the individual with a fistula must include the volume and characteristics of the output, the contours of the abdominal wall and fistula opening, and indicators of progress toward or impediments to spontaneous closure.

BOX 18-2 DOCUMENTATION FOR THE WOC NURSE

Focused Assessment
- Fistula source (see **Table 18-1**)
- Pain
- Fistula opening
  - Location
  - Length and width
  - Height (retracted, skin level, protruding)
- Perifistular skin integrity
  - Intact
  - Impaired (erythema, maceration, candidiasis, denudement)
- Abdominal contours and proximity of fistula to scars, skin folds, bony prominences, drains, or ostomies
- Output/effluent
  - Volume
  - Consistency
  - Color
  - Odor
- Containment system and frequency of changes

Interventions
- Emotional support
- Changes in containment method/procedure with rationale (if any change required)
- Education of patient/family
  - Normal versus impaired skin
  - Signs of infection
  - Containment procedure

Evaluation
- Indicators of progress in closure (or impediments, such as pseudostoma formation)
- Effectiveness of containment system
  - Wear time without leakage
  - Perifistular skin intact or improved
  - Odor control
  - Effects on patient mobility
  - Ease of care
- Patient/family response to interventions
  - Patient satisfaction
  - Comfort
  - Level of activity
  - Learning

Follow-up Plan
- Approximate day of next visit
- Instruction for staff between visits (including what to do if questions/concerns arise)

BOX 18-3 FACTORS THAT PREVENT SPONTANEOUS CLOSURE

- Compromised distal suture line/anastomosis (i.e., tension on suture line, improper suturing technique, inadequate blood supply to anastomosis)
- Distal obstruction
- Foreign body in fistula tract or suture line
- Epithelium-lined tract contiguous with skin (pseudostoma)
- Presence of tumor or disease in site
- Previous irradiation to site
- Crohn's disease
- Abscess
- Hematoma

Adapted from Bryant, R., & Best, M. (2015). Management of draining wounds and fistulas. In R. Bryant & D. Nix (Eds.), *Acute and chronic wounds: Current management concepts* (5th ed.). St. Louis, MO: Mosby. (In Print.)

Skin contours should be noted, and the abdomen should be inspected for irregular skin surfaces that are created by scars, creases, bony prominences, or other obstacles such as sutures/staples, incisions (dehisced or intact), or stomas. The location of the fistula should be identified, and visible openings should be measured (length and width in cm) and documented. The level at which the fistula empties in relation to the skin (or wound) surface is of critical importance. The fistula opening may be retracted (lower than skin level), level with the skin, above the level of the skin, or in a deep wound (see **Fig. 18-2**). If the fistula empties directly onto the skin and is level with the skin, a convex pouching system is usually required; in contrast, a fistula that has undergone mucosal maturation (pseudostoma formation) and that protrudes above the level of the skin may enable a better pouch seal. The opening might also contain a drain, as seen in **Figure 18-1**, for drainage of an abscess.

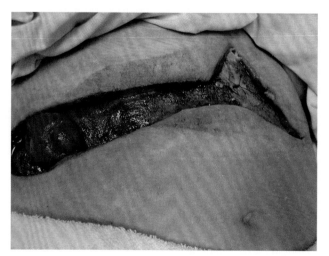

FIGURE 18-2. Pseudostoma in Deep Wound.

Abdominal Contours and Fistula Opening

The fistula opening and abdominal contours should be assessed while the patient is standing, sitting, and lying down if possible. If the pannus is large, more positions may be necessary to observe the changes in perifistular contours that occur with shifts in position of the pannus.

Assessment of all these parameters will help determine the level of skin protection required, as well as the flexibility, size, and shape of adhesive barrier needed for effective protection of the perifistular skin and avoidance of any areas that could compromise the adhesion of the pouching system or cause discomfort to the patient.

Effluent Characteristics

Assessment of fistula effluent (source, volume, odor, consistency, composition) influences topical management selection by providing insight into the degree of risk for perifistular skin breakdown and odor as well as the type of pouch closure needed. For example, an odorous fistula producing effluent with semiformed consistency is most likely originating from the left transverse or descending colon. Effluent from the transverse or descending colon will be less damaging to the skin than is output from the small intestine or stomach. (See **Fig. 18-1** for illustration of skin damage related to small bowel drainage.) Thus, the primary goals of topical management for that patient would be containment of effluent and odor control.

Fistula output volumes >100 mL over 24 hours usually require a pouch or suction or both. In contrast, the fistula with minimal output can often be managed with the application of a perifistular moisture barrier and an absorptive dressing. However, in the presence of odor, even the patient with a low-output fistula may prefer a containment pouch for odor control. It should be noted that odor may originate from numerous sources, including fecal drainage, exudate, necrotic or infected tissue, soiled dressings, and/or chemicals used during treatment.

Consistency of effluent is particularly important to selection of a pouching system because it influences the type of skin barriers needed as well as the type of drainage outlet required to efficiently empty the pouch. For example, liquid effluent is much more corrosive than is thick effluent and is much more likely to result in premature erosion of the skin barrier; thus, liquid effluent requires the most durable skin barrier/protectant. Liquid

effluent is easier to empty from a spout rather than clamp-type closure.

Constant exposure of the epidermis to moisture, enzymes, extremes in pH, and mechanical trauma frequently leads to perifistular skin damage. Denudation of perifistular skin is a common complication in fistula patients and often is present when the patient is first seen with the fistula. Perifistular skin is also at risk for fungal infection as a consequence of moisture entrapment against the skin and antibiotic precipitated changes in the normal skin flora. Candidiasis is a common secondary perifistular skin complication and requires treatment with a topical antifungal agent. See Chapter 16 to learn more about moisture-associated skin damage (MASD).

In addition to visual inspection, valuable information can be obtained from the patient and nursing staff. For example, patient reports of burning or stinging sensations around the fistula commonly indicate denudation or erosion of the epidermis, and the patient who requires frequent dressing or pouch changes is at risk for skin damage from mechanical injury in addition to damage from exposure to the effluent.

INTERVENTIONS AND CONTAINMENT STRATEGIES

Fistulas can be managed with skin protection and either dressings or containment devices (pouches, suction, negative pressure). There are a wide number of products available, and the appropriate selection is based on patient assessment. Principles of management warrant repetition: begin with the easiest approach based on assessment and sound rationale, reassess frequently and be flexible, and expect that needs will change. Interventions should be based on established principles and rationale, should include measures for skin protection and containment as well as patient and family support and education, and should be thoroughly documented (see **Box 18-2**). **Tables 18-2** and **18-3** present factors to consider when selecting containment methods.

Skin Protectants and Barriers

Skin protectant products are available in many types and forms (**Table 18-2**). Major types include moisture barrier skin protectant creams, ointments, or pastes; solid pectin-based adhesive wafers, rings, or strips; hydrocolloid or karaya-formulated rings; barrier (ostomy) paste formulated with or without alcohol; barrier powder; and liquid

TABLE 18-2 FISTULA PRODUCTS AND THEIR INDICATIONS

PRODUCT/ACCESSORY	ACTION	INDICATIONS
Liquid skin barrier wipes, wands, or sprays	Provides a protective film to skin	**Low-output fistulae**—provides protective layer to skin. Used in combination with dressings **High-output fistulae**—used in combination with pouches, suction systems, and NPWT to protect against adhesive trauma
Moisture barrier creams, ointments, or pastes	Repels moisture and protects skin	**Low-output fistulae**—provides protection to skin around fistula. May be used in combination with dressings **High-output fistulae**—not indicated. Does not provide enough protection with high-output effluent. Contraindicated with the use of any adhesive products (i.e., pouches), as creams will not allow products to adhere to skin
Skin barrier rings, strips, and pastes	Provides physical barrier to effluent/stool	**Low-output fistulae**—provides skin protection against effluent **High-output fistulae**—used to fill in uneven surfaces for pouching or as a part of the pouching system
Pouches	Contain effluent/stool and odor from fistula	**Low-output fistulae**—where odor is a problem or the patient prefers to change pouch as opposed to dressings **High-output fistulae**—used to contain stool and odor
Suction systems	Contain effluent in combination with low intermittent suction and dressings or pouches	**Low-output fistulae**—not indicated **High-output fistulae**—where pouching systems to gravity drainage are not effective due to large amounts of liquid effluent. Not a long-term solution
NPWT	Direct pressure closure	**Low-output fistulae**—not indicated **High-output fistulae**—where closure is a possibility. No abscess can be present. The patient must receive bowel rest and nutritional support, e.g., TPN. There should be no evidence of epithelial cells on opening of fistula (no evidence of pseudostoma formation)
Dressings	Absorb drainage	**Low-output fistulae**—used in combination with other skin protectants such as liquid skin barrier wipes, barrier creams and pastes, and skin barrier wafers **High-output fistulae**—not indicated

NPO, nothing by mouth; NPWT, negative pressure wound therapy; TPN, total parenteral nutrition.

barrier film products (previously known as skin sealant), which are available as wipes, wands, and sprays with or without alcohol. As previously stated, product selection must always be based on assessment and a clear under-standing of the patient's needs and the properties and indications for use of the various products. For example, moisture barrier products are appropriate only for low-output fistulas managed with dressings. Pectin-based barrier

TABLE 18-3 FISTULA CONTAINMENT OPTIONS BASED ON OUTPUT AND NEED FOR ACCESS

OUTPUT VOLUME	<100 mL	<100 mL	>100 mL OR DRESSING CHANGE > EVERY 4 h	>100 mL OR DRESSING CHANGE > EVERY 4 h
Need for odor control	No	Yes	Yes or no	Yes or no
Need for frequent access	Yes/no	Yes/no	Yes	No
Containment options	Absorptive dressings and perifistular skin protectant (e.g., ointment, paste barrier)	Charcoal cover dressing (placed over absorptive dressings) with environmental deodorants and frequent dressing changes OR Ostomy pouch	Wound management system with window, emptied frequently or attached to a dependent bedside drainage collector OR Two-piece ostomy pouch emptied frequently Two-piece urostomy pouch emptied frequently or attached to a dependent bedside drainage collector (urinary or fecal spout)	Pouching systems OR Closed systems with suction or attached to straight drainage NPWT

wafers, rings, strips, and paste are widely used to protect the skin and improve adhesion of pouching systems and NPWT systems. Barrier powder is used to treat denuded skin. Liquid barrier film products are primarily used to protect the skin against adhesive trauma. **Table 18-2** provides indications and contraindications for use of each type of barrier product.

KEY POINT

Moisture barrier products are used to protect the skin against moisture and drainage but are appropriate only for low-output fistulas managed with absorptive products; barrier films are used primarily to protect against adhesive trauma; and pectin-based pouches, rings, and pastes are used to promote an effective pouching system and to protect the skin against enzymatic drainage.

Pectin-Based Barrier Products

Most containment pouches have an integrated solid skin barrier attached to the pouch by the manufacturer. Barrier pastes, strips, or rings are frequently needed accessory products that are used to fill skin defects and create a flat pouching surface, add convexity, or provide caulking to ensure an effective pouch seal. If the skin is denuded and moist, a barrier powder may be lightly applied (sprinkled on the skin, gently rubbed in, and the excess brushed off) (as shown in **Fig. 18-3**) to absorb moisture and improve adhesion of the barrier and pouch to the damaged skin. It is important to realize that application of excessive amounts of powder will impair adhesion. When the skin is extremely denuded, application of the powder can be followed by application of an alcohol-free liquid barrier film; these steps can be repeated up to three times to create a dry surface or crust. This technique is known as "crusting." When applied and removed

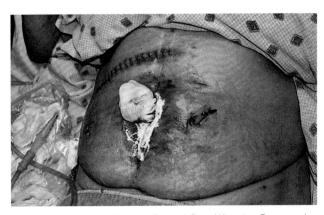

FIGURE 18-3. Pectin Powder Dusted Onto Weeping Damaged Skin; Excess Powder Removed to Avoid Compromised Adhesion of Pouch. (Reproduced with permission from Davis, M., Dere, K., & Hadley, G. (2000). Options for managing an open wound with draining enterocutaneous fistula. *Journal of Wound, Ostomy & Continence Nursing, 27*(2), 118–123.)

appropriately, most of these pectin barrier products are safe to use on damaged skin. It should be noted that liquid barrier films must be allowed to dry so solvents can escape before other products are applied. Some barrier films and barrier pastes contain alcohol and can cause great discomfort when used on damaged skin. Clear protocols and ongoing staff education are essential to assure that alcohol-free products are the "standard of care" for damaged skin. Great care must be taken to prevent medical adhesive–related skin injury (MARSI) as described in Chapter 16.

KEY POINT

Skin barrier powder can be dusted onto areas of denuded skin to create a gummy protective layer; avoid excessive powder application, to prevent interference with pouch adhesion.

Absorptive Dressings and Moisture Barriers

Fistulas that are nonodorous with low-volume output (<100 mL/day) or located in deep creases or anatomical locations that make pouching impossible may require management with dressings and moisture barriers. In these situations, the perifistular skin maybe protected with a liquid barrier film or a moisture barrier ointment (petrolatum, dimethicone, or zinc oxide–based ointment or paste) or solid skin barrier, over which absorptive dressings are applied. The frequency of changes and reapplication of dressings and barriers is determined by the volume of drainage and the specific products being used. Absorptive dressings include gauze (sponges or strip packing), alginates, hydrofibers, foams, and combinations. When packing is required (e.g., wounds with depth, tunnels, or undermined areas), a dressing must be selected that can be completely retrieved from the wound. If the volume of drainage is such that the dressing must be changed more frequently than every 4 to 8 hours, pouching or closed suction should be considered.

Closed Suction

Closed suction systems can provide skin protection, drainage containment, and odor control and have been used for years as a reliable and cost-effective method for managing high-output fistulas or fistulas that are too difficult to pouch (Jeter et al., 1990; Jones & Harbit, 2003; Kordasiewicz, 2004). The wound and surrounding skin are gently cleansed; the periwound skin is then protected with a liquid barrier film and/or hydrocolloid barrier strips. Any major skin defects adjacent to the wound can be filled with barrier strips or paste to improve adhesion of the dressing. The wound base is covered by several layers of moistened gauze to prevent damage to the wound surface by the suction catheter; the suction catheter is then placed near the fistula orifice and stabilized with additional layers of moistened

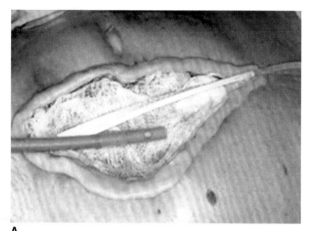

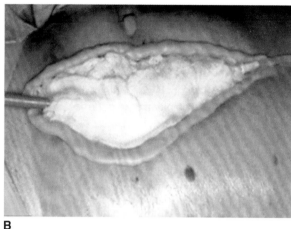

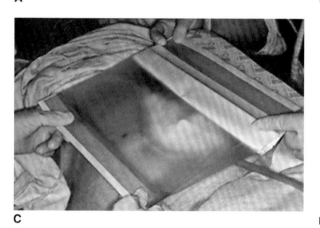

FIGURE 18-4. A–C. Closed Suction Procedure.

gauze. The entire wound is then covered with a transparent adhesive dressing, and paste is applied around the suction catheter where it exits the wound, if needed to obtain a secure seal. The suction catheter is connected to wall suction at a low level of continuous suction (see **Fig. 18-4A–C**). A Hemovac can provide the suction for short periods to increase the patient's mobility. Effluent must be liquid if suction is to be effective; thick or particulate effluent will occlude the catheter. Typically, these systems are changed every 2 to 3 days to prevent leakage and to permit wound assessment.

KEY POINT

Closed suction may be a good option for the patient who is not a candidate for pouching; it provides effective drainage containment and skin protection but is used only short term because it severely limits patient mobility.

It must be emphasized that a catheter that is inserted into the fistula tract will act as a foreign body and may interfere with healing and even increase fistula output. On the other hand, a catheter coiled in a defect above the orifice or in the open wound surrounding the fistula opening will not inhibit closure. Because firm tubes can

injure fragile tissue, only soft, flexible suction catheters should be used with fistulas. Suction systems should be considered a short-term intervention because of the limitations placed on patient mobility and the time-intensive nature of the care (Dearlove, 1996; Nishide, 1997; Pontieri-Lewis, 2005).

KEY POINT

A catheter inserted into the fistula tract acts as a foreign body and prevents wound closure.

Negative Pressure Wound Therapy
NPWT incorporates foam or gauze and subatmospheric pressure (suction) to promote closure of fistula tracts, the removal and containment of effluent, and/or wound healing. The mechanisms involved in promotion of wound healing include reduction in edema (with associated improvement in perfusion) and mechanical deformation of cells, which has been shown to stimulate the wound repair process. NPWT systems have built-in sensors to alert caregivers to potential and actual breaches in the integrity of the system.

Although there are no large studies comparing NPWT fistula management with traditional pouching techniques, its use with fistula management is widespread because surgeons are familiar with the technology from the use with problematic wounds. Wainstein and colleagues (2008) reported their 10-year experience with a vacuum-assisted device in management of 179 fistulas in 91 patients. Forty-two patients (46%) achieved spontaneous closure within 90 days of initiating vacuum-assisted therapy. Among the others, the closure rate after operation was 84%. Overall mortality rate was 16%.

NPWT can be used with fistulas located in open wounds so long as the following conditions are met: the fistula exhibits the potential for spontaneous closure (i.e., no evidence of pseudostoma formation); there is no evidence of exposed bowel in the wound base; and there is no evidence of abscess or distal obstruction. Caution should be used to prevent any additional fistula formation, that is, a contact layer or the nonporous "white" foam should be used in contact with the wound bed. If the effluent is too thick for suction, or if the fistula has "stomatized" but the wound still needs NPWT for promotion of granulation tissue formation, there are techniques and devices that segregate the fistula for management with pouching while permitting continued use of NPWT for promotion of wound healing (Bruhin et al., 2014; Heineman et al., 2015; Reed et al., 2006; Reider, 2017) (see **Box 18-4**; **Fig. 18-5**). The NSWOCC (2018) Nursing Best Practice Recommendations for ECF and EOF presents pictorial step-by-step procedures for isolating fistulas with and without the use of commercially available devices and can be accessed at http://nswoc.ca/ecf-best-practices/. Further information about the application and use of NPWT is presented in Chapter 12 of the wound core curriculum.

KEY POINT

NPWT can be used to promote wound healing and fistula closure so long as there are no impediments to spontaneous closure; a contact layer or nonporous foam should be used in contact with the wound bed to prevent any additional trauma.

Pouching Systems

Fistula pouches, ostomy pouches (pediatric or adult), retracted penis pouches, and fecal incontinence collectors have all been used for fistula management. Most are attached to a skin barrier. Additional skin barrier products may be required to caulk edges, fill creases, and/or add convexity (see **Table 18-2**).

When the fistula is located adjacent to an incision, the skin barrier of the pouch sometimes needs to be placed over the incision to prevent leakage onto the incision. When applied and removed appropriately, these products will protect rather than harm an incision. A simple strategy for protection of the incision is to place Steri-Strips or tape strips over the suture line or staple line prior to application of the pouching system.

BOX 18-4 PROCEDURE FOR ISOLATING A FISTULA FOR NPWT

1. Assemble equipment: Ostomy pouch and supplies, NPWT supplies, skin barrier ring, skin barrier paste, transparent dressing.
2. Prepare ostomy/fistula pouch as described in Box 18-5. Apply bead of paste to back of pouch around opening.

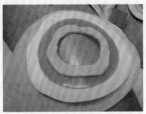

3. Cut a ring out of NPWT sponge dressing material slightly larger than the stomatized fistula; place into wound bed around fistula opening.

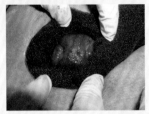

4. Optional: Place skin barrier ring right around fistula and over the NPWT sponge ring; apply bead of paste directly around fistula to caulk area between fistula and barrier ring.
5. Proceed to dress the wound utilizing NPWT procedure/protocol. Initiate suction and assure secure seal.

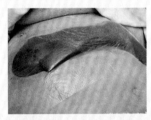

6. Cut an opening in the transparent dressing over fistula.

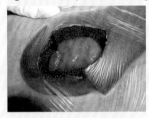

7. Apply the pouch over the fistula on top of the NPWT dressing; close the end of the pouch.

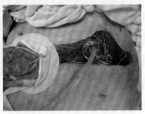

Photos courtesy of: Terri Reed and Diana Economon

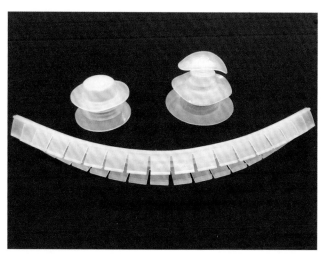

FIGURE 18-5. Example of a Commercially Available Device for Isolating a Fistula, Stoma, or Drain to Diverting Effluent Away From Wounds. One-piece devices are compressible and customizable for different sizes and number of fistulas. (Photo courtesy of Mary Anne Obst.)

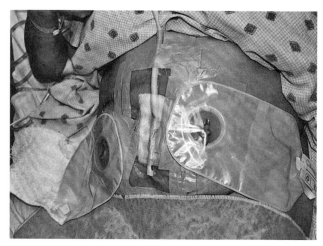

FIGURE 18-6. Two Pouches Used for Separate Fistulas. (Reproduced with permission from Davis, M., Dere, K., & Hadley, G. (2000). Options for managing an open wound with draining enterocutaneous fistula. *Journal of Wound, Ostomy & Continence Nursing, 27*(2), 118–123.)

Strategies to promote adhesion of the pouch to the perifistular skin include assurance of a dry surface; a moist surface will impair pouch adhesion. Skin barrier powders (NOT talc or corn starch) may be used to absorb moisture from denuded skin and to create a dry surface that supports pouch adherence. The amount of skin barrier powder used should be just enough to absorb the moisture and create a gummy or dry surface; too much powder will impair the adhesion of the pouch. Severely denuded skin may benefit from the "crusting" procedure, as described previously.

KEY POINT

If a pouching system or NPWT dressing extends over the suture or staple line, Steri-Strips or tape strips may be placed over the incision for protection prior to application of the dressing or pouching system.

Medical adhesive products approved for the skin should be used according to manufacturers' instructions and only when needed. Medical adhesives can be used to enhance the tack of an existing adhesive, to extend the adhesive surface on a pouch, or to compensate for the reduced adhesion caused by the application of skin barrier powder onto denuded perifistular skin. Medical adhesives are formulated as liquids/cements, medical adhesive sprays, and adhesive strips, rings, and sheets. Some adhesive products contain potential irritants or allergens, such as latex and/or alcohol; therefore, it is critical for the WOC nurse to carefully evaluate any adhesive product being considered for use in terms of indications, contraindications, and guidelines for use. Adhesive liquids and sprays must be allowed to dry completely in

order for solvents to evaporate and the adhesive product to become tacky (Bryant, 1992; Bryant & Best, 2015).

If two drainage/fistula sites are too far apart to be included in one pouching system, two pouches may be necessary (see **Fig. 18-6**) (Davis et al., 2000). When the fistula is located in a deep wound (see **Fig. 18-2**), it may be helpful to select a pouching system with an integrated window/access cap that facilitates adjunct use of wound filler dressing such as an alginate or antimicrobial or saline-moistened gauze. A pattern and procedure for preparation, removal, and application of the pouching system should be created, dated, and kept in the patient's room with instructions and supplies. **Figure 18-7** and **Box 18-5** present examples of a pattern and pouch change procedure.

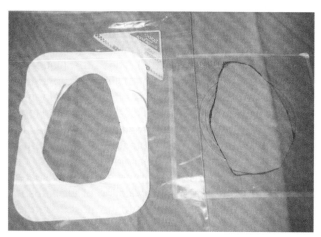

FIGURE 18-7. Pattern for Fistula Pouch. (Reproduced with permission from Davis, M., Dere, K., & Hadley, G. (2000). Options for managing an open wound with draining enterocutaneous fistula. *Journal of Wound, Ostomy & Continence Nursing, 27*(2), 118–123.)

BOX 18-5 FISTULA POUCH CHANGE PROCEDURE

1. Assemble equipment: Pouch with integrated skin barrier, pattern, skin barrier paste, scissors, closure device or attachment for bedside bag, water, soft gauze.
2. Prepare pouch.
   a. Trace pattern onto skin barrier surface of pouch. Note: the pattern should provide at least ¼ inch "clearance" of the wound edges (to prevent undermining of drainage under edge of pouch).
   b. Pull the anterior pouch surface away from posterior surface to avoid accidentally cutting hole in pouch surface.
   c. Cut out skin barrier surface according to tracing.
   d. Remove protective backing(s) from the pouch.
3. Remove and apply the pouch.
   a. Remove the pouch, using "push–pull" technique; gently press down on skin with one hand while pulling up on the pouch with the other.
   b. Discard the pouch and save closure clip or attachment device for bedside bag.
   c. Control any discharge with soft gauze.
   d. Clean the skin with water or gentle skin cleanser (without emollients that may impair adhesion of the pouch).
   e. Dry gently and thoroughly.
   f. Position the patient so abdomen has minimal wrinkles and folds (usually supine).
   g. Apply paste around the fistula. Fill in any uneven skin surfaces with paste, barrier rings, or skin barrier strips as needed.
   h. Apply a new pouch, centering fistula/wound site in opening.
   i. Close the bottom of the pouch with clip or attach to bedside bag.

Pouching System Adaptations

There are situations in which adaptations of standard pouching techniques are required. Pouching system adaptations (e.g., bridging, saddle bagging, and troughing) have been previously described and illustrated by Bryant (1992) and are recognized internationally over two decades later (NSWOCC, 2018). These techniques will be briefly described and illustrated (Figs. 18-8 to 18-10).

Troughing (**Fig. 18-8**) is a very effective management technique when the fistula is located within an open wound and routine pouching procedures are ineffective. The periwound skin is first protected with overlapping strips of skin barrier or hydrocolloid sheets and/or barrier paste. The wound is then covered with a transparent adhesive dressing; prior to application of the transparent dressing, an opening is cut into the most dependent portion of the dressing and a pouch is applied over the opening. The opening in the pouch/transparent dressing unit must be placed at the junction between the skin and the inferior aspect of the wound and must be wider than the diameter of the wound at that point. Since most wounds for which the trough procedure is required are very large, it is helpful to apply the transparent adhesive dressing in overlapping strips. (Typically, the strips are applied from "bottom" to "top"; the bottom strip is the one with the opening and the pouch.) Since most of these fistulas are high output, it is helpful to select a pouch with a spout that can be connected to gravity drainage (or to wall suction if needed) (Bryant, 1992; Hoedema & Suryadevara, 2010).

Troughing can frequently be used to provide effective skin protection and containment of effluent for patients in whom a secure pouch seal cannot be maintained. A common concern in management of fistulas located within open wounds and managed either by pouching or troughing is the impact of small bowel drainage on the healing process. Fortunately, the enzymes in small bowel fluid do not attack the newly formed collagen and blood vessels that comprise granulation tissue, and the very low bacterial counts in small bowel fluid minimize the risk of infection. Clinicians observe that wounds with fistulas continue to heal at the expected rate despite exposure to small bowel effluent.

Bridging (**Fig. 18-9**) may be used when the fistula is located at the inferior aspect of a long vertically oriented wound or at the most lateral aspect of an extensive horizontally oriented wound. The goal is to isolate the fistula from the remainder of the wound so that the fistula can be managed with pouching or troughing and the wound can be managed with moist wound healing or packing. Steps in the bridging procedure are as follows: (1) Identify a point slightly above (or medial to) the fistula at which the bridge will be "built." (2) Apply 1-inch strips of skin barrier or hydrocolloid wafer in layers to create a structure that fills the wound at that point and extends slightly above skin level. (The white foam used for NPWT therapy can also be used to create a bridge that fills the wound and extends slightly above the skin surface.) (3) Cut a strip of skin barrier or hydrocolloid wafer that is 1 inch wide (to match the width of the bridge) and long enough to cover the diameter of the wound and 2 inches of skin on either side of the wound. Place the covering strip over the bridge and onto the surrounding skin. (4) Proceed with pouching or troughing of the fistula and management of the remaining wound according to moist wound healing principles (Bryant, 1992, Hoedema & Suryadevara, 2010).

KEY POINT

Wounds continue to heal at the expected rate despite exposure to small bowel effluent.

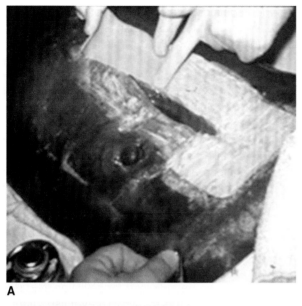

A

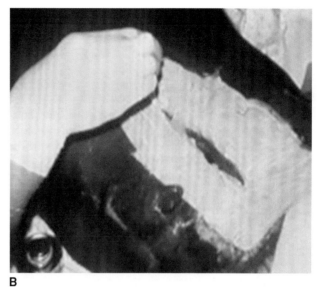

B

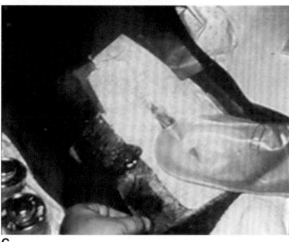

C

FIGURE 18-8. **A–C.** Troughing Procedure.

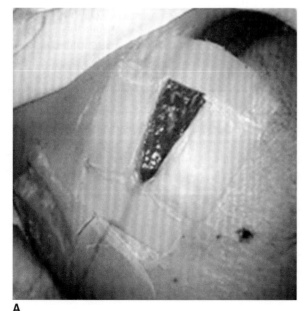

A

FIGURE 18-9. **A, B.** Bridging.

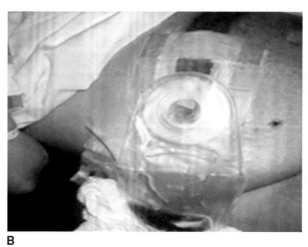

B

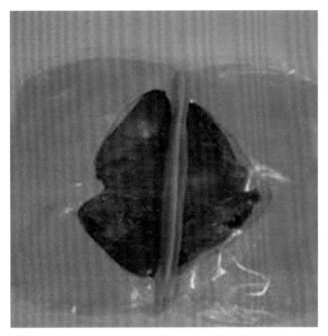

FIGURE 18-10. Saddlebagging: Example of Two Fistula Pouches Connected Together Along the Adhesive Surface to Make One Larger Adhesive Surface.

Saddlebagging (Fig. 18-10) is a technique in which two pouches are attached at the skin barrier adhesive edges of each pouch to create one pouch with a larger adhesive surface than standard pouches (Bryant, 1992; Bryant & Best, 2015). This technique may be necessary for larger fistulas or fistulas within a large wound that need to be pouched.

EDUCATION AND EMOTIONAL SUPPORT

The development of a fistula is associated with a significant reduction in the health-related quality of life for the patient and family (Hoeflok et al., 2015). Education and emotional support are critical aspects of the plan of care and its effectiveness. Patients report feelings of loss of control, frustration, embarrassment, hopelessness, isolation, and demoralization due to prolonged hospitalization, financial concerns, alterations in body image, and uncertain outcomes (Kaushal & Carlson, 2004; Kozell & Martins, 2003; Lloyd et al., 2006; Renton et al., 2006). Feelings may be exacerbated by the inability to eat normally, the possibility of additional procedures, the trial and error process so often required to achieve adequate skin protection and containment of effluent, and the prolonged care trajectory (Kozell & Martins, 2003).

KEY POINT

Education and emotional support are critical aspects of care for the patient with a fistula and his/her family.

Open communication with the patient and family will decrease anxiety, increase trust, and facilitate independence (Cobb & Knaggs, 2003; Kaushal & Carlson, 2004; Kozell & Martins, 2003). Education should be individualized based on goals of care, specific management approaches, and the patient's needs and learning style. Whenever possible, the patient should learn by participating in his/her care to gain back his/her independence and sense of control. It is important for the WOC nurse to help the patient and family to establish realistic goals and expectations, and to understand that fistula management and educational needs change over time (Burch & Buchan, 2004; Kozell & Martins, 2003).

SURGICAL CLOSURE

Given few fistulas close spontaneously, surgical intervention is required for closure of most fistulas. Surgical procedures may also be indicated for palliation (Nussbaum & Fischer, 2006). Factors known to prevent spontaneous closure are listed in Box 18-3 (Bryant & Best, 2015).

A systemic review and meta-analysis conducted by de Vries and colleagues (2017) found that postponing surgery for enteric fistula closure is associated with lower recurrence. Because of the wide range of time to definitive surgery within each study, optimal timing of surgery could not be defined. Researchers estimate that between 6 and 12 months after the last laparotomy may be needed to resolve abdominal infection, restore nutritional state and homeostasis, soften adhesions, and provide adequate wound care and muscle strength. This bridging-to-surgery approach has become standard practice in intestinal failure (IF) centers (ESCP, 2016; de Vries et al., 2017).

Surgical interventions for ECF and EAFs either divert the fecal stream (without resection of the fistula) or provide definitive resection of the fistula tract. Diversion techniques divert the stool away from the fistula site without removal of the fistula by creating a stoma proximal to the fistula or by anastomosing (end-to-end or side-to-side) the two segments of bowel on each side of the fistula. This approach is required when resection of the fistula is not possible or appropriate, such as in the presence of extensive or recurrent malignancy or inadequate perfusion in the vicinity of the fistula due to previous surgery, scar formation, or prior irradiation. The process of resection involves removal of the diseased tissue and fistula tract followed by end-to-end anastomosis of the intestine. To protect the anastomosis, diversion of the fecal stream through a temporary stoma may be indicated. If the fistula involves the colon and the distal colon and rectum are not suitable for anastomosis or the anal sphincters are not competent, a permanent stoma with a Hartmann's pouch may be the safest procedure. Enteric fistulas communicating with the urinary tract will always require diversion of the fecal stream proximal to the fistula site to prevent urinary tract infections and pyelone-phritis. Timing of surgery depends on the patient's status. Surgery for a type 1 fistula (see **Table 18-1**) is appropriate when the patient is nutritionally and metabolically stable, the fistula tract has been free of infection for 6 to 8 weeks, and the abdominal wall and peritoneal cavity have returned to a relatively soft, supple, pliable state; the goal is to maximize the potential for successful closure of the fistula and to minimize the potential for additional complications, including recurrent fistula formation. Judicious timing is warranted for surgical closure of complex type 2 fistulas (see **Table 18-1**); surgery is usually delayed for 3 to 6 months, which is extremely frustrating for the patient and family. It is important to be able to explain to the patient and family that the extensive intra-abdominal infection associated with the original bowel perforation or anastomotic breakdown resulted in formation of extensive scar tissue within the abdominal cavity (obliterative peritonitis) and that it takes a number of months for the scar tissue to soften enough for the surgeon to separate the loops of bowel and remove the fistula tract without risking additional injury to the bowel and additional fistula formation. Nutritional, metabolic, and immunologic status should be restored prior to surgery (Wong et al., 2004); for the patient with an ECF or EAF, this usually means that TPN will be required until the fistula is closed. However, the restrictions on oral intake are usually liberalized once it is clear that the fistula will not close spontaneously and that surgical intervention will be required; typically, patients are allowed to eat and drink small amounts for pleasure and to keep the bowel mucosa healthy, as discussed earlier.

KEY POINT

Surgical closure is required for fistulas with known impediments to healing and for those that "fail" medical management (i.e., fail to close within 5 to 6 weeks of comprehensive management); surgical intervention is usually delayed for several months to permit softening of intra-abdominal adhesions.

 ## VESICOVAGINAL, RECTOVAGINAL, OR ENTEROVAGINAL FISTULAS

While the vast majority of fistulas involve openings between two loops of bowel or between the bowel and the skin, fistulous openings can also develop between the bladder, rectum, or small bowel and the vagina. Vesicovaginal fistulas (between the bladder and vagina) are typically managed initially by urinary diversion with indwelling urethral or suprapubic catheter or nephrostomy tubes, followed by surgery to close the fistula tract. The urine draining continually from the vagina is usually managed with absorptive pads; alternatively, a balloon-tipped catheter can be placed in the vagina and connected to a leg bag. (If the diameter of the vaginal

vault exceeds the diameter of the inflated balloon, causing the catheter to constantly slip out of place, the catheter can be threaded through a baby nipple so that the tip of the catheter rests just above the base of the nipple; the baby nipple/catheter unit is then folded and gently inserted into the vagina so that the base of the nipple rests within the introitus to minimize leakage.) This technique can also be used for management of enterovaginal fistulas; because the drainage is thicker, it is necessary to use a large diameter catheter. Rectovaginal fistulas are typically managed by fecal diversion to permit healing of the fistula tract. For the patient who is not a candidate for surgical intervention, the focus of management should be measures to minimize vaginal contamination, specifically, titration of fiber and fluid intake to maintain soft formed stool that will not pass through the narrow fistulous tract. The patient can also be counseled to use mild antiseptics approved for intravaginal use to reduce or eliminate odor (e.g., Trimo-San).

 ## CONCLUSIONS

Caring for a patient with a fistula is one of the most challenging, and rewarding, situations the WOC nurse will encounter. Effective management requires a clear understanding of the anatomy of the fistula tract and plan of care, ongoing assessment regarding progress in closure or evidence of failure to close, creativity in developing an effective strategy for containment of effluent and odor, and consistent support and education for the patient and family. The key ingredients to positive outcomes when managing a patient with a fistula are patience; persistence; interdisciplinary collaboration; close surveillance; excellent communication with the patient, family, and colleagues; and a little ingenuity.

REFERENCES

Arebi, N. & Forbes, A. (2004). High output fistula. *Clinics in Colon and Rectal Surgery, 7*(2), 89–98.

Bailey, E. H., & Glasgow, S. C. (2016). Challenges in the medical and surgical management of chronic inflammatory bowel disease. *Surgical Clinics of North America 95*, 1233–1244.

Bryant, R. (1992). Management of drain sites and fistulas. In R. Bryant (Ed.), *Acute and chronic wounds: Nursing management*. St. Louis, MO: Mosby.

Bryant, R., & Best, M. (2015). Management of draining wounds and fistulas. In R. Bryant & D. Nix (Eds.), *Acute and chronic wounds: Current management concepts* (5th ed.). St. Louis, MO: Mosby.

Bruhin, A., Ferreira, F., Chariker, M., et al. (2014). Systematic review and evidence based recommendations for the use of negative pressure wound therapy in the open abdomen. *International Journal of Surgery, 12*(10), 1105–1114.

Burch, J., & Buchan, D. (2004). Support and guidance for failure and enterocutaneous fistula care. *Gastrointestinal Nursing, 2*(7), 25–32.

Causey, M. W., Rivadeneira, D. E., & Steele, S. R. (2012). Historical and current trends in colon trauma. *Clinics in Colon and Rectal Surgery, 25*(4), 189–199.

Chamieh, J., Prakash, P., & Symons, W. J. (2018). Management of destructive colon injuries after damage control surgery. *Clinics in Colon and Rectal Surgery, 31*(1), 36–40. doi:10.1055/s-0037-1602178.

Cobb, A., & Knaggs, E. (2003). The nursing management of enterocutaneous fistulae: A challenge for all. *British Journal of Community Nursing, 8*(9), S32–S38.

Coetzee, E., Rahim, Z. et al. (2014). Refedding enteroclysis as an alternative to parenteral nutrition for enteric fistula. *Colorectal Disease, 16*(10), 823–830.

Collier, B., Guillamondegui, O., Cotton, B., et al. (2007). Feeding the open abdomen. *JPEN. Journal of Parenteral and Enteral Nutrition, 31*(5), 410–415.

Coughlin, S., Roth, L., Lurati, G., et al. (2012). Somatostatin analogues for the treatment of enterocutaneous fistulas: A systematic review and meta-analysis. *World Journal of Surgery, 36*(5), 1016–1029.

Davis, M., Dere, K., Hadley, G., et al. (2000). Options for managing an open wound with draining enterocutaneous fistula. *Journal of Wound, Ostomy, and Continence Nursing, 27*(2), 118–123.

Davis, K. G., Johnson, E. K. (2013). Controversies in the care of the enterocutaneous fistula. *Surgical Clinics of North America, 93*, 231–250.

Dearlove, J. L. (1996). Skin care management of gastrointestinal fistulas. *Surgical Clinics of North America, 76*(5), 1095–1109.

de Vries, F. E. E., Reeskamp, L. F., van Ruler, O., et al. (2017). Systematic review: pharmacotherapy for high output enterostomies or enteral fistulas. *Alimentary Pharmacology and Therapeutics, 46*(3), 266–273.

Draus, J. M. Jr, Huss, S. A., Harty, N. J., et al. (2006). Enterocutaneous fistula: Are treatments improving? *Surgery, 140*(4), 570–576; discussion 576–578.

Dubose, J., & Lundy, J. (2010). Enterocutaneous fistulas in the setting of trauma and critical illness. *Clinics in Colon and Rectal Surgery, 23*(3), 182–189.

ESCP Intestinal Failure Group; Vaizey, C. J., Maeda, Y., Barbosa, E., et al. (2016). ESCP consensus on the surgical management of intestinal failure in adults. *Colorectal Disease 18*, 535–548.

Gribovskaja-Rupp, I., & Melton, G. (2016). Enterocutaneous fistula: Proven strategies and updates. *Clinics in Colon and Rectal Surgery, 29*(2), 130–137.

Haack, C. I., Galloway, J. R., & Srinivasan, J. (2014). Enterocutaneous fistulas: A look at causes and management. *Current Surgery Reports, 2*, 71.

Heimroth J., Chen E., & Sutton E. (2018). Management approaches for enterocutaneous fistulas. [Review] *American Surgeon, 84*(3), 326–333.

Heineman, J. T., Garcia, L. J., Obst, M. A., et al. (2015). Collapsible enteroatmospheric fistula isolation device: a novel, simple solution to a complex problem. *Journal of the American College of Surgery, 221*, e7–e14.

Hoedema, R. & Suryadevara, S. (2010). Entrostomal therapy and wound care of the fistula patient. *Clinic Colon Rectal Surgery, 23*(3), 161–168.

Hoeflok, J., Jaramillo, M., Li, T., et al. (2015). Health-related quality of life in community-dwelling persons living with enterocutaneous fistulas. *Journal of Wound, Ostomy, and Continence Nursing, 42*(6), 607–613.

Hollington, P., Maurdsley, J., Lim, W., et al. (2004). An 11 year experience of enterocutaneous fistulae. *British Journal of Surgery, 91*, 1046–1051.

Irrgang, S., Bryant, R. (1984). Management of the enterocutaneous fistula (continuous education credit). *Journal of Enterostomal Therapy, 11*(6), 211–228.

Jeter, K. F., Tintle, T. E., & Chariker, M. (1990). Managing draining wounds and fistulae: New and established methods. In D. Krasner (Ed.), *Chronic wound care: A clinical source book for healthcare professionals* (pp. 240–246). King of Prussia, PA: Health Management.

Jones, E. G., & Harbit, M. (2003). Management of an ileostomy and mucous fistula located in a dehisced wound in a patient with morbid obesity. *Journal of Wound, Ostomy, and Continence Nursing, 30*(6), 351.

Juárez-Oropeza, M. A., & Román-Ramos, R. (2012). Factors predictive of recurrence and mortality after surgical repair of enterocutaneous fistula. *Journal of Gastrointestinal Surgery, 16*(1), 156–163, discussion 163–164.

Kassis, E. S., & Makary, M. A. (2008). Enterocutaneous fistula. In J. S. Cameron (Ed.), *Current surgical therapy* (9th ed.). St. Louis, MO: Mosby.

Kaushal, M., & Carlson, G. L. (2004). Management of enterocutaneous fistulae. *Clinics in Colon and Rectal Surgery, 17*(2), 79–87.

Knechtges, P., & Zimmermann, E. M. (2009). Intra-abdominal abscesses and fistulas. In T. Yamada, et al. (Eds.), *Textbook of Gastroenterology, Vol II* (6th ed.). Philadelphia, PA: Lippincott Williams & Wilkins.

Kordasiewicz, L. M. (2004). Abdominal wound with fistula and large amount of drainage status after incarcerated hernia repair. *Journal of Wound, Ostomy, and Continence Nursing, 31*(3), 150.

Kozell, K., & Martins, L. (2003). Managing the challenges of enterocutaneous fistulae. *Wound Care Canada, 1*(1), 10–14.

Kumpf, V. J., de Aguilar-Nascimento, J. E., Diaz-Pizarro Graf, J. I., et al. (2017). ASPEN-FELANPE clinical guidelines. *JPEN Journal of Parenteral and Enteral Nutrition, 41*(1), 104–112.

Li, P. H., Tee, Y. S., Fu, C. Y., et al. (2018). The Role of noncontrast CT in the evaluation of surgical abdomen patients. *The American surgeon, 84*(6), 1015–1102.

Lloyd, D. A. J., Gabe, S. M., & Windsor, A. C. J. (2006). Nutrition and management of enterocutaneous fistula. *British Journal of Surgery, 93*, 1045–1055.

Lynch, A. C., Delaney, C. P., Senagore, A. J., et al. (2004). Clinical outcome and factors predictive of recurrence after enterocutaneous fistula surgery. *Annals of Surgery, 240*(5), 825–831.

Makhdoom, Z. A., Komar, M. J., & Still, C. D. (2000). Nutrition and enterocutaneous fistulas. *Journal of Clinical Gastroenterology, 31*(3), 195.

Mehta, N. Y., Copelin, II E. L. [Updated 2019 Jul 31]. Abdominal abscess. In *Stat Pearls [Internet]*. Treasure Island, FL: Stat Pearls Publishing. Retrieved from https://www.ncbi.nlm.nih.gov/books/NBK519573

Neutzling, C. B., Lustosa, S. A. S., Proenca, I. M., et al. (2017). Stapled versus handsewn methods for colorectal anastomosis surgery. *Cochrane Database of Systematic Reviews*, (2), CD003144. DOI: 10.1002/14651858.CD003144.pub2.

Nishide, K. (1997). Development of closed-suction pouch drainage for giant fistulae: A report on two cases. *WCET Journal, 17*(1), 16–19.

Nurses Specialized in Wound, Ostomy and Continence Canada (NSWOCC) (formally CAET). (2018). *Nursing best practice recommendations: Enterocutaneous fistulas (ECF) and enteroatmospheric fistulas (EAF)* (2nd ed.). Ottawa. Retrieved 15 December, 2019, from http://nswoc.ca/ecf-best-practices.

Nussbaum, M. S., & Fischer, D. R. (2006). Gastric, duodenal and small intestinal fistulas. In C. J. Yeo, et al. (Eds.), *Shackelford's surgery of the alimentary tract* (6th ed.). St. Louis, MO: Saunders.

Parli, S. E., Pfeifer, C, Oyler, D. R., et al. (2018). Redefining "bowel regimen": Pharmacologic strategies and nutritional considerations in the management of small bowel fistulas. [Review] *American Journal of Surgery, 216*(2), 351–358.

Polk, T. M., & Schwab, C. W. (2012). Metabolic and nutritional support of the enterocutaneous fistula patient: A three-phase approach. *World Journal of Surgery 36*(3), 524–533.

Pontieri-Lewis, V. (2005). Management of gastrointestinal fistulae: A case study. *Medical-Surgical Nursing, 14*(1), 68–72.

Quinn, M., Falconer, S., McKee, R. F. (2017). Management of enterocutaneous fistula: Outcomes in 276 patients. *World Journal of Surgery, 41*(10), 2502–2511.

Rahman, F. N., & Stavas, J. M. (2015). Interventional radiologic management and treatment of enterocutaneous fistulae. [Review] *Journal of Vascular and Interventional Radiology: JVIR, 26*(1), 7–19.

Rahbour, G., Sci, B. M., & Siddiqui, M. R. (2012). Systematic review and meta analysis a meta-analysis of outcomes following use of somatostatin and its analogues for the management of enterocutaneous fistulas. *Annals of Surgery, 256*(6), 946–954.

Reed, T., Economon, D., & Wiersema-Bryant, L. (2006). Colocutaneous fistula management in a dehisced wound: A case study. *Ostomy/Wound Management, 52*(4), 60–64, 66.

Reider, K. (2017). Fistula isolation and the use of negative pressure to promote wound healing: A case study. *Journal of Wound, Ostomy, and Continence Nursing, 44*(3), 293–298.

Renton, S., Robertson, I., & Speirs, M. (2006). Alternative management of complex wounds and fistulae. *British Journal of Nursing, 15*(16), 851–853.

Rolstad, B., & Wong, W. D. (2004). Nursing considerations in intestinal fistulas. In P. A. Cataldo, & J. M. MacKeigan (Eds.), *Intestinal stomas: Principles, techniques, and management* (2nd ed.). New York, NY: Marcel Dekker.

Samad, S., Anele, C., Akhtar, M., et al. (2015). Implementing a pro- forma for multidisciplinary management of an enterocutaneous fistula: a case study. *Ostomy/Wound Management 61*(6), 46–52.

Schecter, W. P., Hirshberg, A., Chang, D. S., et al. (2009). "Enteric fistula" principles of management. *Journal of the American College of Surgeons, 209*(4), 484–491.

Stevens, P., Foulkes, R. E., Hartford-Beynon, J. S., et al. (2011). Systematic review and meta-analysis of the role of somatostatin and its analogues in the treatment of enterocutaneous fistula. *European Journal of Gastroenterology & Hepatology, 23*(10), 912–922.

Teixeira, P. G., Inaba, K., Dubose, J., et al. (2009). Enterocutaneous fistula complicating trauma laparotomy: A major resource burden. *The American Surgeon, 75*(1), 30–32.

Telem, D. A., Chin, E. H., Nguyen, S. Q., et al. (2010). Risk factors for anastomotic leak following colorectal surgery: A case–control study. *Archives of Surgery, 145*(4), 371–376.

Tran, N. A., & Thorson, A. G. (2008). Rectovaginal fistula. In J. L. Cameron (Ed.), *Current surgical therapy* (9th ed.). St. Louis, MO: Mosby.

Wainstein, D. E., Fernandez, E., Gonzalez, D., et al. (2008). Treatment of high output enterocutaneous fistulas with a vacuum-compaction device. A ten-year experience. *World Journal of Surgery 32*, 430–435.

Wercka, J., Cagol, P. P., Melo, A. L., et al. (2016). Epidemiology and outcome of patients with postoperative abdominal fistula. *Revista do Colégio Brasileiro de Cirurgiões, 43*(2), 117–123.

Whelan, J. F. Jr, & Ivatury, R. R. (2011). Enterocutaneous fistulas: an overview. *European Journal of Trauma and Emergency Surgery, 37*(3), 251–258.

Willcutts, K., Mercer, D., & Ziegler, J. (2015). Fistuloclysis: An interprofessional approach to nourishing the fistula patient. *Journal of Wound, Ostomy, and Continence Nursing, 42*(5), 549–553.

Williams, L. J., Zolfaghari, S., & Boushey, R. P. (2010). Complications of enterocutaneous fistulas and their management. *Clinics in Colon and Rectal Surgery, 23*(3), 209–220.

Wong, W. D., et al. (2004). Management of intestinal fistulas. In P. A. Cataldo & J. M. MacKeigan (Eds.), *Intestinal stomas: Principles, techniques, and management* (2nd ed.). New York, NY: Marcel Dekker.

Zelga, P., Tchórzewski, M., Zelga, M., et al. (2017). Radiation-induced rectovaginal fistulas in locally advanced gynecological malignancies-new patients, old problem? *Langenbeck's Archives of Surgery, 402*(7), 1079–1088.

QUESTIONS

1. The WOC nurse suspects that a patient's surgical wound is developing a fistula. Which of the following is the definitive indicator of an enterocutaneous fistula?
   A. Fever and infection in the wound bed
   B. Abdominal pain and wound dehiscence
   C. Blood migrating from a wound bed to the gastrointestinal tract
   D. Passage of gastrointestinal secretions or urine into an open wound bed

2. A patient is diagnosed with an enterocutaneous fistula with a high-output volume. Which statement correctly defines this diagnosis?
   A. A passage is created from the Intestine to the skin, and the volume is >500 mL/24 h.
   B. A passage is created from the colon to the vagina, and the volume output is >500 mL/24 h.
   C. A passage is created from the bladder to the vagina, and the volume output is 200 to 500 mL/24 h.
   D. A passage is created from the colon to the skin, and the volume output is <200 mL/24 h.

3. The WOC nurse is assessing the wound of a patient diagnosed with a type 1 complex fistula. What data regarding the fistula would the nurse document in the patient record?
   A. Fistula with a short direct tract, no abscess, no other organ involvement
   B. Fistula with an abscess, with multiple organ involvement
   C. Fistula that opens into the base of the wound
   D. Fistula with a tract that is contained within the body

4. What is the etiology of the majority of enterocutaneous fistulas (ECFs)?
   A. Bowel disease
   B. Diverticulitis
   C. Surgical procedures
   D. External trauma

5. The WOC nurse is planning care for a patient with an enterocutaneous fistula (ECF). What is a key initial step in managing a patient with ECF?
   A. Administer H$_2$ antagonists to decrease ECF closure time.
   B. Use a 2-week trial of octreotide to reduce fistula output.
   C. Limit oral or enteral intake to amount keeping intestinal mucosa healthy.
   D. Force fluids to decrease gastric, biliary, and pancreatic secretions.

6. A patient is diagnosed with an intra-abdominal abscess following a CT scan. What is the initial management of choice for this patient?
   A. CT-guided drainage
   B. Surgical intervention
   C. Pharmacological management
   D. Keeping the patient NPO for 3 days

7. Which of the following assessment findings indicates that the patient will require surgical closure?
   A. Output exceeding 750 mL/24 h.
   B. Evidence of mucosal eversion/pseudostoma formation.
   C. History indicates fistula has been present >14 days.
   D. Hypertrophic granulation tissue in wound bed.

8. The WOC nurse is recommending products for patients with fistulas. Which product is used correctly?
   A. Moisture barrier cream for a high-output fistula
   B. Negative pressure wound therapy (NPWT) for a low-output fistula
   C. Suction system for a low-output fistula
   D. Pouch for a high- or low-output fistula

9. A patient presents with a fistula that has an output volume <50 mL with a need for odor control. What would be a good containment option for this patient?
   A. Wound management system with window emptied frequently
   B. Closed system with suction
   C. Charcoal dressings over dressings with environmental deodorants
   D. Absorptive dressings (e.g., calcium alginate dressings)

10. The WOC nurse is teaching a patient how to change a fistula pouch. Which of the following is a recommended step in this procedure?
   A. Trace the pattern onto the skin barrier surface of the pouch providing at least ¼ inch clearance of wound edges.
   B. Trace the pattern onto the skin barrier of the pouch being careful to size the opening to match the contours of the wound exactly.
   C. Remove the pouch by pulling off the skin quickly while applying gentle pressure on skin with one hand.
   D. Clean the skin with an alcohol wipe or skin cleanser with an emollient and dry gently and thoroughly.

ANSWERS AND RATIONALES

1. D. Rationale: Fever, infection, abdominal pain, wound dehiscence, and blood migrating from a wound bed to the gastrointestinal tract may occur with a fistula. However, passage of gastrointestinal secretions or urine into an open wound bed is a definitive indicator.

2. A. Rationale: An enterocutaneous fistula is a passage from the GI or GU tract to the skin; a passage from the GI or GU tract to the vagina is called a colo- or vesicovaginal fistula. High-output volume is defined as >500 mL/24 h.

3. B. Rationale: A simple fistula does not involve abscess or organ, while a complex fistula type 1 involves abscess and multiple organs or opens to the wound base.

4. C. Rationale: ECFs can occur spontaneously, as a result of inflammatory bowel disease, cancer, or diverticulitis. However, they most commonly develop postoperatively, due to anastomotic breakdown.

5. C. Rationale: Reduced oral/enteral intake minimizes fistula output by decreasing luminal contents, GI stimulation, and pancreaticobiliary secretions. H_2 receptors have not been shown to affect either the number of ECFs that close spontaneously or the time to ECF closure. Octreotides decrease intestinal output in some situations and may be appropriate as a short-term adjunctive therapy.

6. A. Rationale: CT-guided drainage is the initial management of choice in patients presenting with spontaneous or postoperative intra-abdominal abscess. This can obviate the need for early operative intervention.

7. B. Rationale: A fistula with high output or duration >14 days can spontaneously close under the right conditions. Evidence of mucosal eversion/pseudostoma formation, however, will not close spontaneously and will require surgical closure.

Hypertrophic granulation tissue in wound bed does not impact fistula closure.

8. D. Rationale: The high-output fistula is best managed with pouches, suction systems, or NPWT. Moisture barrier creams provide skin protection for the low-output fistula.

9. C. Rationale: Charcoal dressings are better designed for odor control than other absorbent dressings and can manage the low-output fistula with the proper skin protection and change frequency. A wound management system with a window emptied frequently or a closed system with suction may control odor but is indicated for the high-output fistula.

10. A. Rationale: Prepare a fistula pouch by tracing the pattern onto the skin barrier surface of the pouch providing at least ¼ inch clearance of wound edges; matching contours of the wound exactly does not allow enough adhesive surface. Pulling adhesive off the skin quickly can cause skin injury. Alcohol can be caustic to perifistula skin. Skin cleanser with emollient can impair adhesion of the pouch.

CHAPTER 19

NURSING MANAGEMENT OF THE PATIENT WITH PERCUTANEOUS TUBES

Jane Fellows and Michelle Rice

OBJECTIVE

Apply assessment and nursing management techniques to address the complex care needs of a patient with percutaneous tubes.

TOPIC OUTLINE

Introduction **304**

Gastrostomy and Jejunostomy Tubes **304**
 Comparative Complication Rates   306
 Routine Tube Care   306
 Managing Skin Complications   307
 Hypertrophic Granulation   307

Tube Replacement   311
 Pediatric Considerations   312
Nephrostomy Tubes **312**
Biliary Tubes **313**
Conclusions **313**

INTRODUCTION

Percutaneous tube placement into body organs or spaces is a means for drainage of fluids, maintaining an opening into an organ where obstruction exists, or providing for instillation of fluids, medication, or feeding through the tube. The tubes are usually placed by a health care provider in surgery, via endoscopy or interventional radiology. The WOC nurse is often consulted for management of these tubes and the complications that may occur with them. Knowledge of the location, purpose, and desired outcome of the tube placement is essential to effectively manage the care of patients with these tubes. The use of percutaneous tubes is common in the adult and pediatric patient populations across acute care, long-term care, and home care settings. Increasingly, they are being used for pain relief and symptom management in palliative care (Requarth,

2011). Common types of these tubes are gastrostomy, jejunostomy, biliary, and nephrostomy.

GASTROSTOMY AND JEJUNOSTOMY TUBES

Nasogastric tubes (NGT) are the simplest to insert in the gastrointestinal (GI) tract and the least invasive, but they carry a higher risk for dislodgment and aspiration leading to pneumonia (Boullata et al., 2017). When feeding through the tube or decompression of the GI tract is needed for more than a few weeks, a percutaneous tube is inserted. NGT are indicated for short-term use. Common indications for gastrostomy tube (GT) insertion are obstructing head and neck cancer, benign and malignant esophageal disease, neurologic dysfunction, trauma, and respiratory failure.

GTs have been reported in the literature since the 1800s. Dr. Martin Stamm developed a surgical procedure for placement of a tube directly into the stomach, which is still used today. The standard Stamm gastrostomy involves circumferential purse-string sutures to stabilize the tube within the lumen of the stomach and affix the stomach to the anterior abdominal wall. A later technique developed by Witzel involves creating a serosal tunnel as well as an abdominal wall tunnel through which the tube passes. This is useful when the stomach has been altered so that it cannot be secured to the abdominal wall such as after a gastric bypass surgery or resection of esophageal cancer. Variations on these open surgical procedures remained the standard of care for feeding or gastric decompression until the 1980s when a procedure for percutaneous endoscopic gastrostomy (PEG) was developed. PEG is a method of placing a tube into the stomach through the skin, aided by endoscopy (**Fig. 19-1**). A PEG with a jejunal extension tube can be placed through a preexisting PEG to facilitate more distal feeding while also providing an avenue for gastric decompression when necessary.

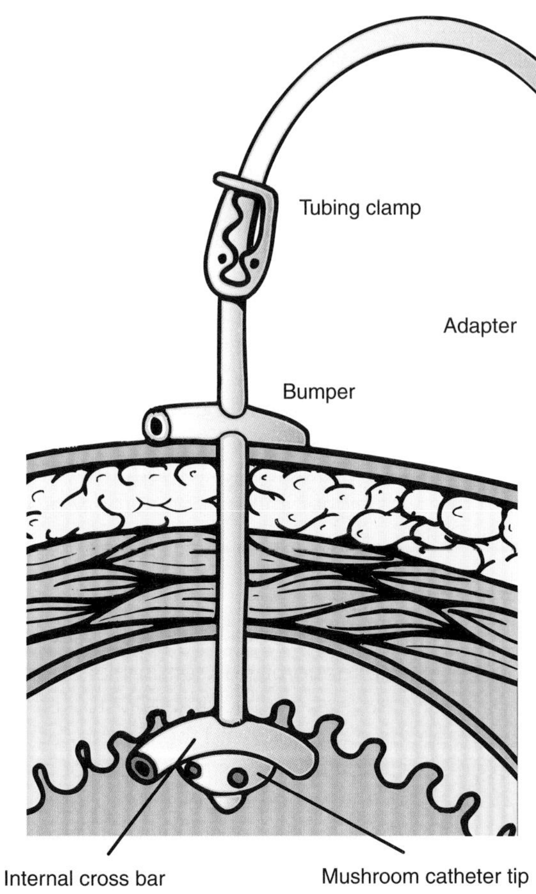

PEG is often considered the method of choice for enteral access due to the simplicity, effectiveness, and lower cost of the procedure, but it is important to do a complete assessment of the patient's GI anatomy and comorbid conditions before deciding which type of enteral access will be best for the patient (Boullata et al., 2017). PEG is not always clinically appropriate, and some of the possible contraindications include the following:

- Uncorrected coagulopathy or thrombocytopenia
- Upper tract obstruction or malformation
- Severe ascites
- Hemodynamic instability
- Sepsis
- Intra-abdominal perforation
- Active peritonitis
- Abdominal wall infection at the selected site of placement
- Gastric outlet obstruction (if PEG tube is being placed for feeding)
- Severe gastroparesis (if PEG tube is being placed for feeding)
- History of total gastrectomy

When a PEG is not feasible for the patient, radiologic placement is a possible alternative. This was first described in the literature in the mid-1980s (Kim et al., 2010) and avoids the use of an endoscope and is not contraindicated in the presence of upper tract obstruction. It uses fluoroscopy and ultrasound to identify the stomach, and a GT with a balloon is secured against the gastric mucosa with an external bumper on the skin (**Fig. 19-2**). If gastroesophageal reflux or delaying gastric emptying is a problem, another feeding tube option is a percutaneous gastrojejunal tube (**Fig. 19-3**). This tube has a balloon and an external skin bumper. There is an extension that is guided through the duodenum and into the jejunum for feeding. These tubes will have a gastric port that can be used for medication or fluid

Tubing clamp

Adapter

Bumper

Internal cross bar

Mushroom catheter tip

FIGURE 19-1. PEG Tube with Internal and External Bumper. (Published in Potter, P. A., Perry A. G., Stockert, P., Hall, A. (2015). *Essentials for nursing practice* (8th ed., p. 926), copyright Elsevier.)

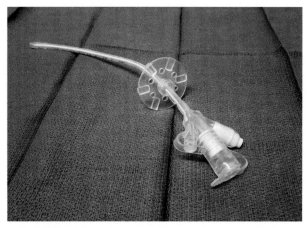

FIGURE 19-2. Balloon-Tipped Gastrostomy Tube. Courtesy of Jane Fellows, MSN, RN, CWOCN.

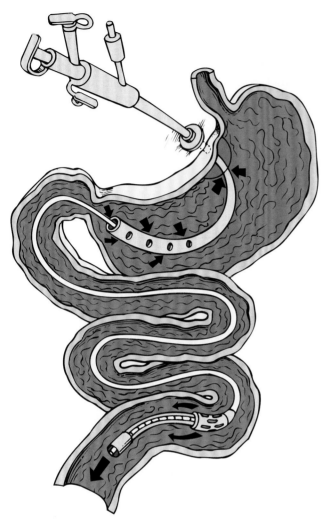

FIGURE 19-3. PEG with Jejunal Extension. Published in Potter, P. A., Perry, A. G., Stockert, P., Hall, A. (2015). *Essentials for nursing practice* (8th ed., p. 926), copyright Elsevier.

administration or decompression of the stomach and one port for the jejunal feeding. A study of 124 patients requiring conversion from a GT to gastrojejunal tube showed a significantly higher success rate using the radiologic placement procedure rather than nonradiologic procedures (Kim et al., 2010). These radiologic procedures require providers with training in interventional radiology, which is not always an option in all facilities.

Both the PEG and radiologic procedures can be done with sedation rather than anesthesia making the procedure safer for the patient, and the time for initial feedings is not delayed. If feeding in the stomach is not possible due to surgical absence of the organ, severe gastroparesis, or gastric outlet obstruction, radiologic intervention is used to place a feeding tube directly into the jejunum. This tube is initially secured with a stabilizer sutured to the skin.

For those patients who are not candidates for PEG or radiologic procedures, surgical approaches offer the advantage of direct visualization of tube placement

into the intended organ (stomach or jejunum). An open laparotomy or laparoscopy is done by a surgeon in the operating room, and the patient receives general anesthesia. During the surgical approach, the stomach or jejunum is identified following a laparotomy incision or insertion of the laparoscope. The laparoscopic approach offers smaller incision size, less pain, and decreased risk of incisional hernia (Mizrahi et al., 2014). The appropriate feeding tube is secured within the lumen of the targeted organ and brought out through a separate stab incision. If a patient is scheduled for an open or laparoscopic abdominal surgery and it is expected that a feeding tube may be needed, it should be placed at the time of the surgery.

COMPARATIVE COMPLICATION RATES

There are many potential complications with these procedures, and most of the patients are malnourished and have significant comorbidities. However, the complication rates are relatively low. The complication rates reported in the literature vary, but it seems generally accepted to be 1% to 3% for PEG placement, 8% to 10% with radiologic procedures, and 7% to 15% with surgical procedures (Miller et al., 2014). Complications associated with percutaneous endoscopic approaches include endoscopic trauma and perforation of the GI tract, bleeding, skin and soft tissue infection, injury to intra-abdominal viscera such as the liver or colon, tube dislodgment, and fistula creation. Radiologic placement has many of the same risks as do endoscopically placed tubes, but there is no risk of upper tract trauma from the endoscope. Surgically placed tubes are associated most commonly with skin and soft tissue infection, incisional hernia, bleeding, inadvertent removal of the tube, and complications associated with general anesthesia. Issues with inadvertent injury to surrounding intra-abdominal viscera are very rare due to the better visibility during the procedure. In a study comparing laparoscopic versus open laparotomy, the laparoscopic surgery took longer to perform, but the complication rate was higher in the open surgery group (Mizrahi et al., 2014).

ROUTINE TUBE CARE

Following placement of percutaneous gastric tubes, the external bolster should generally be left in place for at least 4 days. After 4 days, there should be 1/2 to 1 cm of laxity left between the entry point and the bumper of the tube to prevent ulceration of the gastric mucosa or pressure injury to the skin under the bumper. Due to the possibility of edema at the tube site, positioning of the tube should be observed frequently for the first 48 hours after insertion (Miller et al., 2014). Evidence for most effective site care is lacking, but patient education materials recommend that the site be washed with mild soap and water, rinsed well with water, and dried daily. One gauze drain sponge may be placed under the bumper unless it sutured in place to absorb any drainage from the site. The use of a dressing after the first week is optional if there is no drainage around the tube site. It is important to know how much fluid was put into the balloon at the time of placement (if the tube is a balloon tube) and what manufacturer made the tube. The manufacturer's Web sites have specific information about their tubes and recommendations about how often to check the fluid levels in the balloon. If leakage is a problem, check the balloon for fluid and refill the balloon to the level placed at the time of the tube insertion. Use sterile water, not saline, to fill the balloon to avoid salt encrustation (Roveron and Antonini, 2018).

KEY POINT

If there is crusting around the opening, use a water-moistened cotton-tipped applicator to gently remove.

The time before the tube can be used for feeding varies with the procedure performed and the preference of the provider. When feeding is allowed, it is important to routinely flush the tube to prevent clogging from occurring. It should be flushed with 30 mL water before and after each feeding and every 4 to 6 hours when the patient has continuous feedings. If it is possible for a patient to swallow medication, this is the preferred route of administration. If the medication must be given per tube, use 15 mL water to flush before and after giving each medication. Each medication should be given separately and not be mixed into the enteral feeding. Consult with a pharmacist about extended release medications or enteric coated medications as these should not be crushed. Use of liquid medication should also be discussed with a pharmacist as additives or dosages may need to be adjusted depending on the patient's needs (Boullata et al., 2017).

If the tube does become clogged, try the following:

- Be sure the tube is not kinked.
- Flush the tube with lukewarm water using a 60-mL catheter-tipped syringe and a push-pull motion to loosen the obstruction.
- If it is still clogged, repeat the above step with one pancreatic enzyme tablet and one sodium bicarbonate tablet crushed and mixed in 5 to 10 mL of water (Roveron & Antonini, 2018).
- If the tube cannot be unclogged, contact the health care provider. Instrumentation or replacement may be necessary.
- Do not use soda or cranberry juice as this may actually cause more obstruction to occur (Roveron & Antonini, 2018).

MANAGING SKIN COMPLICATIONS

There are many types of possible complications with enteral feeding tubes. The most serious adverse effects, such as abscess or necrotizing infection in the skin around the tube; buried bumper syndrome, where the internal tube bumper becomes imbedded in the gastric mucosa; or hemorrhage at the tube site, are uncommon. Complications that may require a consult for the WOC nurse are those that involve skin breakdown (**Table 19-1**). The most common cause of skin breakdown around the tube site is leakage of gastric contents on the skin. This is caused by movement of the tube that may enlarge the opening in the skin. To stabilize the tube, gently pull up on the tube until the internal anchoring device (bumper) or balloon is against the wall of the stomach and then slide the external stabilizer down to rest comfortably on the skin without excess tension. If there is an external stabilizer sutured to the skin with a jejunostomy and the sutures are no longer intact, it may be necessary to have these replaced. This tube is not secured with an internal bumper or a balloon, so it will migrate if sutures are not present. If there are sutures in the bumper of a PEG tube stabilizer, they may impede the ability to care for the skin and prevent skin complications such as irritant dermatitis and device-related pressure injuries. It is appropriate to ask if these can be removed after healing has taken place. If there is no external bumper, the use of a commercial stabilizing device to secure the tube (**Fig. 19-4**) or taping the tube in place may prevent movement. With a balloon-tipped tube, loss of water in the balloon will cause migration of the tube. Replacing a leaking tube with a larger diameter tube in the hopes of obtaining a better seal is not effective and is contraindicated (Boullata et al., 2017). This will further enlarge and distort the leaking tube tract. In rare cases of persistent leakage, the tube must be removed and placed in a different site allowing the original site to close.

KEY POINT

It is recommended that the amount of water in the balloon is checked weekly and replaced with the correct amount. Consider teaching the patient or family to weekly check the fluid and replace when needed.

HYPERTROPHIC GRANULATION

It is thought that a poorly secured tube or one that migrates easily in and out of the skin opening may be a causative factor in the development of hypertrophic granulation tissue or hypergranulation around an enteral tube. Leakage of fluid, use of hydrogen peroxide, and poor fitting low-profile GT may also contribute to this overgrowth of tissue. The tissue itself is moist and often

TABLE 19-1 COMPLICATIONS ASSOCIATED WITH ENTERAL TUBES

TYPE	CONTRIBUTING FACTORS	MANAGEMENT
Irritant dermatitis	Leakage of gastric secretions Tube displacement Improper balloon inflation Inadequate tube stabilization Recent weight loss Increased abdominal pressure related to chronic cough, constipation, hypertonicity/spasticity Presence of granulation tissue/hyperplasia Inability to decompress gastric content (i.e., burp) Delayed gastric motility Body structure changes (spinal stenosis, scoliosis) Failure of tract closure related to inadequate wound healing	1. If balloon-tipped tube is in place, check for proper inflation of balloon and add fluid if amount is inadequate 2. Check balloon volume weekly 3. Stabilize the tube by gently pulling up on the tube until the internal bumper or balloon is against the stomach wall, slide the external stabilizer down to rest comfortably on the skin without tension 4. Apply barrier ointment, such as zinc oxide or alcohol-free liquid skin barrier to irritated skin 5. Use light gauze, or foam dressings to absorb fluid and change whenever wet 6. If unable to stop leakage, consider pouching with nipple device to bring the tube through the front of the pouch (**Box 19-1**)
Medical device–related pressure injury	Excess tension of the bumper against the skin Failure to rotate bumper after initial insertion Location of tube in a skin fold Weight gain or increased girth Sutured bumpers	1. Ensure the stabilizer rests comfortably against the skin without excess tension 2. Rotate bumper daily if appropriate 3. Consider eliminating the need for the bumper by utilizing a tube anchoring device 4. Depending on the characteristics of the injury, consider the following: 5. Skin barrier powder, sheet hydrocolloid, or absorptive dressing 6. Ask health care provider if suture removal (if present) is an option
Fungal infection	Chronic moisture in the area of the tube Deep skin fold around the tube On systemic antibiotics Receiving immunosuppressive medications	1. Keep the skin dry 2. Use moisture barrier creams or alcohol-free liquid skin barrier 3. Apply topical antifungal powder twice daily and continue for 2 wk after rash is resolved 4. Recommend systemic treatment if topical is not effective
Cellulitis	Invasive procedure Immunosuppression Diabetes Inappropriate or excessive handling of tube Chronic steroid use	1. Observe the skin for erythema, induration, purulent drainage 2. Assess pain with palpation 3. Recommend a systemic antibiotic if indicated by assessment
Hypertrophic granulation tissue	Moist friable tissue at the site where the tube enters the abdomen. Tissue is composed of connective tissue and tiny blood vessels and bleeds easily	1. Stabilize the tube if the etiology is felt to be a tube that is not secured 2. Consider use of silver nitrate cautery, topical steroid, or antimicrobial foam

is friable, which contributes to leakage of formula and enteral fluid round the tube creating a cycle of leakage being both cause and effect. In some cases, it is painful to touch and may bleed easily. The presence of this tissue is not considered a serious complication, but there are reports in the literature linking it to wound infection and cellulitis around the tube (Pars & Cavusoglu, 2019). A wide variety of treatment options from the application of topical antimicrobial agents, steroids or silver impregnated thin foams, cauterization with silver nitrate, and surgical removal have been described in the literature, but the evidence is anecdotal. Nurses in one community health district in the United Kingdom described a care routine for those persons (n = 25) in homes or care facilities with GTs and an overgrowth of granulation tissue around them. They used an antimicrobial cleanser and an antimicrobial foam dressing around the tube for 6 weeks and checked on them at 2-week intervals. At the

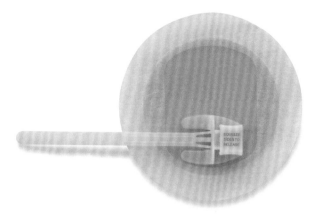

FIGURE 19-4. Drain Tube Attachment Device. Courtesy of Hollister Incorporated.

end of the first 2 weeks, one third (*n* = 8) of the patients no longer had hypergranulation present. At the end of 6 weeks, the problem was resolved in six additional patients. The remaining patients received a silver alginate under a foam dressing, and if that did not resolve the hypergranulation, a steroid cream was applied (Warriner & Spruce, 2014). When hypergranulation tissue is present, it is important to stabilize the tube to reduce movement of the tube in the tract. Silver nitrate applicator sticks should be used with care to avoid getting the silver nitrate on intact skin as this may cause a burning sensation. More than one application may be needed. In extreme cases, surgical excision of the tissue may be required (Roveron & Antonini, 2018).

BOX 19-1   PROCEDURE FOR POUCH APPLICATION AROUND THE GASTROSTOMY TUBE

Equipment:

Ostomy pouch: One piece
Scissors
Skin barrier powder
Wet and dry cloths
No sting skin prep
Cotton-tipped applicators
Gloves
Catheter holder device
Water-resistant tape

Directions:

1. Clamp tube and turn off feeding.
2. Remove the pink tape from around the tube where it exits the pouching system and gently remove the pouch using adhesive remover or warm water. Be careful not to pull or dislodge the tube.
3. Clean the skin with water and pat dry. Cleanse the area under the tube bumper by inserting a cotton-tipped applicator between sutures. Sprinkle skin barrier powder under the bumper to protect the skin.
4. If there is any skin breakdown (**A**), sprinkle skin barrier powder on the skin, rub in, and seal with alcohol-free liquid skin barrier.
5. Cut an opening in the skin barrier of the one-piece pouching system to fit around the bumper. Cut an X-shaped opening on the front of the pouch so the gastrostomy tube can be pulled through (**B**).

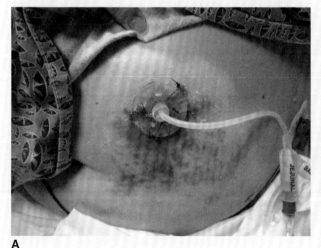

A

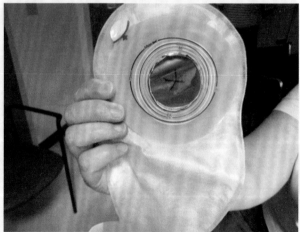

B

BOX 19-1   PROCEDURE FOR POUCH APPLICATION AROUND THE GASTROSTOMY TUBE (*Continued*)

6. Place catheter holder device over X cut in front of the pouch to secure the tube and avoid leakage (**C**). Instructions come with each device. Cut a hole in the nipple large enough to pull the tube through (**D**).

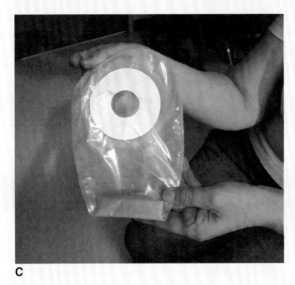

C

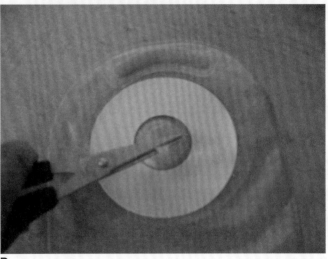

D

7. Pull tube through the opening and place the pouch on the skin. Make sure the skin is dry before placing the pouch (**E**). Use water resistant tape around the tube where it exits the pouch to seal the opening in the nipple (**F**).

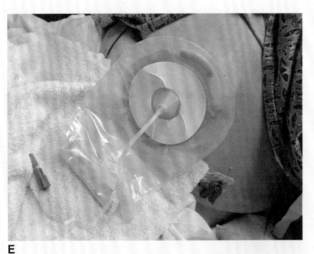

E

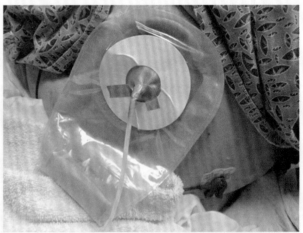

F

TUBE REPLACEMENT

GTs may become accidentally dislodged for a variety of reasons. The stabilizer may have loosened, water may have leaked from the balloon, inadvertent traction is placed on the tube, or the patient may have pulled it out. The latter cause is usually secondary to an altered mental state. In these patients, a low-profile tube may be appropriate (**Fig. 19-5**). The low-profile tube may also be used as a replacement tube when the patient wishes to have one for convenience and ease of concealing the tube under clothing. It is required to measure the stoma tract; there are measuring devices that determine the size tract for low-profile tube needed. This is especially important in pediatric patients as a child is growing and may need to have another size tube. GT replacement may be done by a nurse, but verification of workplace policies and regulations of the state board of nursing should guide the decision to do this. In a healthy person, the tract in which the GT is placed would be healed in 2 to 3 weeks. The patients requiring enteral access for feeding are usually malnourished and have chronic conditions that may interfere with healing, so it is advisable to wait 4 to 6 weeks before a nurse should attempt tube replacement (Boullata et al., 2017). There is a risk of inserting the tube in the peritoneum if the tract is not healed. When a tube is dislodged unexpectedly after 6 weeks from original placement, it must be replaced as soon as possible before the tract and the opening in the skin begins to close (**Box 19-2**). For patients at home, a

FIGURE 19-5. Low-Profile Gastrostomy Tube. MIC-KEY™ G Feeding Tube is a Registered Trademark or Trademark of Halyard Health, Inc. or its affiliates. Image copyright © 2014 HYH. All rights reserved.

BOX 19-2	**PROCEDURE FOR CHANGING A GASTROSTOMY TUBE**

Equipment:
  Gastrostomy tube of the same size as the one being removed
  Water-based lubricant
  Empty 10-mL syringe
  10-mL syringe filled with water
  60-mL catheter-tipped syringe
  Gauze pads
  Gloves

Directions:
1. Inform the patient of the purpose of the procedure.
2. Place the patient in supine position or elevate the head 30 degrees, as the patient prefers.
3. Test the balloon on the new tube by filling it with water and ascertain that there is no leak. Remove the water from the balloon.
4. Slide the bumper up the tube to make sure it moves easily.
5. If the old tube is in place (i.e., it has not been inadvertently removed), use an empty syringe to remove the water from the balloon through the aspiration port. Reaspirate to be sure the balloon is empty.
6. Pull the tube gently out. Note the length of the tube from skin level to the tip.
7. Use gauze to wipe away any gastric contents that come out with the tube. The insertion site and 5 cm beyond the site should be cleansed with normal saline and dried well.
8. Lubricate the replacement tube. Do not use a petroleum-based lubricant.
9. Insert the lubricated tube into the stoma opening a couple of centimeters past the length of the tube that was removed.
10. Fill the balloon with the required amount of water.
11. Pull the tube up until you feel resistance against the stomach wall.
12. Slide the bumper down the tube so that there is only 2 to 3 mm of space between the bumper and the skin. No dressing is required. The tube should be able to be turned around freely in the opening. Rotate the tube 360 degrees to confirm the tube has free rotation.
13. Use the 60-mL syringe to aspirate gastric contents to affirm correct placement.
14. If no gastric contents can be aspirated, connect the tube to a bedside drainage bag and wait 20 minutes to see if the contents drain.
15. If there is no drainage in 20 minutes, tube placement should be confirmed with an abdominal radiograph in the oblique position using contrast.
16. Do not start feeding or flush the tube until there is confirmation of intragastric placement.
17. Document the size of tube and the amount of water that was used to inflate the balloon.

---

family member may be taught to do this to avoid loss of access. Placing a tube into the opening will solve the immediate problem of maintaining the tract, but the tube should not be used until proper placement has been ascertained by radiographic study or return of gastric fluid through the tube (Boullata et al., 2017). Replacement of GTs is preferred, but a Foley catheter may be used temporarily if a GT is not available. The only reason for using a tube not designed for the GI tract is to keep the tract open until a GT can be obtained and inserted. (Boullata et al., 2017)

KEY POINT

The patient should understand that when the tube falls out, they should replace the tube immediately or seek medical attention for replacement.

PEDIATRIC CONSIDERATIONS

The use of enteral feeding tube is a widely used, effective, and standard means of meeting the nutritional needs of child with a dysfunctional GI tract or who is unable to take oral nutrition. Enteral tubes are common in pediatric patients with neurological disorders as well as diseases resulting in malnutrition including cancer, short gut syndrome, cystic fibrosis, and cardiac and metabolic illnesses (Pars & Cavusoglu, 2019). The procedure is considered minimally invasive, and patients are discharged a short time after the procedure (Rollins et al., 2013). However, the procedure is not without risks and complications. A review of the literature demonstrates that patients with GTs have significant number of complications and emergency department (ED) visits for nonurgent tube issues. According to Pars and Cavusoglu (2019), the frequency of common minor complications ranges from 2% to 55% and includes tube blockage, dislocation, and peristomal skin infections. Major complications including aspiration, bleeding, pneumoperitoneum, and peritonitis range in frequency from 5% to 25%. Other common complications include leakage, peristomal skin breakdown, enlarged tracts, medical device–related pressure injuries, and hypergranulation tissue.

The management of these complications is the same as for adult patients with a feeding tube. Tube dislodgment may be decreased with a low-profile tube, and these are used frequently in pediatric patients. A retrospective study by Novotny et al. (2009) of 223 young children who received a standard PEG (n = 110) versus a low-profile PEG (n = 113) showed a significant decrease in tube dislodgment with the low-profile tube and no difference in infection rate. There was also a significantly decreased length of hospital stay in the low-profile tube group. There was not a difference in ED visits for minor complications with the tubes. Use of a silicone foam dressing can be used as a pressure injury prevention strategy for patients at risk. Silver impregnated moisture wicking fabric can also be used for moisture management and treatment of hypergranulation tissue. It is important to wrap the fabric upward around the tube if the goal is moisture management. This will allow the moisture to be wicked away from the skin (Singh, 2016). According to a 4-year prospective study by Goldberg et al. (2010), infection developed in 37% of patients with the majority of infections occurring during the first 15 days after placement. Hypergranulation tissue was noted in 68% of children with a recurrence in 17% of patients after receiving treatment. A 2009 retrospective cross-sectional descriptive study by Saavedra et al. (2009) showed that over a 23-month period, 77 patients had 181 ED visits for complaints related to the GT. Dislodgment of the GT occurred in 62% of the patients, and 75% of the visits were for GT replacement. In a study of 247 patients treated at a tertiary children's hospital, Correa et al. (2014) found that 20% of patients accounted for 44 ED visits within the first 30 days of discharge for complaints of leaking, mild clogs, and hypergranulation (hyperplasia) tissue. During the time period of 31 to 365 days post discharge, 40 additional patients returned to the ED a total of 71 times for potentially avoidable visits.

It is clear that care of these children creates substantial stress for family caregivers specific education on recognizing potential complications and how to manage them must be provided to the patients and their families in order to decrease the number of avoidable visits to the clinic and ED or rehospitalizations. It is important to assess the learning style of the family, engage an interdisciplinary approach, and incorporate multimedia into family education. Families that are confident in their knowledge and ability to provide needed care may have a decrease in anxiety and increase in satisfaction (Schweitzer et al., 2014). In addition, the use of patient messaging and uploading of patient's photos via the electronic health record (HER) is a secure way for families to obtain answers and a plan of care for minor issues. This is an area in which a WOC nurse can have tremendous impact on patient and caregiver quality of life.

⬤ NEPHROSTOMY TUBES

Percutaneous nephrostomy tubes are inserted through the skin and into the renal pelvis of the kidney. The purpose of percutaneous nephrostomy tubes is to facilitate drainage of urine after a partial or complete obstruction has occurred or if a urine leak is present (diverting the urine away from the leak to allow healing). Indications for use include tumors, strictures, dilations, and kidney stone removal. The tube exits through the flank and is connected to extension tubing and drains into a leg or bedside drainage bag. Important factors in the management of this tube include tube stabilization to prevent pulling, kinking, or dislodgment; possible tube flushing with MD order; prevention of skin irritation; and signs of infection (Martin & Baker, 2019).

Tube stabilization can be accomplished with the use of a commercial catheter holder. Tape may also be used if commercial devices are not available. When securing the tube, consider the tube angle to prevent kinking.

In some instances, flushing of the tube may be needed if there is an absence of urine; persistent flank pain; or presence of clots, debris, or sediment (Seladi-Shulman, 2018). Consult facility protocols and/or health care provider guidelines for this practice. Generally, 5 to 10 mL of sterile, normal saline is flushed into the tube. Do not force the saline into the tube. After saline is instilled, reconnect to straight drainage. If unable to instill saline, the health care provider must be notified.

During the first 2 weeks post procedure, sterile gauze nephrostomy dressings should be kept dry and be changed daily and as needed for drainage. For sensitive skin, consider the use of adhesive remover or releaser to loosen the dressing. If a sterile transparent dressing is in use, it must be changed every 3 days. After the initial 2-week period, the dressing should be changed twice per week and if wet or lifting off (Martin & Baker, 2019). If skin irritation occurs, consider the use of an alcohol-free liquid skin barrier to protect the area. If a fungal rash appears to be present, use an antifungal powder rather than an ointment or cream. If there appears to be sensitivity to the adhesive, consider a dressing with a silicone backing.

Patient and family education includes how to flush the tube if ordered by health care provider, signs of infection, skin care, how to use and care for a leg or bedside drainage bag, and how often the nephrostomy tube will be changed (usually every 2 to 3 months).

 BILIARY TUBES

Biliary tubes are necessary when an alternate method of draining bile from the hepatobiliary system is needed. Often, the bile ducts are blocked, resulting in a buildup of bile in the liver that can lead to jaundice, nausea, vomiting, itching, fever, dark urine, and infection; see **Box 19-3**. Blockages are caused by tumors, strictures, and gallstones. The thin tube is inserted through the skin into the bile ducts by an interventional radiologist and is connected to a small drainage bag.

BOX 19-3 SIGNS AND SYMPTOMS OF BILIARY TUBE BLOCKAGE

Leakage at exit site
Decrease in bile drainage output
Inability to flush the tube
Fever, chills, nausea, and increased jaundice
(Memorial Sloan Kettering Cancer Center (MSKCC) (2017) About your biliary drainage catheter. https://www.mskcc.org/cancer-care/patient-education/about-your-biliary-drainage-catheter.)

Management of the biliary tube includes adequate securement of the tube to prevent kinking or dislodgment, flushing of the tube with MD order, dressing changes, and keeping the drain bag below the waist to facilitate proper drainage (MSKCC, 2017).

Dressing changes should be done weekly and whenever wet or soiled. For sensitive skin, consider the use of adhesive remover or releaser to loosen the dressing. If skin irritation develops, an alcohol-free liquid skin barrier may be used to protect the area. Flushing the tube is done twice daily with 10 mL or other prescribed amount of sterile saline. Never force the saline into the tube. If there is inability to instill, pain occurs, or leakage at the exit site occurs, the health care provider must be notified (MSKCC, 2017).

KEY POINT

Patient and caregiver education must include routine care of the catheter, assessment of catheter integrity, signs of infection, and signs and symptoms of a blockage.

 CONCLUSIONS

The provision of adequate nutrition support in the hospital setting is the standard of care. The use of the GI tract for feeding that is provided through enteral access is preferred to the use of parenteral nutrition whenever possible (Boullata et al., 2017). It carries benefits physiologically for the patient as well as decreases the significant risks associated with parenteral nutrition. Patients with higher acuity are candidates for enteral access through endoscopic, radiologic, and surgical techniques available in various care settings. The WOC nurse must know what procedures may be done in his or her practice setting to be prepared for managing the care of these patients and those with other types of percutaneous tubes. Caregiver support and patient education are essential for those patients leaving the hospital with percutaneous tubes, and the WOC nurse can play an important role in preparing both patients and caregivers for discharge (see Care of Feeding Tubes, Appendix I).

REFERENCES

Boullata, J., Correra, A., Harvey, L., et al. (2017). ASPEN safe practices for enteral nutrition therapy. *Journal of Parenteral and Enteral Nutrition, 41*(1), 15–103.

Correa, J. A., Fallon, S. C., Murphy, K. M., et al. (2014). Resource utilization after gastrostomy tube placement: Defining areas of improvement for future quality improvement projects. *Journal of Pediatric Surgery, 49*(11), 1598–1601. doi: http://dx.doi.org/10.1016/j.jpedsurg.2014.06.015.

Goldberg, E., Barton, S., Xanthopoulos, M. S., et al. (2010). A descriptive study of complications of gastrostomy tubes in children. *Journal of Pediatric Nursing, 25*(2), 72–80. doi: 10.1016/j.pedn.2008.07.008.

Kim, C. Y., Patel, M. B., Miller, M. J., et al. (2010). Gastrostomy-to-gastrojejunostomy tube conversion: Impact of the method of original gastrostomy tube placement. *Journal of Vascular Interventional Radiology: JVIR, 21*(7), 1031–1037.

Martin, R., Baker, H. (2019). Nursing care and management of patients with a nephrostomy. *Nursing Times [online], 115*, 11, 40–43.

Memorial Sloan Kettering Cancer Center (MSKCC). (2017). About your biliary drainage catheter. Retrieved from https://www.mskcc.org/cancer-care/patient-education/about-your-biliary-drainage-catheter

Miller, K. R., McClave, S. A., Kiraly, L. N., et al. (2014). A tutorial on enteral access in adult patients in the hospitalized setting. *JPEN: Journal of Parental and Enteral Nutrition, 38*(3), 282–294.

Mizrahi, I., Garg, M., Divino, C. M., et al. (2014). Comparison of laparoscopic vs open approach to gastrostomy tubes. *JSLS: Journal of the Society of Laparoendoscopic Surgeons, 18*(1), 28–33.

Novotny, N. M., Vegeler, R. C., Breckler, F. D., et al. (2009). Percutaneous endoscopic gastrostomy buttons in children: Superior to tubes. *Journal of Pediatric Surgery, 44*(6), 1193–1196.

Pars, H., & Cavusoglu, H. (2019). A literature review of percutaneous endoscopic gastrostomy. *Gastroenterology Nursing, 42*(4), 351–359.

Requarth, J. (2011). Image-guided palliative care procedures. *Surgical Clinics of North America, 91*(2), 367–402.

Rollins, H., Nathwani, N., & Morridson, D. (2013). Optimizing wound care in a child with an infected gastrostomy exit site. *British Journal of Nursing, 22*, 1275–1279.

Roveron, G, & Antonini, M. (2018). Clinical practice guidelines for nursing management of percutaneous endoscopic gastrostomy and jejunostomy (PEG/PEJ) in adult patients. *Journal of Wound, Ostomy, and Continence Nursing, 45*(4), 326–334.

Saavedra, H., Loske, J. D., Shanley, L., et al. (2009). Gastrostomy tube related complaints in the pediatric emergency department identifying opportunities for improvement. *Pediatric Emergency Care, 25*(11), 728–732.

Schweitzer, et al., 2014. Evaluation of a discharge education protocol for pediatric patients with gastrostomy tubes. *Journal of Pediatric Health Care, 28*(5), 420–428.

Seladi-Shulman, J. (2018). Caring for your nephrostomy tube. Retrieved from https://www.healthline.com/health/nephrostomy-tube-care

Singh, C. D. (2016). Use of a moisture wicking fabric for prevention of skin damage around drains and parenteral access lines. *Journal of Wound, Ostomy, and Continence Nursing, 43*(5), 551–553.

Warriner, L., & Spruce, P. (2014). Managing over granulation tissue around gastrostomy sites. *British Journal of Nursing, 21*(5), S20–S25.

QUESTIONS

1. The nurse is assessing a patient who has a nasogastric tube (NGT) in place following gastric surgery. What complication should the patient be monitored for?
   A. Fluid and electrolyte imbalance
   B. Aspiration pneumonia
   C. Constipation
   D. Gastroesophageal reflux

2. A patient is scheduled for placement of a feeding tube in interventional radiology. What potential complication is avoided by using this method instead of the endoscopic method?
   A. Bleeding
   B. Soft tissue infection
   C. Upper tract trauma
   D. Liver trauma

3. What intervention is most likely to prevent hypergranulation tissue from forming around a gastrostomy tube?
   A. Cleaning the area around the tube with hydrogen peroxide
   B. Stabilizing the tube to reduce movement of the tube in the tract
   C. The use of several gauze pads to absorb drainage
   D. Maintenance of the external bumper at least one inch above the skin

4. The nurse is teaching a patient routine tube care for a newly placed percutaneous endoscopic gastrostomy (PEG) tube. What statement follows recommended guidelines for this care?
   A. Following placement of the tube, the external bolster will be left in place for 1 week.
   B. A water-resistant dressing should be placed over the tube and insertion site and left in place for 48 hours.
   C. The site of the tube should be washed with mild soap and water, rinsed well with water, and dried daily.
   D. One gauze drain sponge may be placed under the bumper of a tube that is sutured in place to absorb any drainage from the site.

5. The nurse is providing care for a patient with a gastrostomy tube. What is a recommended intervention when using the tube to administer medication?
   A. Flush the tube with 15 mL water before and after each medication.
   B. Flush the tube with 60 mL water before giving medication.
   C. Cut tablets in half before administering through the tube.
   D. Do not give any medications that do not come in liquid form.

6. What would be the first intervention when a feeding tube becomes clogged?
  A. Insert a brush into the tube to remove any mechanical obstruction.
  B. Aspirate fluid from the tube and instill 20 mL of cranberry juice into the tube.
  C. Use pancreatic enzymes and sodium bicarbonate tablets crushed and mixed in water.
  D. Use a 60-mL catheter-tipped syringe filled with lukewarm water and pull back and forth on the plunger to dislodge the obstruction.

7. If a G tube leaks with feedings, what is the most common skin complication that is likely to occur?
  A. Irritant dermatitis
  B. Candidiasis
  C. Cellulitis
  D. Allergic reactions

8. When using a low profile G tube, it is important to measure the tract to select the correct G tube length. Ongoing monitoring of the size is especially important in which population of patients?
  A. Geriatric
  B. Terminally ill
  C. Pediatric
  D. Young adults

9. A patient has a percutaneous nephrostomy tube. Which condition describes the most likely reason it was placed?
  A. It is an alternative to dialysis for urinary drainage.
  B. The patient has experienced frequent urinary tract infections.
  C. The patient has urinary incontinence.
  D. Urine cannot pass into the bladder because of an ureteral obstruction.

10. A patient has a percutaneous biliary tube for malignant obstruction of the bile duct. The caregiver reports a 24-hour history of leakage of bile fluid around the tube that has saturated several 4 × 4 gauze pads. There is very little fluid in the drainage bag. What is the first action the nurse should take to resolve this problem?
  A. Protect the skin from the bile drainage with a skin barrier cream.
  B. Flush the tube to see if there is blockage causing the fluid to leak around the tube.
  C. Call the health care provider to arrange for removal of the tube.
  D. Instruct the caregiver to change the dressings more frequently to avoid contact of the fluid with the skin.

ANSWERS AND RATIONALES

1. B. Rationale: Dislodgement of the tube could result in fluid going into the lungs causing aspiration pneumonia.

2. C. Rationale: There is no need for the use of an endoscope to ascertain placement with the radiologic procedure, so the upper GI tract is not at risk for trauma.

3. B. Rationale: A tube that is not stabilized can move in the tract, can damage the tissue around the tube thus stabilizing the tube may prevent hypertrophic granulation tissue formation.

4. C. Rationale: While evidence for care is lacking, the generally accepted standard for tube site care is daily cleansing with mild soap and water.

5. A. Rationale: 15 mL of water is adequate to ensure patency of the tube and clear the tube of residual medication after completing administration.

6. D. Rationale: Using a push-pull technique with warm water in a catheter tip syringe is the first method used to dislodge a tube blockage.

7. A. Rationale: If leakage occurs around the tube, the fluid may contain both the formula mixed with the gastric fluid. Gastric fluid and formula will cause skin breakdown, irritant dermatitis.

8. C. Rationale: The tube length is critical for a good fit of the low profile tube and because pediatric patients frequently have low profile tubes, and as they grow, the length between the skin and the stomach will change necessitating a new tube length.

9. D. Rationale: Nephrostomy tubes are used to prevent hydronephrosis resulting from the inability of the kidney to drain into the bladder due to ureteral obstruction.

10. B. Rationale: Obstruction of the tube is the most likely cause of this problem. Skin protection is very important but, first, the tube function needs to be assessed. The health care provider will need to be notified if the tube is unable to be flushed, but exchange, not removal of the tube, would be the likely result.

Surgical Procedures

SURGICAL PROCEDURE	ANATOMICAL RESECTION	INDICATIONS FOR
Abdominal perineal resection	Sigmoid colon, rectum, and anus; closure of the perineum; and creation of end colostomy	Distal rectum cancers in which distal negative margins cannot be achieved, those with direct extension into levator muscles, or patients with preoperative fecal incontinence
Total pelvic exenteration	**Women:** removal of all pelvic organs; rectum, distal sigmoid colon, urinary bladder with distal ureters, internal iliac vessels, pelvic node dissection, uterus, ovaries, tubes, and vagina **Men:** bladder, prostate, urethra, seminal vessels, vas deferens, rectum and lower colon, pelvic node dissection A urinary diversion, either continent diversion or ileal conduit, and descending colostomy will be created.	Advanced or recurrent cancer of the pelvis, rectal tumors with invasion to adjacent pelvic structures, or gynecologic or urinary malignancies with involvement of the rectum
Anterior exenteration	Removal of female or male reproductive organs, bladder along with pelvic nodes, the colon and rectum remain. A urinary diversion, either continent diversion or ileal conduit, will be created.	
Posterior exenteration	Removal of rectum, lower colon, anus along with pelvic node dissection. The urinary tract is spared. This results in a colostomy.	
Segmental colectomy	Partial removal of colon with ileorectal anastomosis (small intestine or colon to rectum), if the rectum has no disease	Crohn's disease
Total abdominal colectomy with Hartmann's	Removal of the entire colon; the remaining rectum and anus remain with the top of the rectal stump closed with sutures; anus remains open	Colon cancer, ulcerative colitis; other indications may include ischemic colitis, diverticular disease
Ileocecostomy	With the removal of terminal ileum and cecum, two ends of the bowel are brought together in side–side or side–end anastomosis	Crohn's disease
Subtotal colectomy	Resection of part of the diseased colon	Crohn's disease Perianal disease and sepsis of rectum and anus
Total proctocolectomy	Removal of colon and rectum Permanent ileostomy	Ulcerative colitis, Crohn's disease, familial polyposis

(Continued)

SURGICAL PROCEDURE	ANATOMICAL RESECTION	INDICATIONS FOR
Ileal pouch anal anastomosis	Removal of entire colon and rectum; preserving anal sphincter, ileal pouch is created from the small intestine Performed in one, two, or three steps One step: Removal of colon and rectum, creation of ileal pouch, connected to anus: no fecal diversion Two steps: Step one: removal of colon and rectum, creation of IPAA and connected to anus and temporary loop ileostomy; Step two: closure of stoma Three steps: Step one: removal of colon (colectomy) creation of end ileostomy; Step two: take down of stoma, creation of ileal pouch with anastomosis; Step three: take down of ileostomy and bowel continuity is restored	Ulcerative colitis, familial polyposis
Kock pouch	Internal reservoir is made from small bowel and nipple valve created as continence device	UC, familial polyposis
Ileal conduit	Removal of the bladder (cystectomy), in males the prostate and lymph nodes, in females the posterior wall of the vagina, uterus, ovaries, and lymph nodes. 10–15 cm of ileum, proximal to ileocecal valve, is resected. Proximal end is closed and the distal end is used to create stoma. Ureters are anastomosed into the ileal segment.	Bladder cancer Neurogenic bladder Pyocystis Refractory cystitis Urinary cystitis
Cystectomy with Indiana pouch	Removal of bladder (cystectomy) Internal reservoir constructed with 10–12 cm of ileum (catheter channel), ileocecal valve (continent mechanism), and right colon (reservoir)	Bladder cancer
Cystectomy with neobladder (orthotropic)	Removal of bladder (cystectomy) Segment of ileum is used to create reservoir. Ureters implanted, and distal portion is connected to urethra to allow voiding	Bladder cancer
Vesicostomy	Bladder is externalized to the abdominal wall	Myelomeningocele (spina bifida)
Mitrofanoff	An abdominal catheterizable channel constructed between the bladder and the skin utilizing appendix or bowel as a conduit	For patients who are unable to catheterize their own urethra.

American Cancer Society www.cancer.org	Mission: To save lives. Web site provides basic information about cancer and its causes to in-depth information on specific cancer types—including risk factors, early detection, diagnosis, and treatment options.
American College of Gastroenterology www.patients.gi.org	Mission: To enhance the ability of members to provide world-class care to patients with digestive disorders and advance the profession through excellence and innovation. Resources include guidelines and other education tools.
American College of Surgeons www.fasc.org	Mission: To improve the care of the surgical patient and to safeguard standards of care in an optimal and ethical practice environment. Among other products is the Ostomy Home Skills Kit, which supports patients with educational and simulation materials to learn and practice the skills needed for optimal postoperative recovery. The kit can be used to prepare a patient anticipating ostomy surgery. There is also a pediatric version that can aid in the education of parents whose infant/child is facing ostomy surgery.
American Gastroenterological Association www.gastro.org	Mission: To empower clinicians and researchers to improve digestive health. Colorectal Cancer Guidelines, IBD and Bowel Disorders Guidelines, as well as patient info are available on the site.
American Society of Colorectal Surgeons www.fascrs.org	Mission: A community of health care professionals who are dedicated to advancing the understanding, prevention, and treatment of disorders of the colon, rectum and anus. Available resources: Clinical Guidelines covering ERAS, colorectal cancers, bowel preps, etc.
Bladder Cancer Awareness Network Bcan.org	Mission: National advocacy organization devoted to advancing bladder cancer research and supporting those impacted by the disease. Tool kits for patient and resources for patients dealing with bladder cancer including treatment options
Crohn's and Colitis Foundation https://www.crohnscolitisfoundation.org/	Mission: To cure Crohn's disease and ulcerative colitis, and to improve the quality of life of children and adults affected by these diseases. Clinician and patient resources, support group information
Cystic Fibrosis Foundation www.cff.org	Mission: To cure cystic fibrosis and to provide all people with CF the opportunity to lead long, fulfilling lives by funding research and drug development, partnering with the CF community, and advancing high-quality, specialized care. Treatment and therapies and living with CF as well as colorectal cancer are covered.
GIKids www.kidsibd.org	Mission: Working to reach out directly to families, kids, and teens who live with digestive conditions to provide them with the information they need to understand and improve their digestive health, work with their health care providers, live a more independent life, and understand what works in plain language instead of medical jargon. IBD information is available on the site. Resources include nutrition guides, podcasts with various topics, videos, and PDFs.
International Foundation for Functional Gastrointestinal Disorders www.iffgd.org	Mission: To inform, assist, and support people affected by gastrointestinal (GI) disorders and support or encourage research. Topics covered include constipation, IBD, gastroparesis, incontinence, and GI mobility.
Just like me IBD http://www.justlikemeibd.org/join-the-community/	Mission: Web site offered by Crohn's and Colitis Foundation for teens and young adults. Describes living and coping with IBD and various topics of interest to young adults

(Continued)

Pull-Thru Network www.pullthrunetwork.org	Mission: Providing information, education, support, and advocacy for families, children, teens, and adults who are living with the challenges of congenital anorectal, colorectal, and/or urogenital disorders and any of the associated diagnoses. Access to articles, care guides, handouts, quarterly newsletters
Quality of Life Association www.qla-ostomy.org	Mission: Educate on advances in ostomy options; empower through information and support. To be a resource for individuals, as well as the medical community seeking information about continent ostomies. Information on continent ostomies, management, and troubleshooting
Short Gut Support www.shortgutsupport.com	Mission: To provide parents and families of children with short gut syndrome with support and resources to help them to become better advocates and caregivers for their children through discussion and education about short gut syndrome, treatments, and therapies. Online community, support, and resources on living with short gut syndrome
The J Pouch Group www.j-jpouch	Mission: Dedicated to the ileoanal anastomosis or J pouch operation. Support and information regarding the ileoanal anastomosis, forums, and information regarding the J pouch operation
United Ostomy Associations of America www.ostomy.org	Mission: Supports, empowers, and advocates for people who have had or who will have ostomy or continent diversion surgery. Provides ostomy information, support, and advocacy
Wound Ostomy and Continence Nurses Society www.wocn.org	Mission: Professional community dedicated to advancing the practice and delivery of expert health care to individuals with wound, ostomy, and continence care needs. Support of members' practice through advocacy, education, and research. Resources include ostomy clinical guidelines, best practice documents, and tools for peristomal assessment and treatment.
Youth Rally www.youthrally.org	Mission: To provide an environment for adolescents living with conditions of the bowel and bladder that encourages self-confidence and independent living. Every year hosts a rally for kids and teens living with conditions of the bowel and bladder at a college campus for a 5-day camp experience.

Selected Ostomy Product Suppliers and Manufacturers

Suppliers stock a large selection; most have toll-free numbers, free shipping, online catalogs with online ordering, and staff who are able to give advice regarding management problems.

Byram Healthcare: www.byramhealthcare.com

Edgepark Medical Supplies: www.edgepark.com

Liberator Medical Supply Inc: www.liberatormedical.com/ostomy-supplies

Liberty Medical: www.libertymedical.com/ostomy/products

Parthenon Co Inc: www.parthenoninc.com

SGV Medical: http://sgvmedical.com

Shield Healthcare: www.shieldhealthcare.com/products/ostomy

Cymed: http://cymedostomy.com

Coloplast: www.us.coloplast.com

ConvaTec: www.convatec.com

Genairex: http://genairex.com

Hollister Inc: www.hollister.com/us/ostomy

Marlen International: www.marlen.com

Nu-Hope Laboratories Inc: www.nu-hope.com

Perma-Type Co Inc: www.perma-type.com

Torbot: www.torbot.com

DISCLAIMER

Brand names/manufacturers are representative examples of ostomy accessories. This list is not inclusive of all products available in the category, nor is it intended to be a recommendation of listed products.

Most major manufacturers of ostomy products will send free samples if requested. Many also have an ostomy nurse on staff

Catheterization of an Ileal or Colon Conduit Stoma: Best Practice for Clinicians

ACKNOWLEDGMENTS

Catheterization of an Ileal or Colon Conduit Stoma: Best Practice for Clinicians

This is an update to the 2012 document Procedure for Obtaining a Urine Sample from a Urostomy, Ileal Conduit, and Colon Conduit: Best Practice for Clinicians, originally developed by the WOCN Society's Clinical Practice Ostomy Committee. Updates to this document were done in 2018. Date Submitted for Initial Review: June 2018.

ORIGINATED BY:

Wound, Ostomy, and Continence Nurses Society's (WOCN) Clinical Practice Ostomy Committee in 2012.

UPDATED/REVISTED: 2018

CONTRIBUTOR:

Mary F. Mahoney, MSN, RN, CWON, CFCN, Chair
Wound and Ostomy Nurse
UnityPoint at Home
Des Moines, Iowa

INTRODUCTION

The number of people in America with a urostomy is not clearly known; reports estimate the range from 150,000 to 250,000 (Turnbull, 2003). One of the most common complications following a radical cystectomy is urinary tract infection (UTI; Kim et al., 2016). According to Mano et al. (2018), the median time for patients with ileoconduits to develop UTI after initial surgery is 11 months. Due to the small number of people with a urostomy, clinicians may not be familiar with the correct technique to obtain a urine sample from a stoma to test for a UTI. Incorrect sampling techniques may lead to inaccurate culture results and inappropriate diagnosis and treatment. This document provides a quick and easy resource for correct technique with and without use of a catheter.

PURPOSE

To obtain an uncontaminated urinary specimen from the stoma for laboratory analysis:

- A clean uncontaminated specimen is necessary for accurate laboratory analysis (urine culture; Faller & Lawrence, 1994; Hampton & Bryant, 1992).

MANAGEMENT

- Specimens from the urostomy sample often have bacteria. Ensure that the specimen obtained is not contaminated during the collection of the sample.
- The sample collection will take several minutes because the ileoconduit serves only as a passageway for the urine, not a reservoir.
- Specimens for culture should never be obtained directly from an existing urostomy pouch or bedside drainage bag (Pagana & Pagana, 2007).
- One small random controlled trial indicated no significant difference between samples obtained directly from the stoma via clean catheterization, obtained by allowing urine to drip into a sterile specimen cup, or obtained from a clean urostomy pouch (Vaarala, 2018).
- Expert opinion is that the best method to obtain the urine specimen from the urostomy is sterile catheterization or clean catch drip collection method.

POUCH CONSIDERATIONS

- Patient with one-piece pouching system: The urostomy pouch system is completely removed, the specimen is collected, and a new pouching system is placed.
- Patient with two-piece pouch systems: One of the following options may be chosen:

- The urostomy pouch is removed from the skin barrier flange (wafer), the specimen collected, and the pouch replaced.
- The urostomy pouching system is completely removed, the specimen collected, and a new pouching system placed.

PROCEDURE WHEN CATHETER IS AVAILABLE

Supplies

- Cleansing solution. Follow institution policy. Further research is needed on the use of antiseptic solutions versus sterile water or saline for cleaning prior to catheter insertion. Some of the solutions recommended are Betadine, chlorhexidine, and soap and water (Gould et al., 2009; Unlu et al., 2007).
- Sterile 4 × 4 gauze.
- Straight catheter for drainage. Faller and Lawrence (1994) suggest the use of a 16-Fr catheter to allow for mucous drainage.
- Water-soluble lubricant.
- Sterile specimen container with lid, label, and laboratory specimen bag.
- Sterile and clean gloves.
- New pouch or pouching system.
- Soft paper towels and/or washcloths for cleaning prior to replacing pouch.

Procedure

- Explain the procedure to the patient.
- Wash hands and use standard precautions.
- Don clean gloves.
- Drape a towel or absorbent pad under the stoma for privacy and absorption if needed.
- Open the supplies; maintain sterility.
- Remove pouch or pouching system and dispose per institutional policy.
- Wash hands.
- Don sterile gloves.
- Use sterile technique.
- Cleanse the stoma with cleansing solution, using a circular motion from stoma opening outward (Faller & Lawrence, 1994).
- Blot the stoma with sterile gauze.
- Place the open end of catheter into the specimen container.
- Lubricate the catheter with a small amount of water-soluble lubricant. Gently insert the catheter tip no more than 2 to 3 inches (5.0 to 7.5 cm) into the stoma (never force—if resistance is detected, rotate catheter until it slides in; Faller & Lawrence, 1994; Hampton & Bryant, 1992).
- Hold catheter in position until urine begins to drip. Collect approximately 5 to 10 mL of urine before removing catheter. Collecting a sufficient amount of urine may take 5 to 15 minutes.
- Clean and dry the stoma and peristomal skin.
- Apply pouching system.
- Discard supplies according to institution policy.

PROCEDURE FOR CLEAN CATCH DRIP COLLECTION METHOD SUPPLIES

- Cleansing solution. Follow institution policy. Further research is needed on the use of antiseptic solutions versus sterile water or saline for cleaning prior to catheter insertion. Some of the solutions recommended are Betadine, chlorhexidine, and soap and water (Gould et al., 2009; Unlu et al., 2007).
- Sterile 4 × 4 gauze.
- Sterile specimen container with lid, label, and laboratory specimen bag.
- Sterile and clean gloves.
- Soft paper towels and/or washcloths for cleaning prior to replacing pouch.
- New pouching system.

Procedure

- Explain the procedure to the patient.
- Wash hands and use standard precautions.
- Don clean gloves.
- Drape a towel or absorbent pad under the stoma for privacy and absorption if needed.
- Open the supplies; maintain sterility.
- Remove pouch and dispose per institutional policy.
- Wash hands.
- Don sterile gloves.
- Use sterile technique.
- Cleanse the stoma with cleansing solution, using a circular motion from stoma opening outward (Faller & Lawrence, 1994).
- Blot the stoma with sterile gauze.
- Discard the first few drops of urine by allowing urine to drip onto sterile gauze.
- Hold the sterile specimen cup under the stoma. Collect approximately 5 to 10 mL of urine. Collecting a sufficient amount of urine may take 5 to 15 minutes.
- Clean and dry the stoma and peristomal skin.
- Apply new pouching system.
- Discard supplies according to institutional policy.

PROCEDURE IF STENTS** ARE PRESENT IN THE UROSTOMY STOMA

- Cleansing solution: Follow institution policy. Further research is needed on the use of antiseptic solutions versus sterile water or saline for cleaning prior to catheter insertion. Some of the solutions recommended are Betadine, chlorhexidine, and soap and water (Gould et al., 2009; Unlu et al., 2007).

- Sterile 4 × 4 gauze.
- Sterile specimen container with lid, label, and laboratory specimen bag.
- Sterile and clean gloves.
- Soft paper towels and/or washcloths for cleaning prior to replacing pouch.
- New pouching system.

Procedure

1. Explain the procedure to the patient.
2. Wash hands and use standard precautions.
3. Don clean gloves.
4. Drape a towel or absorbent pad under the stoma for privacy and absorption if needed.
5. Open the supplies; maintain sterility.
6. Remove pouch and dispose per institutional policy. There may be a collection of mucus where the stents exit the stoma. Use a piece of dry gauze to gently remove the mucus without dislodging the stents.
7. Wash hands.
8. Don sterile gloves.
9. Use sterile technique.
10. Cleanse the outside ends of the stents with cleansing solution.
11. Blot the stents with sterile gauze.
12. Discard the first few drops of urine by allowing urine to drip onto sterile gauze.
13. Hold the sterile specimen cup under the stents. Collect approximately 5 to 10 mL of urine. Collecting a sufficient amount of urine may take 5 to 15 minutes.
14. **Do not insert a catheter to obtain specimen when stents are present.**
15. Clean and dry the stoma and peristomal skin.
16. Apply the pouching system.
17. Discard supplies according to institutional policy.

AFTERCARE

- Place lid on specimen container. Apply patient identification label on container with a note that the specimen is from a urostomy stoma and put in a laboratory specimen bag for transport to the laboratory.
- Transport specimen to lab within 1 hour. In the home care setting, if unable to transport specimen in 1 hour, refrigerate the specimen and transport within 24 hours.
- Document in patient's record:
  - Procedure and observations.
  - Instructions given to patient/caregiver.

ANTIBIOTIC THERAPY CONSIDERATIONS

- Use caution when considering antibiotics to treat urinary infection for patients with a urostomy: "Patients should only commence antibiotic therapy if they are symptomatic" (Spraggon, 2008, p. 26).
- Asymptomatic bacteriuria should not be treated, unless history of recurrent pyelonephritis. Patients with a

history of recurrent pyelonephritis may warrant prophylactic antibiotic treatment (Falagas & Vergidis, 2005).
- "In the case of ileal conduit or continent urinary diversion, bacteriuria is practically always present, and measurements taken to eradicate the bacterial carriage are fruitless" (Wullt et al., 2004, p. 192).
- "The detection of urinary infection in these patients is difficult because the ileal loops are almost always colonized. Asymptomatic bacteriuria in the presence of a ureteroileal conduit should not be treated and prophylactic antibiotics are not recommended. Positive urine cultures associated with physical findings of fever, chills, and flank pain should prompt initiation of appropriate bactericidal antibiotics" (Schrier, 2007, p. 884).

RECOMMENDATIONS FOR FUTURE RESEARCH

- Further research is needed on the use of antiseptic solutions versus sterile water or saline for cleaning of the stoma prior to catheterization of the urinary stoma.
- Replication of the small randomized controlled trial comparing the three urinary collection methods (Vaarala, 2018) using a larger sample and more robust crossover methodology.

SUMMARY

- The recommended method for collecting a urine specimen from the urinary ostomy is via sterile catheterization.
- If sterile catheterization cannot be accomplished, the secondary method for obtaining a urine specimen from the urinary ostomy is via clean catch drip collection method using a sterile urine collection container.
- If urinary stents are present in the urinary ostomy, the urine specimen should be collected via clean catch drip collection method using a sterile urine collection container.
- Urinary specimens should never be collected directly from an existing pouching system or the bedside drainage bag.
- Antibiotic therapy should be initiated with caution in patients with urinary ostomies and based on physical findings rather than asymptomatic bacteriuria.

PATIENT EDUCATION

- Educate patients regarding appropriate urine specimen collection methods from their urinary ostomy as they may need to advise health care providers on appropriate collection methods.

GLOSSARY

Bacteriuria presence of bacteria in the urine (Carmel et al., 2015).

Colon conduit type of urinary diversion whereby ureters are implanted into a section of dissected colon (large intestine) that is sutured closed on one end, while the other end is brought through the abdominal wall to create a stoma.

Ileal conduit type of urinary diversion whereby ureters are implanted into a section of dissected ileum that is sutured closed on one end, while the other end is brought through the abdominal wall to create a stoma.

Stent small tube inserted from the stoma into the kidney during surgery to allow drainage of the urine during healing of the ureters and conduit.

Urostomy an opening into the urinary system that can be constructed from the small or large intestine. The term urostomy describes that there is an opening that drains urine and the type of stoma will be an ileal or colon conduit, or an ureterostomy. An ileal or colon conduit uses the ileum or colon to make a passage for the urine to exit the body.

REFERENCES

Carmel, J. E., Colwell, J. C., Goldberg, M. T., et al. (2015). *WOCN Society Core Curriculum: Ostomy Management*. Philadelphia, PA: Wolters Kluwer.

Falagas, M. E., & Vergidis, P. I. (2005). Urinary tract infections in patients with urinary diversions. *American Journal of Kidney Diseases, 46*(6), 1030–1037.

Faller, N. A., & Lawrence, K. G. (1994). Obtaining a urine specimen from a conduit urostomy. *AJN The American Journal of Nursing, 94*(1), 37.

Gould, C. V., Umscheid, C. A., Agarwal, R. K., et al. (2009). Guideline for prevention of catheter-associated urinary tract infections. Retrieved November 9, 2011, from https://www.cdc.gov/infectioncontrol/guidelines/CAUTI/index.html

Hampton, B. G., & Bryant, R. A. (1992). *Ostomies and continent diversions: Nursing management* (1st ed.). St. Louis, MO: Mosby.

Kim, K. H., Yoon, H. S., Yoon, H., et al. (2016). Febrile urinary tract infection after radical cystectomy and ileal neobladder in patients with bladder cancer. *Journal of Korean Medical Science, 31*(7), 1100–1104.

Mano, R., Goldberg, H., Stabholz, Y., et al. (2018). Urinary tract infections after urinary diversion-different occurrence patterns in patients with ileal conduit and orthotopic neobladder. *Urology, 116*, 87–92.

Pagana, K. D., & Pagana, T. J. (2007). *Mosby's diagnostic and laboratory test reference* (8th ed.). St. Louis, MO: Mosby Elsevier.

Schrier, R. W. (2007). *Diseases of the kidney and urinary tract* (8th ed.). Philadelphia, PA: Lippincott Williams & Wilkins.

Spraggon, E. (2008). The management of ileal conduit urinary diversions. *Continence UK, 2*(1), 17–28.

Turnbull, G. B. (2003). Ostomy statistics: The $64,000 question. *Ostomy/Wound Management, 49*(6), 22–23.

Unlu, H., Sardan, Y. C., & Ulker, S. (2007). Comparison of sampling methods for urine cultures. *Journal of Nursing Scholarship, 39*(4), 325–329. doi: 10.1111/j.1547-5069.2007.00188.x.

Vaarala, M. H. (2018). Urinary sample collection methods in ileal conduit urinary diversion patients: A randomized control trial. *Journal of Wound, Ostomy, and Continence Nursing, 45*(1), 59–62. doi: 10.1097/WON.0000000000000397.

Wullt, B., Agace, W., & Mansson, W. (2004). Bladder, bowel and bugs—Bacteriuria in patients with intestinal urinary diversion. *World Journal of Urology, 22*(3), 186–195. doi: 10.1007/s00345-004-0432-x.

STATEMENT ACKNOWLEDGING CONTENT VALIDATION

This document was reviewed in the consensus-building process of the Wound, Ostomy, and Continence Nurses Society known as Content Validation.

UROSTOMY URINE SAMPLE COLLECTION INSTRUCTION CARD

UROSTOMY

A urostomy (also known as ileoconduit or colon conduit) is a surgically created opening on the abdomen that drains urine. An ostomy pouch is used to collect the urine. During waking hours, the pouch is drained into the toilet. At nighttime, the pouch is connected to a larger collection system to allow for uninterrupted sleep and to prevent reflux into kidneys.

URINARY TRACT INFECTION

Due to the changes in your body following surgery, there is higher risk for urinary tract infection (UTI). The signs and symptoms of UTI may be different than before surgery.

SIGNS AND SYMPTOMS OF UTI WHEN YOU HAVE A UROSTOMY

- Cloudy urine
- Dark or bloody urine
- Urine with bad odor
- Extra mucus (it is normal for the urine from a urostomy to have small shreds of mucus)
- Fever
- Back pain/flank pain
- Abdominal pain
- Nausea or vomiting
- Diarrhea

URINE SAMPLE

A urine sample is needed to check for UTI. The sample should not be taken directly from the used urostomy pouch. The correct procedure should be followed to avoid contamination of the urine sample. Contamination can result in incorrect culture results and improper use of antibiotics.

INSTRUCTIONS

Please give these instructions to the person collecting the urine specimen.

NOTE

This entire procedure may take 20 to 30 minutes. Collecting a sufficient amount of urine may take 5 to 15 minutes.

SUPPLIES

- Cleansing solution. Follow institution policy (e.g., Betadine or soap/water)
- Sterile 4 × 4 gauze
- Sterile specimen container
- Sterile and clean gloves
- Soft paper towels

If available:
- *16-Fr catheter*
- *Water-soluble lubricant*
- Pouch—may need new pouching system to replace if current pouch is not able to be reused.

PROCEDURE

1. Explain procedure to patient.
2. Wash hands and use standard precautions.
3. Don clean gloves.
4. Drape a towel or absorbent pad under the stoma for privacy and absorption if needed.
5. Open the supplies; maintain sterility.
6. Remove pouch or pouching system and dispose per institutional policy.
7. Wash hands.
8. Don sterile gloves.
9. Use sterile technique.
10. Cleanse the stoma with cleansing solution, using a circular motion from stoma opening outward.
11. Blot the stoma with sterile gauze.
12. Place the open end of catheter into the specimen container.
13. Lubricate the catheter with a small amount of water-soluble lubricant. Gently insert the catheter tip no more than 2 to 3 inches (5.0 to 7.5 cm) into the stoma (never force—if resistance is detected, rotate catheter until it slides in).
14. Hold catheter in position until urine begins to drip. Collect required amount of urine per institutional policy before removing catheter.
15. Clean and dry the stoma and peristomal skin.
16. Apply pouching system.
17. Discard supplies according to institution policy.

If catheter is not available, follow steps 1 to 11. Then complete the collection using these steps:
12. Discard the first few drops of urine by allowing urine to drip onto sterile gauze.
13. Hold the sterile specimen cup under the stoma. Collect required amount of urine per institutional policy.
14. Clean and dry the stoma and peristomal skin.
15. Apply new pouching system.
16. Discard supplies according to institutional policy.

AFTERCARE

Follow institutional policy for urine specimen collection labeling, ordering, and transport.

For full citations and references, please refer to: Catheterization of an Ileal or Colon Conduit Stoma: Best Practice for Clinicians.

Colostomy and Ileostomy Products and Tips

Best Practice for Clinicians

ACKNOWLEDGMENTS

Colostomy and Ileostomy Products and Tips: Best Practice for Clinicians.

This document was developed by the WOCN Society's Clinical Practice Ostomy Committee between April 2011 and April 2012.

Ginger Salvadalena, Chair, PhD, RN, CWOCN
Senior Clinical Research Scientist
Hollister Incorporated
Libertyville, IL

Carole Bauer, MSN, RN, ANP-BC, OCN, CWOCN
Wound, Ostomy, and Continence Nurse Practitioner
The Barbara Ann Karmanos Cancer Center
Detroit, MI

Kathryn Baxter, MS, RN, FNP, CWOCN
Nurse Practitioner, Colon/Rectal Surgery
St. Luke's Roosevelt Hospital
New York, NY

Cathy P. Downey, BSN, RN, CWOCN
Program Coordinator, OP/BCT
University Medical Center
Las Vegas, NV

Kay Durkop-Scott, BSN, RN, CWOCN
Wound Ostomy Continence RN
Porter Adventist Hospital
Denver, CO

Mary F. Mahoney, BSN, RN, CWON
WOC Nurse
Iowa Health Home Care
Des Moines, IA

Barbara Metzger, BSN, RN, CWOCN
WOC Nurse
University of Kentucky Medical Center—Good Samaritan
Lexington, KY

Jacqueline Perkins, MSN, FNP-C, CWOCN
Wound/Ostomy Nurse Practitioner
VA Central Iowa Health Care System
Des Moines, IA

Michelle Rice, MSN, RN, CWOCN
Ostomy Clinical Nurse Specialist
Duke University Hospital
Durham, NC

Victoria Schafer, MSN, RN, CWON, CCRA
Ostomy Care
Associate Director, Medical & Scientific Liaison
Medical Affairs North America
ConvaTec
Skillman, NJ

Shirley Tyler, MS, RN, CWOCN
Wound Care Specialist
Home Care
Mattoon, IL

INTRODUCTION

A colostomy or ileostomy is a surgically created opening (stoma) on the abdomen to allow the draining of feces/effluent. The ostomy drainage is typically managed by wearing a pouch over the stoma. The pouch is either changed or emptied into the toilet usually when it is 1/3 to 1/2 full.

This document is for nurses and other health care providers. This document provides an overview of the features of the different types of products, pouching systems, and accessories used to manage a colostomy or ileostomy, along with advantages and disadvantages. It concludes with helpful tips for emptying drainable colostomy or ileostomy pouches.

POUCHING SYSTEMS

DESCRIPTION	ADVANTAGES	DISADVANTAGES
Disposable Pouching System		
• System designed to be thrown away after removal. Typically made of lightweight plastic film, which is available in transparent or opaque material. Disposable pouches can be closed-end, or drainable, and part of either one-piece or two-piece pouching systems. May have plastic or fabric backing	• Odor resistant • May be worn in bath, shower, and swimming pool • Cleaning usually not necessary • Drainable pouches are typically changed every 3–7 days. Closed pouches are discarded and replaced when 1/3–1/2 full of feces/effluent. • Convenient, easy to carry and dispose • Various sizes/capacities	• May be more expensive than reusable pouching systems over time • May require removing stool and then cleaning the end "tail" of pouch for odor control
Reusable Pouching System		
• Pouch that can be washed and reapplied multiple times. Typically made of vinyl or thick plastic film. Reusable pouches can be closed-end (if used with a liner), or drainable. May be a one-piece or two-piece system composed of a pouch, also referred to as a skin barrier or wafer	• Washable • Able to be reused multiple times • Some can be used without an adhesive.	• Can retain odors • Limited number of manufacturers • Initial cost may be more expensive than that of disposable pouching system. • May require more time to clean • Might require a belt and/or adhesive
One-Piece Pouching System		
• The skin barrier and pouch are attached together during manufacturing. Available in drainable and closed styles, with and without filters	• Many styles are flexible and conform to abdominal contours. • Low profile • No chance for leakage between skin barrier and pouch as in two-piece systems • May be less costly than a two-piece system • May be easier to learn to use • Often used when abdominal plane contours are uneven, as it can provide greater flexibility than a two-piece system	• Cannot reposition once applied • Cannot burp for gas • Cannot change the pouch without changing the entire system • Some have less support for loose peristomal skin.
Two-Piece Pouching System		
• The skin barrier and pouch are made separately with rigid to semirigid rings or with an adhesive coupling system that allows the pouch to be attached to the skin barrier.	• Can provide support to loose peristomal skin • Can switch between drainable and closed-end pouches without removing the skin barrier • Can change position of the pouch with patient's position changes (especially for bed-bound patients) to facilitate better drainage	• Need dexterity and strength to assure attachment of pouch to skin barrier • Higher profile • More costly than a one-piece pouch • Less flexible than a one-piece pouching system and does not mold well to the body contours
Pouching System with Adhesive Flange		
• The skin barrier and pouch are made separately and designed to stick together without a rigid flange.	• Can change pouch for disposal, emptying or rinsing without removing the skin barrier • Low profile • Flexibility similar to a one-piece system • May be easier to apply than pouching systems with a flange, for those with poor dexterity • May be used when abdominal plane contours are uneven, such as with a peristomal hernia	• Less support for flabby peristomal skin • Limited number of times pouch can be reattached (dependent on manufacturer) • Must have the coordination to apply properly on the skin barrier • Cannot reuse pouch if adhesive area becomes soiled • May be more difficult for visually impaired to use

TYPES OF POUCHES

DESCRIPTION	ADVANTAGES	DISADVANTAGES
Transparent Pouch		
• Pouch made of clear film	• Can see stoma for easy application of pouching system • Able to monitor stoma and effluent appearance, especially in the early postoperative period	• Appearance of feces/effluent in the pouch may be unpleasant for the patient and/or the significant other.
Opaque Pouch		
• Pouch made of colored film (typically white or beige)	• Cosmetically appealing; unable to see stoma or stool • More discreet under light-colored clothing	• May be more difficult to apply when part of a one-piece pouching system
Drainable Pouch		
• Pouch with an opening at the bottom. A clamp or integrated closure is used to keep the pouch closed until it is time to empty.	• Able to empty frequently • Cost effective • Long and shorter lengths are available. • Available with and without filter for gas release	• Risk of spillage. Can require some skill to drain successfully without spillage of stool • Need dexterity and strength to manage various closures • Some versions may be too long for comfort or body size. • Rinsing/cleaning of the pouch may be needed or preferred by some patients.
Closed-End Pouch		
• Also called a closed or nondrainable pouch. A pouch without an opening or clamp. It must be removed/discarded when 1/3–1/2 full.	• Low profile • More discreet for intimate situations • Generally shorter than drainable pouches • May be easier to use than drainable for some people • See section on disposable liners. • Available with and without filters for gas release	• Smaller pouch capacity • Not practical if having frequent stools or large amounts of fecal/effluent output
High-Output Pouch		
• A drainable pouch that accommodates larger amounts of output. Has a drainage spout at the end of the pouch	• Used for frequent or high-volume fecal output • Does not need to be emptied as often • If stool is liquid, it can be attached to a bedside drainage bag/container.	• More expensive than smaller drainable pouches, but insurance reimbursement is available • Larger size may make it difficult to conceal. • When connected to bedside drainage bag, tubing and/or pouch can potentially twist and kink, so the tubing should be anchored well and monitored to ensure adequate drainage.
Colostomy Irrigation Pouch		
• Long, sleeve-type pouch used during colostomy irrigation. Allows containment of the stool and allows irrigation fluid to flow through the sleeve into the toilet. Some have flanges to use with two-piece system. Some have self adhesive. Pouch size varies by manufacturer.	• Use of colostomy irrigation allows a person with a colostomy to control when he or she has a bowel movement. May be used to administer an ostomy bowel prep. May eliminate the need for a drainable pouching system between irrigations • Extra long drain directs effluent into the toilet • Top opening pouch accommodates a stoma cone. • May be rinsed with cool water for reuse • May be used as high-capacity pouch for short periods of time	• Irrigation process requires time and appropriate toileting facility. • Pouch is not odor proof.

(Continued)

TYPES OF POUCHES (*Continued*)

DESCRIPTION	ADVANTAGES	DISADVANTAGES
Stoma Cap		
• A small closed pouch, usually <4 inches in diameter, with an absorbent pad inside the pouch. Covers stoma when periods of inactivity can be anticipated, such as after a stoma irrigation. Some are available with a vent or filter for gas release.	• More discreet for intimate situations or under clothes • Easier to apply than a dressing or bandage-type cover	• No capacity to contain stool • Only indicated for use between colostomy irrigations in persons with descending or sigmoid colostomy
Pouch with Integrated Closure		
• A drainable pouch that has an attached closure at the bottom of the pouch. The closure is part of the drainable pouch, attached during the manufacturing process.	• No clamp/clip to lose • May be more comfortable • May be easier to manipulate for those with limited hand dexterity	• Individuals who have used clips for a long time need instruction and reassurance. • May be harder to remove feces/effluent in order to keep clean and odor free
Filter		
• A feature available on some pouches that allows gas (but not odor) to escape from the pouch. Filters may be integrated in the pouch during manufacturing or purchased separately and added to a pouch.	• Venting of gas is passive (requires no action on the part of the user). • Low risk of accidental spillage	• Ineffective if it becomes wet. Newer versions have a barrier film to prevent wetness from entering from either inside or outside the pouch. • May be an added expense • Add-on filters can become dislodged. • If stool is liquid, may leak through filter and render charcoal ineffective.
Belt Loops		
• A feature on a pouch or skin barrier that allows for use of an elastic belt with a one-piece or two-piece pouching system	• Belt loops on the skin barrier allow the pouch to be applied and removed without disturbing the belt. • Belt loops on the pouch can add security to the connection between pouch and skin barrier flange.	• Presence of belt loops may make the skin barrier more rigid. • The belt loops may be uncomfortable against the body, and wearing a belt too tightly may lead to a pressure ulcer.

SKIN BARRIERS

The skin barrier is the part of a pouching system that is applied directly to the skin. Adhesive skin barriers are typically made from pectin, karaya gum, and/or synthetic materials. A nonadhesive skin barrier is made from silicone or rubber.

DESCRIPTION	ADVANTAGES	DISADVANTAGES
Flat Skin Barrier		
• A skin barrier that has a level or flat appearance • May be part of a one-piece or two-piece pouching system	• Used when the peristomal skin surface is flat and the stoma is well budded (protruding at least 1/2 inch above the abdominal wall surface)	• If the peristomal skin surface is not flat and/or the stoma is not well protruded, accessories such as paste or barrier rings may be needed to achieve a better seal around the base of the stoma. • Requires scissors and dexterity to create a cut-to-fit opening.
Convex Skin Barrier		
• A skin barrier that has a rounded "inverted bowl shape" surface on the side that adheres to the skin used when the stoma is at skin level/flushed or retracted/below skin level • May be part of a one-piece or two-piece pouching system.	• Used for peristomal skin surface that is concave • Used for soft peristomal skin surface with a flush or short stoma • Convexity can be rigid/firm or somewhat flexible and can be useful for stomas that have different depths/degrees of stoma retraction.	• May need to add an ostomy belt to provide added security/support by keeping wafer/barrier in place • May lift from the skin with body movement and position changes or cause pressure damage if the convexity is too stiff/rigid • Neither an ostomy belt nor a firm convex barrier should be used in the immediate postoperative period to avoid tension on the suture line of the stoma and to prevent mucocutaneous separation.

SKIN BARRIERS (*Continued*)

DESCRIPTION	ADVANTAGES	DISADVANTAGES
Moldable, Shapeable, or Stretchable Skin Barrier		
• A skin barrier that allows the opening for the stoma to be shaped with fingers rather than using scissors.	• Available flat or convex • Moldable skin barrier has "shape memory," which provides a constant, self-adjusting fit around the base of the stoma • No scissors needed • Useful for those with poor hand dexterity or poor eyesight, which would make cutting barrier to size difficult	• May not work consistently with flush, partially flush stomas, or retracted stomas. • May need some dexterity to shape • Can move over stoma opening over time, leading to leakage • Option currently only available with a two-piece pouching system
Skin Barrier with Floating Flange		
• A skin barrier with a flange that does not adhere to the base of the barrier	• A skin barrier used in a two-piece pouching system. A floating flange allows the pouch to be snapped onto the skin barrier while minimizing the pressure to the patient's abdomen. • Available flat or convex	• Higher profile than nonfloating flange
Skin Barrier with Locking Flange		
• A skin barrier with a system to lock the pouch to the flange • A skin barrier used in a two-piece pouching system	• Available flat or convex • May require less dexterity to attach pouch to flange • Designed for individuals with limited eye–hand coordination • Allows the pouch to be snapped onto the skin barrier without adding pressure to the abdomen	• Higher profile than nonlocking flange • May require more dexterity to attach pouch to flange or coupling mechanism
Skin Barrier with Smooth Flange		
• A skin barrier with a docking area for the pouch to adhere • A skin barrier used in a two-piece pouching system	• The pouch adheres to the skin barrier plate with an adhesive ring. • Available flat or convex • Can be detached and reapplied • More flexible than the locking or floating flange	• Adhesive surface must be dry for good adherence.
Tape Border		
• A skin barrier with adhesive tape attached to the edges of the barrier	• Some skin barriers have a tape border around the outside of the barrier, which makes the skin barrier more flexible and lower profile. • Patients may feel more secure with a tape border.	• Patients may have sensitivity to adhesives leading to allergic/contact dermatitis.

ACCESSORIES

DESCRIPTION	ADVANTAGES	DISADVANTAGES
Pouch Lubricant		
• A lubricant added to the pouch to facilitate the ease of emptying stool from the pouch	• Pouch sides less likely to stick together • Stool less likely to stick to sides of pouch • May also contain an odor eliminator • Unlike household products, such as mineral oil, nonstick cooking spray, and liquid soap, commercial lubricant will not damage the film of the pouch.	• Extra step and expense

(*Continued*)

ACCESSORIES (Continued)

DESCRIPTION	ADVANTAGES	DISADVANTAGES
Gas Vent/Filter		
• Vent added to a pouch to allow wearer to have control over when they release gas	• Decreases risk of spillage compared to burping or releasing gas from the tail end • Control when gas is vented • Accessory filter may also be used.	• Will not deodorize gas without a charcoal filter • Extra steps are required to apply separate gas vent/filter if it was not integrated into pouch by the manufacturing process. It must be applied 24 h in advance of using. • Requires dexterity • Added cost • May leak liquid effluent from the filter or around connection on pouch • Gas venting not automatic. Gas vent needs to be manually opened to release gas.
Pouch Liners		
• Placed inside a two-piece pouch and held in place when the pouch is snapped to the flange of the skin barrier. After bowel movement, the used liner is removed and flushed and a new liner is placed inside the same pouch.	• Keeps pouch clean—same pouch can be used multiple times • Wear time of pouch can be extended with use of disposable liners • May be more discreet for the user because they can be flushed rather than disposed in trash • Compatible with pouches with or without gas filter	• Not covered by insurance • Not compatible with septic systems • Not compatible with two-piece systems using the Adhesive Coupling Technique • May adversely affect the security of the pouch adhering to the barrier • Learning to remove the liner from the pouch without spillage can take time, dexterity, and practice
Clamp		
• The removable plastic clip used on a drainable pouch	• Can be cleaned • Reusable • Available with curved shape to fit thigh for lower profile • Several options are available: individuals can often find one that they can handle with their limitations.	• The clamp can break. • Can be dropped or lost when emptying the pouch • Higher profile (more visible) than integrated pouch closures • Some styles are difficult for people with limited dexterity. • Added cost if needed to be replaced
Pouch Cover		
• Cloth envelope-like sleeve to place over ostomy pouch while it is on the body	• Cosmetically appealing; stoma or stool cannot be seen • Can reduce sweating, skin irritation, and provide a more comfortable surface against the skin • May help reduce noise from vinyl or plastic pouch • May be integrated within available disposable pouches	• Added expense with fabric material already covering some pouches
Skin Sealant		
• Plasticizing agent such as copolymer; some may contain isopropyl alcohol. Available as wipe, spray, gel, liquid, and roll-on	• Provides a thin protective film to the skin surface. Helps to prevent stripping of the epidermis during adhesive removal and also acts as a moisture barrier • If applying stoma powder to skin irritation, skin sealant may be added to provide a surface for skin barrier adherence.	• Sealants may not be recommended under some skin barriers because the protective film may reduce the adherence of the barrier. • Skin sealants that contain alcohol can cause pain when applied to irritated skin.

ACCESSORIES (*Continued*)

DESCRIPTION	ADVANTAGES	DISADVANTAGES
Adhesive Remover		
• Solvent available as gel, wipe, or liquid	• Aids in the removal of tape, skin adhesives, and residue. May be helpful to the patient with sensitive skin to reduce trauma from removal of pouching system	• Rinsing is typically required to remove residue before pouch application to prevent chemical dermatitis or nonadherence of next pouch.
Skin Adhesive		
• Adhesive made of silicone or latex	• Used to increase adhesion of an adhesive pouching system or to provide adhesion for a reusable (nonadhesive) system	• Need to teach patient to allow adhesive to dry to prevent chemical irritation • May be flammable
Paste		
• Pectin-based product used to help prevent leakage of stoma drainage under the skin barrier	• Can be used use to fill in uneven areas and/or as a caulking around the inner edge of the skin barrier to prevent leakage under the skin barrier • Used to increase the seal of skin barrier to contours of the abdominal surface • Fills in small creases and depressions and evens out skin contours under a skin barrier • Used appropriately, will offer a quick seal for the pouching system until the skin barrier adhesive is pressed into place	• Patients often think this is adhesive paste and use it inappropriately. • Patients often use too much. • Requires dexterity for application to either peristomal skin or skin barrier. May sting when applied to irritated peristomal skin • May help with improving the fit of barrier • Is not substantial enough to fill in large creases. Does not hold up well when exposed to urinary or ileal effluent
Skin Barrier Rings		
• Pectin or sodium carboxymethylcellulose–based product that is soft and moldable; used as a washer around the base of the stoma to help prevent effluent drainage under the skin barrier	• Used to increase the seal of skin barrier to contours of the abdominal surface. Can be used to enhance the pouching system seal • Alternative to paste. To help with fitting over contours • Can be stretched and molded to create custom shapes • Can be used straight from the package or molded into desired shape to fill in areas that need to be leveled out • Can be cut, bent, and stacked together to improve the fit of the skin barrier • For individuals with sensitive skin or limited dexterity • May prolong skin barrier wear time • Convex barrier rings can be used to adjust skin barrier thickness for deeper convexity or used to create oval-shaped convexity.	• Requires dexterity for application to either peristomal skin or skin barrier • Added cost • Added step
Stoma Powder		
• Pectin- or karaya-based powder used to protect peristomal skin and mucocutaneous separation from exposure to stoma discharge	• Aids healing and protection • Helps protect open, weeping skin against stoma discharge. Absorbs moisture or exudate from skin prior to placing a skin barrier on peristomal skin for added protection • May be sealed to the skin by applying a layer of skin sealant before the pouching system is applied	• If applied improperly, may prevent adhesion of skin barrier

(*Continued*)

ACCESSORIES (*Continued*)

DESCRIPTION	ADVANTAGES	DISADVANTAGES
Strip Paste		
• Pectin-based product used to help prevent leakage of stoma drainage under the skin barrier	• Used to increase the seal of skin barrier to contours of the abdominal surface. Can be used to enhance the pouching system seal • Can be cut, bent, and stacked together to improve the fit of the skin barrier • Conforms to irregular skin folds/creases • Soft and moldable	• Requires dexterity for application to either peristomal skin or skin barrier • Added cost • Added step
Odor Control Products		
• Air sprays, pouch deodorants, oral deodorants, charcoal filters • Some sprays have a fragrance that covers up the odor. • Some sprays act by eliminating the odor.	• May decrease odor when emptying pouch	• Extra step and expense • May not be effective • May trigger chemical sensitivities on the stoma or skin • Oral deodorizers may have side effects. • Diet changes can also be helpful.

TIPS FOR EMPTYING DRAINABLE POUCHES

DESCRIPTION	ADVANTAGES	DISADVANTAGES
Prevention of Splashing		
• Place a layer of toilet paper on the water in the toilet before emptying a drainable pouch.	• Can muffle the sound of stool hitting the water • Can prevent being splashed with toilet water	• May not work depending on the amount and consistency of stool
Cuff the End of the Drainable Pouch		
• This technique can be used to empty a drainable pouch without integrated closure. • Hold tail end of pouch up so that stool will not spill out. • Roll tail end of pouch up forming a cuff. • Direct the end of the pouch down and empty. • Clean edge of rolled cuff with toilet paper or moistened paper towel. • Unroll pouch and reclamp.	• Intended to keep end of pouch and clamp clean, which prevents odor accumulation and soiling of clothing and/or skin • Enables patient to empty with less risk of soiling hands • Can reduce time involved in emptying because the inside of the end of the pouch isn't soiled and doesn't need to be cleaned	• Requires some dexterity • Difficult when pouch is fairly full or stool is liquid • Not recommended with pouches that have integrated closure mechanisms

ACKNOWLEDGMENT ABOUT CONTENT VALIDATION

This document was reviewed in the consensus-building process of the Wound, Ostomy, and Continence Nurses Society known as Content Validation, which is managed by the Center for Clinical Investigation.

WOCN Society and AUA Position Statement on Preoperative Stoma Site Marking for Patients Undergoing Urostomy Surgery

ORIGINATED BY:

Wound, Ostomy, and Continence Nurses Society's (WOCN®) Stoma Site Marking Task Force in collaboration with the American Urological Association (AUA) in 2009 (AUA & WOCN, 2009).

UPDATED/REVISED BY:

WOCN Society's Stoma Site Marking Task Force in collaboration with the American Society of Colon and Rectal Surgeons (ASCRS) and the AUA.

CONTRIBUTING AUTHORS:

Task Force Chair

- **Ginger Salvadalena, PhD, RN, CWOCN**, Principal Scientist, Global Clinical Affairs, Hollister Incorporated, Libertyville, Illinois

Task Force Members

- **Samantha Hendren, MD, MPH**, Associate Professor of Surgery, University of Michigan, Ann Arbor, Michigan
- **Linda McKenna, MSN, RN, CWOCN**, Ostomy & Wound Specialist, Memorial Medical Center, Springfield, Illinois
- **Roberta Muldoon, MD, FACS**, Assistant Professor of Surgery, Vanderbilt University Medical Center, Nashville, Tennessee
- **Debra Netsch, DNP, RN, CNP, FNP-BC, CWOCN**, Mankato Clinic, Ltd, Mankato, Minnesota
- **Ian Paquette, MD**, Assistant Professor of Surgery, University of Cincinnati College of Medicine, Cincinnati, Ohio
- **Joyce Pittman, PhD, ANP-BC, FNP-BC, CWOCN**, Team Lead Wound/Ostomy Adjunct Assistant Professor, Indiana University School of Nursing, Indiana University Health Methodist, Indianapolis, Indiana
- **Janet Ramundo, MSN, RN, CWOCN**, WOC Nurse, Houston Methodist Hospital, Houston, Texas
- **Gary Steinberg, MD**, The Beth and Bruce White Family Professor and Director of Urologic Oncology; Vice Chairman Section of Urology, The University of Chicago Medicine, Chicago, Illinois

DATE COMPLETED:

June 2014

DATE APPROVED BY THE WOCN BOARD OF DIRECTORS:

November 12, 2014

THE WOCN SOCIETY SUGGESTS THE FOLLOWING FORMAT FOR BIBLIOGRAPHIC CITATIONS:

Wound, Ostomy, and Continence Nurses Society. (2014). *WOCN Society and AUA Position Statement on Preoperative Stoma Site Marking for Patients Undergoing Urostomy Surgery.* Mt. Laurel, NJ: Author.

STATEMENT OF POSITION:

Ostomy education and stoma site selection should be performed preoperatively for all patients when an ostomy is a possibility (AUA & WOCN, 2009). Multiple studies indicate that patients who have their stoma site marked preoperatively by a trained clinician have fewer ostomy-related complications (Gulbiniene et al., 2004; Millan et al., 2010; Park et al., 1999; Parmar et al., 2011; Pittman et al., 2008; WOCN, 2010). An appropriate stoma site may decrease ostomy related complications such as leakage of the pouching system and peristomal dermatitis. It may also influence the predictability of a pouch's wear time and ability of the patient to adapt to the ostomy and become independent, and may even help control health care costs. Preoperatively marking the stoma site allows assessment of the patient's abdomen in multiple positions, which promotes selection of the optimal stoma site. In addition, this preoperative session promotes a patient-centered approach respecting the individuality, values, and information needs of the patient and family. The session may allow time to provide information regarding ostomy management, including pouching options, and provide psychosocial support. While preoperative stoma site marking is strongly supported, it is acknowledged that intraoperative circumstances may not allow for the optimal stoma site to be used in all situations. The final stoma site is chosen by the surgeon after the abdominal cavity is entered and the condition of the bowel is determined.

Urologists and certified ostomy nurses are the optimal clinicians to select and mark stoma sites, as this skill is a part of their education, practice, and training. However, these providers are not always available in emergency situations. All physicians who are called on to choose ostomy sites should familiarize themselves with the principles of proper stoma site selection, including placement of the stoma within the rectus abdominis muscle, use of multiple patient positions to identify appropriate stoma sites, avoidance of folds and scars, and consideration of the clothing/beltline.

PURPOSE (RATIONALE FOR POSITION):

The WOCN Society in collaboration with the AUA and ASCRS developed the following educational guide to assist clinicians (especially those who are not surgeons or WOC nurses) in selecting an effective stoma site. Marking the optimal location for a stoma preoperatively enhances the likelihood of a patient's independence in stoma care, predictable pouching system wear times, and resumption of normal activities.

RECOMMENDATIONS:

A. Key points to consider

1. The stoma site should be located within the rectus abdominis muscle.
2. Positioning issues: Contractures, posture, mobility (e.g., wheelchair confinement, use of a walker, etc.).
3. Physical considerations: Large/protruding/pendulous abdomen, abdominal folds, wrinkles, scars/suture lines, other stomas, rectus abdominis muscle, waist line, iliac crest, braces, pendulous breasts, vision, dexterity, and the presence of a hernia.
4. Patient considerations: Diagnosis, age, occupation, prior experience with a stoma, and preferences about the stoma's location.
5. Surgical considerations: Surgeon's preferences, type of surgery/stoma planned, segment of intestine used, and whether an incontinent versus a continent catheterizable diversion is planned.
6. Multiple stoma sites: If a fecal stoma is also present or planned, consider marking the urinary and fecal stoma sites on different horizontal planes/lines in the event that an ostomy belt is required.

B. Stoma site marking procedure

1. Gather items needed for the procedure: Marking pen, surgical marker, transparent film dressing, and flat skin barrier (i.e., according to the surgeon's preference and/or the facility's policy).
2. Explain the stoma site marking procedure to the patient, and encourage the patient's participation and input.
3. Carefully examine the patient's abdominal surface. If possible, begin with the patient fully clothed in a sitting position with both feet on the floor.
   - Observe the presence of belts, braces, and any other ostomy pouches.
   - Individuals with spinal cord injuries are optimally marked in their usual position, as this will facilitate fitting and care of the pouching system (Cataldo, 2008).
   - If the patient uses a wheelchair, it is best to position the patient in his or her own chair and allow time for the body to relax into the usual habitus before marking (Hocevar & Gray, 2008).
4. Have the patient completely remove any clothing that is placed over the abdomen, rather than just moving it out of the way. Waistbands and elastic can create or obscure skin folds that may or may not be present when the clothing is completely removed.
5. Examine the patient's exposed abdomen in various positions (e.g., standing, lying, sitting, and bending forward) to observe for creases, valleys, scars, folds, skin turgor, and contour.
6. Consider an imaginary line where the surgical incision will be located. If possible, choose a point at least 2 inches from the surgical incision where 2 to 3 inches of a flat adhesive skin barrier can be placed.
7. With the patient lying on his or her back, identify the rectus abdominis muscle. This can be done by having the patient do a modified sit-up (i.e., raise the head up and off the bed) or by having the patient cough. Palpate the edge of the rectus abdominis muscle. Expert opinion suggests that placement of the stoma within the rectus abdominis muscle may help prevent a peristomal hernia and/or a prolapse (AUA & WOCN, 2009).
8. Mark a spot on the skin of the abdomen that is located within the rectus abdominis muscle, in the appropriate quadrant for the planned surgery, and within the patient's visual field.
   - Care should be taken to avoid scars or creases; the priority is a flat pouching surface.
   - Individuals who use a wheelchair or have a large, rounded abdominal contour may benefit from having the stoma site marked in an upper quadrant (Hocevar & Gray, 2008).

- Choose an area that is visible to the patient, and if possible below the belt line to conceal the pouch.

9. If the abdomen is protuberant, choose the apex of the abdominal contour, or if the patient is extremely obese, consider marking the site in an upper abdominal quadrant (Colwell, 2014). In many obese patients the adipose layer is not as thick in the upper abdominal quadrants as compared to the lower quadrants, which may allow better visualization of the stoma (Cataldo, 2008; Colwell, 2014).

10. The mark should initially be made with a sticker or ink pen that can be removed if this is not the optimal spot.

   - It may be desirable to mark sites on the right and left sides of the abdomen to prepare for a change in the surgical outcome, and number the first choice as #1.
   - Have the patient assume sitting, bending, and lying positions to assess and confirm the best choice.

- It is important to have the patient confirm he or she can see the site. However, the critical consideration should be a flat pouching surface.

11. After the optimal site is chosen, clean the desired site with alcohol and allow it to dry. Then proceed with marking the selected site with a surgical marker or pen. If desired, cover the site with a transparent film dressing to preserve the final mark. Ensure that any other stray marks have been removed.

C. Examples of stoma site marking

1. See **Figure 1**: Example of marking a stoma site for a female with a protuberant abdomen, creases, and folds.
2. See **Figure 2**: Example of marking a stoma site for a male with a protuberant abdomen.

Step 1
Look at the profile of the patient. Notice where the abdomen curves back under toward the body. The underside of the abdomen is not visible to the patient. Avoid this area.

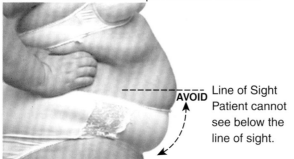

Line of Sight
Patient cannot see below the line of sight.

AVOID

Step 2
While patient is seated, look for skin folds and creases. Note and avoid skin folds and creases.

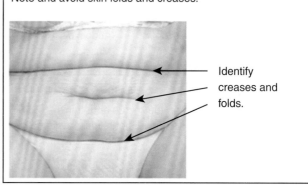

Identify creases and folds.

Step 3
Identify and target the rectus abdominis muscle below the ribs.

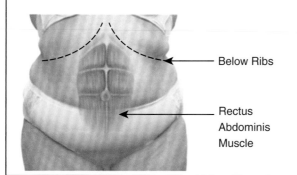

Below Ribs

Rectus Abdominis Muscle

Step 4
Mark optimal stoma sites on the rectus abdominis, that are in patient's line of sight, while avoiding creases and skin folds.

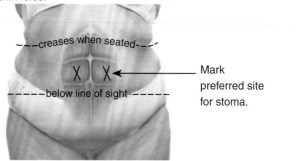

creases when seated

X X

Mark preferred site for stoma.

below line of sight

FIGURE 1 Stoma Site Marking for a Female with a Protuberant Abdomen. (Images used with permission: **Step 1**, female photograph © milk122/veer; **Step 2**, female photograph © SeDmi/veer; **Steps 3 and 4**, female photograph © kokhanchikov/shutterstock, and muscle overlay © Randall Reed Photography/veer.)

Step 1

Look at the profile of the patient. Notice where the abdomen curves back under toward the body. The underside of the abdomen is not visible to the patient. Avoid this area.

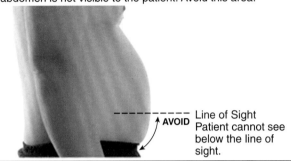

AVOID — Line of Sight Patient cannot see below the line of sight.

Step 2

Identify and target the rectus abdominis muscle below the ribs.

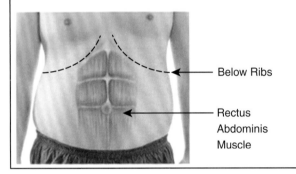

← Below Ribs

← Rectus Abdominis Muscle

Step 3

Mark optimal stoma sites on the rectus abdominis muscle, that are in patient's line of sight, while avoiding creases and skin folds.

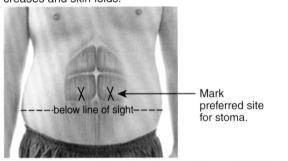

X X

----below line of sight----

← Mark preferred site for stoma.

FIGURE 2 Stoma Site Marking for a Male with a Protuberant Abdomen. (Images used with permission: **Steps 1, 2, and 3**, male photograph © sirastock/shutterstock; **Steps 2 and 3**, muscle overlay © Randall Reed Photography/veer.)

SUMMARY:

Stoma site selection should be a priority during the pre-operative visit. Marking the site for a stoma preoperatively provides an opportunity to select the optimal site, which can help reduce postoperative problems such as leakage, peristomal dermatitis, and difficulty with self-care of the ostomy. Whenever possible, ostomy education and stoma site selection should be performed preoperatively when an ostomy is a possibility.

ACKNOWLEDGMENT

The task force wishes to acknowledge Christina Augustyn, Industrial Designer, Innovation Management Office, Hollister Incorporated, Libertyville, Illinois, for her contribution in the selection and development of the images.

REFERENCES

AUA & WOCN Society. (2009). AUA and WOCN joint position statement on the value of preoperative stoma marking for patients undergoing creation of an incontinent urostomy. *Journal of Wound, Ostomy, and Continence Nursing, 36*(3), 267–268.

Cataldo, P. A. (2008). Technical tips for stoma creation in the challenging patient. *Clinics in Colon and Rectal Surgery, 21*(1), 17–22. doi: 10.1055/s20081055317.

Colwell, J. C. (2014). The role of obesity in the patient undergoing colorectal surgery and fecal diversion: A review of the literature. *Ostomy Wound Management, 60*(1), 24–28.

Gulbiniene, J., Markelis, R., Tamelis, A., et al. (2004). The impact of preoperative stoma siting and stoma care education on patient's quality of life. *Medicina (Kaunas, Lithuania), 40*(11), 1045–1053.

Hocevar, B., & Gray, M. (2008). Intestinal diversion (colostomy or ileostomy) in patients with severe bowel dysfunction following spinal cord injury. *Journal of Wound, Ostomy, and Continence Nursing, 35*(2), 159–166. doi: 10.1097/01.WON.0000313638.29623.40.

Millan, M., Tegido, M., Biondo, S., et al. (2010). Preoperative stoma siting and education by stomatherapists of colorectal cancer patients: A descriptive study in twelve Spanish colorectal surgical units. *Colorectal Disease, 12*(7 Online), e88–e92. doi: 10.1111/j.14631318.2009.01942.x.

Park, J. J., Del Pino, A., Orsay, C. P., et al. (1999). Stoma complications: The Cook County Hospital experience. *Diseases of the Colon and Rectum, 42*(12), 1575–1580.

Parmar, K. L., Zammit, M., Smith, A., et al. (2011). A prospective audit of early stoma complications in colorectal cancer treatment throughout the Greater Manchester and Cheshire colorectal cancer network. *Colorectal Disease, 13*(8), 935–938. doi: 10.1111/j.14631318.2010.02325.x.

Pittman, J., Rawl, S. M., Schmidt, C. M., et al. (2008). Demographic and clinical factors related to ostomy complications and quality of life in veterans with an ostomy. *Journal of Wound, Ostomy, and Continence Nursing, 35*(5), 493–503. doi: 10.1097/01.WON.0000335961.68113.cb.

Wound, Ostomy, and Continence Nurses Society (WOCN). (2010). *Management of the patient with a fecal ostomy: Best practice guideline for clinicians.* Mount Laurel, NJ: WOCN Society.

WOCN Society and ASCRS Position Statement on Preoperative Stoma Site Marking For Patients Undergoing Colostomy or Ileostomy Surgery

ORIGINATED BY:

Wound, Ostomy, and Continence Nurses Society's (WOCN®) Stoma Site Marking Task Force in collaboration with the American Society of Colon and Rectal Surgeons (ASCRS) in 2007 (ASCRS & WOCN, 2007).

UPDATED/REVISED BY:

WOCN Society's Stoma Site Marking Task Force in collaboration with the ASCRS and the American Urological Association (AUA).

CONTRIBUTING AUTHORS:

Task Force Chair

- **Ginger Salvadalena, PhD, RN, CWOCN**, Principal Scientist, Global Clinical Affairs, Hollister Incorporated, Libertyville, Illinois

Task Force Members

- **Samantha Hendren, MD, MPH**, Associate Professor of Surgery, University of Michigan, Ann Arbor, Michigan
- **Linda McKenna, MSN, RN, CWOCN,** Ostomy & Wound Specialist, Memorial Medical Center, Springfield, Illinois
- **Roberta Muldoon, MD, FACS**, Assistant Professor of Surgery, Vanderbilt University Medical Center, Nashville, Tennessee
- **Debra Netsch, DNP, RN, CNP, FNP-BC, CWOCN**, Mankato Clinic, Ltd, Mankato, Minnesota
- **Ian Paquette, MD**, Assistant Professor of Surgery, University of Cincinnati College of Medicine, Cincinnati, Ohio
- **Joyce Pittman, PhD, ANP-BC, FNP-BC, CWOCN**, Team Lead Wound/Ostomy Adjunct Assistant Professor, Indiana University School of Nursing, Indiana University Health Methodist, Indianapolis, Indiana

- **Janet Ramundo, MSN, RN, CWOCN**, WOC Nurse, Houston Methodist Hospital, Houston, Texas
- **Gary Steinberg, MD**, The Beth and Bruce White Family Professor and Director of Urologic Oncology; Vice Chairman Section of Urology, The University of Chicago Medicine, Chicago, Illinois

DATE COMPLETED:

June 2014

DATE APPROVED BY THE WOCN BOARD OF DIRECTORS:

November 12, 2014

THE WOCN SOCIETY SUGGESTS THE FOLLOWING FORMAT FOR BIBLIOGRAPHIC CITATIONS:

Wound, Ostomy and Continence Nurses Society. (2014). *WOCN Society and ASCRS Position Statement on Preoperative Stoma Site Marking for Patients Undergoing Colostomy or Ileostomy Surgery*. Mt. Laurel, NJ: Author.

STATEMENT OF POSITION:

Ostomy education and stoma site selection should be performed preoperatively for all patients when an ostomy is a possibility (ASCRS & WOCN, 2007). Multiple studies indicate that patients who have their stoma site marked preoperatively by a trained clinician have fewer ostomy-related complications (Gulbiniene et al., 2004; Millan et al., 2010; Park et al., 1999; Parmar et al., 2011; Pittman et al., 2008; WOCN, 2010).

An appropriate stoma site may decrease ostomy-related complications such as leakage of the pouching system and peristomal dermatitis. It may also influence the predictability of a pouch's wear time and ability of the patient to adapt to the ostomy and become independent, and may even help control health care costs. Preoperatively marking the stoma site allows assessment of the patient's abdomen in multiple positions, which promotes selection of the optimal stoma site. In addition, this preoperative session promotes a patient-centered approach respecting the individuality, values, and information needs of the patient and family. The session may allow time to provide information regarding ostomy management, including pouching options, and provide psychosocial support. While preoperative stoma site marking is strongly supported, it is acknowledged that intraoperative circumstances may not allow for the optimal stoma site to be used in all situations. The final stoma site is chosen by the surgeon after the abdominal cavity is entered and the condition of the bowel is determined.

Colon and rectal Surgeons and certified ostomy nurses are the optimal clinicians to select and mark stoma sites, as this skill is a part of their education, practice, and training. However, these providers are not always available in emergency situations. All physicians who are called on to choose ostomy sites should familiarize themselves with the principles of proper stoma site selection, including placement of the stoma within the rectus abdominis muscle, use of multiple patient positions to identify appropriate stoma sites, avoidance of folds and scars, and consideration of the clothing/beltline.

PURPOSE (RATIONALE FOR POSITION):

The WOCN Society in collaboration with the ASCRS and the AUA developed the following educational guide to assist clinicians (especially those who are not surgeons or WOC nurses) in selecting an effective stoma site. Marking the optimal location for a stoma preoperatively enhances the likelihood of a patient's independence in stoma care, predictable pouching system wear times, and resumption of normal activities.

RECOMMENDATIONS:

A. Key points to consider

1. The stoma site should be located within the rectus abdominis muscle.
2. Positioning issues: Contractures, posture, mobility (e.g., wheelchair confinement, use of a walker, etc.).
3. Physical considerations: Large/protruding/pendulous abdomen, abdominal folds, wrinkles, scars/suture lines, other stomas, rectus abdominis muscle, waist line, iliac crest, braces, pendulous breasts, vision, dexterity, and the presence of a hernia.
4. Patient considerations: Diagnosis, age, occupation, prior experience with a stoma, and preferences about the stoma's location.

5. Surgical considerations: Surgeon's preferences, type of surgery/stoma planned, segment of intestine used, and whether an incontinent versus a continent catheterizable diversion is planned.
6. Multiple stoma sites: If a urinary stoma is also present or planned, consider marking the fecal and urinary stoma sites on different horizontal planes/lines in the event that an ostomy belt is required.

B. Stoma site marking procedure

1. Gather items needed for the procedure: Marking pen, surgical marker, transparent film dressing, and flat skin barrier (i.e., according to the surgeon's preference and/or the facility's policy).
2. Explain the stoma site marking procedure to the patient, and encourage the patient's participation and input.
3. Carefully examine the patient's abdominal surface. If possible, begin with the patient fully clothed in a sitting position with both feet on the floor.
   - Observe the presence of belts, braces, and any other ostomy pouches.
   - Individuals with spinal cord injuries are optimally marked in their usual position, as this will facilitate fitting and care of the pouching system (Cataldo, 2008).
   - If the patient uses a wheelchair, it is best to position the patient in his or her own chair and allow time for the body to relax into the usual habitus before marking (Hocevar & Gray, 2008).
4. Have the patient completely remove any clothing that is placed over the abdomen, rather than just moving it out of the way. Waistbands and elastic can create or obscure skin folds that may or may not be present when the clothing is completely removed.
5. Examine the patient's exposed abdomen in various positions (e.g., standing, lying, sitting, and bending forward) to observe for creases, valleys, scars, folds, skin turgor, and contour.
6. Consider an imaginary line where the surgical incision will be located. If possible, choose a point at least 2 inches from the surgical incision where 2 to 3 inches of a flat adhesive skin barrier can be placed.
7. With the patient lying on his or her back, identify the rectus abdominis muscle. This can be done by having the patient do a modified sit-up (i.e., raise the head up and off the bed) or by having the patient cough. Palpate the edge of the rectus abdominis muscle. Expert opinion suggests that placement of the stoma within the rectus abdominis muscle may help prevent a peristomal hernia and/or a prolapse (ASCRS & WOCN, 2007).

8. Mark a spot on the skin of the abdomen that is located within the rectus abdominis muscle, in the appropriate quadrant for the planned surgery, and within the patient's visual field.

   • Care should be taken to avoid scars or creases; the priority is a flat pouching surface.

   • Individuals who use a wheelchair or have a large, rounded abdominal contour may benefit from having the stoma site marked in an upper quadrant (Hocevar & Gray, 2008).

   • Choose an area that is visible to the patient, and if possible below the belt line to conceal the pouch.

9. If the abdomen is protuberant, choose the apex of the abdominal contour, or if the patient is extremely obese, consider marking the site in an upper abdominal quadrant (Colwell, 2014). In many obese patients, the adipose layer is not as thick in the upper abdominal quadrants as compared to the lower quadrants, which may allow better visualization of the stoma (Cataldo, 2008; Colwell, 2014).

10. The mark should initially be made with a sticker or ink pen that can be removed if this is not the optimal spot.

   • It may be desirable to mark sites on the right and left sides of the abdomen to prepare for a change in the surgical outcome, and number the first choice as #1.

   • Have the patient assume sitting, bending, and lying positions to assess and confirm the best choice.

   • It is important to have the patient confirm he or she can see the site. However, the critical consideration should be a flat pouching surface.

11. After the optimal site is chosen, clean the desired site with alcohol and allow it to dry. Then proceed with marking the selected site with a surgical marker or pen. If desired, cover the site with a transparent film dressing to preserve the final mark. Ensure that any other stray marks have been removed.

C. Examples of stoma site marking

1. See **Figure 1**: Example of marking a stoma site for a female with a protuberant abdomen, creases, and folds.

2. See **Figure 2**: Example of marking a stoma site for a male with a protuberant abdomen.

Step 1
Look at the profile of the patient. Notice where the abdomen curves back under toward the body. The underside of the abdomen is not visible to the patient. Avoid this area.

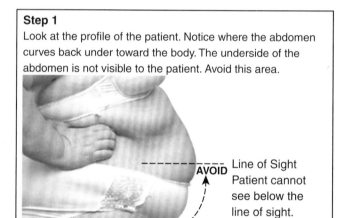

AVOID — Line of Sight Patient cannot see below the line of sight.

Step 2
While patient is seated, look for skin folds and creases. Note and avoid skin folds and creases.

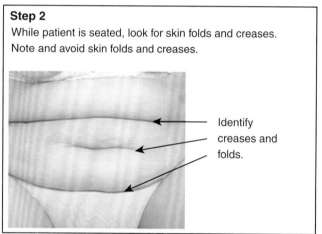

Identify creases and folds.

Step 3
Identify and target the rectus abdominis muscle below the ribs.

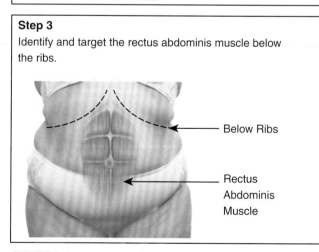

Below Ribs

Rectus Abdominis Muscle

Step 4
Mark optimal stoma sites on the rectus abdominis, that are in patient's line of sight, while avoiding creases and skin folds.

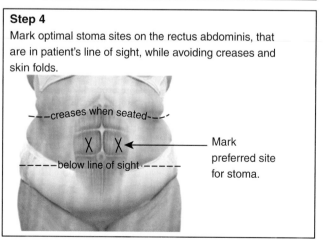

creases when seated

below line of sight

Mark preferred site for stoma.

FIGURE 1 Stoma Site Marking for a Female With a Protuberant Abdomen. (Images used with permission: **Step 1**, female photograph © milk122/veer; **Step 2**, female photograph © SeDmi/veer; **Steps 3 and 4**, female photograph © kokhanchikov/shutterstock, and muscle overlay © Randall Reed Photography/veer.)

Step 1

Look at the profile of the patient. Notice where the abdomen curves back under toward the body. The underside of the abdomen is not visible to the patient. Avoid this area.

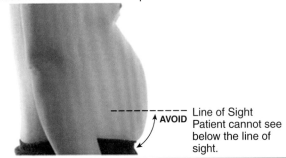

↑ **AVOID**

Line of Sight
Patient cannot see below the line of sight.

Step 2

Identify and target the rectus abdominis muscle below the ribs.

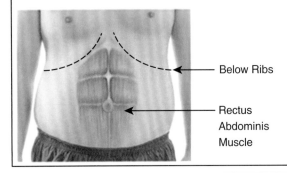

← Below Ribs

← Rectus Abdominis Muscle

Step 3

Mark optimal stoma sites on the rectus abdominis muscle, that are in patient's line of sight, while avoiding creases and skin folds.

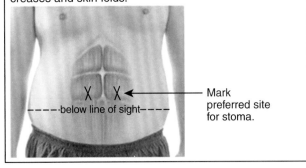

X X ← Mark preferred site for stoma.

----below line of sight----

FIGURE 2 Stoma Site Marking for a Male with a Protuberant Abdomen. (Images used with permission: **Steps 1, 2, and 3**, male photograph © sirastock/shutterstock; **Steps 2 and 3**, muscle overlay © Randall Reed Photography/veer.)

SUMMARY:

Stoma site selection should be a priority during the pre-operative visit. Marking the site for a stoma preoperatively provides an opportunity to select the optimal site, which can help reduce postoperative problems such as leakage, peristomal dermatitis, and difficulty with self-care of the ostomy. Whenever possible, ostomy education and stoma site selection should be performed preoperatively when an ostomy is a possibility.

ACKNOWLEDGMENT

The task force wishes to acknowledge Christina Augustyn, Industrial Designer, Innovation Management Office, Hollister Incorporated, Libertyville, Illinois, for her contribution in the selection and development of the images.

REFERENCES

American Society of Colon and Rectal Surgeons Committee Members & Wound Ostomy Continence Nurse Society Committee Members. (2007). ASCRS and WOCN joint position statement on the value of preoperative stoma marking for patients undergoing fecal ostomy surgery. *Journal of Wound, Ostomy, and Continence Nursing, 34*(6), 627–628.

Cataldo, P. A. (2008). Technical tips for stoma creation in the challenging patient. *Clinics in Colon and Rectal Surgery, 21*(1), 17–22. doi: 10.1055/s-2008-1055317.

Colwell, J. C. (2014). The role of obesity in the patient undergoing colorectal surgery and fecal diversion: A review of the literature. *Ostomy Wound Management, 60*(1), 24–28.

Gulbiniene, J., Markelis, R., Tamelis, A., et al. (2004). The impact of preoperative stoma siting and stoma care education on patient's quality of life. *Medicina (Kaunas, Lithuania), 40*(11), 1045–1053.

Hocevar, B., & Gray, M. (2008). Intestinal diversion (colostomy or ileostomy) in patients with severe bowel dysfunction following spinal cord injury. *Journal of Wound, Ostomy, and Continence Nursing, 35*(2), 159–166. doi: 10.1097/01.WON.0000313638.29623.40.

Millan, M., Tegido, M., Biondo, S., et al. (2010). Preoperative stoma siting and education by stomatherapists of colorectal cancer patients: A descriptive study in twelve Spanish colorectal surgical units. *Colorectal Disease, 12*(7 Online), e88–e92. doi: 10.1111/j.1463-1318.2009.01942.x.

Park, J. J., Del Pino, A., Orsay, C. P., et al. (1999). Stoma complications: The Cook County Hospital experience. *Diseases of the Colon and Rectum, 42*(12), 1575–1580.

Parmar, K. L., Zammit, M., Smith, A., et al. (2011). A prospective audit of early stoma complications in colorectal cancer treatment throughout the Greater Manchester and Cheshire colorectal cancer network. *Colorectal Disease, 13*(8), 935–938. doi: 10.1111/j.1463-1318.2010.02325.x.

Pittman, J., Rawl, S. M., Schmidt, C. M., et al. (2008). Demographic and clinical factors related to ostomy complications and quality of life in veterans with an ostomy. *Journal of Wound, Ostomy, and Continence Nursing, 35*(5), 493–503. doi: 10.1097/01.WON.0000335961.68113.cb.

Wound, Ostomy and Continence Nurses Society (WOCN). (2010). *Management of the patient with a fecal ostomy: Best practice guideline for clinicians.* Mount Laurel, NJ: WOCN Society.

APPENDIX H

Urostomy Products and Tips

Best Practice for Clinicians

ACKNOWLEDGMENTS

Urostomy Products and Tips: Best Practice for Clinicians
  This document was developed by the WOCN Society's Clinical Practice Ostomy Committee between February 2012 and July 2013.

Mary Mahoney, Chair, BSN, RN, CWON
Wound and Ostomy Nurse
Iowa Health Home Care
Urbandale, IA

Kathryn Baxter, RN, FNP, CWOCN
Nurse Practitioner
St. Luke's Roosevelt Hospital
New York, NY

Joanna Burgess, BSN, RN, CWOCN
Wound, Ostomy, and Continence Nurse
WakeMed Health and Hospitals
Cary, NC

Carole Bauer, MSN, RN, ANP-BC, OCN, CWOCN, MSN, RN, ANP-BC, OCN, CWOCN
Wound, Ostomy, and Continence Nurse Practitioner
Karmanos Cancer Center
Detroit, MI

Cathy Downey, BSN, RN, CWOCN
Program Coordinator
University Medical Center
Las Vegas, NV

Janet Mantel, MA, RN-BC, APN, CWOCN
Advanced Practice Nurse
Englewood Hospital & Medical Center
Englewood, NJ

Jacqueline Perkins, MSN, ARNP, FNP, CWOCN
Wound/Ostomy Nurse Practitioner
VA Central Iowa Health Care System
Des Moines, IA

Michelle Rice, MSN, RN, CWOCN
Ostomy Clinical Nurse Specialist
Duke University Hospital
Durham, NC

Ginger Salvadalena, PhD, RN, CWOCN
Senior Clinical Research Scientist
Hollister Incorporated
Libertyville, IL

Vickie Schafer, MSN, RN, CWON, CCRA
Associate Director, Medical & Scientific Liaison
Medical Affairs North America
Skillman, NJ

Shirley Sheppard, MSN, RN, CWON
Wound Ostomy Skin Care Nurse
University of Illinois Hospital and Health Sciences System
Chicago, IL

INTRODUCTION

A urostomy (e.g., ileal conduit or colon conduit) is an opening on the abdomen that is surgically created to drain urine. The urine is typically managed by wearing a pouch on the abdomen. The pouch is drained into the toilet. Additional products are available to accommodate an increased volume of drainage, such as leg bags and bedside drainage collectors.

This document was developed as a resource for nurses and other health care providers who care for patients with urostomies. It provides a brief description of the features of different types of pouching systems (i.e., pouch and skin barrier) and accessories. This overview also includes advantages, disadvantages, and special considerations for the use of different types of pouching systems. Additionally, it includes tips for routine pouch care including emptying the pouch, plus attaching, detaching, and cleaning of drainage collection containers.

POUCHING SYSTEMS

PRODUCT DESCRIPTION	ADVANTAGES	DISADVANTAGES	SPECIAL CONSIDERATIONS
Disposable Pouching System			
• The pouching system is designed to be discarded upon removal after wearing for a period of time, which varies according to the product or a patient's preference. • Pouches are typically made of lightweight plastic, which is available in transparent or opaque material, and may have a plastic or fabric backing. • Disposable pouches can be part of one-piece or two-piece pouching systems, and are available in various sizes/capacities.	• Odor resistant • May be worn during a bath, shower, in the swimming pool, and during other water-related activities • Cleaning is not usually necessary. • Pouches are typically changed every 3–7 days.	• Over time, disposables may be more expensive than reusable pouching systems.	
Reusable Pouching System			
• It may be a one-piece or two-piece system, composed of a pouch with a skin barrier, or a pouch and a silicone ring. The pouch and barrier or rings are made of material that can be cleaned for reuse, and are available in various sizes/capacities. • Pouches are commonly made of vinyl or thick plastic. Rubber products are available. • Barriers are commonly plastic or rubber.	• Can reuse/reapply multiple times with appropriate care and cleansing (length of use dependent on manufacturer) • Some can be used without an adhesive. • Some styles may be removable for daily bathing.	• Can retain odors • Limited number of manufacturers • Initial cost may be more expensive than a disposable pouching system. • More time involved with cleaning the system • Might require use of a belt or adhesive	
One-Piece Pouching System			
• The skin barrier and pouch are fused together during manufacturing.	• Many styles are flexible and conform to abdominal contours. • Low profile • No chance for leakage between the skin barrier and pouch, which can occur in two-piece systems • May be less costly than a two-piece system • May be easier to learn to use than a two-piece system	• Cannot reposition the pouch once it is applied • Cannot change the pouch without changing the entire system	

POUCHING SYSTEMS (*Continued*)

PRODUCT DESCRIPTION	ADVANTAGES	DISADVANTAGES	SPECIAL CONSIDERATIONS
Two-Piece Pouching System with Interlocking Flange			
• The skin barrier and pouch are made separately and have rigid to semirigid rings, which allow the user to attach the two parts together.	• Can change the angle of the pouch to accommodate changes in a patient's position. • Can detach the pouch from the barrier to obtain a urine sample from the stoma • Can detach the pouch from the barrier to change the pouch without removing the barrier	• Higher profile than a one-piece system • Less flexible than a one-piece system, and does not mold as well to the body's contours	• Requires manual dexterity and strength to assure attachment of the pouch to the skin barrier
Two-Piece Pouching System with Flexible Adhesive Flange			
• The skin barrier and pouch are made separately and designed to adhere together without a rigid flange.	• Can change the pouch for disposal or emptying without removing the skin barrier • Extremely low profile • Flexibility of a one-piece system • May be easier to apply for those with poor manual dexterity	• Limited number of times the pouch can be reattached to the skin barrier (dependent on the manufacturer) • May be difficult to reuse or reattach the pouch if the adhesive area becomes wet • May be more difficult for visually impaired patients to use	• Must have good hand–eye coordination to properly attach the pouch's adhesive area to the skin barrier
Nonadhesive Pouching System			
• The system is reusable and is composed of a pouch, a nonadherent silicone O-ring seal, and a belt. The silicone O-rings are available in different sizes and thickness. Pouches are available in different sizes and designed with the stoma opening either on the right or left side. • With adequate tension of the belt, the pliable silicone O-ring creates a secure seal between the pouch and abdomen.	• Can reuse/reapply multiple times with appropriate care and cleansing (length of use dependent on manufacturer) • Useful for individuals with allergies to adhesive skin barriers or with other significant skin conditions in the area of the pouch adhesive	• Nonadhesive systems may not seal well with flush or retracted stomas, or with deep skin folds/creases near the stoma.	• If additional compression is needed to obtain an adequate seal for patients with a softer abdomen or with skin folds, the thicker (taller) O-ring may be needed. • Peristomal skin should be monitored for signs of damage if the belt is worn tightly.

TYPES OF POUCHES

PRODUCT DESCRIPTION	ADVANTAGES	DISADVANTAGES	SPECIAL CONSIDERATIONS
• Urostomy pouches have a valve, cap, or plug at the bottom to keep the pouch closed until it is time to empty the pouch or attach to a drainage collection container.	• Urostomy pouches are specifically designed to drain urine. • Most urostomy pouches have an antireflux feature to prevent backflow of urine onto the stoma.		• Requires manual dexterity and strength to manage the various valves or plugs for emptying. • It is not recommended to use fecal pouches for a urostomy.

(*Continued*)

TYPES OF POUCHES (*Continued*)

PRODUCT DESCRIPTION	ADVANTAGES	DISADVANTAGES	SPECIAL CONSIDERATIONS
Transparent Pouch			
• Pouch is made of clear lightweight plastic.	• Can see the stoma through the pouch for easy application of the pouching system, if applying as a one-piece • Can see the stoma while the pouch is in place to monitor the color and appearance of the stoma • Can see the urine while it is inside the pouch to monitor the color and clarity of the urine	• May be unpleasant for the patient or the patient's spouse/partner to see the stoma or urine inside the pouch	
Opaque Pouch			
• Pouch is made of colored lightweight plastic (typically white or beige).	• Cosmetically appealing: cannot see the stoma or urine in the pouch • More discreet under light-colored clothing	• May be more difficult to apply when part of a one-piece pouching system because of the inability to visualize the stoma through the pouch for placement	

TYPES OF SKIN BARRIERS

PRODUCT DESCRIPTION	ADVANTAGES	DISADVANTAGES	SPECIAL CONSIDERATIONS
• Skin barriers: The part of the pouching system that is attached or placed against the skin. Adhesive skin barriers are made from pectin, karaya gum, or synthetic materials. A nonadhesive barrier is made from silicone or rubber. • Skin barriers are available with presized openings (precut) or can be sized to the patient's stoma (cut-to-fit or shapable).			
Flat Skin Barrier			
• A skin barrier that is completely level.	• Useful for flat peristomal skin surfaces	• May need to add accessories to obtain a better seal if the peristomal skin is not flat	
Convex Skin Barrier			
• A skin barrier that has a rounded surface on the back (skin contact side) of the barrier. • Convex skin barriers can be rigid or flexible.	• Useful for a peristomal skin surface that is concave or with a flush or retracted stoma	• May need to add an ostomy belt to enhance the seal • Barrier may lift from the skin if the convexity is too rigid. • May be more expensive than a flat skin barrier	
Shapable Skin Barrier			
• The barrier's stomal opening can be molded to fit. • Available flat or convex	• Allows the opening for the stoma to be stretched and shaped with fingers rather than using scissors to cut the opening	• May not seal consistently with flush or partially flush stomas • The barrier can expand over the stomal opening, leading to leakage and decreased wear time.	

TYPES OF SKIN BARRIERS (*Continued*)

PRODUCT DESCRIPTION	ADVANTAGES	DISADVANTAGES	SPECIAL CONSIDERATIONS
Skin Barrier with Stationary Flange			
• A skin barrier used in a two-piece pouching system with a flange that is secured to the barrier • Available flat or convex	• Lower profile than a floating flange	• Snapping the pouch to a barrier that is already attached on the patient's abdomen may cause discomfort.	
Skin Barrier with Floating Flange			
• A skin barrier used in a two-piece pouching system with a flange that rises above the barrier, allowing a person's fingers to fit between the barrier and the flange. • Available flat or convex	• A floating flange allows the pouch to be snapped onto the skin barrier without adding pressure to the abdomen.	• Higher profile than a nonfloating flange	
Skin Barrier with Locking Flange			
• A skin barrier used in a two-piece pouching system • Available flat or convex	• The pouch can be locked into place. • May require less manual dexterity to attach the pouch to the flange • Allows the pouch to be snapped onto the skin barrier without applying pressure to the abdomen	• Higher profile than a nonlocking flange	
Skin Barrier with Plastic Surface			
• A skin barrier used in a two-piece pouching system. The pouch adheres to the skin barrier's plastic surface with an adhesive ring. • Available flat or convex	• Pouch can be detached and reapplied. • Low profile	• Pouch does not stick well if the adhesive surface gets wet.	
Skin Barrier with Tape Collar			
• Skin barrier has a wide collar of tape around the outside of the barrier.	• A skin barrier with the tape collar has more flexibility and a lower profile than solid barriers.	• Potential tape sensitivity (rare) • Potential for epidermal skin stripping with tape removal	

SILICONE RING BARRIER

PRODUCT DESCRIPTION	ADVANTAGES	DISADVANTAGES	SPECIAL CONSIDERATIONS
• A nonadhesive ring used instead of a skin barrier • Rings are available in different sizes to use with disposable or reusable pouches that are available in various shapes/sizes to accommodate individual needs or preferences.	• The nonadhesive quality is helpful for people with allergies, or for people who want to remove the system on a daily basis.	• Need to wear a belt to hold in place • May not seal well in certain abdominal contours (i.e., deep creases or folds), or with flush or retracted stomas	

OTHER POUCH/SKIN BARRIER FEATURES

PRODUCT DESCRIPTION	ADVANTAGES	DISADVANTAGES	SPECIAL CONSIDERATIONS
Belt Loops			
• A feature on a pouch or skin barrier that allows for use of an elastic belt	• Belt loops on the skin barrier allow the pouch to be applied and removed without disturbing the belt. • Belt loops on the pouch can add security to the connection between the pouch and skin barrier flange.	• Presence of belt loops may make the skin barrier more rigid. • The belt loops may be uncomfortable against the body and can result in skin damage.	
Adapters (Connectors)			
• Devices specifically designed to allow for attachment of urostomy pouches to other drainage systems	• Adapters securely connect the pouch outlet to tubing for attachment of a drainage collection container, such as a bedside drainage container or a leg bag. • Adapters are designed to be more secure than pieces of latex or silicone tubing.	• Adapters are not interchangeable between the brands.	• Requires manual dexterity and strength to attach the adapter • An adapter is replaced when the drainage collection container is replaced.
Drainage Collection Container			
• Consists of a container, which is either a soft plastic container (i.e., leg bag or bedside drainage bag) or a hard plastic jug, and tubing that connects to the regular pouch with an adapter	• Connecting the pouch to a drainage collection container increases capacity of the pouch and decreases the frequency of emptying. • Extending the frequency of emptying prevents overfilling of the pouch during times when the pouch cannot be emptied, and allows the person the time to rest through the night.	• Patient will need a place to store the collection container when it is not in use. • Tubing may kink.	• To prevent kinking of the tubing, position the tubing down the patient's leg or toward the foot of the bed securing the tubing with leg straps or tape. • Teach the patient to clean the collection container to decrease bacteria and control odor. • There are different methods of cleansing the collection container: follow agency or manufacturer's protocol. • Soft drainage collection containers are replaced twice a month or according to facility or agency policy. • Hard plastic jug containers are replaced every 3 months.

ACCESSORIES

PRODUCT DESCRIPTION	ADVANTAGES	DISADVANTAGES	SPECIAL CONSIDERATIONS
Pouch Cover			
• Cloth, envelope-like sleeve to place and wear over the ostomy pouch while it is on the body	• Cosmetically appealing, cannot see the stoma or urine inside the pouch • Easily applied by slipping over pouch while it is on the body • Provides a comfortable surface against the skin to help prevent perspiration, chafing, or allergies • May help reduce noise from a vinyl or plastic pouch • May be integrated within available disposable pouches	• Added expense if fabric material is already covering the backing (skin side) of a pouch • If integrated into the pouch, may take time to dry after bathing, showering, or swimming	

ACCESSORIES (*Continued*)

PRODUCT DESCRIPTION	ADVANTAGES	DISADVANTAGES	SPECIAL CONSIDERATIONS
Skin Sealant			
• Plasticizing agent made of ingredients such as silicone or a copolymer • Contains variable amounts of isopropyl alcohol • Available as a wipe, spray, gel, liquid, or roll-on	• Provides a thin protective film to the surface of the skin • Helps to prevent stripping of the epidermis during adhesive removal, and some also act as a moisture barrier	• Sealants may not be recommended under some skin barriers because the protective film may reduce the adherence of the skin barrier. • Many sealants contain alcohol that causes pain when applied to irritated skin, and in such situations, an alcohol-free product is needed.	• If applying stoma powder to skin irritation, a skin sealant applied over the powder and dried provides a dry, smooth surface for adherence of the skin barrier. • May be used to seal antifungal powder when needed to treat peristomal candidiasis
Skin Adhesive			
• Adhesive products made of silicone or latex	• Can be used to strengthen the adhesion of an adhesive pouching system, or to provide adhesion for a reusable (nonadhesive) system	• May cause pain and further irritation to already denuded skin. Recommend "crusting technique" prior to application to denuded skin. • May be flammable	• Teach the patient to allow the adhesive to dry prior to application of the pouch to prevent chemical irritation.
Adhesive Remover			
• Available as a wipe, spray or liquid	• Aids in the removal of tape, skin adhesives, and other residue on the skin • May be helpful to the patient with sensitive skin to reduce trauma from removal of the pouching system	• Cleaning the skin with mild soap and water is typically required to remove any of the solvent's residue before application of the next pouching system to prevent chemical dermatitis or nonadherence of the pouching system.	• A silicone-based, alcohol-free adhesive remover may not require additional cleansing.
Paste			
• Pectin-based or karaya products	• Can be used to fill in uneven areas or as caulking around the inner edge of the skin barrier to prevent stomal drainage getting beneath the skin barrier • Fills in small creases and depressions and evens out skin/abdominal contours under a skin barrier to increase the fit and adherence of the skin barrier • Used appropriately, will offer a quick seal for the pouching system until the skin barrier adhesive is pressed into place • Not commonly used for patients with a urostomy, but some patients find it helpful	• Most pastes contain some alcohol and may sting when applied to irritated peristomal skin. • Paste is not substantial enough to fill in large creases, as it will wash out. • Patients often think the paste is an "adhesive" and use it inappropriately (i.e., spread the paste like a glue over a large surface area on the skin or skin barrier). • Patients often use excessive amounts of paste, resulting in poor adherence of the pouch and leakage. • Karaya products melt easily when exposed to urine.	• Requires manual dexterity to squeeze paste from the tube and for application of paste to the peristomal skin or skin barrier

(Continued)

ACCESSORIES (*Continued*)

PRODUCT DESCRIPTION	ADVANTAGES	DISADVANTAGES	SPECIAL CONSIDERATIONS
Skin Barrier Rings			
• Pectin or sodium carboxymethylcellulose based product that is soft and moldable formed by the manufacturer into a flat or convex ring • Available in different sizes and flat or convex	• Prevent leakage of stomal drainage under the skin barrier • Increase the seal of skin barriers by molding into contours of the abdominal surface • May be used as an alternative, or in addition, to paste • Can be used in their original shape and form, or stretched and molded to create custom shapes to fill in uneven areas • Can be cut, bent, or stacked together to improve the fit of the skin barrier • May prolong a skin barrier's wear time • Leave less residue than paste on the skin after removal • Conform to irregular skin folds • Alcohol free and may be used on irritated skin	• Added cost • Added step in the application technique	Requires manual dexterity for application to the peristomal skin or skin barrier
Skin Barrier Strip Paste			
• Pectin-based product in soft, moldable, flexible strips	• Prevents leakage of urine under the skin barrier • Increases the seal of a skin barrier by molding into contours of the abdominal surface • May be used as an alternative to paste • Can be used in the original shape and form, or stretched and molded to create custom shapes to fill in uneven areas • Can be cut, bent, or stacked together to improve the fit of the skin barrier • May extend skin barrier wear time • Leaves less residue than paste on the skin after removal • Conforms to irregular skin folds • Alcohol free and may be used on irritated skin	• Added cost, and may not be covered by insurance • Added step in the application process	• Requires manual dexterity for application to the peristomal skin or skin barrier
Stoma Powder			
• Pectin or karaya-based powder used to protect peristomal skin and areas of mucocutaneous separation from exposure to stomal discharge	• Aids in healing of open, irritated peristomal skin • Absorbs moisture or exudate from the peristomal skin prior to placing a skin barrier for added protection and enhanced adherence of the skin barrier	• Karaya powder may sting when applied to irritated peristomal skin. • If applied improperly (i.e., excessive amounts), powder may prevent adhesion of the skin barrier.	• Powder may be sealed to the skin by applying a layer of skin sealant over the powder and allowing it to dry, before applying the pouching system, to provide a smooth, dry surface for adherence of the pouching system.

ACCESSORIES (*Continued*)

PRODUCT DESCRIPTION	ADVANTAGES	DISADVANTAGES	SPECIAL CONSIDERATIONS
Elastic Barrier Strip			
• Elastic material designed to be placed around the edges of the ostomy skin barrier to hold it securely in place	• Strips are a skin-friendly alternative to tape. • Use supports longer wear time by decreasing the roll-up on the edges of the barrier. • Due to the elasticity, strips move with the body to hold the skin barrier firmly in place during movement.	• Added cost may not be covered by insurance.	• Store strips in a cool, dry location (away from direct sunlight). • Apply strips while they are at room temperature.
Ostomy Belt			
• Elastic belt with hooks to fasten to the belt loops on the pouch or skin barrier to hold the pouching system firmly in place • Belts are available in varying sizes and widths, and are adjustable. Most belts are latex free.	• Adds stability and security to the ostomy pouching system • Often used with convex skin barriers for added security • Belts are washable and reusable.	• Ostomy belts may be uncomfortable for some patients. • Added cost, and may not be covered by insurance	• Requires manual dexterity to attach the belt • Attaching the belt so it lies evenly on the abdomen and is level with the belt loops helps prevent the belt from riding up or down on the abdomen and possibly dislodging the pouching system (American Cancer Society, 2011; American College of Surgeons, n.d.a). • It is important that the tightness of the belt be adjusted so that it does not leave deep grooves or cuts in the skin (American Cancer Society, 2011; American College of Surgeons, n.d.a). • Belt will get wet during showering, bathing, and swimming, which may affect the fit/security of the belt. • It is important for individuals with latex allergies to verify that their chosen belts are latex free.
Ostomy Support Belt			
• Wide, binder-type, belts are designed to support the abdominal muscles or peristomal hernias, or provide pouch support. • Support belts are available in various sizes, widths, and fabrics. Most support belts are latex free. • The belts can be customized for the location and size of the opening for the pouch.	• Support belts can increase the comfort and security of the pouching system to increase wear time. • Can help manage peristomal hernias, or support pendulous, bulging abdomens • Belts are washable and reusable.	• Support belts may be uncomfortable for some patients. • Added cost, and may not be covered by insurance • If not fitted correctly, the support belt may dislodge the pouching system.	• Requires manual dexterity to apply the belt • Manufacturer's directions for measuring and selection of the size and type of support belt must be carefully followed. • For best results with hernias, apply and fasten the support belt in a flat-lying position. • Prolapsed stomas are not common in patients with a urostomy, but prolapse overbelt attachments are available to help manage prolapsed stomas. • It is important for individuals with latex allergies to verify that their chosen support belts are latex free.

TIPS FOR EMPTYING THE POUCH

PRODUCT DESCRIPTION	ADVANTAGES	DISADVANTAGES	SPECIAL CONSIDERATIONS
• Teach the patient to empty the pouch when it is one-third to one-half full. • Teach the following steps for emptying the pouch (American Cancer Society, 2011; American College of Surgeons, n.d.b): • Sit on toilet with the pouch between the legs or stand in front of/or alongside the toilet. • Place a layer of toilet paper in the toilet to reduce splashing. • Point the end of the pouch into the toilet and open the closure on the spout at the end of the pouch to drain the urine. • Wipe the end of the pouch/spout with toilet paper. • Close the spout on the pouch. • Wash hands.	• Regular emptying of the pouch: • Minimizes exposure of the stoma to urine in the pouch • Prevents excess weight and volume in the pouch to prevent dislodging the skin barrier or pouch • Prevents bulging of the pouch, to maintain a low profile		• Requires mobility and manual dexterity • Requires adaptation of the emptying technique for patients with visual, physical, and other mobility or functional limitations (e.g., bedbound, wheelchair bound, hemiplegia, paraplegia, blindness, severe arthritis in hands)

TIPS FOR ATTACHING THE POUCH TO A DRAINAGE COLLECTION CONTAINER (DRAINAGE COLLECTOR)

PRODUCT DESCRIPTION	ADVANTAGES	DISADVANTAGES	SPECIAL CONSIDERATIONS
• Teach the patient to use the correct adapter for the brand of pouch he or she is using when connecting to a drainage collector. • Steps in connecting to a drainage collector (American Cancer Society, 2011; American College of Surgeons, n.d.a; United Ostomy Associations of America, Inc., n.d.): • Leave a small amount of urine in the pouch prior to attaching the drainage collector to prevent creating a vacuum in the system. • Wash hands. • Attach the adapter to the tubing or spout on the drainage collector. • Connect the end of the pouch to the adapter on the drainage collector. • Open the closure on the pouch's drainage spout to allow the urine to flow. • Position the drainage collector below the level of the urostomy pouch.	• A drainage collector adds capacity to the ostomy pouch.	• Needs to be rinsed and kept clean/dry • Takes extra time to care for the drainage collection container • Additional cost, and may not be covered by insurance	• Requires manual dexterity to attach

TIPS FOR DETACHING AND CLEANING A DRAINAGE COLLECTION CONTAINER (DRAINAGE COLLECTOR)

PRODUCT DESCRIPTION	ADVANTAGES	DISADVANTAGES	SPECIAL CONSIDERATIONS

• Teach the patient how to detach and clean the drainage collector.
• Steps in detaching the drainage collector (American College of Surgeons, n.d.a):
  1. Wash hands.
  2. Close the spout of the urostomy pouch to prevent leakage.
  3. Detach the drainage collector along with the adapter from the urostomy pouch.
  4. Empty the urine from the drainage collector and rinse with cool water.
  5. Clean the drainage collector (tubing and adapter) daily or every other day with a vinegar and water solution (1 part white vinegar and 3 parts water); or according to agency or manufacturer's protocol (American Cancer Society, 2011; Einstein Healthcare Network, n.d.; United Ostomy Associations of America, Inc., n.d.).
  6. Instill the vinegar and water solution through the tubing or spout into the container and let it sit for an hour; then empty and rinse with cool water (Einstein Healthcare Network, n.d.).
  7. Allow the drainage collector to air dry with the closure open.
	• Regular rinsing and cleansing reduces odor of the drainage collector.		• Requires manual dexterity to detach and clean the drainage collector
			• Requires a space to hang the collector to dry when it is not in use

REFERENCES

American Cancer Society. (2011). *Urostomy: A guide*. Retrieved July 2013, from http://www.cancer.org/acs/groups/cid/documents/webcontent/002931-pdf.pdf

American College of Surgeons. (n.d.a). *Empty the pouch SKILL*. Retrieved July 2013, from http://www.facs.org/patienteducation/skills/empty-pouch.pdf

American College of Surgeons. (n.d.b). *What is a urostomy?* Retrieved July 2013, from http://www.facs.org/patienteducation/skills/your-urostomy.pdf

Einstein Healthcare Network. (n.d.). *Urostomy: Using a night drainage system*. Retrieved July 2013, from http://www.einstein.edu/einstein healthtopic/?articleId=89997&articleTypeId=3&healthTopicid=-I&h ealthTopicName=HealthSheets

United Ostomy Associations of America, Inc. (n.d.). *Urostomy guide*. Retrieved July 2013, from http://www.ostomy.org/ostomy_info/pubs/UrostomyGuide.pdf

ACKNOWLEDGMENT ABOUT CONTENT VALIDATION

This document was reviewed in the consensus-building process of the Wound, Ostomy, and Continence Nurses Society known as Content Validation, which is managed by the Center for Clinical Investigation.

APPENDIX I

Care of Feeding Tubes

INTRODUCTION

There are many reasons why people need feeding tubes. Some need feeding tubes for a short while, and others need them for a lifetime. The choice to place a feeding tube can be difficult.

This document is designed to help you make the choice that is best for you and your family. These pages show the proper care of a feeding tube. Please note that while this document was put together as a general guide for those caring for a feeding tube, there may be information in it that does not apply to you or may be slightly different than what your health care provider has told you. Please use this tool as a reference and always consult your primary provider.

MY FEEDING TUBE

Date of procedure: _____

Health care provider performing the procedure: _____

Procedure: _____
Contact information: _____
Current feeding tube type:
☐ Gastrostomy tube or G-tube or PEG tube
Type: _____
☐ Gastrojejunostomy tube or G-J tube
Type: _____
☐ Jejunostomy tube or J tube
Type: _____
For balloon-retained feeding tubes:
Amount of water in balloon: _____mL
Some tubes have to be removed by the doctor in the operating room. Some tubes can be removed in a clinic setting.
☐ Your tube: Can be removed in a clinic setting
☐ Must be removed in the operating room

Health care provider managing my tube feeds: _____

Contact information: _____
My primary physician: _____
Contact information: _____
Home health agency: _____
Contact information: _____
Home care supplies: _____
Contact information: _____

Why Do I Need a Feeding Tube?

Your body needs food and drink to heal, have energy, and help you feel better. Since you have trouble swallowing or cannot eat enough calories, giving you food and liquids through the tube in your stomach or intestines helps your body to get the food and water it needs.

What Is a Feeding Tube?

A *feeding tube* is a tube used to provide food and water directly into your stomach or intestines. The tube is placed by a doctor. An opening is made in your skin, and the tube is put through this opening into your stomach or intestines.

What Are the Different Types of Feeding Tubes?
Gastrostomy Tube

A gastrostomy tube is a tube that goes through your skin and abdominal wall into your stomach. It is also called "G-tube" or "PEG tube."

PEG stands for:

P = percutaneous (Going through the skin)

E = endoscopic (Looking into your body with a camera and light)

G = gastrostomy (An opening put in your stomach by a doctor)

The tube may be inserted in the endoscopy department, radiology, or the operating room.

The gastrostomy tube can be used to put liquid food into the stomach. It can also be used to pull out air and liquid if the stomach isn't working properly and needs to be emptied of extra pressure. Liquid or crushed medications can also be given through the tube.

Gastrojejunostomy Tube

This tube is often called a "GJ-tube." The "J" stands for jejunum, which is a part of the small intestine. A GJ tube is actually made of two different tubes that are combined together—one that leads from the outside of your body into the stomach (a G-tube), and an extension that goes into your intestines. A GJ tube has two openings or "ports." One goes into the stomach (G-port), and one goes into the intestine (J-port). The G-port can be used just like a G-tube, as described above. The J-port can only be used for liquid nutrition. If you need to use the J-tube for medications, then the medications or crushed pills should be the same consistency as formula. Typically, medications are not given through the J-tube; however, there may be times when this is the only option for you. Prior to using the J-tube for medication, you should talk with your provider. Crushed pills can clog the tube.

Jejunostomy Tube

This tube is also called a "J-tube." This tube goes through the skin directly into the intestine (the jejunum). A J-tube is very small and can only be used for liquid nutrition. Crushed pills should NOT be put into the J-tube as they could clog the tube. Suction should never be applied to the J-tube.

What Are the Parts of a Feeding Tube?

Here are the parts of your tube you will need to know so you can use and care for your tube:

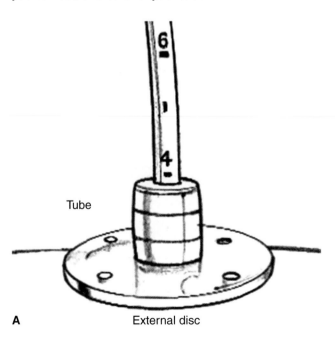

Tube

A   External disc

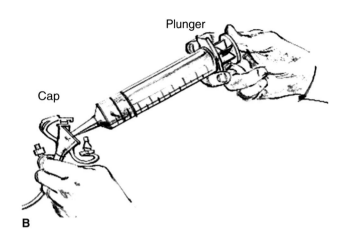

Plunger

Cap

B

Cap—The cover to the opening of the tube where the feeding goes in

Tube—Plastic or silicone tubing that may have numbers on it

External disc—Also called an "external bumper" or "bolster." This is a plastic disc outside of your skin that helps keep the tube secure

G-tubes and GJ-tubes often have an internal "bumper" or a balloon attached to the tube on the inside of the stomach to help hold it in place.

T-fasteners—In some cases, your doctor will use these to help perform the surgery. You may see one or more little "buttons" made of hard plastic or cotton, which are stitched to your skin.

Syringe—A 60-mL (2 ounces) tube with a plunger. It is used:

• As a funnel for feedings
• To flush the tube with water
• To give yourself liquid or crushed medicines

Low-profile button is a feeding tube that sits closer to the skin and attachments are needed for use

Extension sets are the tubes used with low-profile buttons for feeding and venting

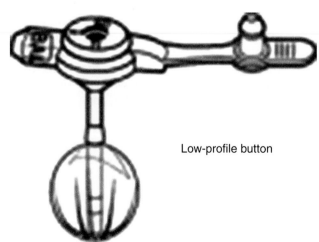

Low-profile button

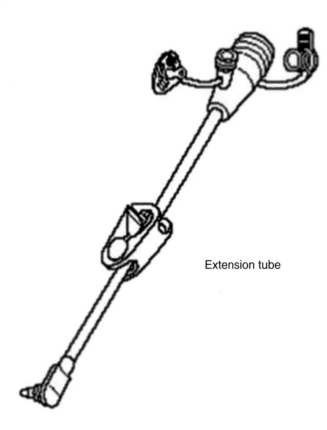

Extension tube

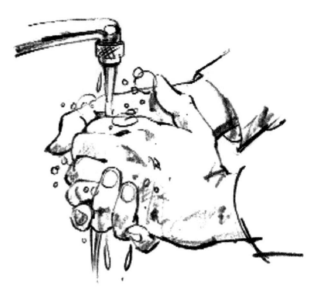

Call your health care provider's office if you have these signs of infection.

Always wash your hands very well with soap and warm water before you touch the tube. Keep the supplies that you use to care for your tube clean. Wash your hands after you finish caring for your tube or feeding yourself.

How Does the Feeding Tube Stay In?
The type of tube determines how the tube is secured. There may be a balloon on the end of the tube in your stomach that will keep it from coming out. Sometimes, the feeding tube is stitched to your skin. Your provider will explain how and when those sutures will be removed.

How Do I Protect the Tube?
• Keep the tube inside your waist band or attached to your clothes.
• Do not pull on the tube.
• Be gentle with it.
• Do not let anyone else pull out the tube.

When Should I Return to the Doctor?
Depending on the type of tube put in, you may need to come to the doctor's clinic. If so, the appointment will be made before you leave the hospital. It is often 1 week after your surgery if you have stitches that need to be removed. You may feel discomfort when the stitches are removed. Removing stitches is quick, and your skin will feel better without them.

Next Appointment: _____

What Are Signs That the Area Around the Tube May Be Infected?
• Increasing redness of the skin
• Thick yellow or green drainage around the tube that has an odor different from normal yellow-green mucus drainage
• Increasing tenderness or soreness
• Fever

How Do I Take Care of My Skin Around the Tube?
For the first few weeks, you may notice a small amount of bloody or pale yellow drainage around the tube site. The fluid may be stomach juices. This is normal and should not alarm you.

• Clean around the base of the tube two times every day. Use a Q tip or regular wash cloth with soap and water to wash around the site. Cleaning around the feeding tube site will help remove any dried crust and fluid. It will also keep your skin clean while healing.
• If needed after each cleaning, put one small gauze square around the base of the tube. Cut a T-shape in the middle of the gauze. This helps the gauze fit around the base of the tube.

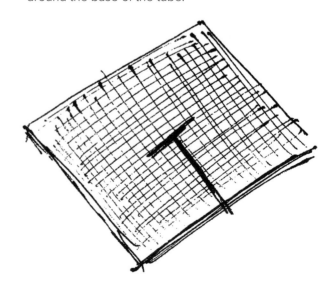

- You may also cleanse your skin in the shower.
- Depending on your normal drainage you may want to continue to place one gauze square around the base of the tube. This helps collect drainage that may occur.

My Nutrition

My current weight: _____

My current height: _____

My goal weight: _____

Nutrition instructions:

Your feeding plan should be provided by the dietician. Name of formula/feeds recommended:

_____

☐ Continuous Feeds   ☐ Bolus Feeds

Amount of Formula Daily: _____mL OR _____ cans

Amount of Water Flushes: _____mL

Amount of Additional Water: _____mL

Special Instructions: _____

_____

_____

How Do I Do a Bolus Feeding Through the Tube?

1. Take the formula from the refrigerator. Allow it to come to room temperature. This is less likely to cause stomach upset.
2. Always wash your hands well before you touch the tube or can.
3. Pour 30 mL (1 ounce) of lukewarm water into a clean measuring cup.

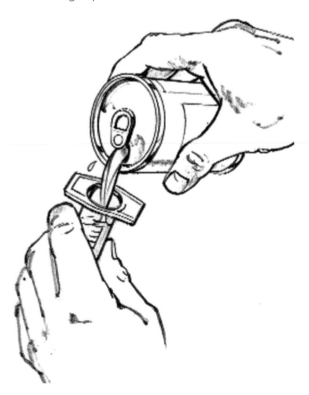

4. If you are using a can or bottle of formula:
   a. Check the expiration date on the can or bottle and discard if it has expired.
   b. Shake the can or bottle well.
   c. Rinse top of can or bottle before opening.
   d. Measure the amount of formula that is ordered for your feeding into a measuring cup.
   e. Cover and refrigerate any extra formula.
   f. Throw away any open cans or bottles of formula after 24 hours.
5. If you are being fed into a G-tube, sit with your head raised to about a 45-degree angle (approximately two pillows) as shown in the picture below.
6. This prevents fluid from entering your lungs (aspiration).

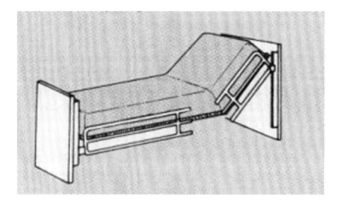

7. Clamp feeding tube. This prevents air from entering your stomach. Air causes too much fullness. It also prevents the fluid in your stomach from leaving your stomach.
8. Remove the plunger from the syringe. You do not need the plunger to feed yourself.
9. Put the tip of the syringe into tube.
10. Fill the syringe with the water. Unclamp the tube and allow the water to flow in by gravity. The flow goes more slowly if you lower the syringe. It goes more quickly if you raise the syringe.
11. Pour the formula into syringe when most of the water has gone in the stomach. This prevents air from entering your stomach.
12. After taking the right amount of formula, flush tubing with another 30 mL (1 ounce) of water. This helps prevent the feeding tube from clogging.
13. Remove the syringe and replace the plug in the end of the tube.
14. Wash your syringe and measuring cups with dish soap and warm water. Leave them on a clean towel to dry.
15. Keep your head up for 60 minutes after feeding is completed.

Note

- Do not put hot or cold liquids through the feeding tube. Hot liquids may hurt the stomach lining. Cold liquids tend to upset the stomach.
- Do not add medicine to the formula unless you have discussed this with your health care provider.

How Do I Get Water?

Water is important in taking care of yourself and your tube. You may put water through the feeding tube. The nutritionist will tell you how much water you need each day. Besides the water you use to flush the tube, this extra water prevents you from being:

- Too dry (dehydrated) in your mouth and skin and bowels
- Too thirsty (dry mouth)
- Constipated or irregular with your bowel movement

Flushing water through your tube before and after each feeding keeps it clean and open. Put 30 mL of luke-warm water through the tube **before and after** every use each day.

How Do I Take My Medicines?

Some medicines can be put through your feeding tube. *Check with your doctor* and pharmacist before putting any medicines through your tube. Your pharmacist can also talk to you about what types of medicines can be crushed or come in liquid form. Use liquid medicines when possible; crush pills well and mix with lukewarm water.

How Do I Check for Residuals?

Your doctor may ask you to "check residuals." This is to measure how much fluid is still in your stomach from the last feeding. You check for residuals before giving yourself a feeding. Checking residuals assures that the formula is being emptied by the stomach.

If you have recently taken any food by mouth, wait approximately 60 minutes before checking residuals.

1. Unclamp and open your feeding tube.
2. Attach the syringe with the plunger.

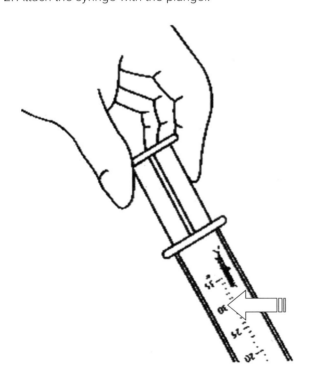

3. Slowly pull back on the plunger until it is harder to pull. The stomach contents will enter the syringe. If the stomach is empty, there may be no formula that comes back.
4. If the stomach is not empty, you may draw up some stomach juices. You may also draw up some formula from an earlier feeding. This is normal.
5. Check the numbers on the side of the syringe to determine the amount of residual. (If you withdraw more than the 60 mL of residual, you may need to empty this into a measuring cup until all of the residual is obtained and measured.)
6. **Inject the residuals back into the stomach**. It is very important to return the gastric residuals back into the stomach. The gastric juices contain chemicals (enzymes and electrolytes) that your body needs to digest the feedings.
7. If the stomach residual is >150 mL, wait 30 to 60 minutes, and check again before administering more formula. If you continually draw up high residuals (more than 150 mL), call your health care provider.

REMEMBER—When the Tube Is Not in Use

Curl it up and tuck it into your clothing or clip it to your clothing.

What Are Some Problems I Might Have with Tube Feedings?
Clogged Tubes

- To prevent a clogged tube, always flush with at least 30 mL (1 ounce) of warm water after a feeding.
- Do not put whole pills or capsules into the tube. Crush all medicines until they are powder and dissolve in water. Ask your home care nurse or your health care provider for hints.
- If the tube gets clogged, try to loosen it by putting 30 mL of warm water in the tube. Then pull back and forth on the plunger.
- For tough clogs, call the doctor's office for advice.

Aspiration

Aspiration happens when food or fluids enter the lungs. Signs of aspiration include: coughing, gagging, change in skin color, increased temperature, rapid pulse, and noisy breathing. If this occurs: STOP the feeding and notify the doctor's office. To prevent aspiration:

- Sit or lie upright at a 30- to 45-degree angle (two pillows) during the feedings.
- Remain in this position for 1 hour after feedings.
- Administer feedings slowly.

Feeling Sick

Nausea or bloating happens when formula:

- is given too fast
- is too concentrated
- is too cold

To prevent feeling sick:

- Feed slowly over 20 minutes.
- Relieve gas or bloating by allowing air out through the tube. Lie flat. Carefully open the cap and let the gas out. Massaging the belly will help get the air to the tube so that it can come out. Stomach contents may come out too.
- If nausea, bloating, or vomiting happens often with feedings, contact the doctor.

Leaking Tube

The most common complication of a feeding tube is leakage of stomach or intestinal contents around the tube. This is usually caused by a failure to secure the tube to prevent movement. A small amount of clear or pale yellow drainage around the tube can be normal.

You may have larger amounts of leakage if:

- The surrounding skin and tissues are not healing well
- The tube is in the wrong position
- The intestines are blocked
- The tube is not secured

Always make sure your tube is secured so it will not move side to side or in and out. Some tubes that do not have an external disc can be secured with a commercial tube stabilization device available from a medical supply company.

If your tube is leaking, you will need to protect your skin. Apply a layer of "diaper cream" containing zinc oxide before placing the gauze dressing. Wipe the drainage off the top of the cream and change the dressing whenever it is wet.

Hyperplasia

Hyperplasia is an overgrowth of red, raw tissue where the tube exits the skin. It can cause pain or bleeding. This tissue needs to be treated and can be treated with silver nitrate or a steroid cream. Ask your home health nurse or health care provider to help you with this.

Diarrhea

If you have loose stools for more than 3 days after beginning the tube feedings, contact your doctor.

- Diarrhea is common when starting new formula.
- It may also be a side effect of some medicines.

Constipation

Constipation happens when:

- physical activity is limited
- you take in too little water
- you take certain medications

Ask for advice from your home health nurse or health care provider. You may need to take a laxative or stool softener. More fiber in your feeding may also be needed.

How Can I Do a Feeding Using a Pump?

Some people cannot tolerate bolus feedings that go in relatively fast. They will need a pump that will provide the feeding over several hours or continuously. This will allow a slower controlled rate. Below are the instructions for pump feeding. You will be trained to use your particular pump by the home health nurse or medical supply company. The instructions vary by manufacturer of the pumps.

- Gather your supplies and equipment.
- Wash your hands.
- Check the expiration date of the formula.
- Clean the top of the can.
- Vent or open your G-tube to allow air to come out (typically 1 to 2 minutes).
- Clamp the feeding bag.
- Pour formula into the feeding bag.
- Prime the feeding set—unclamp and allow the feeding to flow all the way to the end of the set. Then clamp.
- Place tubing into pump. Set pump rate.
- Attach the tubing to your tube.
- Unclamp the feeding set. Start the machine.
- When feeding is finished, flush tubing with water. Then disconnect.
- Some people require venting after feeding to help reduce excess air in belly.

Important Information

- If you have nausea or vomiting or are very uncomfortable with the feeding, **STOP** the pump or the bolus feeding. Clamp off the feeding tube. Call your health care provider.
- Cover and refrigerate open cans.
- Throw away opened cans after 24 hours.
- Change feeding bags every 24 hours. Stop and vent periodically.

NOTES
FEEDING TUBE FEEDING ROUTINE

TIME	FLUSH (mL) BEFORE	FORMULA (CANS)	MECHANICAL PUMP RATE (mL per hour)	FLUSH (mL) AFTER

FEEDING TUBE MEDICINE ROUTINE

TIME	FLUSH (mL) BEFORE	MEDICINE (CRUSHED)	MEDICINE (LIQUID)	FLUSH (mL) AFTER

Ostomy Products HCPCS Codes (Healthcare Common Procedural Coding System)

HCPCS CODES:

GROUP 1 CODES:

CODE	DESCRIPTION
A4331	Extension drainage tubing, any type, any length, with connector/adaptor, for use with urinary leg bag or urostomy pouch, each
A4357	Bedside drainage bag, day or night, with or without antireflux device, with or without tube, each
A4361	Ostomy faceplate, each
A4362	Skin barrier; solid, 4 × 4 or equivalent, each
A4363	Ostomy clamp, any type, replacement only, each
A4364	Adhesive, liquid or equal, any type, per ounce
A4366	Ostomy vent, any type, each
A4367	Ostomy belt, each
A4368	Ostomy filter, any type, each
A4369	Ostomy skin barrier, liquid (spray, brush, etc.), per ounce
A4371	Ostomy skin barrier, powder, per ounce
A4372	Ostomy skin barrier, solid 4 × 4 or equivalent, standard wear, with built-in convexity, each
A4373	Ostomy skin barrier, with flange (solid, flexible or accordion), with built-in convexity, any size, each
A4375	Ostomy pouch, drainable, with faceplate attached, plastic, each
A4376	Ostomy pouch, drainable, with faceplate attached, rubber, each
A4377	Ostomy pouch, drainable, for use on faceplate, plastic, each
A4378	Ostomy pouch, drainable, for use on faceplate, rubber, each
A4379	Ostomy pouch, urinary, with faceplate attached, plastic, each
A4380	Ostomy pouch, urinary, with faceplate attached, rubber, each
A4381	Ostomy pouch, urinary, for use on faceplate, plastic, each

HCPCS CODES:

GROUP 1 CODES:

CODE	DESCRIPTION
A4382	Ostomy pouch, urinary, for use on faceplate, heavy plastic, each
A4383	Ostomy pouch, urinary, for use on faceplate, rubber, each
A4384	Ostomy faceplate equivalent, silicone ring, each
A4385	Ostomy skin barrier, solid 4 × 4 or equivalent, extended wear, without built-in convexity, each
A4387	Ostomy pouch, closed, with barrier attached, with built-in convexity (1 piece), each
A4388	Ostomy pouch, drainable, with extended wear barrier attached (1 piece), each
A4389	Ostomy pouch, drainable, with barrier attached, with built-in convexity (1 piece), each
A4390	Ostomy pouch, drainable, with extended wear barrier attached, with built-in convexity (1 piece), each
A4391	Ostomy pouch, urinary, with extended wear barrier attached (1 piece), each
A4392	Ostomy pouch, urinary, with standard wear barrier attached, with built-in convexity (1 piece), each
A4393	Ostomy pouch, urinary, with extended wear barrier attached, with built-in convexity (1 piece), each
A4394	Ostomy deodorant, with or without lubricant, for use in ostomy pouch, per fluid ounce
A4395	Ostomy deodorant for use in ostomy pouch, solid, per tablet
A4396	Ostomy belt with peristomal hernia support
A4397	Irrigation supply; sleeve, each
A4398	Ostomy irrigation supply; bag, each
A4399	Ostomy irrigation supply; cone/catheter, with or without brush
A4402	Lubricant, per ounce
A4404	Ostomy ring, each

HCPCS CODES:

GROUP 1 CODES:

CODE	DESCRIPTION
A4405	Ostomy skin barrier, non–pectin based, paste, per ounce
A4406	Ostomy skin barrier, pectin-based, paste, per ounce
A4407	Ostomy skin barrier, with flange (solid, flexible, or accordion), extended wear, with built-in convexity, 4 × 4 inches or smaller, each
A4408	Ostomy skin barrier, with flange (solid, flexible, or accordion), extended wear, with built-in convexity, larger than 4 × 4 inches, each
A4409	Ostomy skin barrier, with flange (solid, flexible, or accordion), extended wear, without built-in convexity, 4 × 4 inches or smaller, each
A4410	Ostomy skin barrier, with flange (solid, flexible, or accordion), extended wear, without built-in convexity, larger than 4 × 4 inches, each
A4411	Ostomy skin barrier, solid 4 × 4 or equivalent, extended wear, with built-in convexity, each
A4412	Ostomy pouch, drainable, high output, for use on a barrier with flange (2-piece system), without filter, each
A4413	Ostomy pouch, drainable, high output, for use on a barrier with flange (2-piece system), with filter, each
A4414	Ostomy skin barrier, with flange (solid, flexible or accordion), without built-in convexity, 4 × 4 inches or smaller, each
A4415	Ostomy skin barrier, with flange (solid, flexible or accordion), without built-in convexity, larger than 4 × 4 inches, each
A4416	Ostomy pouch, closed, with barrier attached, with filter (1 piece), each
A4417	Ostomy pouch, closed, with barrier attached, with built-in convexity, with filter (1 piece), each
A4418	Ostomy pouch, closed, without barrier attached, with filter (1 piece), each
A4419	Ostomy pouch, closed, for use on barrier with nonlocking flange, with filter (2 piece), each
A4420	Ostomy pouch, closed, for use on barrier with locking flange (2 piece), each
A4421	Ostomy supply; miscellaneous
A4422	Ostomy absorbent material (sheet/pad/crystal packet) for use in ostomy pouch to thicken liquid stomal output, each
A4423	Ostomy pouch, closed, for use on barrier with locking flange, with filter (2 piece), each
A4424	Ostomy pouch, drainable, with barrier attached, with filter (1 piece), each
A4425	Ostomy pouch, drainable, for use on barrier with nonlocking flange, with filter (2-piece system), each
A4426	Ostomy pouch, drainable, for use on barrier with locking flange (2-piece system), each

HCPCS CODES:

GROUP 1 CODES:

CODE	DESCRIPTION
A4427	Ostomy pouch, drainable; for use on barrier with locking flange, with filter (2-piece system), each
A4428	Ostomy pouch, urinary, with extended wear barrier attached, with faucet-type tap with valve (1 piece), each
A4429	Ostomy pouch, urinary, with barrier attached, with built-in convexity, with faucet-type tap with valve (1 piece), each
A4430	Ostomy pouch, urinary, with extended wear barrier attached, with built-in convexity, with faucet-type tap with valve (1 piece), each
A4431	Ostomy pouch, urinary, with barrier attached, with faucet-type tap with valve (1 piece), each
A4432	Ostomy pouch, urinary, for use on barrier with nonlocking flange, with faucet-type tap with valve (2 piece), each
A4433	Ostomy pouch, urinary, for use on barrier with locking flange (2 piece), each
A4434	Ostomy pouch, urinary, for use on barrier with locking flange, with faucet-type tap with valve (2 piece), each
A4435	Ostomy pouch, drainable, high output, with extended wear barrier (1-piece system), with or without filter, each
A4450	Tape, nonwaterproof, per 18 square inches
A4452	Tape, waterproof, per 18 square inches
A4455	Adhesive remover or solvent (for tape, cement, or other adhesive), per ounce
A4456	Adhesive remover, wipes, any type, each
A5051	Ostomy pouch, closed, with barrier attached (1 piece), each
A5052	Ostomy pouch, closed, without barrier attached (1 piece), each
A5053	Ostomy pouch, closed, for use on faceplate, each
A5054	Ostomy pouch, closed, for use on barrier with flange (2 piece), each
A5055	Stoma cap
A5056	Ostomy pouch, drainable, with extended wear barrier attached, with filter (1 piece), each
A5057	Ostomy pouch, drainable, with extended wear barrier attached, with built-in convexity, with filter (1 piece), each
A5061	Ostomy pouch, drainable, with barrier attached (1 piece), each
A5062	Ostomy pouch, drainable, without barrier attached (1 piece), each
A5063	Ostomy pouch, drainable, for use on barrier with flange (2-piece system), each
A5071	Ostomy pouch, urinary, with barrier attached (1 piece), each

HCPCS CODES:

GROUP 1 CODES:

CODE	DESCRIPTION
A5072	Ostomy pouch, urinary, without barrier attached (1 piece), each
A5073	Ostomy pouch, urinary, for use on barrier with flange (2 piece), each
A5081	Stoma plug or seal any type
A5082	Continent device; catheter for continent stoma
A5053	Continent device; stoma-absorptive cover for continent stoma
A5093	Ostomy accessory; convex insert
A5102	Bedside drainage bottle with or without tubing, rigid or expandable, each
A5120	Skin barrier, wipes, or swabs, each

HCPCS CODES:

GROUP 1 CODES:

CODE	DESCRIPTION
A5121	Skin barrier, solid, 6 × 6 or equivalent, each
A5122	Skin barrier, solid, 8 × 8 or equivalent, each
A5126	Adhesive or nonadhesive; disk or foam pad
A5131	Appliance cleaner, incontinence and ostomy appliances, per 16 ounce
A6216	Gauze, nonimpregnated, nonsterile, pad size 16 square inches or less, without adhesive border, each dressing
A9270	Noncovered item or service

Retrieved March 25, 2020, from https://www.cms.gov/medicare-coverage-database/details/lcd-details.aspx?LCDId=33828&amp%3bver=14&amp%3bDate&amp%3bDocID=L33828&amp%3bbc=iAAAABAAAAAAAA%3d%3dhow

APPENDIX K

Ostomy-Related Items

The purpose of this list is to provide a sampling of ostomy-related products and is not meant to be inclusive or indorsed by the Society. Check the Web sites for additional information.

- **Concealment and Security.** Designed to support and conceal an ostomy pouching system. The pouching system is contained in the belt. For additional information, please visit https://www.stealth-belt.com/stealth-belt-pro?gclid=EAIaIQobChMlqafqzbTM5gIVRNbACh18pA1KEAQYASABEgI7CvD_BwE. (Used with permission from Stealth Belt.)

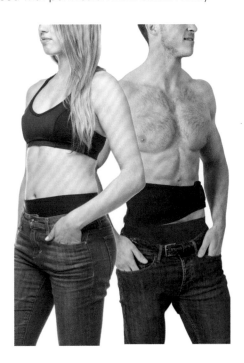

- **Stoma and Pouch Protection.** Stoma guard for impact protection prevents seat belt or firm, hard items such as a tool belt from harming stoma and prevents pressure from clothing belts. For additional information, please visit https://stomaplex.com/?gclid=EAIaIQobChMlxNfYxbXM5gIVDvDACh3pWgYCEAAYASAAEgI2ffD_BwE. (Used with permission from Stomaplex LLC.)

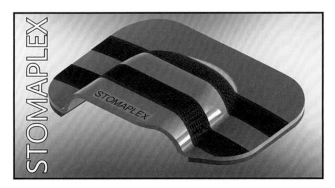

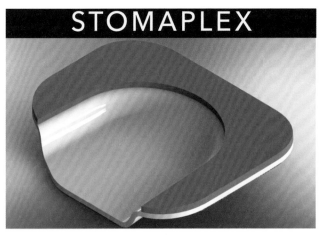

- **Stoma Shield.** Stoma shield prevents seat belt or firm, hard items such as a tool belt from harming stoma and prevents pressure from clothing belts. For additional information, please visit https://www.stomagear.com/. (Used with permission from StomaGear.)

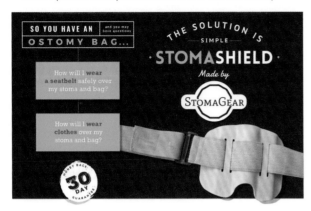

- **StomaDome.** StomaDome protects against daily impacts and seat belts with piece of adhesive Velcro attached to any ostomy pouch. For additional information, please visit https://stomadome.com/#about-stomalite-section. (Used with permission from StomaLite, LLC.)

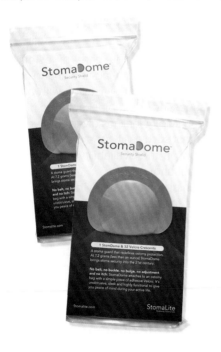

- **StomaTuck.** StomaTuck provides protection from waistline of pants and/or belt (to prevent pouch or stoma compression). For additional information and images, please visit https://www.stomatuck.com/the-product
- **Concealment and Support.** Unisex Wraps. Purpose:
  - Keeps ostomy pouch supported and flat
  - Completely covers the pouch
  - Supports the weight of the pouch as it fills
  - Prevents pouch from "swinging" under clothing

For additional information and images, please visit https://www.ostomysecrets.com/unisex-wraps

- **Belly Bands.** Provides support for pouching system, keeps pouch flattened and concealed. Manufactured by many companies; search ostomy pouch concealment bellyband, frequently found under maternity bellybands. For additional information and images, please visit https://pouchwear.com/
- **Maternity Band.** For additional information and images, please visit https://www.target.com/s/maternity+pants+extender
- **Ostomy Undergarments.** Products that have a standard higher waist and inner pocket and that conceal the pouch provide extra security. For additional information and images, please visit https://www.ostomysecrets.com/basic-panty-grey
- **Pouch Covers.** Covers pouch; used for coverage under clothing, to act as a layer between skin and pouch (decreases moisture) as well as during intimacy. For additional information and images, please visit https://www.ostomysecrets.com/women-s-ostomy-illusion-wrap-black. For additional information and images that demonstrate the styles and types of pouch covers available in patterns, in materials, and as lingerie, please visit http://cspouchcovers.com/

DISCLAIMER

Brand names/manufacturers are representative examples of ostomy accessories. This list is not inclusive of all products available in the category, nor is it intended to be a recommendation of listed products.

United Ostomy Associations of America: You Matter! Know What to Expect and Know Your Rights: Ostomy and Continent Diversion Patient Bill of Rights©

The Ostomy and Continent Diversion Patient Bill of Rights is a tool for patients to advocate for their own care. It is meant to empower those who live with an ostomy (temporary or permanent) or a continent diversion. It identifies the needs and expectations for those needing this type of surgery and for the community of people who are currently living with an ostomy or continent diversion. In order to achieve a desirable quality of life, a person undergoing ostomy or continent diversion surgery must have access to high-quality care in all health care settings. Counseling and care in the patient bill of rights should be provided by a trained medical professional such as a Certified Wound Ostomy Continence Nurse (WOCN), Ostomy Nurse, Ostomy Management Specialist (OMS), or Ostomy Care Associate (OCA). The patient shall be involved in all phases of the surgical experience except in emergent situations and shall:

RECEIVE PREOPERATIVE COUNSELING THAT MUST INCLUDE:

- Preoperative stoma site marked by a medical professional following Standards of Care (established by the Wound, Ostomy, and Continence Nurses Society, American Society of Colon and Rectal Surgeons and American Urological Association position statement)
- Explanation of surgical procedure and the rationale for surgery
- Discussion of ostomy/continent diversion management
- Impact of surgery on activities of daily living such as physical adaptation, clothing choices, exercise, possible changes in sexual activity and treatment, and dietary needs
- The opportunity to talk with someone who has been through ostomy or continent diversion surgery
- The opportunity to discuss the emotional impact of surgery
- Counseling in a language and at a level of understanding that is comfortable for the patient

RECEIVE DURING THE OPERATIVE PHASE:

- A stoma that can be fitted with a quality functioning pouching system
- A stoma that is appropriately positioned for the patient's unique body, needs, and comfort (if medical condition allows)

Receive postoperative nursing care specific to ostomy/continent diversion type and include the patient as well as the patient's designated advocate (if any). Preparation for discharge will include:

- Individual instruction in care of ostomy including demonstration of emptying and changing pouch
- Ways to troubleshoot difficulties with basic skin and stoma issues including blockage and hernias
- Dietary and fluid guidelines given both verbally and in a written format such as UOAA's Ostomy Nutrition Guide
- Information on the availability of a variety of supply and product choices
- Information about the supply ordering process
- Resources for obtaining supplies specific to patient circumstances (e.g., uninsured/underinsured)
- Concierge services through ostomy manufacturers
- Resources to organizations who support and advocate for patients living with an ostomy or continent diversion
- Educational materials (such as UOAA's New Ostomy Patient Guide)

Receive during the lifetime of the ostomy or continent diversion the patient/designated advocate will benefit from ongoing support and care to include:

- Access to health care professionals with knowledge specific to the care of an ostomy or continent diversion in the outpatient setting
- Recognition of the need for reevaluation of care with the changes caused by aging and change in medical status

If you believe your rights are not being met, speak up—be a force for change!

Pouching Infants/Children and Pediatric Pouches

POUCHING INFANTS/CHILDREN

- Gently remove pouching system using "push/pull" technique:
  - Use a silicone-based adhesive remover/releaser to take off the pouching system.
  - Avoid using alcohol-based or oil-based solvents/adhesive removers/releasers for low birth weight infants or neonates (i.e., birth to 28 days of life for term infants) due to the risk of absorption and toxicity from chemicals in the solvents; use of solvents should only be considered in situations where an aggressive adhesive would strip off the epidermis upon removal.
  - Schedule routine changes of the pouching system.
- Assess the stoma and pouch fit.
  - If the stoma is budded, fit the skin barrier at the stoma skin junction.
  - Assess the peristomal skin and abdominal contours in sitting and lying positions to determine the best shape of the skin barrier and the use of accessory product so if the stoma is flat or retracted, add convexity.
  - Consider the use of extended-wear skin barriers; may need to use an adult pouch because there are no pediatric extended-wear options.
  - Consider use of an ostomy belt.
  - Use skin barrier powder and an alcohol-free skin barrier/sealant to treat denuded peristomal skin.
  - Use alcohol-free skin barrier paste, skin barrier rings, and/or strip paste to fill creases or folds or even out the peristomal skin.
- Assess clothing options.
  - Onesies for infants and toddlers can prevent the child from pulling at the pouch.
  - Tubular netting can be made into a bodysuit to help secure the pouch and prevent the child from pulling and dislodging the pouching system.

VESICOSTOMY

- Use a large diaper or an absorbent pad to cover the stoma. Change the diaper frequently.

- Gently cleanse the skin with water and pat dry.
- Use a protective skin barrier cream/ointment around the vesicostomy opening to protect the skin.
- Routine complete removal of the barrier cream/ointment is not necessary and may irritate skin.
- Removal of the cream may be done by soaking the area with warm water and gentle cleansing using cotton balls or a soft cloth and mineral or baby oil.

NONPOUCHING OPTIONS FOR THE PATIENT WITH A FECAL STOMA

- Protect the peristomal skin from the effluent anytime a pouch is not used.
  - At each change after gentle cleansing of the peristomal skin, apply a moisture barrier ointment for skin protection.
  - If the peristomal skin is denuded, apply skin barrier powder to denuded skin, gently rub into the skin, and seal with an alcohol-free liquid skin barrier; then apply a protective skin preparation (e.g., zinc oxide–based moisture barrier, petrolatum).
  - Do not use skin barrier paste or a hydrocolloid on the peristomal skin as a barrier to effluent.
- Fluffed gauze, a diaper, or an absorbent dressing may be placed around the stoma to absorb the effluent.
  - Return to a pouching system as soon as possible.
- Consider double diapering. Apply one small diaper over the stoma and then a larger diaper in the normal diapering method.
- Change the diaper frequently (e.g., every 1 to 3 hours and as needed).

POUCHING MULTIPLE STOMAS

- Stomas in close proximity may be pouched within the same pouch:
  - When possible, create a pattern with two openings to adequately protect the skin bridge between the stomas.
  - The use of moldable strip paste or small pieces of skin barrier rings between the stomas adds protection to the skin bridge.

- If a starter hole is present in the skin barrier, and the opening in the skin barrier will not include the precut opening, it can be covered with a piece of skin barrier or a hydrocolloid.
- Patients with an imperforate anus who have a double-barrel stoma should have the mucous fistula pouched separately from the functioning stoma to prevent crossover of stool to the distal limb of the bowel. However, this is not always possible if the stomas are very close.
- The mucous fistula may produce large amounts of mucus and may need to be pouched separately, or a foam cover dressing may be used.

- Consider "picture framing" the edges of the skin barrier of the pouch with silicone tape, a hydrocolloid dressing, transparent film dressing, or waterproof tape to prevent moisture from an adjacent mucous fistula, gastrostomy tube, or wound from loosening the seal.
- Choose adhesive products that cause the least amount of trauma to the tissue upon removal (when possible) such as silicone tape, strips of a hydrocolloid dressing, or a transparent film dressing.

Adapted from Wound, Ostomy and Continence Nurses Society. (2011). *Pediatric ostomy care: Best practice for clinicians*. Mt. Laurel, NJ: Author.

PEDIATRIC POUCHES

Coloplast Corporation, Minneapolis, MN	One-piece pediatric pouch Two-piece pediatric pouch
Convatec, Princeton, NJ	Little Ones ActiveLife One-Piece Little Ones Sur-Fit Natura Two-Piece
Cymed Ostomy Co., Berkeley, CA	One-piece Drainable-Mini (Pediatric), w and w/o wafer
Dansac A/C, Fredensborg, Denmark	CombiMicro Mini Infant Soft D
Hollister Inc., Libertyville, IL	Pouchkins One-Piece Pediatric Pouch Pouchkins Two-Piece Pediatric Pouch
Marlen Manufacturing & Development Co., Bedford, OH	"Ultra" Pedi-Ileostomy Pouch
Nu-Hope Laboratories, Inc., Pacoima, CA	Neonatal Pouch Systems Nu-Flex Mini Round-Mini Drainable Nu-Flex Mini Oval-Mini Drainable
Perma-Type Company, Inc., Plainville, CT	Nondisposable Infant Standard One-Piece and Two-Piece Appliance, absolute flat and three levels of convexity

From Wound, Ostomy and Continence Nurses Society. (2016). *Pediatric ostomy complications: Best practice for clinicians*. Mt. Laurel, NJ: Author.

DISCLAIMER

Brand names/manufacturers are representative examples of ostomy accessories. This list is not inclusive of all products available in the category, nor is it intended to be a recommendation of listed products.

Emergency Staff Procedure: Ileostomy Obstruction

Symptoms: No stomal output; cramping abdominal pain; nausea and vomiting; abdominal distention; stomal edema; absent or faint bowel sounds.

1. Contact the patient's surgeon or WOC nurse to obtain history and request orders.
2. Start IV fluids (lactated Ringer solution/normal saline).
3. Obtain flat abdominal x-ray or CT scan to rule out volvulus and determine the site/cause of the obstruction. Check for local blockage (peristomal hernia or stomal stenosis) via digital manipulation of the stoma lumen.
4. Evaluate fluid and electrolyte balance via appropriate laboratory studies.
5. If an ileostomy lavage is ordered, it should be performed by a surgeon or ostomy nurse using the following guidelines:
   - Gently insert a lubricated, gloved finger into the lumen of the stoma. If a blockage is palpated, attempt to gently break it up with your finger.
   - If available, attach a colostomy irrigation set sleeve to the patient's two-piece pouching system. Many brands of pouching systems have Tupperware-like flanges onto which the same size diameter irrigation sleeve can be attached. If the patient is not wearing a two-piece system, remove the one-piece system and attach a CI sleeve to an elastic belt and place it over the stoma.
   - If colostomy irrigation set is not available, leave the pouching system in place and cut a hole just above the stoma that will allow the red rubber catheter to be inserted into the stoma.
   - Another option: cut a hole over the stoma if they have a one-piece pouching system and do the irrigation and then change the pouch.
   - Working through the pouch opening or CI sleeve insert a lubricated soft catheter (#14 to 16 Fr) into the lumen of the stoma until the blockage is reached. Do not force the catheter.
     Note: Slowly instill 30 to 50 mL NS into the catheter using a bulb syringe. Remove the catheter and allow for returns into the irrigation sleeve. Repeat this procedure instilling 30 to 50 mL at a time until the blockage is resolved. This can take 1 to 2 hours.
6. Once the blockage has been resolved, a clean, drainable pouch system should be applied. Because the stoma may be edematous, the opening in the barrier should be slightly larger than the stoma.

Adapted from United Ostomy Associations of America | WWW. OSTOMY.ORG. How To Treat Ileostomy Blockage. Copyright © 2020 UOAA. Reprinted with permission.

APPENDIX O

Diagnosis and Management Algorithm for Acute Pouchitis

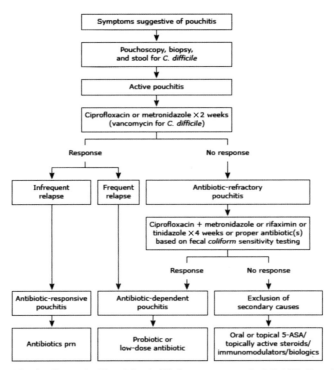

C. difficile, *Clostridioides* (formerly *Clostridium*) *difficile*; prn, as needed; 5-ASA, 5-aminosalicylic acid. (From Quinn KP, Lightner AL, Faubion WA, et al. (2019). A comprehensive approach to pouch disorders. *Inflammatory Bowel Diseases, 25*(3), 460–471. doi: 10.1093/ibd/izy267. Inflamm Bowel Dis | © 2018 Crohn's & Colitis Foundation. Oxford University Press. https://academic.oup.com/journals/pages/open_access/funder_policies/chorus/standard_publication_modelBo Shen)

Abdominal perineal resection (APR): a surgical procedure that includes the resection of the sigmoid colon, rectum, and anus; closure of perineum; and creation of end colostomy.

Anorectal malformation (ARM): a spectrum of congenital defects potentially occurring in the bowel and urinary and reproductive systems.

Anti–tumor necrosis factor (anti-TNF) antibodies: a drug that suppresses response to tumor necrosis factor (TNF), which is part of the inflammatory response.

Body image: a subjective picture of one's own physical appearance, usually based upon self-observation and by gauging the reactions of others.

Carcinoid tumors: a type of neuroendocrine tumor originating from the crypts of Lieberkühn.

Chromoendoscopy: use of dye instilled into the GI tract via endoscopy to identify tissue type or pathology.

Colonic inertia: a motility disorder, in which muscles or nerves in the colon fail to operate normally, preventing fecal matter from progressing normally through the colon.

Colostomy: a surgically created opening into any section of the colon.

Convex skin barrier: the interface between the skin and pouch of the pouching system that has curvature varying between a minimal amount of curvature (light convexity) and a maximum amount of curve (deep convexity).

Crohn's disease: an inflammatory bowel disease in which the inflammation may occur anywhere within the GI tract, from the mouth to the anus, and may be continuous or patchy. The most commonly affected area is the terminal ileum, and many of those patients have cecal and/or right colonic involvement.

Diverticular disease: pockets that develop in the colon wall, usually in the sigmoid or left colon, but may involve the entire colon. Diverticulosis describes the presence of these pockets. Diverticulitis describes inflammation or complications of these pockets.

Diverting fecal stoma: a diversion that allows the fecal stream to be diverted from the diseased or injured portion of bowel.

Duodenoduodenostomy: surgery for duodenal atresia; side-to-side anastomosis technique to bypass obstructive segment of duodenum.

Elastic skin barrier strip: a piece of hydrocolloid with elastic used to secure the outer seal of the pouching system.

End stoma: a stoma that is created by dividing the intestine, bringing the proximal end of the intestine through the abdominal wall, and maturing the stoma once outside of the abdominal wall to attach to the skin.

Enteroatmospheric fistula: an abnormal connection between the GI tract and atmosphere; for example fistula in an open surgical wound.

Extraintestinal manifestations: inflammatory-type involvement of areas outside of the gastrointestinal tract found in some patients with ulcerative colitis or Crohn's disease.

Familial adenomatous polyposis (FAP): a condition caused by mutations in the oncogene *APC* and inherited in an autosomal dominant pattern with a 100% risk of developing colon cancer by age 40 years. Individuals with FAP develop hundreds to thousands of adenomatous polyps in the colon and in the duodenum and stomach.

Familial benign chronic pemphigus, also known as Haley-Haley disease: vesicular or erythematous plaque formation occurring commonly in groin, axillae, and inframammary area.

Finney stricturoplasty: a type of stricturoplasty (see below) that is performed for longer strictures up to 15 cm.

Fistula: an abnormal connection between two epithelium-lined surfaces (i.e., two hollow organs or hollow organ and skin).

Folliculitis: hair follicle inflammation, develops when there is inflammation due to injury or infection of skin; the mechanism of injury may be multidirectional shaving or pulling of hair when the adhesive skin barrier is removed.

Gardner syndrome: an inherited polyposis syndrome that, in addition to colonic polyposis, is associated with osteomas, epidermoid cysts, soft tissue tumors, fibromas, and/or desmoid tumors. Skin manifestations of Gardner syndrome include epidermoid cysts, trichilemmal hybrid, or pilomatrixomas developing on the face, scalp, or limbs of patients.

Gastroschisis: birth defect of the abdominal wall; intestines are found outside the abdomen, exiting from an opening near the umbilicus.

Hamartomas: noncancerous (benign) masses of normal tissue that build up in the intestines or other places. These masses are called polyps if they develop inside a body structure, such as the intestines.

Hartmann's pouch: consists of the anus and rectum that remain in place with the top of the rectum sewn closed as a defunctionalized segment.

Heineke-Mikulicz stricturoplasty: a type of stricturoplasty (see below) that is performed for short strictures up to 10 cm.

Hereditary mixed polyposis syndrome: a hereditary condition that is associated with an increased risk of developing polyps in the digestive tract.

Hirschsprung disease (HD): the absence of intraneural ganglion cells and hypertrophic nerves of the bowel, which have created a functional partial or full obstruction. With the lack of ganglion cells, peristalsis does not occur and the stool cannot be pushed through the intestines properly and leads to a blockage.

HNPCC (Lynch syndrome): a type of colorectal cancer inherited by mutations in one of several mismatch repair genes (*MLH1*, *MSH2*, *MSH6*, and *PMS2*) leading to microsatellite instability. It is estimated that HNPCC accounts for 5% of colorectal cancers with a lifetime risk of developing CRC at a rate of 70% to 90%.

Ileal conduit: a type of urinary diversion whereby ureters are implanted into a section of dissected ileum that is sutured closed on one end, while the other end is brought through the abdominal wall to create a stoma.

Ileal pouch anal anastomosis (IPAA): the removal of the entire colon and rectum while preserving the anal sphincter and the creation of an ileal pouch to serve as an internal pelvic reservoir of intestinal contents.

Ileocecectomy: the removal of the terminal ileum and the cecum.

Ileostomy: an opening into the last portion of the small intestine, the ileum.

Indiana pouch: a continent catheterizable urinary diversion that is created from 10 to 12 cm of ileum (catheterizable channel), the ileocecal valve (continence mechanisms), and the right colon (reservoir).

Inspissated: thick abnormal meconium that adheres to mucous membrane of the distal small bowel.

Intussusception: the process, more common in children, in which the intestine telescopes back on itself. The resulting blockage can result in bowel necrosis if left untreated.

Jejunostomy: a surgically created opening into the jejunum.

Juvenile polyposis syndrome (JPS): a hereditary condition characterized by the presence of hamartomatous polyps in the digestive tract. The term "juvenile polyposis" refers to the type of polyp (juvenile polyp), not the age at which people are diagnosed. Most juvenile polyps are noncancerous, but there is an increased risk of cancer of the digestive tract (such as stomach, small intestine, colon, and rectum cancers) in families with JPS.

Kock pouch: a high-volume, low-pressure intra-abdominal reservoir constructed from the terminal ileum that allows patients to maintain continence of stool and flatus without the need for an external pouching system. The internal pouch is emptied by intermittent self-catheterization when increasing volume of intestinal contents cause the pouch to expand, giving the sensation of fullness to indicate it should be emptied.

Learner readiness: the degree to which a person is "ready to learn" and willingness to participate in behavior change.

Liquid skin barrier: an acrylate copolymer or a cyanoacrylate clear film that can be placed on the peristomal skin to provide skin protection from stoma effluent and adhesive stripping.

Loop stoma: a stoma that is created in the small or large intestine by mobilizing the side of the intestine up through the abdominal wall, making a transverse incision on the intestine, and maturing the mucosa. A supporting rod can be placed under the stoma to prevent stoma retraction. The stoma will have two lumens, proximal and distal.

Loop-end stoma: the intestine is transected from the lower bowel. After closing this end with a stapler, a loop of intestine approximately 10 cm proximal to this stapled end is brought to the abdominal surface. Externally, there is no difference in how a loop or loop-end stoma looks. With loop-end construction, the distal lumen leads to a blind pouch. The blind segment is usually not very long and will produce mucus as the bowel is viable. Loop-end construction is used in bowel stomas when the person has a thick abdominal wall, shortened mesentery, or a combination, and there is concern about adequate blood supply to the distal end of the stoma.

Maturation: the eversion of the bowel segment to expose the mucosa.

Michelassi side-to-side isoperistaltic stricturoplasty: a type of stricturoplasty (see below) used for extensive and/or strictures occurring sequentially over long intestinal segments.

Mucocutaneous junction: intersection between the bowel mucosa and the skin.

Mucocutaneous separation: the detachment of stomal tissue from the surrounding peristomal skin of the stoma and mucocutaneous junction.

Mucosal transplantation: seeding of viable intestinal mucosa along the suture line onto the peristomal skin.

Mucous fistula: the end of a section of defunctionalized bowel brought through the abdominal wall when a stoma is created.

Neobladder (also called an orthotopic urinary diversion): the creation of a low-pressure, high-volume intestinal reservoir that is anastomosed to the urethra. Patients rely on their urinary sphincter for continence and void by relaxing their sphincter and pelvic floor in combination with increasing intra-abdominal pressure by performing Valsalva or Credé maneuver.

Neurogenic bladder: bladder dysfunction caused by neurologic impairment of the central and peripheral nervous system, which innervates the bladder.

One-piece pouching system: a solid skin barrier and the pouch as one unit; the pouch is heat sealed onto the skin barrier.

Orthotopic urinary diversion (also called a neobladder): the creation of a low-pressure, high-volume intestinal reservoir that is anastomosed to the urethra. Patients rely on their urinary sphincter for continence and void by relaxing their sphincter and pelvic floor in combination with increasing intra-abdominal pressure by performing Valsalva or Credé maneuver.

Parastomal (peristomal) hernia: a defect in abdominal fascia that allows the intestine to bulge into the parastomal area.

Percutaneous endoscopic gastrostomy (PEG): a tube placed into the stomach through the skin, aided by endoscopy.

Percutaneous nephrostomy tubes: tubes that are inserted through the skin and into the renal pelvis of the kidney to facilitate drainage of urine after a partial or complete obstruction has occurred.

Peristomal allergic contact dermatitis: an inflammatory skin response resulting from hypersensitivity to chemical elements.

Peristomal fungal/candidiasis infection: a fungal rash that can occur beneath the skin barrier and/or beneath tape-bordered pouching systems.

Peristomal moisture–associated skin damage: an inflammation and erosion of the skin adjacent to the stoma, associated with exposure to effluent such as urine or stool.

Peristomal psoriasis: a chronic inflammatory and autoimmune disorder with many clinical variants. Peristomal and periwound skin is particularly vulnerable for patients with psoriasis because of the Koebner phenomenon, in which a flare of the disorder occurs in an area of localized skin trauma.

Peristomal varices: enlarged blood vessels caused by portal hypertension. The varices may be visible as dilated veins in the submucosal area (referred to as caput medusa), bluish discoloration of the skin in the stoma area. These may also present as spontaneous bleeding from the mucocutaneous junction without any visible skin changes.

Peutz-Jeghers syndrome: a condition characterized by the development of noncancerous growths called hamartomatous polyps in the gastrointestinal tract (particularly the stomach and intestines) and a greatly increased risk of developing certain types of cancer.

Permission, Limited Information, Specific Suggestions, Intensive Therapy (PLISSIT): four levels of response to issues with sexual health that encourages the nurse to intervene at the level at which he or she is most comfortable to provide counseling.

Pouching system: products used to collect the stoma effluent, which provide a secure predictable seal and protect the peristomal skin.

Prebiotics: plant fibers that promote healthy bowel flora growth.

Probiotics: probiotic bacteria that arrive to the bowel in an active state. They interact with epithelial and immune cells boosting systemic immune activity and epithelial function.

Proctocolectomy with permanent end ileostomy: the entire colon, rectum, and anus are removed and an end ileostomy is created.

Prune belly syndrome (PBS): a severe congenital malformation with absence of abdominal musculature that presents with wrinkly appearance of the abdominal skin and urinary tract anomalies.

Pseudoverrucous lesion: an exuberant growth of benign papules that occur around a stoma when urine or stool irritates the skin; a type of chronic irritant contact dermatitis.

Pyoderma gangrenosum: a neutrophilic dermatosis characterized by recurrent, painful ulcerations that present as pustules that enlarge and open into partial- or full-thickness wounds, sometimes with dark-colored, irregular borders and purulent exudate. These painful undermined ulcerations progress rapidly.

Radiation enteritis: inflammation of the intestines that may occur after radiation therapy. Progressive loss of cells, villous atrophy, and cystic crypt dilation occur in the ensuing days and weeks. Occurs mostly in people receiving radiation to the abdomen and pelvic areas.

Recanalize: formation of a new channel.

Retraction: the disappearance of stoma tissue protrusion in line with or below skin level.

Skin barrier paste: an adhesive hydrocolloid mixture available in a tube, used to enhance the seal of the pouching system by caulking the edge of the skin barrier closest to the stoma to help to prevent undermining of the seal. Also used to fill in uneven areas around and near the stoma to facilitate the seal of the solid skin barrier.

Skin barrier powder: a hydrocolloid that is used to absorb moisture that can be utilized on denuded peristomal skin.

Skin barrier ring: an adhesive hydrocolloid washer used around a stoma to enhance the seal by providing additional solid skin barrier and/or to level out the area around the stoma.

Skin barrier strip paste: a band of adhesive hydrocolloid used to fit around a stoma to enhance the seal or to fill in uneven peristomal area.

Solid skin barrier: the interface between the skin and the pouch of the pouching system that provides the seal (adhesion) and protects the peristomal skin.

Stamm gastrostomy: a surgically placed tube into the stomach that involves circumferential purse-string sutures to stabilize the tube within the lumen of the stomach and affix the stomach to the anterior abdominal wall.

Stomal necrosis: death of the stoma tissue resulting from impaired blood flow.

Stomal prolapse: the telescoping of the intestine through the stoma.

Stomal stenosis: the impairment of effluent drainage due to narrowing or contracting of the stoma tissue at the skin or fascial level.

Stomal trauma: an injury to the stomal mucosa often related to pressure or physical force.

Stricture: a narrowing of the bowel lumen caused by prolonged inflammation that can lead to scarring.

Stricturoplasty: the creation of a longitudinal incision through the narrowed area of the intestine while closing the incision transversely, which widens the intestinal lumen used for the treatment of fibrotic strictures in Crohn's disease.

Synbiotics: synergistic combinations of both probiotics and prebiotics.

TNM classification: a cancer staging system that describes the following: tumor invasion, spread to lymph nodes, and distant metastatic spread.

Total pelvic exenteration: a surgical procedure that includes the resection of pelvic structures including uterus, vagina, bladder, urethra, and rectum. This is indicated for rectal tumors with invasion to adjacent pelvic structures or gynecologic or urinary malignancies with involvement of the rectum.

Two-piece pouching system: a solid skin barrier with a mechanism that accepts the pouch.

Ulcerative colitis: an inflammation of the large bowel limited to the superficial mucosal lining of the bowel that follows a characteristic pattern: the rectum is always involved, and it extends proximally to include part of the colon or the entire colon.

Ureterostomy: an opening in which the ureters may be each brought to the skin in two separate stomas or one ureter anastomosed to the other and a single ureter brought out as a stoma.

Urostomy: is an opening into the abdominal wall through which urine will pass through a stoma. This can be constructed from small or large intestine. The type of urinary diversion will be an ileal or colon conduit, or an ureterostomy. An ileal or colon conduit uses the ileum or colon to make a passage for the urine to exit the body.

Vesicostomy: an opening is created above the symphysis pubis, the bladder opened, and the bladder mucosa approximated to the skin, generally seen in the pediatric population.

Volvulus: a twisting of a portion of the gastrointestinal tract that can cause a blockage, impair blood flow, and damage part of the intestine.

Witzel gastrostomy technique: surgical placement of a tube that involves creating a serosal tunnel as well as an abdominal wall tunnel through which the tube passes.

Note: Page numbers followed by "*f*" refer to figures; page numbers followed by "*t*" refer to tables; page numbers followed by "*b*" refer to boxes.

A

Abdominal cavity organs and
 peritoneum, 16–26
 anal canal, 23–24
 colon segments, 22–23
 duodenum, 20
 ileocecal valve, 18*f*, 21
 ileum, 21
 intestinal bacteria, 24
 jejunum, 20–21
 large intestine (colon), 21–22, 22*f*
 omentum and mesentery, 16, 17*f*
 rectum, 23, 23*f*
 small intestine, 18–20, 18*f*
 stomach, 17–18, 17*f*
Abdominal/pelvic trauma
 clinical presentation, 109
 etiology, 109
 medical management, 109
 surgical management, 109–110
Abscess, 62
 peristomal, 260–261, 260*f*
Acute pouchitis, diagnosis and
 management algorithm for, 370,
 370*f*
Adaptations, rehabilitation, and long-
 term care management issues
 chemotherapy
  antiemetic, 215
  for bladder and colon cancer, 216,
   216*t*
  classification, 215
  mucositis/stomatitis, 216
  oxaliplatin, 215–216
  pouch system, 215
  side effects, 215
 cognitive deficits, 215
 colostomy
  bowel prep, 206
  constipation, prevention and
   management of, 205–206, 205*t*
  contraindications to colostomy
   irrigation, 204*b*
  diarrhea, prevention and
   management of, 206
  irrigation, 203–204, 203*f*

  irrigation procedure, 204, 204*b*
  irrigation tips, 204, 204*b*
  odor and flatus management,
   204–205, 205*b*
  patient selection, 203–204, 204*b*
 cultural, religious, and spirituality
  diversity, 217–218
  language barriers, 218
  long-term issues with ostomy, 218
 end of life, 214–215
 ileal conduit, 208–209
 ileostomy
  bowel prep, 208
  dehydration, 206
  diet, 207–208
  food blockage, 207, 207*b*
  high output and hospital
   readmissions, 206–207
  medications, 208
 morbid obesity, 214
 ostomy impact
  adaptation process, 210
  age/developmental stage, 212
  family or significant others, 211
  health care team/WOC nurse, 211
  ostomy visitor, 211–212
  past experiences with ostomy/
   expectations, 211
  self-efficacy, 211
  self-esteem/coping skills, 211
 pelvic exenteration (PE), 209
 physical and mental limitations, 217
  hearing deficit, 217
  spinal cord injury, 217
  visually impaired, 217
 pregnancy, 213–214
  contraception, 214
 psychomotor assessment, 215
 radiation therapy, 215–216
 sexual function
  counseling models, 213
  ostomy, body image/sexual
   relationships, 213
  pelvic dissection impact on, 212
 temporary fecal diversions,
  202–203, 202*b*

Adenomatous polyps, 101
Administrator, 5
Advanced practice registered nurses
 (APRNs), 3
Adventitia (serosa), 14–15
Allergic contact dermatitis (ACD),
 256–257, 257*f*
Anal canal, 23–24
Anorectal malformation (ARM)
 assessment, 230
 incidence, 229
 management, 230
 perineal fistulas and rectovestibular
  fistulas, 230
 presentation, 229–230
 rectourethral fistulas or cloaca,
  230–231
 VACTERL association, 229, 229*t*
Antegrade continence enema (ACE),
 243
Appendicovesicostomy (APV), 244,
 244*f*
Appendix, colon segments, 22
ARM. *See* Anorectal malformation (ARM)
Ascending colon, 22
Attenuated FAP (AFAP), 101
Autoimmune skin disease
 atypical presentations, 263–264
 bullous pemphigoid, 264, 264*f*, 265*t*
 epidermolysis bullosa acquisita, 265,
  265*t*
 familial benign chronic pemphigus,
  265, 265*t*, 265*f*
 malignancy, 265–266
 pemphigus vulgaris, 264–265, 265*t*,
  265*f*
 peristomal psoriasis, 263–264,
  263*f*–264*f*

B

Bacteroides, 24
Balloon-tipped gastrostomy tube,
 305–306, 305*f*–306*f*
Biliary tubes, 313, 313*b*
Biopsy-proven mucosal implantation,
 261–262, 261*f*

Bladder cancer
  diagnostic considerations, 118–120
  histopathology, 118, 119f
  management, 120
  presentation, 118
  risk factors, 118
Bullous pemphigoid (BP), 264, 264f,
    265t

C

Candida albicans, 257–258
Caput medusae, 259
Carcinoid tumors, 52
CD. *See* Crohn's disease (CD)
Cecostomy, 137
Certification, 8, 8t
Certified Wound Ostomy Continence
    Nurse (CWOCN), 3
Chemotherapy
  antiemetic, 215
  for bladder and colon cancer, 216,
    216t
  classification, 215
  mucositis/stomatitis, 216
  oxaliplatin, 215–216
  pouch system, 215
  side effects, 215
CI. *See* Colostomy irrigation (CI)
Clean intermittent catheterization (CIC),
    243
Clostridium perfringens, 24
Colon, 21–22. *See also* Large intestine
  ascending, 22
  descending, 23
  sigmoid, 23
  transverse, 22
Colon cancer
  adjuvant treatment algorithm for,
    49f–50f
  segmental colon resection for, 48f
Colon conduit, 123
  complications, 123–124
  postoperative care, 123
  surgical procedure, 123
Colon polyps, 101
Colon segments, 22–23
Colonic atresia, 227
Colonic inertia, 111–112
Colorectal adenocarcinoma
  adjuvant treatment, 50f, 51
  advanced disease, 51
  cancer screening, 45–46
  etiology, 44–45
  neoadjuvant therapy, 49–51,
    49f–50f
  presentation/workup, 46, 46t
  primary prevention, 45
  risk assessment and patient
    stratification, 45
  risk factors, 45
  surgical management

colon cancer, 47–49, 47f–48f
    rectal cancer, 49–51, 49f–50f
  treatment algorithms, 47
Colorectal cancer (CRC), 44, 55
Colorectal neoplasia, stoma
    formation for
  low anterior resection syndrome, 54,
    55f
  permanent stoma, 53–54, 53f–54f
  surveillance, 54–55
  temporary stoma, 52–53
    colostomies/loop ileostomies,
      52–53, 53f
    defunctionalize/protect distal
      anastomosis, 53
    timing to reverse, 53
Colostomy, 137, 138f, 339
  long-term care management issues
    bowel prep, 206
    constipation, prevention and
      management of, 205–206, 205t
    contraindications to colostomy
      irrigation, 204b
    diarrhea, prevention and
      management of, 206
    irrigation, 203–204, 203f
    irrigation procedure, 204, 204b
    irrigation tips, 204, 204b
    odor and flatus management,
      204–205, 205b
    patient selection, 203–204, 204b
  products and tips, 327
Colostomy irrigation (CI), 203–204,
    203f, 204b
Constipation, prevention and
    management of, 205–206, 205t
Consultant, 5
Continence specialty, 4
Continent ileostomy, 90–94
  catheter care, management of, 92–93
  complications with, 92
  contraindications, 91
  diet, 93
  indications, 90
  pregnancy and childbirth, 93–94,
    93b, 94b
  stoma care, 93
  surgical procedure, 91–92, 91f, 92f
Continent urinary diversion
  cutaneous catheterizable urinary
    diversion, 124
  Indiana pouch
    complications, 126
    outcome, 126
    patient considerations, 124–125
    physician considerations, 124
    postoperative care, 125–126
    preoperative considerations, 125
    surgical procedure, 125, 125f
  Miami pouch, 126
Counseling models, 213

Crohn's disease (CD), 238
  assessment, 238
  incidence, 238
  management, 238–239
  medical management, 60, 66–67
    diet, 65
    differential diagnosis, 61, 61t
    epidemiology, 60
    etiology, 60
    extraintestinal manifestations, 65
    fistulizing disease, 64–65
    inflammation, 62–63
    medication class, 63, 63t
    overview, 61, 61t
    strictures, 65
  preoperative preparation, 72–79
    abdominal imaging studies, 73
    immunosuppressive/biologic
      therapy, 72–73
    mechanical bowel preparation
      combined with antibiotics, 73
    medical optimization, 72
    ostomy site selection/patient
      education, 73
    venous thromboembolism
      prophylaxis, 73
  presentation, 238
  surgical management
    bowel resection, 73–77
    ileocecectomy, 73–74, 74f
    indications, 72, 72b
    Kono-S anastomosis, 74–75, 75f
    laparoscopic *vs.* open approach,
      73
    nonhealing perineal wound,
      77–78, 78b
    operative management, 72
    potential complications, 77–79,
      78b
    proctocolectomy with ileostomy,
      77, 77f
    segmental colectomy, 75–76, 75f
    stricturoplasty, 78–79, 79f–80f
    subtotal colectomy, 76–77, 76f
    urinary and sexual function, 77–78
Cutaneous ureterostomy, 124, 124f

D

Deep enteroscopy, 62–63
Descending colon, 23
Diarrhea, prevention and management
    of, 206
Digestive organs
  colon, 22–23
  esophagus, 16
  ileum, 21
  mouth, 15–16
Diverticular disease, 104–107
  acute, 104
  clinical presentation, 105
  etiology, 105

medical management, 105–106
surgical management, 106–107
Duhamel technique, 235, 235f
Duodenal atresia and stenosis,
    224–226
  assessment, 226
  incidence, 225
  management, 226
  presentation, 225–226
  types, 225f
Duodenostomy, 136
Duodenum, 20

E

Educator, 4–5
Elastic skin barrier strip, 181, 181f
Electrolyte balance
  acid–base balance, 39
  calcitonin, 39
  calcium regulation, 39
  endocrine function, 40
  erythropoietin (EPO), 40
  fluid and, 37–38
  magnesium regulation, 39
  phosphate regulation, 39
  potassium regulation, 38–39
  and renin–angiotensin–aldosterone
      system, 40
  vitamin D, 39
  vitamin D$_3$, 40
Emergency staff procedure, 369
End loop ileostomy, 167
End loop urinary stoma, 167
End stoma, 165, 166f
Enhanced recovery after surgery
    (ERAS) program, 189–190
Enteroatmospheric fistula (EAF), 284
Enterobacter aerogenes, 24
Enterocolitis, signs and symptoms,
    236b
Enterocutaneous fistula (ECF), 261, 284
Enterostomal therapy (ET) program, 2
Epidermolysis bullosa acquisita (EBA),
    265, 265t
Erythropoietin (EPO), 30, 40
Escherichia coli, 24
Esophagus
  function, 16
  structure, 16
Exocrine pancreas, 25–26
Ex-PLISSIT model, 213

F

Familial adenomatous polyposis (FAP)
    syndrome, 45
  clinical presentation, 101–102
  etiology, 101
  medical management, 102
  surgical management, 102
Familial benign chronic pemphigus,
    265, 265t, 265f

Familial polyposis syndromes
  assessment, 240
  incidence, 239
  management, 240
  presentation, 240
FAP syndrome. *See* Familial
    adenomatous polyposis (FAP)
    syndrome
Fecal diversions
  abdominal/pelvic trauma
    clinical presentation, 109
    etiology, 109
    medical management, 109
    surgical management, 109–110
  colonic inertia, 111–112
  diverticular disease, 104–107
    acute, 104
    clinical presentation, 105
    etiology, 105
    medical management, 105–106
    surgical management, 106–107
  formation of, 101
  intussusception, 111
  management issues (*see*
      Adaptations, rehabilitation, and
      long-term care management
      issues)
  obstruction, 110
  patient education (*see* Postoperative
      patient education)
  pediatric patient
    pediatric pouching, techniques
        and indications for, 240–241
    refeeding ostomy output, 241
  polyposis syndromes
    familial adenomatous polyposis
        (FAP) syndrome, 101–102
    Gardner's syndrome, 102–103
    Peutz–Jeghers syndrome (PJS),
        103–104
  radiation enteritis, 107–109
    clinical presentation, 107
    effects of, 107
    etiology, 107, 107t
    medical management, 108
    surgical management, 108–109
  volvulus, 110
Fecal immunochemical test (FIT), 46
Fecal occult blood test (FOBT), 46
Fecal stoma
  assessment parameters, 164t
  colon and rectum, cancers of
    carcinoid tumors, 52
    gastrointestinal stromal tumors
        (GISTs), 52
    lymphoma, 52
    melanoma, primary and metastatic,
        52
    sarcoma, 52
  colorectal adenocarcinoma
    adjuvant treatment, 50f, 51

advanced disease, 51
colon cancer, surgical
    management, 47–49, 47f–48f
etiology, 44–45
neoadjuvant therapy, 49–51,
    49f–50f
presentation/workup, 46, 46t
primary prevention, 45
rectal cancer, surgical
    management, 49–51, 49f–50f
risk assessment and patient
    stratification, 45
risk factors, 45
screening, 45–46
TNM classification, 46, 46t
treatment algorithms, 47
  colorectal neoplasia, stoma
      formation for
    permanent stoma, 53–54,
        53f–54f
    quality of life with or without stoma
        after low anterior resection,
        54–55, 55f
    temporary stoma, 52–53, 53f
    timing to reverse temporary
        stoma, 53
Fecal stoma, nonpouching for patient
    with, 367
Fecal stoma construction
  anatomic classification
    cecostomy, 137
    colostomy, 137, 138f
    duodenostomy, 136
    ileostomy, 136
    jejunostomy, 136
    mucous fistula, 137–138, 138f
  stoma classifications, 132, 132t
  stoma construction types, 133t
    end stoma, 132–133, 133f
    loop stoma, 133–135, 134f–135f
    loop–end stoma, 135–136, 135f
  stoma maturation, 132, 133f
Feeding tubes, 354, 355f–356f
  bolus feeding through, 357
  check residuals, 358
  complication of, 358–359
    aspiration, 358
    clogged tubes, 358
    constipation, 359
    diarrhea, 359
    feeling sick, 358–359
    hyperplasia, 359
    leaking tube, 359
  definition, 354
  feeding routine, 360
  health care management, 354
  infections, 356
  medicine routine, 360
  medicines through, 358
  necessity of, 354
  nutrition instructions, 357

Feeding tubes (*Continued*)
    parts of, 355
    postoperative care, 356
    protection, 356
    secured in skin, 356
    skin protection, 356–357
    tool, 354–358
    types, 354–355
    using pump, 359
    water requirement, 358
Finney stricturoplasty, 78–79, 79*f*
Fistula, peristomal, 260*f*, 261*f*
Fistula management, 283–303
    assessment, for WOC nurse,
        288–290
        abdominal contours and fistula
            opening, 286*f*, 289–290, 289*f*
        documentation, 288, 289*b*
        effluent characteristics, 286*f*, 290
        progress toward and impediments
            to spontaneous closure, 288,
            289*b*, 289*f*
    clinical presentation and
        classification, 284, 285*t*
    definition, 284
    education and emotional support,
        298
    enterovaginal fistulas, 299
    etiologic factors, 284–285
    interprofessional approach, 284
    interventions and containment
        strategies, 290–298
        absorptive dressings, 292–293
        closed suction systems, 292–293,
            293*f*
        containment methods, 290, 291*t*
        moisture barriers, 292–293
        negative pressure wound therapy,
            293–294, 294*b*, 295*f*
        pectin-based barrier products,
            292, 292*f*
        pouching system adaptations,
            296–298, 297*f*, 298*f*
        pouching systems, 294–295, 295*f*,
            296*b*
        products and indications,
            290, 291*t*
        skin protectants and barriers,
            290–292, 291*t*
    medical management, 285–288
        control of infection, 286, 286*f*
        fistula tract, definition of, 286,
            298–299
        fluid and electrolyte balance,
            286–287
        minimize fistula output, 287–288
        nutritional support, 287
        skin protection and containment,
            288, 288*b*
    mortality rates, 284
    rectovaginal fistulas, 299

    surgical closure, 285*t*, 298–299
    vesicovaginal fistula, 299
Folliculitis, 258–259, 258*f*–259*f*
Fungal/candidiasis skin infection,
    257–258, 258*f*

G

Gallbladder, 25
Gardner's syndrome
    clinical presentation, 103
    etiology, 103
    medical management, 103
    surgical management, 103
Gastrointestinal stromal tumors (GISTs),
    52
Gastrointestinal (GI) tract
    abdominal cavity organs and
        peritoneum
        anal canal, 23–24
        colon segments, 22–23
        duodenum, 20
        ileocecal valve, 18*f*, 21
        ileum, 21
        intestinal bacteria, 24
        jejunum, 20–21
        large intestine (colon), 21–22, 22*f*
        rectum, 23, 23*f*
        small intestine, 18–20, 18*f*
        stomach, 17–18, 17*f*
    accessory organs, 24–26
        exocrine pancreas, 25–26
        gallbladder, 25
        liver, 25
    anatomy of, 13, 14*f*
    digestive organs
        esophagus, 16
        mouth, 15–16
    digestive processes, 13, 15–16
    histologic characteristics
        mucosa, 13
        muscularis, 14
        serosa or adventitia, 14–15
        submucosa, 13
    layers of, 13, 15*f*
Gastrojejunostomy tube, 355
Gastrostomy and jejunostomy tubes
    balloon-tipped gastrostomy tube,
        305–306, 305*f*–306*f*
    biliary tubes, 313, 313*b*
    comparative complication
        rates, 306
    hypertrophic granulation, 307–309
    managing skin complications, 307,
        308*t*, 309*b*, 309*f*
    pediatric considerations, 312
    percutaneous endoscopic
        gastrostomy (PEG) tube
        with internal and external bumper,
            305, 305*f*
        with jejunal extension, 305–306,
            306*f*

    routine tube care, 306–307
    tube replacement, 311–312,
        311*b*, 311*f*
Gastrostomy tube, 354–355
GISTs. *See* Gastrointestinal stromal
    tumors (GISTs)
Granuloma, 259–260, 260*f*
Gut-associated lymphoid tissues
    (GALTs), 21

H

Hailey-Hailey disease (HHD), 265,
    265*t*, 265*f*
HD. *See* Hirschsprung's disease (HD)
Health care reimbursement, 7–8
Heineke-Mikulicz stricturoplasty,
    78–79
Hereditary nonpolyposis colon cancer
    (HNPCC), 45
Hirschsprung's disease (HD), 233–236
    assessment, 233–235, 234*f*
    incidence, 233
    management, 235
        Duhamel technique, 235, 235*f*
        Soave endorectal pull-through,
            235–236, 236*t*, 236*b*, 236*f*
        Swenson technique, 235, 235*f*
    presentation, 233, 233*f*
HNPCC. *See* Hereditary nonpolyposis
    colon cancer (HNPCC)
Hydrocephalus, 243

I

IBD. *See* Inflammatory bowel diseases
    (IBD)
Ileal conduit, 121, 139, 139*f*
    complications, 123
    long-term care management issues,
        208–209
    outcomes, 123
    patient considerations, 121
    physician considerations, 121
    postoperative care, 122–123
    preoperative considerations, 121
    surgical procedure, 121–122, 122*f*
Ileal pouch–anal anastomosis (IPAA)
    complications of, 87–90, 89*f*
    function and expected outcomes, 87,
        87*t*, 88*b*
    loop ileostomy, 85–86
    perianal skin irritation, 86–87
    pouchitis management and
        prevention, 88–90
    stool frequency, 86–87
Ileocecal valve, 18–19, 18*f*, 21
Ileostomy, 136, 339
    long-term care management issues
        bowel prep, 208
        dehydration, 206
        diet, 207–208
        food blockage, 207, 207*b*

high output and hospital readmissions, 206–207
medications, 208
obstruction, emergency staff procedure, 369
products and tips, 327
Ileovesicostomy, 244
Ileum, 21
Indiana pouch
  complications, 126
  outcome, 126
  patient considerations, 124–125
  physician considerations, 124
  postoperative care, 125–126
  preoperative considerations, 125
  surgical procedure, 125, 125f
Inflammatory bowel diseases (IBD), 60, 66–67. See also Crohn's disease (CD); Ulcerative colitis (UC)
  cancer risk, 65
  continent ileostomy, 90–94
  diet in, 65
  differential diagnosis, 61, 61t
  epidemiology, 60
  etiology, 60
  extraintestinal manifestations, 65
  ileal pouch–anal anastomosis (IPAA)
    complications of, 87–90, 89f
    function and expected outcomes, 87, 87t, 88b
    loop ileostomy, 85–86
    perianal skin irritation, 86–87
    restorative proctocolectomy, 80, 82
    stool frequency, 86–87
    total proctocolectom, 93–94
  laparoscopic-assisted restorative proctocolectomy, ulcerative colitis, 85
  medical management
    Crohn's disease (CD), 62–65
    ulcerative colitis, 61–64, 61t–63t
  nutrition in, 65–66
    micronutrient deficiencies, 66
    protein and caloric malnutrition, 66
    supportive care, 66
    wound healing, 66
  pediatric patient, 238
  proctocolectomy with ileostomy, 77
    Crohn's disease (CD), 77
    ulcerative colitis, 77f, 81–82, 81t
  surgical management
    Crohn's disease (CD), 72, 72b, 77–79, 79f–80f
    ulcerative colitis, 79–85, 80t–81t, 83f, 84t, 84f
    total proctocolectomy, ulcerative colitis, 79, 93–94
Inflammatory polyps, 101
Integrity, 2

Interstitial cystitis, 120
Intestinal atresia and stenosis, 224
Intestinal bacteria, 24
Intestinal nonrotation, 227–229, 228f
Intestinal obstruction, 110
Intestinal urinary diversion, 118
  colon conduit, 123
  continent urinary diversion
    cutaneous catheterizable urinary diversion, 124
    Indiana pouch (see Indiana pouch)
  cutaneous ureterostomy, 124, 124f
  incontinent and continent, 119t
  indications for
    bladder cancer, 118–120
    gynecologic malignancy, 120
    interstitial cystitis, 120
    neurogenic bladder, 120
    radiation cystitis, 120
    rectal malignancy, 120
    trauma, 121
  surgical procedures, incontinent urinary diversion, 121–128, 122f
Intussusception, 111
IPAA. See Ileal pouch–anal anastomosis (IPAA)

J
Jejunal conduit, 139
Jejunoileal atresia and stenosis, 226–227
  assessment, 227
  classification, 226, 227f
  incidence, 226
  management, 227
  presentation, 226–227
Jejunostomy, 136, 164
Jejunostomy tube, 355
Jejunum, 20–21
Juvenile polyposis syndrome (JPS), 101

K
Kidney, 30f
  function of, 36–37
    urine concentration and volume, 37
    urine formation, 36–37
    urine pH, 37
  location and structure, 30–31, 30f, 31f
Koch pouch, 91, 91f, 126. See also Continent ileostomy

L
Lactobacillus bifidus, 24
Large intestine
  blood supply, 21–22, 22f
  function, 22
Leadership, 2
Liquid skin barrier, 181–182
Liver, 25

Loop stoma, 166
Loop–end ileal conduit, 139, 139f
Low anterior resection syndrome (LARS), 54
Lower urinary tract
  adjacent organs, 36
  adrenal glands, 36
  pelvic floor, 35–36, 35f
  pelvis, 35
  urethra, 34–35
  urinary bladder, 33–34, 34f
Lymphoma, 52
Lynch syndrome, 45

M
Maceration, 254, 254f
Malignancy, 265–266
Malrotation and volvulus, 227–229
  assessment, 228
  incidence, 228
  management, 228–229
  presentation, 228
  of sigmoid colon, 228, 228f
Mechanical damage, 254–255
  medical adhesive–related skin injuries, 255, 256f
  pressure injuries, 251, 256, 256f
Meconium ileus (MI)
  assessment, 237, 237f
  CFTR variants, 236
  incidence, 236–237
  management, 237–238
  nonoperative treatment, 236
  presentation, 237
Medical adhesive–related skin injuries, 255
Melanoma, primary and metastatic, 52
Metastatic melanoma, 52
Michelassi side-to-side isoperistaltic stricturoplasty (SSIS), 78–79, 79f–80f
Mitrofanoff procedure, 244, 244f
Moisture-associated skin damage (MASD), 290
Mouth, function
  digestion, 16
  ingestion, 16
  speech, 16
  swallowing, 16
Mucocutaneous junction, 168
Mucocutaneous separation
  assessment, 272, 272f
  etiology/incidence, 272
  management, 272
  presentation, 272
Mucosa, 13
Mucous fistula, 137–138, 138f, 167, 167f
Muscularis, 14
Myelomeningocele, 242–243, 243f
  assessment, 242
  etiology, 242

Myelomeningocele (*Continued*)
  incidence, 242
  management, 242–243
  neural tube defects, 242
  presentation, 242
  symptoms, 242

N
Nasogastric tubes (NGT), 304
National Comprehensive Cancer
    Network (NCCN), 45
Necrotizing enterocolitis (NEC), 224,
    231–233
  assessment, 231
  incidence, 231
  management, 231–233
  presentation, 231
  schematic representation, 231, 232*f*
Negative pressure wound therapy
    (NPWT), 285, 291*t*, 293–294,
    294*b*, 295*f*
Neobladder. *See* Orthotopic urinary
    diversion
Nephrostomy tubes, 312–313
Neural tube defects (NTDs), 242
Neurogenic bladder, 120
Node-negative tumors (T1N0), 49
NPWT. *See* Negative pressure wound
    therapy (NPWT)

O
Obstruction, 110
Orthotopic urinary diversion
  complications, 128
  outcomes, 128
  patient considerations, 126–127
  physician considerations, 126
  postoperative care, 127–128
  preoperative consideration, 127
  surgical procedure, 127, 127*f*
Ostomy
  continent diversion patient bill of
      rights, 366
  HCPCS CODES, 361
  product suppliers and manufacturers,
      321
  -related products, 364, 364*f*–365*f*
    belly bands, 365
    concealment and security, 364
    concealment and support, 365
    maternity band, 365
    ostomy undergarments, 365
    pouch covers, 365
    stoma and pouch protection, 364
    stoma shield, 365
    stomadome, 365
    stomatuck, 365
  support resources, 319
  surgical procedures, 317
Ostomy impact
  adaptation process, 210

factors affecting ability to adapt,
    210–212
  age/developmental stage, 212
  family or significant others, 211
  health care team/WOC
      nurse, 211
  ostomy visitor, 211–212
  past experiences with ostomy/
      expectations, 211
  self-efficacy, 211
  self-esteem/coping skills, 211
Ostomy pouches. *See also* Pouching
    systems
  drainable pouch for
    fecal stoma management, 183–184,
        184*f*
    urinary stoma management, 183*f*, 184
  gas management, 185
  nondrainable pouches, 183*f*, 184
  one-piece pouching system, 175*f*,
      182–183
  pouch films, 183*f*, 184
  pouch length, 183*f*, 184
  two-piece pouching system,
      182*f*–184*f*, 183
Ostomy specialty, 4

P
Pancreas, 25–26
Parastomal hernia
  assessment, 278
  etiology/incidence, 277–278
  management, 278–279, 279*t*
  presentation, 278, 278*f*
Patient assessment, fecal/urinary
    diversion, 146–148
  cognitive, 147
  diagnosis, 146
  family, 146–147
  learning style/learning level, 147–148,
      148*b*
  ostomy, type of, 146*t*
  patient's support system, 148
  physical abilities, 147
  planned procedure, 146
  prognosis, 146
  psychological stress, 147
  self-care, 147
  surgical procedure, 146*t*
  treatment plan, 146
  typical location, 146*t*
  understanding fears, 147
PBS. *See* Prune belly (Eagle-Barrett)
    syndrome (PBS)
Pediatric patient
  fecal diversions
    pediatric pouching, techniques
        and indications for, 240–241
    refeeding ostomy output, 241
  pathology and management
      conditions

anorectal malformation (ARM),
    229–231, 229*t*, 229*f*
  colonic atresia, 227
  Crohn's disease, 238–239
  duodenal atresia and stenosis,
      224–226, 225*f*
  familial polyposis syndromes,
      239–240
  Hirschsprung's disease (HD),
      233–236, 233*f*, 234*f*, 235*f*, 236*t*,
      236*b*, 236*f*
  inflammatory bowel disease (IBD),
      238
  intestinal atresia and stenosis, 224
  jejunoileal atresia and stenosis,
      226–227, 227*f*
  malrotation and volvulus, 227–
      229, 228*f*
  meconium ileus (MI), 236–238, 237*f*
  necrotizing enterocolitis (NEC),
      231–233, 232*f*
  pediatric trauma, 240
  ulcerative colitis, 239
pediatric urinary diversions
  appendicovesicostomy, 244, 244*f*
  ileovesicostomy, 244
  vesicostomy, 243–244, 244*f*
rehabilitative issues
  adolescent (13 to 18 years), 246
  premature infant/full-term infant,
      245, 245*f*–246*f*
  school age (6 to 12 years),
      245–246
  support and education, for child
      and family, 244–245
  toddler (12 months to 3 years) and
      preschool (3 to 5 years), 245
urinary diversion, pathology and
    management conditions
  myelomeningocele, 242–243,
      243*f*
  Prune belly syndrome (PBS),
      241–242, 242*f*
Pediatric pouches, 368
Pediatric trauma
  assessment, 240
  incidence, 240
  management, 240
  presentation, 240
Pelvic exenteration (PE), 209
Pelvic floor, 35–36
  anal sphincter, 36
  endopelvic fascia, 36
  female, 35–36, 35*f*
  levator ani, 36
  male, 35*f*, 36
  perineal body, 36
  perineal membrane, 36
Pelvis, 35
Pemphigus vulgaris (PV), 264–265,
    265*t*, 265*f*

Percutaneous endoscopic gastrostomy (PEG) tube
  with internal and external bumper, 305, 305f
  with jejunal extension, 305–306, 306f
Peristomal moisture–associated skin damage (PMASD), 252–254, 253f
Peristomal psoriasis, 263–264, 263f–264f
Peristomal pyoderma gangrenosum (PPG), 262–263, 262f
Peristomal skin complications, 168
  allergic contact dermatitis, 256–257, 257f
  assessment guidelines, 251–252
  autoimmune and atypical presentations, 263–264
  bullous pemphigoid, 264, 264f, 265t
  epidermolysis bullosa acquisita, 265, 265t
  fistula, 260f, 261f
  folliculitis, 258–259, 258f–259f
  fungal/candidiasis infection, 257–258, 258f
  granuloma, 259–260, 260f
  guidelines for management, 252
  Hailey-Hailey disease, 265, 265t, 265f
  maceration, 254, 254f
  malignancy, 265–266
  mechanical damage, 255–256, 256f
  mucosal transplantation, 261–263, 261f
  pemphigus vulgaris, 264–265, 265t, 265f
  peristomal abscess, 260–261, 260f
  peristomal moisture–associated skin damage (PMASD), 252–254, 253f
  peristomal psoriasis, 263–264, 263f–264f
  peristomal pyoderma gangrenosum (PPG), 262–263, 262f
  pressure injuries, 256, 256f
  pseudoverrucous lesions, 254–255, 255f
  scope of problem, 250–251
  varices, 259, 259f
Peritoneum, 16, 17f
Permission, Understanding-Limited Information, Specific Suggestions, Intensive Therapy (PLISSIT), 213
Peutz–Jeghers syndrome (PJS), 101
  autosomal dominant inheritance pattern, 103–104
  characteristics, 103
  clinical presentation, 104
  etiology, 104

  medical management, 104
  surgical management, 104
Pittman Ostomy Complication Conceptual Model, 271, 271f
PJS. See Peutz–Jeghers syndrome (PJS)
POLARS (preoperative LARS) score, 54, 55f
Polyposis syndromes, 101–104
  adenomatous polyps, 101
  colon polyps, 101
  familial adenomatous polyposis (FAP) syndrome
    clinical presentation, 101–102
    etiology, 101
    medical management, 102
    surgical management, 102
  Gardner's syndrome
    clinical presentation, 103
    etiology, 103
    medical management, 103
    surgical management, 103
  inflammatory polyps, 101
  Peutz–Jeghers syndrome (PJS)
    autosomal dominant inheritance pattern, 103–104
    characteristics, 103
    clinical presentation, 104
    etiology, 104
    medical management, 104
    surgical management, 104
Postoperative nursing assessment and management
  abdominal drains, presence of, 163
  bowel sounds, 163
  diet, 163
  incisional integrity, 162–163
  pain medication frequency, 163
  postoperative planning, 168–169
  respiratory status assessment, 163
  response to surgery and recovery, 163
  self-care ostomy management, 162
  stoma assessment, 163–168
    anatomic location and function, 163–165, 165f
    patient with new fecal stoma, 164t
    patient with new urinary stoma, 164t
    peristomal skin, 168
    stoma mucosa, 167, 168f
    stoma structure, 168, 168f
  stoma construction/type, 165–167
    end loop ileostomy, 167
    end loop urinary stoma, 167
    end stoma, 165, 166f
    Hartmann's Procedure, 165, 166f
    loop colostomy with plastic stoma bridge, 166, 166f
    loop ileostomy with rubber support bridge, 166, 166f

  loop stoma, 166
  mucous fistula, 167, 167f
  support bridge removal, 166–167
  ureterostomy, 167
  vesicostomy, 167
  urinary catheters, 163
Postoperative patient education, 190
  assessing readiness, 190–191, 191b
  clinical guidelines for ostomy care, 190
  dietary concerns, 196–198
    ileal conduit, 196
    ileostomy and colostomy, 196–197
    odor, 197
    pelvic exenteration, 197
  follow-up care, 197–198
  instruction to family members, 190
  living with stoma
    bathing, 194
    clothing, 194–195
    dietary concerns, 195, 195t–196t
    sexual concerns, 195
    supplies, 194
  medications, 197
  physical activities, 197
  pouching principles, 191–194
    assessing peristomal skin, 193
    emptying a pouch, 191–192, 192b, 192f
    indications for pouch change, 192
    medical attention, 193–194, 194b
    one- and two-piece types of, 191
    peristomal skin cleansing, 193
    pouch change, indications for, 192
    pouching system, placement of, 193
    pouching system, removal of, 193
    preparing equipment, 192–193
    problem identification, 193–194
    stoma measurement, 193
    time to empty, 192
  self-care, 190
  support groups, 198
Pouches
  detaching and cleaning drainage collector, 353t
  drainable pouches, emptying, 334t
  drainage collection container, 352t
  emptying a pouch, 352t
  features, 348t
  types of, 329t–330t, 345t–346t
Pouching infants/children
  multiple stomas, 367–368
  nonpouching for fecal stoma patient, 367
  pediatric pouches, 368
  vesicostomy, 367
Pouching multiple stomas, 367–368
Pouching systems
  accessory products, 331t–334t, 348t–351t

Pouching systems (*Continued*)
absorbent products, 186
adhesive products, 185
belt, 185, 185*f*
elastic skin barrier strip, 181, 181*f*
in-pouch deodorant liquids, 185
liquid skin barrier, 181–182
oral odor eliminators, 186
paste, 180, 180*f*
pouch covers, 185
pouch liners, 185
powder, 180–181, 180*f*
ring, 181, 181*f*
strip paste, 181
adaptations, 296–298
bridging, 296, 297*f*
saddlebagging, 298, 298*f*
troughing procedure, 296, 297*f*
disposable, 328*t*, 344*t*–345*t*
fistula pouches
change procedure, 295, 296*b*
pattern for, 295, 295*f*
two pouches sites, 295, 295*f*
medical adhesive products, 295
nonadhesive, 344*t*–345*t*
one-piece, 328*t*, 344*t*–345*t*
ostomy pouches
fecal stoma management,
drainable pouch for, 183–184,
184*f*
gas management, 185
nondrainable pouches, 183*f*, 184
one-piece pouching system, 175*f*,
182–183
pouch films, 183*f*, 184
pouch length, 183*f*, 184
two-piece pouching system,
182*f*–184*f*, 183
urinary stoma management,
drainable pouch for, 183*f*, 184
postoperative patient education
emptying a pouch, 191–192, 192*b*,
192*f*
indications for pouch change, 192
issues with stoma management,
193–194
medical attention, 194, 194*b*
one- and two-piece types of, 191
peristomal skin assessment, 193
peristomal skin cleansing, 193
placement of, 193
preparing equipment, 192
removal of, 193
stoma measurement, 193
time to empty, 192
removal using "push/pull" technique,
367
reusable, 328*t*, 344*t*–345*t*
skin barrier powders, 295
skin barriers, 174*t*
extended wear barrier, 173

fit of solid skin barrier, 178–180,
178*f*, 179*f*
solid skin barrier, 173–175, 175*f*
solid skin barrier shapes, 175–176, 176*f*
wear time, 175, 175*b*, 176*f*
steri-strips/tape strip, 294
two-piece, 328*t*
with flexible adhesive flange, 328*t*,
344*t*–345*t*
with interlocking flange, 344*t*–345*t*
Practice settings, WOC nursing, 6–7
academia, 6–7
acute care, 6
home health care, 6
industry, 6
long-term/extended care, 6
outpatient care, 6
rehabilitation, 6
research consumer and evidence-
based practice, 7
Preoperative education guidelines,
fecal/urinary diversion
counseling professional, 151
documentation, 158
ostomy visitor, 151
patient assessment, 146–148
barriers to self-care, 147
learning style/learning level,
147–148, 148*b*
patient and family/significant,
146–147
patient support systems, 148
planned procedure, diagnosis,
prognosis, and treatment plan,
146, 146*t*
planned procedure, explanation of
activity, 149
anatomy and physiology, 148
bowel prep, 151–152
clothing, 149
diet, 149
lifestyle modifications, 149
medications, 149
ostomy supplies, obtaining and
paying for, 150
ostomy visitor, 151
peristomal skin management, 150
pouch emptying, 150
pouching systems, 148*b*, 149–150
professional counseling, 151
psychological issues, 150
sexuality, 150
stages of adjustment, 150–151
surgical procedure, 148–149
travel, 149
post discharge education, 145, 145*b*
preoperative ostomy education,
144–145
stoma siting (*see* Stoma siting)
teaching strategies and methods,
144–145, 145*b*

Pressure injuries, 251, 256, 256*f*
Primary melanoma, 52
Prune belly (Eagle-Barrett) syndrome
(PBS)
assessment, 242
characteristics, 241
etiology, 241, 242*f*
incidence, 241
management, 242
presentation, 242
Pseudoverrucous lesions, 254–255, 255*f*

R
Radiation cystitis, 120
Radiation enteritis, 107–109
clinical presentation, 107
effects of, 107
etiology, 107, 107*t*
medical management, 108
surgical management, 108–109
Rectal cancer
adjuvant treatment algorithm for, 50*f*
neoadjuvant therapy and surgical
resection, 49–51, 49*f*–50*f*
treatment algorithm for, 48*f*
Rectum, 23, 23*f*
Regional enteritis. *See* Crohn's
disease (CD)
Registered nurse, WOC, 3
advanced practice registered
nurses, 3
graduate degree, 3
WOCN Educational Programs, 3
Rehabilitation issues
ostomy impact
adaptation process, 210
age/developmental stage, 212
family or significant others, 211
health care team/WOC nurse, 211
ostomy visitor, 211–212
past experiences with ostomy/
expectations, 211
self-efficacy, 211
self-esteem/coping skills, 211
pediatric patient
adolescent (13 to 18 years), 246
premature infant/full-term infant,
245, 245*f*–246*f*
school age (6 to 12 years),
245–246
support and education, for child
and family, 244–245
toddler (12 months to 3 years) and
preschool (3 to 5 years), 245
Renin–angiotensin–aldosterone
system, 40

S
Sarcomas, 52
Saturated skin barrier, 175, 175*f*
Serosa (adventitia), 14–15

Sexual function, 212–218
  counseling models, 213
  ostomy, body image/sexual
    relationships impact, 213
  pelvic dissection impact on, 212
Sigmoid colon, 23
Silicone ring barrier, 347t
Skin barriers, 174t, 330t–331t
  elastic skin barrier strip, 181, 181f
  extended wear barrier, 173
  features, 348t
  fit of solid skin barrier, 178–180, 178f,
    179f
  liquid skin barrier, 181–182
  paste, 180, 180f
  powder, 180–181, 180f
  ring, 181, 181f
  solid skin barrier, 173–175, 175f
  solid skin barrier shapes, 175–176, 176f
  strip paste, 181
  types of, 346t–347t
  wear time, 175, 175b, 176f
Skin–stoma junction, 168
Small intestine, 18–20
  function
    absorption, 15t
    motility, 19
    secretion, 15t, 20
  mesentery of, 18–19, 18f
  submucosal and mucosal layers,
    15f, 19
  villus, 19
Soave endorectal pull-through,
    235–236, 236t, 236b, 236f
Solid skin barrier, 173–175, 175f
  fit of, 178–180, 178f, 179f
  shapes, 175–176, 176f
Spina bifida, 242–243, 243f
Splenic flexure, 23
Spontaneous closure, 285, 288, 289b
Squamous cell cancer (SCC), 265–266
Stent management, 208–209
Stoma assessment, 163–168
  anatomic location and function,
    163–165, 165f
  patient with new fecal stoma, 164t
  patient with new urinary stoma, 164t
  peristomal skin, 168
  stoma mucosa, 167, 168f
  stoma structure, 168, 168f
Stoma complications, 271
  early complications
    mucocutaneous separation, 272,
      272f
    stomal necrosis, 272–273, 273f
    stomal retraction, 273–274
  incidence, 271
  late complications
    parastomal hernia, 277–279, 278f,
      279t
    stomal prolapse, 275–276, 276f
    stomal stenosis, 274–275, 275f

stomal trauma, 276–277, 277f
    Pittman Ostomy Complication
      Conceptual Model, 271, 271f
    symptoms, 271
Stoma construction types, 133t
  end stoma, 132–133, 133f
  loop stoma, 133–135, 134f–135f
  loop–end stoma, 135–136, 135f
Stoma construction/type, 165–167
  end loop ileostomy, 167
  end loop urinary stoma, 167
  end stoma, 165, 166f
  Hartmann's Procedure, 165, 166f
  loop colostomy with plastic stoma
    bridge, 166, 166f
  loop ileostomy with rubber support
    bridge, 166, 166f
  loop stoma, 166
  mucous fistula, 167, 167f
  support bridge removal, 166–167
  ureterostomy, 167
  vesicostomy, 167
Stoma lumen, 168, 168f
Stoma maturation, 132, 133f
Stoma mucosa, 167, 168f
Stoma siting. See also Unique stoma
    marking considerations
  procedure guidelines, 153–158
    marking procedure, 154, 154f, 155f,
      336, 340
    unique stoma marking
      considerations, 154–155
  rationale, 152, 153f
Stoma structure, 168, 168f
Stomach, 17–18, 17f
  columnar epithelial cells in, 17–18
  function, 18
    absorption, 18
    digestion, 18
    ingested bacteria, elimination of,
      18
    secretion, 15t, 18
  muscular layer, 17
  size and shape, 17
Stomal necrosis
  assessment, 273, 273f
  etiology/incidence, 272
  management, 273
  presentation, 272–273
Stomal prolapse
  assessment, 276
  etiology/incidence, 275
  management, 276
  presentation, 275, 276f
Stomal retraction
  assessment, 274
  etiology/incidence, 273–274
  management, 274
  presentation, 274
Stomal stenosis
  assessment, 275
  etiology/incidence, 274

management, 275
  presentation, 274, 275f
Stomal trauma
  assessment, 277
  etiology/incidence, 276
  management, 277
  presentation, 277, 277f
Submucosa, 13
Surgical management, ulcerative colitis
    (UC), 79–85, 80t–81t, 83f, 84t,
    84f
Swenson technique, 235, 235f

T
Temporary fecal diversions,
    management issues, 202–203,
    202b
Temporary stoma, 52–53
Transverse colon, 22
Trauma, 121
Turnbull loop urostomy. See End loop
    urinary stoma

U
Ulcerative colitis (UC)
  colorectal cancer risk in, 65
  medical management, 60, 66–67
    classifications of, 62t
    diet, 65
    differential diagnosis, 61, 61t
    epidemiology, 60
    etiology, 60
    extraintestinal manifestations, 65
    inflammation, 61–62
    medication class, 63, 63t
    mild-to-moderate disease, 63
    moderate-to-severe disease, 64
    overview, 61, 61t
  pediatric patient, 238–239
    assessment, 239
    incidence, 239
    management, 239
    presentation, 239
  surgical management, 79–85
    advantages and disadvantages
      in, 81t
    ileal pouch–anal anastomosis, 79,
      82–85, 83f, 84t, 84f
    indications for surgery, 80, 80t
    laparoscopic surgery, 85
    minimally invasive surgery, 85
    operative management, 80–85, 81t
    proctocolectomy with ileostomy,
      81–82
    robotic surgery, 85
Unique stoma marking considerations
  brace or leg prosthesis, 157
  continent stoma marking, 157
  contractures, 156
  creases and folds, 156
  distension, 156
  infants and children, 157

Unique stoma marking considerations (*Continued*)
  kyphosis, 156
  marking during surgery, 153*f*, 157, 157*b*
  moving the stoma, 155
  pain/limited mobility, 157
  pendulous breasts, 156
  pregnancy, 156
  radiation, 157
  scars, 156
  scoliosis, 156
  special equipment/work belts, 157
  spiritual beliefs, 156
  stoma siting, using computed tomography, 156
  tattoos, 156
  teenagers, 157–158
  thin patient, 155
  two stomas, 155
  wheelchair, 157
United Ostomy Associations of America's (UOAA), 144, 194
Ureteropelvic junction (UPJ), 31–32
Ureterosigmoidostomy, 118
Ureterostomy, 124, 124*f*, 138–139
Ureterovesical junction (UVJ), 31–32
Urethra, 34–35
Urinary bladder, 30*f*, 33–34, 34*f*
Urinary diversions
  management issues (*see* Adaptations, rehabilitation, and long-term care management issues)
  patient education (*see* Postoperative patient education)
  pediatric patient
    appendicovesicostomy, 244, 244*f*
    ileovesicostomy, 244
    myelomeningocele, 242–243, 243*f*
    Prune belly syndrome (PBS), 241–242, 242*f*
    vesicostomy, 243–244, 244*f*
Urinary stoma construction, 138–139
  assessment parameters, 164*t*
  ileal conduit, 139, 139*f*
  jejunal conduit, 139
  types, 138–139
  ureterostomy, 138–139
Urinary tract
  electrolyte balance, 38–40
    acid–base balance, 39
    calcitonin, 39
    calcium regulation, 39
    endocrine function, 40
    erythropoietin (EPO), 40
    fluid and, 37–38
    magnesium regulation, 39
    phosphate regulation, 39

potassium regulation, 38–39
    and renin–angiotensin–aldosterone system, 40
    vitamin D, 39
    vitamin D$_3$, 40
  kidney
    function of, 36–37
    location and structure, 30–31, 30*f*, 31*f*
  lower urinary tract
    adjacent organs, 36
    adrenal glands, 36
    pelvic floor, 35–36, 35*f*
    pelvis, 35
    urethra, 34–35
    urinary bladder, 33–34, 34*f*
  urine, elimination of, 30*f*, 31–33
    ureter clinical and surgical implications, 33
    ureter function, 32–33
    ureters, 31–32
  water regulation, 38
Urine
  concentration and volume, 37
  elimination of, 30*f*, 31–33
    ureter clinical and surgical implications, 33
    ureter function, 32–33
    ureters, 31–32
  formation, 36–37
  pH, 37
Urostomy, 208–209. *See also* Stent management
  products and tips, 343
  urine sample collection instruction card, 326

V
VACTERL Association, 229, 229*t*
Varices, 259, 259*f*
Vesicostomy, 243–244, 244*f*, 367
Video capsule endoscopy (vCE), 62–63
Vitamin D, 39
Vitamin D$_3$, 40
Volvulus, 110

W
WOC Nursing Certification Board (WOCNCB®), 3
Wound, Ostomy, and Continence Nurses Society, 2, 7–8
Wound, Ostomy, and Continence (WOC) nursing, 190, 224, 284
  care coordination and collaboration by, 7
  complex problems, 4
  continuous professional development, 8
  certification, 8, 8*t*

streaming/webcasts sessions, 8
  ethics in, 8–9
  evidenced-based practices, 2–3
  fistula management, 288–290
    abdominal contours and fistula opening, 286*f*, 289–290, 289*f*
    documentation, 288, 289*b*
    education and emotional support, 298
    effluent characteristics, 286*f*, 290
    interventions and containment strategies, 290–298
    progress toward and impediments to spontaneous closure, 288, 289*b*, 289*f*
  health care reimbursement, 7–8
  history and evolution of, 2
  management principles of autoimmune diseases, 265*t*
  nurse roles, 2–5
    administrator, 5
    clinician, 4
    consultant, 5
    dual/multiple roles, 5
    educator, 4–5
    integrity, 2
    knowledge, 2
    leadership, 2
    preceptor, 5
    researcher, 5
  ostomy complications, 271
  populations served by, 5–6
    older adults, 5
    palliative/hospice care, 6
    for pediatric population, 5
  practice settings in, 6–7
    academia, 6–7
    acute care, 6
    home health care, 6
    industry, 6
    long-term/extended care, 6
    outpatient care, 6
    rehabilitation, 6
    research consumer and evidence-based practice, 7
  professional practice goals, 3
  registered nurse, 3
    advanced practice registered nurses, 3
    graduate degree, 3
    WOCN Educational Programs, 3
  specialty, 2
  tri-specialty of, 4
    continence, 4
    ostomy, 4
    wound, 4
Wound Ostomy Continence Nursing Certification Board (WOCNCB), 8
Wound specialty, 4